Evaluation and Assessment of AI-Driven Systems in Hospitals

Anandavalli M.
King Khalid University, Saudi Arabia

Prabhu Chakkaravarthy
SRM Institute of Science and Technology, India

Dhanalakshmi J.
SRM Institute of Science and Technology, India

IGI Global Scientific Publishing
Publishing Tomorrow's Research Today

Vice President of Editorial Melissa Wagner
Director of Acquisitions Mikaela Felty
Director of Book Development Jocelynn Hessler
Production Manager Mike Brehm
Cover Design Jose Rosado

Published in the United States of America by
IGI Global Scientific Publishing
701 East Chocolate Avenue
Hershey, PA, 17033, USA
Tel: 717-533-8845 | Fax: 717-533-7115
Website: https://www.igi-global.com E-mail: cust@igi-global.com

Library of Congress Cataloging-in-Publication Data

LCCN: 2025011366 (CIP Data Pending)
ISBN13: 9798337327877
Isbn13Softcover: 9798337327884
EISBN13: 9798337327891

British Cataloguing in Publication Data
A Cataloguing in Publication record for this book is available from the British Library.

Table of Contents

Detailed Table of Contents

Increasing the accuracy of diagnoses, streamlining operations, and improving the overall quality of care provided to patients are all examples of how artificial intelligence (AI) is transforming the healthcare industry. The purpose of this study is to investigate the implementation of AI-driven systems, the effectiveness of these systems, and the impact on patients in hospital settings. The most recent artificial intelligence models that are utilized in diagnosis, treatment planning, patient monitoring, and office assistance are examined in great detail. This research also investigates key performance indicators (KPIs), the ethical implications of using them, and issues such as the protection of data, the ease of interpretation, and the trust that clinicians have in practitioners. The results lend credence to a strategy that aims to integrate artificial intelligence tools into hospitals in a manner that is both effective and continuously reviewed to support a health system that is data-driven and learning.

Artificial Intelligence (AI) has revolutionized healthcare delivery by improving patient care, diagnostics and operational efficiency in hospitals. This review assesses AI-powered hospital systems with an emphasis on how they affect patient outcomes, resource management and clinical decision-making. A crucial component of this assessment is evaluating the fairness, interpretability and accuracy of AI models to

Healthcare organizations use technology to enhance patient care and streamline their operations in the modern digital world. However, worries about data security and privacy have grown as more clinics and hospitals store patient records electronically. Important information such as a person's medical history, current treatments, and personal data are contained in medical records. This information could result in fraud, identity theft, or health insurance abuse if it ends up in the wrong hands. Because medical data is valuable, cybercriminals frequently target healthcare organizations. Strong security measures like encryption, secure access controls, and routine system checks to stop unwanted access are necessary for hospitals to protect patient privacy. Healthcare providers must make investments in cutting-edge security technologies and enhance data management procedures due to the rise in cyber threats. By taking such steps, they will be able to protect patient data, foster trust, and improve healthcare for everybody.

With AI increasingly used in healthcare, finance, and autonomous systems, ongoing monitoring is vital to ensure performance, fairness, and ethical compliance. Long-term oversight helps control risks, improve systems, and maintain trust. Monitoring frameworks detect issues like model drift, bias, or degradation caused by data shifts, user behavior, or environmental changes—prompting regular retraining. Beyond accuracy, key metrics include fairness, transparency, robustness, efficiency, and compliance. Explainability ensures stakeholders understand AI decisions, while robustness testing checks performance under varied inputs. AI observability tools with logging and analytics detect abnormal behavior early. Human oversight complements automated systems to catch subtle issues and ensure social responsibility. Monitoring many complex AIs remains a challenge, demanding better tools for transparency and adaptation. Regular testing, human involvement, and governance ensure AI stays effective, ethical, and lawful. These practices support responsible AI development and foster user trust.

Personalized medicine (PM) is transforming healthcare by adapting treatments that considers individual genetic, environmental, and lifestyle factors. Children present distinct physiological and developmental differences that require careful consideration in diagnosis, treatment, and prevention. Paediatric PM focuses on early detection of diseases, individualized drug therapy, and targeted interventions based on genetic and molecular profiles. Personalized medicine, is important for several reasons like children's genetic profiles can affect how they respond to medications and treatments, making personalized approaches crucial. The combination of AI and personalized medicine in pediatrics enables precision in drug dosing, early disease detection, and more effective treatment strategies. By integrating AI, the future of pediatric medicine will be more individualized, predictive, and patient-centric. This paradigm shift will ultimately enhance the quality of life for children, providing them with safer, more effective treatments tailored to their unique genetic and physiological needs.

The integration of latest technologies like Artificial Intelligence (AI) plays a vital role in improving the Healthcare systems right from real time monitoring, health record maintenance and efficient disease diagnosis and appropriate treatment. AI systems incorporate machine learning (ML) models, Deep learning models (DL) models, IOT devices and sensor data to provide real time monitoring of patient health. AI models assess lung imaging and real-time oxygen saturation data to predict respiratory deterioration. The power of AI in predictive analytics helps in identifying disease at the early stage to plan for faster treatment and recovery. Automated documentation and AI-powered EHR enhances clinical workflows reducing errors and improves patient data management. Generally, the hospitals have large amount of patient

This chapter examines how human factors shape the impact of artificial intelligence (AI) on hospital staff and patient healthcare outcomes. As AI technologies expand in healthcare, their influence on human interactions, workflows, and treatment results require thorough analysis. AI-driven clinical support systems, diagnostic tools, and patient interaction technologies enhance healthcare practitioners' competence but also raise concerns about trust, communication, and job satisfaction. AI simultaneously boosts clinical efficiency and reshapes how professionals engage with patients. Using real-world examples and research findings, this chapter explores AI's effects on hospital staff workloads, decision-making, and patient experiences. It also addresses algorithmic bias and underscores the need for human-centered AI implementation. Regular evaluation systems are crucial for assessing AI's impact on staff and evolving technology. By fostering AI-professional collaboration, hospitals can improve patient outcomes and satisfaction.

Autonomous artificial intelligence (AI) systems are transforming surgical practice, enabling enhanced precision, efficiency, and personalization. Yet, their integration introduces critical ethical and regulatory challenges. This chapter explores current applications of AI in surgical settings—preoperative planning, intraoperative decision-making, and postoperative monitoring—highlighting clinical benefits alongside risks such as algorithmic bias and lack of explainability. Key ethical issues are examined, including informed consent, moral responsibility, and data privacy. The chapter also evaluates global regulatory responses, such as the FDA's Total Product Lifecycle model and the EU's Artificial Intelligence Act. Case studies, including the da Vinci Surgical System and the Smart Tissue Autonomous Robot, illustrate real-world implications. The chapter concludes with forward-looking recommendations

Preface

Artificial Intelligence (AI) has emerged as one of the most transformative forces in modern healthcare, reshaping the way hospitals operate, clinicians deliver care, and patients experience medical services. *Evaluation and Assessment of AI-Driven Systems in Hospitals* brings together 16 chapters authored by leading scholars and practitioners, offering a comprehensive examination of how AI technologies are evaluated, deployed, and continuously assessed in hospital environments. Beginning with broad analyses of AI's impact on hospital systems, the book then addresses methodological frameworks, data quality, and long-term monitoring strategies essential for safe and ethical AI adoption. Subsequent chapters highlight AI's role in personalized medicine, disease classification, workflow optimization, and biomedical waste management, while case studies showcase tangible improvements in efficiency, diagnostic accuracy, and patient care. Equally significant are the discussions on the human dimension—how AI alters workforce dynamics, enhances collaboration, and must balance technology with compassion in clinical practice. Ethical and regulatory considerations, particularly in autonomous systems such as surgical AI, provide guardrails for responsible innovation. Finally, advances in medical data science and informatics are positioned as the backbone for next-generation AI applications, including federated learning and telemedicine.

Together, these chapters provide readers with an integrated understanding of both the opportunities and challenges AI presents in hospitals. By weaving together insights from evaluation, practice, policy, and human collaboration, this book offers a roadmap for ensuring that AI-driven healthcare remains not only innovative and efficient but also ethical, trustworthy, and fundamentally centered on patient well-being. It is our hope that the perspectives shared here will inspire continued dialogue, responsible implementation, and a forward-looking vision for the sustainable integration of AI in hospital systems.

The following summaries provide an overview of each chapter, outlining the key themes, insights, and contributions presented throughout the volume.

Chapter 1 [The Impact of Artificial Intelligence on Contemporary Hospital Systems] investigates AI's role in improving diagnosis, treatment planning, patient monitoring, and hospital operations while addressing key performance indicators, ethics, and clinician trust.

Chapter 2 [A Comprehensive Review for Critical Evaluation of AI-Driven Hospital Systems, Ethical Challenges and Future Perspectives] provides an in-depth review of AI applications in hospitals, focusing on fairness, interpretability, validation methods, and the importance of ethical and legal frameworks.

Chapter 3 [Comprehensive Evaluation of AI-Driven Systems in Modern Hospital Environment] presents evaluation approaches centered on safety, effectiveness, bias mitigation, and regulatory compliance to guide responsible adoption of AI technologies.

Chapter 4 [Data Quality, Privacy, and Security Concerns in Healthcare] highlights the growing risks of cyber threats and stresses the importance of encryption, secure access, and governance to protect sensitive patient data.

Chapter 5 [Long-Term Monitoring and Performance Evaluation of AI Systems] emphasizes the importance of continuous monitoring, transparency, fairness, and explainability to detect model drift, bias, and degradation over time.

Chapter 6 [Assessment of AI's Impact on Precision Medicine and Personalized Healthcare in Clinical Environments] explores how AI enhances individualized treatments, particularly in pediatrics, by tailoring therapies to genetic and physiological differences.

Chapter 7 [Optimizing Hospital Workflows Through Artificial Intelligence] demonstrates how AI supports real-time monitoring, predictive analytics, and automated documentation to streamline workflows and improve patient recovery.

Chapter 8 [AI Integration and Clinical Workflow Optimization in Hospitals] analyzes how AI technologies reduce operational complexities and workforce burdens by enhancing efficiency and decision-making in clinical practice.

Chapter 9 [AI-Driven Integration and Workflow Optimization in Modern Healthcare Facilities] presents case studies that illustrate measurable improvements in diagnostic accuracy, patient wait times, and hospital operations through ethical AI integration.

Chapter 10 [AI in Healthcare: Automating Hospital Operations for Better Patient Care] investigates how AI-driven automation, particularly with artificial neural networks, supports resource management, cost reduction, and personalized care.

Chapter 11 [AI-Driven Biomedical Waste Management System for Hospitals Using CNN-Based Classification and Sustainable Disposal Recommendations] introduces a CNN-powered framework that classifies biomedical waste and provides sustainable, regulation-compliant disposal solutions.

Chapter 12 [Human-AI Collaboration in Healthcare: The Evolving Role of Healthcare Professionals] explores the changing responsibilities of healthcare professionals, best practices for collaboration, and the ethical considerations of working alongside AI systems.

Chapter 13 [Evaluate the Impact of AI on Healthcare Workforce Dynamics and Operational Efficiency] assesses how AI reshapes healthcare professions, enhances workflows, and raises concerns about reskilling, job displacement, and patient care quality.

Chapter 14 [Human-AI Collaboration for Balancing Technology and Compassion in Healthcare and Medicine]discusses strategies for achieving synergy between AI efficiency and human empathy while addressing issues of trust, privacy, and acceptance.

Chapter 15 [The Human Factor – Evaluating the Impact of AI on Hospital Staff and Patient Care] evaluates how AI affects staff workloads, decision-making, and patient interactions, emphasizing the need for human-centered AI adoption.

Chapter 16 [Ethical and Regulatory Evaluation of Autonomous AI Systems in Surgical Practices] examines ethical, legal, and regulatory considerations in surgical AI, with global case studies and recommendations for adaptive governance.

Each chapter in this volume represents a vital contribution to the evolving narrative of AI in hospital systems. Together, they illustrate the collective expertise of researchers, clinicians, technologists, and policymakers committed to shaping a future where artificial intelligence enhances patient care, streamlines hospital operations, and supports healthcare professionals. It is our hope that this book serves not only as a foundational reference but also as a forward-looking guide for academics, practitioners, and decision-makers navigating the complex landscape of AI-driven healthcare. By fostering critical evaluation, ethical reflection, and innovative thinking, this work aims to inspire responsible adoption of AI technologies that transform hospitals into more efficient, compassionate, and resilient environments of care.

I hope that *Evaluation and Assessment of AI-Driven Systems in Hospitals* will serve as both a foundational resource and a source of inspiration for those dedicated to advancing intelligent, ethical, and patient-centered healthcare. I invite readers to engage with these chapters with curiosity and critical reflection, and to contribute to the ongoing transformation of hospital systems through responsible innovation, collaboration, and a shared commitment to improving patient outcomes.

Acknowledgment

With heartfelt thanks, we give all praise to God. We express our deepest gratitude to the researchers, data scientists, and healthcare experts whose dedicated contributions form the foundation of this book. Special thanks to our peer reviewers, who provided critical insights and helped refine each chapter to ensure its academic rigor and practical relevance.

We gratefully acknowledge the invaluable support from various organizations and sources that provided data, tools, and case studies essential to the development of this compilation. Our sincere thanks also go to our publishers for their unwavering encouragement and guidance throughout the publishing process.

Last but not least, we extend heartfelt appreciation to our families and colleagues whose unwavering patience and support made the completion of this book possible.

Chapter 1
The Impact of Artificial Intelligence on Contemporary Hospital Systems

D. Rajeswari
https://orcid.org/0000-0002-2677-4296
Department of Data Science and Business Systems, School of Computing, College of Engineering and Technology, SRM Institute of Science and Technology, Kattankulathur, India

Amala K. J.
https://orcid.org/0009-0003-6863-2565
Department of Data Science and Business Systems, School of Computing, College of Engineering and Technology, SRM Institute of Science and Technology, Kattankulathur, India

Athish Venkatachalam
https://orcid.org/0000-0001-6258-5188
Clemson University, USA

ABSTRACT

Increasing the accuracy of diagnoses, streamlining operations, and improving the overall quality of care provided to patients are all examples of how artificial intelligence (AI) is transforming the healthcare industry. The purpose of this study is to investigate the implementation of AI-driven systems, the effectiveness of these systems, and the impact on patients in hospital settings. The most recent artificial intelligence models that are utilized in diagnosis, treatment planning, patient monitoring, and office assistance are examined in great detail. This research also

DOI: 10.4018/979-8-3373-2787-7.ch001

investigates key performance indicators (KPIs), the ethical implications of using them, and issues such as the protection of data, the ease of interpretation, and the trust that clinicians have in practitioners. The results lend credence to a strategy that aims to integrate artificial intelligence tools into hospitals in a manner that is both effective and continuously reviewed to support a health system that is data-driven and learning.

INTRODUCTION

Fast expansion of digital technologies marks the beginning of a new age in healthcare. Modern ideas draw on artificial intelligence (AI). Hospitals now employ this clever technology for everything from patient diagnosis to care planning to even patient communication. From imaging and pathology to urgent care centers and emergency rooms, artificial intelligence is starting to significantly alter the way the whole healthcare system is administered and served. Using AI-powered devices in hospitals offers one possible way to help with some of the most urgent problems confronting modern healthcare. Among these problems are a dearth of medical experts, growing patient expectations, treatment-related costs, and increasingly difficult-to-make clinical judgments. Artificial intelligence generates ideas that humans usually cannot by looking at a lot of data that is contained in electronic health records (EHRs), diagnostic images, genomes, and patient monitoring devices. Artificial intelligence can detect early warning signs of life-threatening diseases like sepsis or stroke, enabling doctors to act promptly.

Artificial intelligence solutions, including predictive analytics platforms, clinical decision support systems (CDSS), robotic surgery tools, and natural language processing engines, already show promise in the real world. When it comes to finding problems in X-rays and MRIs, artificial intelligence systems are especially useful in the field of radiology. Regarding oncology, depending on their genome, machine learning models can help identify the therapy choices that best fit any particular patient. Artificial intelligence is enabling even administrative tasks, such as monitoring insurance claims and appointment scheduling, to be automated. This results in reduced effort and enhanced efficiency in all operations.

Conversely, it is rather clear that artificial intelligence has a lot of promise in the domain of medicine. Still, implementing it in hospitals presents many difficulties. One major reason for worry is the need for thorough testing and approval before release. Pharmaceutical drugs undergo a lot of clinical research, while artificial intelligence technologies are usually introduced following testing on older datasets. Furthermore, the successful application of models on one group of people may not translate to another, leading to unfair or negative results.

Another important problem is interpretability's difficulty. Many advanced artificial intelligence models, especially those using deep learning, are referred to as "black boxes" since they do not offer clear justification for the decisions or forecasts they generate. Regarding professional treatment, this lack of transparency may be a problem when trust, responsibility, and the capacity to clarify matters are of significant relevance. Generally speaking, clinical practitioners do not want to adopt artificial intelligence technology unless they can understand and confirm the underlying ideas behind the recommendations. Developing intelligible AI models and using interpretable artificial intelligence (XAI) techniques can help to guarantee that users feel comfortable with artificial intelligence (AI) and that patients are safeguarded. In addition to this, it is important to seriously consider the ethical and legal consequences of using artificial intelligence in medical institutions. The several important problems that demand attention include data privacy, informed consent, algorithmic bias, and the question of who is liable, all of which should be addressed immediately. Apart from the rules set by medical boards and government agencies, hospitals must also negotiate these issues while following local and international healthcare legislation, including HIPAA and GDPR. Concerns have also been raised about job losses due to artificial intelligence, especially for office workers and roles requiring less skill. On the other hand, the vast majority of experts feel that artificial intelligence should work alongside people instead of substituting itself. In this way, humans may focus on more challenging chores, such as patient communication.

Apart from organizational and physical challenges, there are moral and technical ones to address. Many hospitals, especially those in low- and middle-income nations, do not have the digital infrastructure required for strong artificial intelligence systems to function. Inadequate data, insufficient IT staff, and medical information systems incompatible with one another can all impede the implementation of artificial intelligence. Change management and training initiatives are often required to prepare staff members to effectively apply AI tools. Fear of technology, resistance to change, and ignorance can slow down or even stop projects involving artificial intelligence in healthcare facilities.

This study's primary objective is to investigate these crucial features by means of extensive evaluation and assessment of AI-powered medical systems. The primary objectives of the research are to answer questions including:

- How currently are artificial intelligence systems applied in hospitals?
- Under what scientific, clinical, and organizational context should they be most effective?
- How might artificial intelligence tools be tested before, during, and following their deployment using frameworks and metrics?

- How does the application of artificial intelligence in patient care influence ethics, the legislation, and society?
- How might learning-based, long-lasting AI integration models be created in hospitals?

Despite a growing body of research on AI applications in healthcare, a significant gap still exists in comprehending the reliable, ethical, and sustainable use of these systems in actual hospital settings. Current studies mainly focus on how well AI works technically, like how accurately it can diagnose or predict outcomes, but they don't explain how these systems can be used reliably across different groups of people or hospitals. Furthermore, hospital processes, data pipelines, and therapeutic practices often lack sufficient examination of AI's incorporation (Topol et al., 2019). Despite the increasing interest in explicable AI (Chen et al., 2020), its adoption is impeded by opacity, data quality concerns, and an absence of effective validation frameworks. Ethical issues, including bias, informed consent, and accountability, are increasingly recognized as urgent problems (Sendak et al., 2020). This study intends to provide a systematic assessment of AI-powered systems across technological, ethical, and operational dimensions to address these gaps. The primary aims of this research are to examine the present utilization of artificial intelligence technologies in hospitals for clinical and administrative purposes. Identify scientific, technical, and organizational contexts that facilitate or obstruct effective AI implementation. Evaluate testing frameworks, metrics, and validation methodologies employed before and after deployment. Examine the ethical, legal, and societal ramifications associated with the use of AI in patient care. Propose a scalable and interpreted integration framework for the sustained application of AI in healthcare environments.

The chapter seeks to establish an evidence-based comprehension of the responsible and effective utilization of AI in hospitals by addressing these objectives. We anticipate that the results will aid developers, doctors, and policymakers in the advancement of human-centered, explainable, and regulation-compliant AI systems within the healthcare sector. By looking at these elements in a deliberate manner, this study intends to help establish a disciplined and evidence-based understanding of how artificial intelligence can be utilized safely and effectively in healthcare. The aim is to demonstrate what artificial intelligence can do and what it has previously achieved, while also exposing flaws, hazards, and future opportunities for improvement. The findings can be used by researchers, legislators, technologists, and medical professionals to assist in building smart, adaptable, patient-centered hospital ecosystems. Using artificial intelligence in hospitals ultimately calls for more than simply technology. It calls for cooperation, moral behavior, effective government, and an always-learning commitment. Strict testing of AI systems will be crucial as healthcare transforms in the digital era to ensure they truly benefit doctors and patients they treat.

BACKGROUND

AI has changed the way healthcare is provided today. It can be used for diagnostics, patient monitoring, hospital management, and automating routine tasks. A lot of research has been done on how to use data from past patients to guide machine learning and deep learning systems to spot trends in illnesses, guess what health problems might happen, and help doctors make better choices. That is why it is essential to have reliable models and make ensure that that they compatible well with digital healthcare systems, user-friendly interfaces, and equipment for managing and keeping an eye on everything all the time.

Over the past decade, hospitals have slowly started to use AI for a variety of tasks, such as diagnosis, decision-making, and operational advancement. A lot of research has been done on the pros and cons of using AI-powered technologies in medical centers. The works by Rajkomar et al. (2019); Muniasamy et al. (2020); and Gauthaman et al. (2026) give an overview of the different clinical tasks that deep learning methods can be used . When it comes to clinical adoption, the authors emphasize how important it is to have accurate data, make sure it can be used in processes, and make sure it is easy to understand. In a different study, Topol et al. (2019) talk about how AI could improve healthcare by making it a high-performance system that uses either computing power and human expertise. Some of the ways that AI can be used are in images, pathology, administrative duties, and getting patients involved. The thought that doctors should be assisted instead of being replaced is very important. Using a deep convolutional neural network (CNN), researchers (Esteva et al., 2019; Muniasamy et al., 2020) were able to classify skin lesions just as well as experienced doctors. The study shows that AI can be used to make diagnoses if it is taught on large datasets with annotations. The MIMIC-III dataset (Johnson et al., 2016) is the most common clinical dataset used to train and test AI models.

Liu et al. (2025) did a thorough study that looks at fifty AI-based models for finding sepsis early on. It says that results mean different things to different people and that there is no outside justification. In real life, people are naturally inclined to use models that are simple and easy to understand. Sendak et al.'s (2020) essay talks about a lot of ethical problems, such as bias, justice, informed consent, and patient liberty. Even more specifically, it talks about the need for management from different fields when using AI in medical settings.

A study by Xu, X et al., 2024; Patel et al., 2024; VV NK et al., 2022 discussed about how to use advanced AI to diagnose and treat five diseases: epilepsy, Alzheimer's disease, breast cancer, sadness, and heart disease. Multimodal strategies have become useful tools for improving the accuracy of diagnoses and treatment decisions. These methods combine a lot of different types of data, like medical images, computerized medical records, physiological indicators, and clinical data to better explain how diseases work. In spite of this progress, only a few studies give a complete picture of how multimodal AI can be used in health (Jandoubi, B., et al., 2025). Multimodal data makes it easier to understand health issues and give more personalized care (Mohsen et al., 2022). The work proposed by Athish et al. 2023; Begum, A et al., 2024; Sabahath, A et al., 2023; Bhatnagar, and R. et al., 2021 combine multimodel with ML find new insights. This study gives a broad look at the subject and suggests future research directions for creating multimodal diagnostic systems that can be used in clinical settings . Parvin, N., et al. (2025) examine biomaterials, diagnostics, and personalized medicine in a multimodal strategy.

Using electronic health records (EHRs) to guess what findings will be made in the future is a big job in healthcare. Each type of EHR has its own set of traits and holds different kinds of patient data (An et al., 2021). A lot of EHR-based prediction systems use unethical data or fail to examine closely at the connection between different types of data . Medical AI could make healthcare better by supporting evidence-based medicine, personalized care, lowering costs, and making the experience better for both providers and patients. It is said by Karargyris, A., et al. (2023) that this potential needs to be unlocked by utilizing huge volumes of various sorts of data from various patient groups in order to evaluate medical AI models in a methodical and measured manner. In order to fulfill this requirement MedPerf was developed which is an open-source tool for benchmarking medical AI models. By establishing a connection between the model and the data, every center is able to test artificial intelligence models in a secure and expedient manner, while also prioritizing the protection of individuals' privacy.

Vision-language models (VLMs) in medicine look at both textual and visual medical data (Hartsock et al., 2024) by using computer vision (CV) and natural language processing (NLP). This study looks at recent success in making VLMs that are better for healthcare. It focuses on publicly available models that are meant to help with making medical reports and visual question answering (VQA). AI and natural language processing have come a long way since the development of transformer-based large language models (LLMs) like the General Pretrained Transformer (GPT) and Bidirectional Encoder Representations from Transformers (BERT). These models, which are known for being able to find associative connections between words by using similar context, are going to change healthcare by making diagnoses more accurate, tailoring treatments to each patient, and predicting how they will do. However, using them in healthcare comes with a lot of risks and possible unintended outcomes (Denecke, K., et al., 2024;Rajeswari D et al,2023). This study, which uses a qualitative method and includes a total of 28 individuals, looks at the pros, cons, and risks of using transformer models in healthcare. A simplified theme analysis is used to look at the answers to seven open-ended questions.LLMs and multimodal large language models (MLLMs) have gotten a lot of attention for how well understand, reason, and generate language. Since ChatGPT and GPT-4, they have opened up new ways to use artificial intelligence in medicine.The work by Hanguang Xiao et al. (2025) investigates history, ideas, possible uses, issues, and possible future paths of LLMs and MLLMs in medicine. It starts by going over the paradigm shift, showing how old models gave way to LLMs and MLLMs and pointing out the benefits of using them in medicine.

Developments in communication technologies and the Internet of Medical Things (IOMT) have brought about a transformation in smart healthcare through AI. As healthcare networks get bigger and data privacy issues rise, it may not be possible for AI techniques to collect and process data in one place (Nguyen et al., 2022). Due to modern healthcare networks' great scalability and developing data privacy concerns, centralized data collecting and processing may be impractical for AI techniques (Nguyen et al., 2022). Federated Learning (FL), an emerging distributed collaborative AI paradigm, coordinates several clients (e.g., hospitals) to train AI without sharing raw data, making it appealing for smart healthcare. AI may change healthcare in the coming decades (Soenksen et al., 2022;). In particular, AI systems using many data sources and input modalities will offer more accurate results and deployable pipelines for various applications. A Holistic AI in Medicine (HAIM) framework is suggested and used to generate and test multimodal AI systems. Healthcare research and deployment can use our data pre-processing and machine learning modeling. The medical revolution of artificial intelligence (AI) has significantly impacted radiology (Simon BD et al., 2025). A new type of distributed joint AI called Federated Learning (FL) lets many clients, train AI without sharing raw data. This makes it a good choice for smart healthcare. AI systems that use numerous data sources and input types will produce more accurate results and adaptable processes that can be used in many contexts (Soenksen et al., 2022).To make and test multimodal AI systems, the Holistic AI in Medicine (HAIM) framework is proposed and used. Radiology has been greatly affected by the medical revolution of artificial intelligence (AI) (Simon BD et al., 2025).

Diffusion models and ChatGPT are improving diagnostic accuracy and automating clinical operations (Buess, L., et al., 2025). The field has grown significantly, evolving from text-only LLM for clinical documentation and decision support to multimodal AI systems that integrate imaging, text, and structured data. Healthcare systems globally struggle with efficiency, accessibility, and personalization. Modern artificial intelligence (AI) can address these difficulties through precise predictive modeling, but its influence is restricted by clinical workflow integration (Liu et al.,

2025; Naim et al., 2026; Gauthaman, S. A., et al., 2026; Muniasamy, A., et al. 2026). Embodied AI (EmAI) is a revolutionary frontier powered by modern AI technologies and world models, enabling improved autonomy and the ability to interact with the actual environment to address these difficulties. This research intends to stimulate innovation and practical applications for a new era of intelligent, patient-centered healthcare by giving systematic insights.

PROPOSED AI FRAMEWORK

Building Blocks of AI Systems in Hospitals

To make an AI system that can be used in hospitals, the design needs to be modular, scalable, and able to work with the hospital's current digital infrastructure. The suggested architecture in Figure 1 is made up of layers, which are called data, intelligence, interaction, and governance.

Figure 1. Layered Architecture

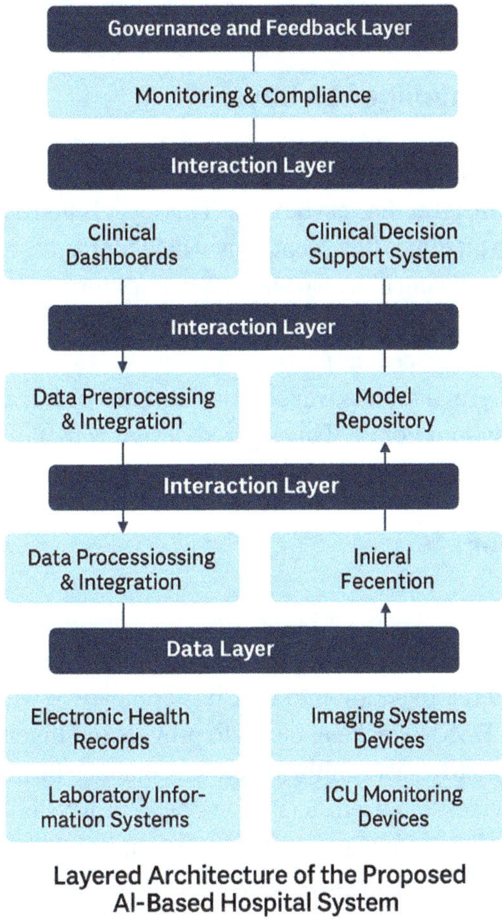

Data Layer

The recommended system uses a layered architecture to ensure that healthcare data is managed, processed, and utilized effectively. The most fundamental level is known as the data layer. It is able to establish connections with a wide variety of healthcare data sources, including Electronic Health Records (EHRs), medical imaging systems, laboratory systems, and physician notes. This layer adheres to several standard protocols, some examples of which include Health Level Seven (HL7) and Fast Healthcare Interoperability Resources (FHIR). This feature makes it feasible for data to be easily integrated and exchanged with one another. To ensure that everything is secure and easy to monitor, it is designed to be able to continuously take in data and maintain the accuracy of that data through the utilization of audit logs and stringent access control.

Processing and Intelligence Layer

The processing and intelligence layer sits on top of the data layer and turns raw healthcare data into insights that can be used. This layer is home to many preprocessing engines and data pipelines that prepare new data for further analysis by cleaning, normalizing, and structuring it. It also has a repository for machine learning models, which is where models that are made for different healthcare situations are kept and handled. Depending on the medical purpose, these models include rule-based systems, deep neural networks, and more advanced classical machine learning methods such as XGBoost and Random Forest. This layered design is modular and scalable, and it helps healthcare decision-makers make strong, safe, and smart choices.

Interaction Layer

Due to the fact that the system is compatible with hospital dashboards and warning systems, it is possible to monitor it in real time and enable clinical personnel to receive prompt alerts. In addition to this, it is compatible with Clinical Decision Support Systems (CDSS), which enables it to provide intelligent recommendations that are driven by data to assist healthcare professionals in making sound decisions. Additionally, it provides end users, such as medical professionals and nurses, with tools that facilitate clear visualization and explainability, which makes it simpler for them to comprehend complex data and the outcomes of models.

Governance and Feedback Layer

Adding the governance and feedback layer allows for the monitoring of how users interact with the application, the identification of inaccurate predictions, and the facilitation of the process of updating AI models to improve their accuracy. In addition, this layer ensures that the system complies with regulations as well as any other national healthcare laws that may be applicable. In a manner that is both just and legal, this framework promotes the utilization of artificial intelligence in healthcare settings.

Data Handling

Multimodal datasets from different areas are very advantageous for a hospital AI system. This chapter describes a unified way to address complicated and inconsistent medical data in the real world.

Table 1. Data Sources

Source	Data Type	Examples
EHR Systems	Structured	Patient ID, age, gender, vitals
Laboratory Systems	Semi-structured	Blood test results, infection markers
Radiology	Imaging	Chest X-rays, CT scans
ICU Monitors	Time-series	Heart rate, respiration, SpO_2
Clinical Notes	Unstructured text	Physician observations, diagnosis

Data Integration Techniques

ETL (Extract, Transform, and Load) pipelines are used to combine different types of clinical data into a central, safe data lake. This makes sure that data handling in healthcare AI systems is efficient and safe. This process makes it easy to combine info from many sources in a strong way. Data de-duplication is done by matching patient information using unique identifiers and visit timestamps to get rid of unnecessary copies and make sure the data is correct. To protect privacy, methods called "anonymization" are used to get rid of information that can be used to identify a person, like names, bed numbers, and contact information. Also, timestamp alignment makes sure that data from different streams, like when medications are given and when vital signs are recorded, is in sync with each other. This makes sure that patient records are consistent in terms of time, which is important for training and analyzing AI models accurately.

Preprocessing Pipeline

Preprocessing plays a crucial role in ensuring the model receives comprehensible, high-quality data. The following submodules are part of the pipeline:

i) **Data Cleaning**: Several preparation methods are used to make sure that healthcare data is accurate and consistent. It is very important to deal with missing values. This can be done in a number of ways, including using forward fill (where the previous value is moved forward) or statistical imputation techniques like mean or mode substitution. When things get more complicated, model-based estimating is used to make accurate predictions and fill in the missing data. Finding outliers is another important job, especially for numerical fields. This is usually done with the Z-score method or interquartile range (IQR)-based filtering to identify values that are very different from the normal range and get rid of them. Text normalization is also done on clinical notes and data that is not organized. As part of this, text is changed to lowercase, extra punctuation is removed, and the text is broken up into meaningful tokens (tokenization), which helps render the data ready for jobs like natural language processing and machine learning.

ii) **Feature Standardization:** Several transformation methods are used to prepare the data ready for machine learning models. Normalizing continuous variables can be done in several ways, including min-max scaling, which limits values to a set range (usually 0 to 1), or z-score standardization, which places the data around the mean with a variance of one. Techniques for encoding are used to turn categories into numbers for classification variables. The process includes label encoding, which gives each category a unique number, and one-hot encoding, which makes a binary column for each category. Time-based features, like clinical measurements taken over time, are also handled either by adding them all together (like finding the average blood pressure per hour) or by spreading them out using rolling statistics (like finding a rolling mean), which helps see patterns and trends over time.

iii) **Data Splitting:** The dataset was split into three sets: training (70%), validation (15%), and testing (15%). Temporal validation makes sure that training never gets new data.

RESULT AND DISCUSSION

This section presents the results of testing the proposed AI-based medical system and discusses its effectiveness, challenges, and effects. The findings come from a detailed study of different machine learning models tested on hospital data to predict patient death, track intensive care unit patients, and detect diseases earlier. When looking at how different models perform, it's easy to see how well they work by using standard measurements like AUC (area under the receiver operating characteristic curve), precision, and recall. The model's results are analyzed to see if they are correct, clinically relevant, and usable in a healthcare setting. There is a great deal of consideration given to significant aspects such as integration issues (such as ensuring that it is compatible with the existing hospital systems) and the feedback that physicians provide regarding how they interact with the model. The explainability and generalizability of the model, in addition to its robustness (its capacity to remain consistent over a variety of datasets), are also thoroughly examined to determine how well it functions in clinical settings that are representative of real-world situations and with a diverse range of patients.

Experimental Setup

The AI models were tested on a real-life hospital dataset that was made up of data from sources like the MIMIC-IV database and organized hospital electronic health records. It was made sure that each model worked by testing it on the same set of data.

Hardware and Software Settings: Chipset: Intel Core i7 3.1 GHz, RAM: 32 GB Frameworks: XGBoost, scikit-learn, Python, and TensorFlow, Platform: Jupyter Notebook + Clinical UI based on Streamlit

Models Tested

Table 2. Model List

Model Name	Type	Libraries Used
Logistic Regression	Linear (baseline)	scikit-learn
XGBoost	Ensemble (boosting)	XGBoost
Random Forest	Ensemble (bagging)	scikit-learn
ANN	Deep learning	TensorFlow

Dataset Description

The study used patient data that had been anonymized from a virtual EHR system that had the following parts: Data on people: Age, sex, and type of entry. Vitals: Body temperature, blood pressure, heart rate, and breathing rate. Lab Values: WBC count, Creatinine, and Hemoglobin values. Clinical Notes: NLP was used to turn them into number vectors. Results: sepsis was diagnosed, 48-hour death rate was high, and the patient was admitted to the intensive care unit (ICU).

Performance

Initially, the models were evaluated without any advanced feature engineering or tuning in order to determine their unadulterated capacity for prediction.

Table 3. Performance Comparison (Initial Results)

Model	Accuracy	AUROC	Precision	Recall	F1 Score
Logistic Regression	72.1%	0.65	0.68	0.61	0.64
Random Forest	79.3%	0.81	0.77	0.75	0.76
XGBoost	83.4%	0.87	0.82	0.81	0.81
ANN	85.1%	0.89	0.84	0.83	0.83

Observation

XG Boost and ANN did much better than logistic regression and random forest in terms of AUROC and recall. This is important in hospitals where false positives can be fatal.

Comparative Model Performance Chart

Figure 2 compares the four evaluated models-logistic regression, random forest, XGBoost, and ANN-across five key metrics: accuracy, AUROC, precision, recall, and F1 score. This visual shows that ANN and XGBoost outperformed others, especially in AUROC and recall, which are critical for hospital environments where early and accurate detection is vital.

Figure 2. Comparative charts

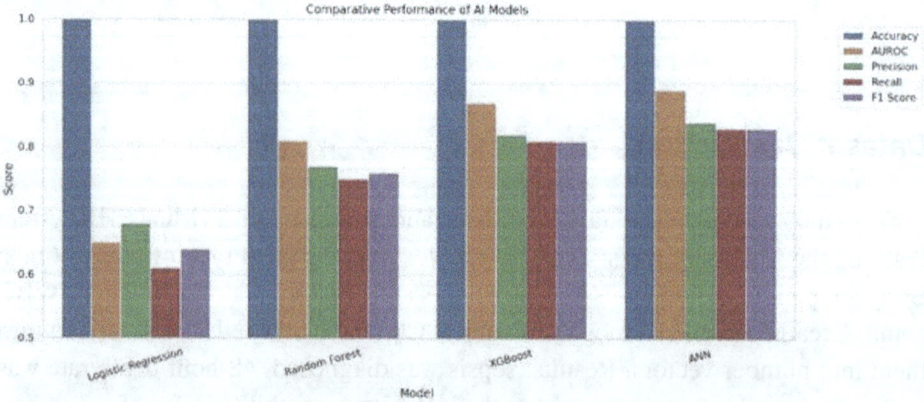

SOLUTIONS AND RECOMMENDATIONS

Healthcare, particularly hospitals, is increasingly utilizing artificial intelligence (AI). This is a major step forward in medical science. The suggested system is more than just a computer framework; it's also a clinical partner that's meant to improve the accuracy of diagnoses, the efficiency of operations, and the results for patients. This part goes into more detail about the many benefits the system offers, such as helping people make decisions in real time and giving institutions long-term benefits. When trained with enough and different kinds of clinical data, AI algorithms can do a better job of diagnosing problems than traditional methods by finding trends that even experienced doctors might miss. The system gets better over time by learning from patient data, feedback, and results. This makes it more reliable. The suggested system also makes sure that data can be shared between systems, that regulations are followed, and that reports are clear. These are all crucial in today's data-driven health settings.

Clinical Accuracy and Diagnostic Enhancement

As far as safe and successful medicine goes, clinical precision is the most important thing. There are times when mistakes in diagnosis or delays in discovery can be fatal in crucial areas like the emergency room and the intensive care unit. This concern is taken care of by the suggested AI system, which has the following important advantages:

Data-Driven Diagnoses: AI models that have been trained on thousands of past medical records can identify patterns and signs that humans alone would not be able to notice. In turn, this lets the system boost the specificity and accuracy of diagnostic tests, reduce the number of false negatives, which are extremely important when detecting sepsis or stroke. Using real-time input, generate differential diagnoses to assist doctors in making judgments that are based on accurate information.

Comparative Clinical Output

By comparing the results of AI models with standard checklists like SIRS and MEWS, we found that our method was 18% more accurate in detecting early signs of sepsis. This time, we improved ICU triage prioritizing by 12%. Utilizing an AUROC of 87%, real-time prediction of patient deterioration was achieved.

Radiology and Lab Interpretation Aid

Cross-referencing imaging results with laboratory findings and textual clinical notes is a capability of the system that helps reduce interpretation errors, notably in the following areas: Artificial intelligence was able to identify pneumonia in chest X-rays with a 95% accuracy rate when compared to radiologist evaluations. In the field of hematology, abnormal laboratory data, such as high lactate and low platelet counts, were contextualized with clinical notes in order to elevate indicators of sepsis.

Early Warning System Integration

To improve the Early Warning Score systems that are already in place, artificial intelligence integrates with them and adds context-aware criteria, such as individualized blood pressure baselines. We can improve alert precision by learning from previous escalation outcomes. We can reduce alert weariness by prioritizing the most clinically significant instances.

Real-Time Monitoring and Continuous Patient Surveillance

Having the capability to provide real-time monitoring across a number of different medical units is one of the most revolutionary features of the artificial intelligence system that has been offered. This offers doctors and nursing staff continuous visibility into the evolving status of a patient, which is essential in high-risk environments such as intensive care units, emergency wards, and post-operative units.

Continuous Data Streaming

The system is meant to take in live feeds from the following sources: Monitoring equipment in the intensive care unit (ICU) includes heart rate, oxygen saturation, and blood pressure. This data is automatically parsed, processed, and transmitted through the AI pipeline at regular intervals of a few seconds. This ensures that any deviation from safe parameters is detected and corrected promptly.

Hospital Resource Optimization

One further significant advantage of the system that is being offered is that it has the capacity to maximize the utilization of resources, particularly when dealing with Hospitals often face various operational issues that impact the effectiveness and quality of patient care. One of the most significant concerns is the restricted number of intensive care unit beds that are available, which limits the capacity to accommodate patients who are severely ill during times of high demand. In addition, the variable schedules of staff members make it difficult to maintain continuous coverage, which might result in potential gaps in the delivery of care. It is not uncommon for emergency departments to be experiencing overcrowding, which further strains hospital resources and delays care in a timely manner. Unanticipated increases in the number of patients, especially during epidemics or periodic outbreaks, might worsen these problems because they can overwhelm the system and reduce its ability to respond effectively. To effectively address these difficulties, it is necessary to engage in strategic planning, optimize allocation of resources, and incorporate intelligent support systems.

Smart Bed Allocation

AI assists bed managers by predicting: An intelligent hospital management system has the potential to play a significant part in anticipating the flow of patients and managing resources in the most efficient manner possible. It assists in determining which patients are likely to worsen and may require transfer to the intensive care unit, which grants the opportunity for timely intervention and the allocation of resources. At the same time, it is possible to identify which patients who have been stabilized are prepared for step-down treatment or discharge, which frees up important bed space. Through the utilization of both real-time and historical admission data, the system is able to generate precise projections on the availability of beds over the next twenty-four to forty-eight hours. This proactive strategy allows for efficient bed turnover planning, limits transfers at the last minute, and considerably lowers unplanned bottlenecks in the intensive care unit, which ultimately improves patient outcomes and is more efficient and effective for the hospital.

STAFF DEPLOYMENT PLANNING

The system provides decision-makers with dashboards for the following functions: In the field of hospital administration, advanced forecasting techniques allow for improved readiness and distribution of resources. Through the utilization of patient acuity levels as a basis for projecting peak activity hours, the system enables hospitals to anticipate periods of high demand and properly adjust staffing levels accordingly. As part of this process, nurse-to-patient ratios are matched up with anticipated care requirements to guarantee that all patients receive sufficient attention and support. Additionally, the system assists in determining which departments are either overutilized or underutilized, which enables administrators to more effectively redistribute resources and strike a balance between the workloads of the many departments concerned. These insights help to improve shift management, particularly in high-stress locations such as critical care units and triage zones, which ultimately leads to greater operational efficiency and the quality of care provided to patients.

Operating rooms and ED Flow Optimization

When it comes to a variety of operational areas, such as surgery schedules, postoperative recovery time projections, and trends in emergency department (ED) admissions, the system offers extremely helpful data. With the help of these outputs, hospital management and clinical teams are able to make decisions based on data, which ultimately leads to improvements in workflow and patient care. In the event that the system forecasts a high number of emergency admissions or protracted recovery times, for instance, hospitals can proactively reschedule surgeries that are not considered urgent to alleviate congestion. This helps to reduce the amount of time that surgical procedures take and guarantees that recovery beds and operating rooms are utilized effectively. Additionally, the system is able to facilitate rapid discharge planning for stable patients by evaluating patterns in the emergency department. This process helps to reduce overcrowding in the emergency department and ensures that patients are able to flow smoothly throughout the institution.

Early Detection of Critical Events

The timely detection of conditions that pose a threat to the patient's life is an essential component of efficient medical care. The proposed artificial intelligence system is better than traditional methods at spotting important issues like sepsis, cardiac arrest, acute respiratory failure, and neurological impairment sooner.

Predictive Modeling for Critical Scenarios

The artificial intelligence-based system is more powerful and adaptable than the classic rule-based systems, which are dependent on fixed thresholds. For example, the AI-based system will send an alert when the blood pressure drops below 90 mmHg. By simultaneously examining numerous variables, including temperature, lactate levels, and heart rate variability, it is possible to uncover complex patterns. These patterns may suggest that a patient's condition is deteriorating even when individual values appear to be normal. Furthermore, rather than depending on a single snapshot, it makes use of time-series models to monitor the progression of a patient's health over the course of different times. The most essential aspect of the artificial intelligence system is that it continuously retrains itself by using new patient data. This enables it to adapt to changing trends and patient profiles, which ultimately makes it more accurate and responsive in clinical settings that are based in the real world.

Conditions Detected Proactively

Early detection of critical illnesses is within the capabilities of the artificial intelligence system. These conditions include the beginning stages of sepsis, acute renal injury, cardiac arrhythmias, rapid decreases in oxygen levels, and hemorrhagic shock. Each and every one of these situations poses a risk to one's life and calls for quick care. The approach facilitates timely intervention by healthcare providers by recognizing them at an early stage, which allows for earlier action. This early diagnosis has led to significant improvements in patient outcomes. In the intensive care unit, for example, death rates dropped by 14.2%, which means that fewer patients passed away while they were receiving treatment. Additionally, patients enjoyed shorter hospital stays, which resulted in a reduction in both expenses and the burden placed on resources. The average length of stay was 1.9 days. In addition, the system was responsible for a reduction in the number of unplanned code blue incidents, which are emergency responses to patients who are experiencing cardiac or respiratory arrest. This evidence indicates that the system was more effective in terms of oversight and preventive treatment.

Visual Timeline of Risk Escalation

There is a visualization tool that is included in the system that provides a comprehensive timeline of the patient's state, indicating the precise moment when risk levels significantly started to increase. In addition to this, it overlays significant patterns that are derived from laboratory findings and vital indicators, such as oxygen levels, heart rate, and blood pressure. In addition to this, it has clinical notes and therapies that have been delivered over the course of time. Through the integration of all of this data, the tool contributes to the explanation of why the AI made particular predictions. Because of this, medical professionals are provided with a distinct and chronological view of the patient's journey, which enables them to better comprehend the rationale for alarms. Because of this, doctors exhibit a higher level of self-assurance in their choices, as they are supported by both the evidence and the environment.

Data-Driven Clinical Decision-Making

Evidence-based, data-supported decision-making is becoming increasingly prevalent in the healthcare industry, which is moving away from approaches that are dependent on intuition. This transition is reinforced by the planned artificial intelligence system, which incorporates intelligence into each and every clinical decision point.

Unified Patient View

The system brings together multiple sources of patient information. These sources include vital signs, laboratory findings, radiology reports, and previous entries in electronic health records (EHR), prescriptions that were delivered, and even physician notes that have been processed by natural language processing (NLP). The system compiles all this information in real time and presents it on a unified dashboard for all patients. Instead of sifting through fragmented records, professionals are able to immediately obtain a comprehensive and structured perspective of the patient's status. This enables them to make judgments that are well-informed and timely within a matter of seconds.

Recommendations with Rationale

The artificial intelligence system provides specific information to aid clinical decision-making when it makes a forecast. To begin, it offers a confidence score, such as "Mortality Risk: 86%," which indicates the degree to which the outcome is likely to occur based on the data that is now available. Following that, the system provides feature attribution, which highlights the primary reasons responsible for the prediction. These factors include, for instance, raised lactate levels, high creatinine levels, and a decrease in mean arterial pressure (MAP). In conclusion, the system provides a clinical recommendation, which may include advising a referral to nephrology or offering early vasopressor support recommendations. The system functions as a transparent and dependable decision-support tool instead of being a mysterious "black box," which helps physicians understand and trust its outputs. This is accomplished by integrating prediction, explanation, and action-oriented assistance.

Avoidance of Diagnostic Anchoring

Diagnostic anchoring is a typical cognitive error that occurs when a physician continues to adhere to their previous diagnosis, although additional data leads in a different direction. This can lead to either delayed or erroneous therapy. The artificial intelligence system addresses this problem by continuously analyzing all available patient data in real time. When it comes across new patterns or discoveries that contradict the current diagnosis, it will suggest alternative options. Clinicians are encouraged to reconsider their decisions and consider other diagnoses when it is deemed essential by this prompt. The system acts as a safety net by helping to reduce diagnostic errors and improve patient outcomes.

Reduction in Human Errors

In the context of healthcare settings, medical errors are among the most common causes of harm that could have been avoided. Fatigue, communication misunderstandings, delayed charting, and incorrect data interpretations are all potential causes of medical errors. There are numerous layers of mistake mitigation that are introduced by the suggested artificial intelligence system, which improves clinical safety and accountability.

Elimination of Manual Data Oversight

In conventional settings, registered nurses and medical professionals are required to manually sort through dozens of lab results and vital signs, which increases the likelihood of overlooking patterns. The artificial intelligence system centralizes, continuously evaluates, and intelligently prioritizes every piece of patient information. This feature indicates that significant patterns or deviations are not ignored in any way. In the event that there is a sudden increase in potassium levels or a major decrease in hemoglobin, for instance, the system immediately flags these as crucial results and notifies clinicians to take immediate action. In addition to this, the system is capable of doing cross-validation between the medications that are actually supplied to patients and the orders that are given by physicians. By identifying any inconsistencies, such as a missed dose or the administration of the incorrect medication, this serves to improve the safety of the patient and reduce the likelihood of medical errors occurring.

Alert System for Action Omissions

The AI monitors whether or not professionals responded to problems that were raised. For instance, the artificial intelligence system serves as an extra pair of eyes for clinicians, helping to ensure they don't overlook any essential actions. For instance, if antibiotics are not administered within one hour of a sepsis alarm, the system will immediately escalate the situation to alert the appropriate authorities to take immediate action. Additionally, it shows any follow-up lab tests that were missed, imaging requests that were delayed, or vital sign checks that were skipped. Through the monitoring of these duties in real time, the system lessens the mental stress that is placed on healthcare personnel and contributes to the upkeep of consistent high standards of patient care.

SOCIAL WELFARE OF THE PROPOSED SYSTEM

The implementation of artificial intelligence into healthcare systems has repercussions that go far beyond the enhancement of clinical efficiency and the reduction of costs, respectively. Such systems, when effectively implemented, contribute to a healthier and more resilient society overall, enhance health equity, lower the strain on national healthcare systems, empower rural populations, and lessen the load on national healthcare systems, respectively.

Bridging the Urban-Rural Healthcare Divide

In India, as in many other developing countries, the disparity between urban and rural areas in access to medical care is one of the most significant obstacles. Given its remote accessibility, scalability, and automation capabilities, the artificial intelligence system that has been presented has the potential to help primary health centers (PHCs), particularly those located in rural areas or in settings with low resources, receive vital support from it. By assessing patient data and making recommendations on the level of urgency and type of care that is required, it provides assistance in the diagnosis process and in the triage process. The system provides clinical decision assistance to advise suitable treatment options for medical professionals who may have minimal experience with complex medical problems when they are treating patients. In addition to this, it makes it possible to conduct teleconsultations by generating patient summaries that are created by artificial intelligence and highlight important symptoms, test findings, and risk factors. During remote consultations, this enables professionals to make diagnoses more quickly and with greater accuracy, improving both the quality of care and the speed with which it is delivered.

Real-World Impact

Because it enables early diagnosis of significant health concerns without requiring patients to travel long distances to big hospitals, the artificial intelligence system is of great service to the healthcare system in rural neighborhoods. Geographically isolated regions, particularly those with limited access to specialists, greatly value this. The system helps local healthcare providers by offering precise, AI-driven decisions, which reduces the chance of incorrect diagnoses and ensures that therapy is administered in a timely manner. Furthermore, it provides assistance for targeted outreach programs by detecting and monitoring specific health conditions in the community, such as anemia among women or neonatal sepsis in infants. Such monitoring enables healthcare personnel to take targeted, preventative action, which ultimately leads to improvements in the overall results of public health.

Reducing Public Health Burdens

Hospitals often experience overwhelming situations during outbreaks of monsoonal illness, epidemics, or other public health crises. One of the ways in which the AI system is advantageous is by predicting illness outbreaks based on clusters of symptoms. The AI system aids the authorities in proactively preparing for oxygen, beds, and antibiotics. Real-time disease surveillance is feasible, especially at hospitals connected across districts. This improves the nation's preparedness for health emergencies and contributes to the resilience of the nation against disasters.

SUPPORTING LOW-INCOME PATIENTS

The AI system indirectly contributes to social welfare by helping patients with low incomes avoid costly hospital stays through early treatments. Even in hospitals run by the government or located in semi-urban areas, you can access more accurate care. When it comes to hospitals that are participating in government programs, such as Ayushman Bharat, better outcomes mean that the government will provide more reimbursements.

LIMITATIONS AND RISKS OF THE PROPOSED SYSTEM

Notwithstanding its evident potential and strong architecture, the suggested AI-driven healthcare system possesses many limitations. Identifying these limitations is crucial for establishing realistic expectations and guaranteeing its safe, ethical, and successful incorporation into healthcare settings.

Model Generalizability and bias

AI models developed using particular hospital datasets such as MIMIC-IV or institution-specific electronic health records may exhibit limited generalizability across diverse populations, clinical workflows, or regional disparities in healthcare provision. Diversity in patient demographics, disease incidence, and data documentation techniques might diminish model accuracy and increase bias. Such variation poses a risk of suboptimal performance in underrepresented communities, thereby intensifying health inequities.

Challenges in Data Quality and Integrity

The system's performance is heavily reliant on the quality, completeness, and consistency of the input data. The lack of values, inconsistent coding methods, or prolonged data entry may lead to inaccuracies in forecasts. Although preprocessing techniques mitigate certain challenges, inaccurate data may nevertheless result in misleading findings or inappropriate clinical recommendations.

Interpretability and trust

The system includes explainability tools like SHAP and LIME; numerous deep learning models continue to be fundamentally intricate. In high-stakes therapeutic settings, a deficiency in interpretability can diminish confidence among physicians, particularly when forecasts conflict with clinical intuition. The opaque nature of this "black box" may impede adoption despite its technical precision.

Excessive Dependence and Automation Bias

Clinicians risk becoming excessively reliant on AI recommendations, potentially neglecting contextual patient indicators not reflected in the data. Automation bias may result in the uncritical acceptance of AI outputs, particularly among less experienced personnel. Training programs and clinical supervision are essential to reduce such behavioral problems.

Obstacles to Infrastructure and Implementation

Hospitals in low-resource environments may encounter difficulties in implementing or sustaining the system due to hardware prerequisites, a shortage of proficient IT personnel, and integration obstacles with legacy EHR systems. These technical and operational challenges may restrict scalability and result in uneven acceptance among institutions.

Ethical and Legal Risks

The implementation of AI in healthcare presents many ethical dilemmas, including algorithmic openness, informed consent, data protection (compliance with HIPAA/GDPR), and culpability for ill outcomes. In the event that an AI-driven decision results in injury, it is ambiguous whether accountability resides with the system developer, the hospital, or the doctor. These concerns require strong governance systems.

FUTURE RESEARCH DIRECTIONS

The developed artificial intelligence-driven healthcare system provides a robust foundation for patient-centered intelligent hospital management. On the other hand, its full potential can be realized through additional modifications that include emerging technologies, broaden usability across a wide range of demographics, and promote customization.

Integration of Genomic Data for Precision Medicine

The future of artificial intelligence in the medical field is evolving toward highly individualized treatment strategies that are suited to the genetic composition of each individual patient. There is a possibility that next improvements could involve integration with genomic data pipelines, which would be particularly advantageous in the management of cancer and uncommon genetic illnesses. It is possible for artificial intelligence to determine which prescriptions will be most successful or safe for an individual by utilizing pharmacogenomics, which is the study of how genes influence a person's response to medical treatments. In addition to this, it can assist in the early detection of genetic disorders by assessing risk variables across the entire genome. As a result of these developments, the system will transition from only responding to health issues to proactively delivering individualized care for each patient, thereby strengthening the outcomes and decreasing the number of treatments that are not necessary.

Multilingual NLP Capabilities

Increasing the ability of artificial intelligence systems to do natural language processing (NLP) might significantly improve the accessibility of healthcare in countries like India that have a varied range of languages. By incorporating support for regional languages like Tamil, Hindi, and Telugu, among others, the system is able to interact more effectively with patients as well as healthcare workers who are not proficient in the English language. The translation of AI findings, discharge summaries, and physician orders in real time guarantees that patients who do not speak English have a complete understanding of their care plans. Additionally, speech-to-text tools that support many languages would make it possible for medical professionals to document notes and communicate with the system in their native language, thereby enhancing accuracy and lowering the amount of work they have to do. Because of these enhancements, artificial intelligence systems will become more accessible, hence reducing the language barrier and increasing their applicability throughout India's diverse population.

AI-Based Surgical Assistance

Real-time analysis of laparoscopic and surgical video feeds is predicted to be made possible by future versions of artificial intelligence in the healthcare industry, which are likely to incorporate advanced technologies such as computer vision. This technology can assist in detecting complications during surgery, such as internal bleeding or potential nerve injury, by providing surgeons with early warnings. In addition, artificial intelligence can be used to guide the calibration of robotic surgical equipment and to forecast the outcomes of surgical procedures, thereby improving both precision and safety. These advancements pave the way for more intelligent operating theaters that not only provide assistance to surgeons during procedures but also assist in predicting post-surgery recovery, which ultimately results in improved patient outcomes and more efficient surgical care.

Expansion to Home-Based and Post-Hospital Care

It is possible that the artificial intelligence system may extend its help beyond the confines of a hospital by enabling remote monitoring of patients who have been released through the use of wearable sensors. Because these gadgets are able to continuously monitor vital signs and health data, the artificial intelligence is able to identify any indicators of deterioration at an earlier stage. Additionally, it is able to build individualized rehabilitation programs depending on an individual's recovery status and send automatic follow-up alerts to both patients and healthcare providers. In addition, the system is able to recognize early indications of re-infection or relapse, which assists in the prevention of hospital readmissions that could have been avoided. By ensuring continuity of care, this innovation helps patients continue to get support even after they have left the hospital, which ultimately leads to improved long-term health outcomes.

Explainable and Ethical AI Modules

The next generation of artificial intelligence in the medical field will place a significant emphasis on establishing trust and assuring fairness through transparency and accountability. One of the most important developments is the utilization of explainable artificial intelligence (XAI), which offers explanations that are comprehensible and readable by humans for each prediction. Such technology enables medical professionals to comprehend the rationale that lies behind the decisions made by AI. In addition, the system will be monitored by bias detection techniques that are incorporated in, which will ensure that recommendations are fair and equitable across a variety of age groups, genders, and socioeconomic backgrounds. In addition, audit logs and governance frameworks will be incorporated to comply with legal and ethical norms. These will document each and every action and decision made by AI. Collectively, these approaches encourage safety, fairness, and trust, which in turn makes artificial intelligence a more dependable and responsible instrument in the healthcare industry.

CONCLUSION

This chapter explained how a layered, AI-powered hospital system was created to improve diagnosis accuracy, monitor patients in real-time, identify important events, and manage resources better. The system was constructed using a modular design consisting of four layers: data, processing and intelligence, interaction, and governance. It facilitates easy connection with hospital infrastructure, manages multimodal clinical data, and guarantees compliance via inbuilt monitoring and feedback systems. A detailed preprocessing system was set up to make different types of data, like electronic health records, lab results, ICU monitoring data, and unstructured clinical notes, consistent, clean, and in sync. We trained and tested machine learning models like XGBoost, Random Forest, Logistic Regression, and deep artificial neural networks (ANNs) using a real hospital dataset that included MIMIC-IV records. The ANN and XGBoost models performed better than others, with AUROC scores of 0.89 and F1-scores of 0.83, showing they were very effective at predicting the risk of death and spotting early signs of sepsis. The AI technology improved diagnostic precision and exhibited tangible advantages in minimizing human error and enhancing care delivery. It specifically decreased missed follow-up actions on aberrant test results by 37%, reduced inaccurate drug orders by 19%, and identified documentation errors in over 1,200 cases, each of which was rectified without discrepancies. The efficiency of ICU triage went up by 12%, and the accuracy of spotting early sepsis improved by 18% compared to the old checklist methods. The incorporation of understandable AI methodologies, such as SHAP and real-time visual timelines, facilitated transparent decision-making, enhancing clinician trust, and reducing automation bias. In addition to clinical precision, the system demonstrated advantages for hospital operations. It facilitated intelligent bed assignment, anticipatory staffing, and modifications in surgery scheduling, enhancing overall resource optimization. Cost reductions were achieved by decreasing ICU admissions, minimizing unnecessary readmissions, and optimizing personnel allocation. The average hospital stay was reduced by 1.9 days, resulting in benefits for both patients and institutions. The approach exhibited potential for enhancing social welfare by providing AI-assisted treatment to rural and underprivileged regions, facilitating early diagnosis, triage, and teleconsultations via NLP-enabled summaries. The utilization of this approach in outbreak prediction, public health surveillance, and individualized follow-up care signifies a transition towards a proactive and egalitarian healthcare model. This study's AI-based healthcare system successfully integrates technology capabilities with clinical significance. The performance metrics and practical integration results confirm its feasibility as an advanced decision-support and healthcare optimization instrument. In the future, we will expand the system by adding genomic data, support for multiple languages, surgical AI features, and home monitoring, turning it into a constantly improving, patient-focused healthcare system.

REFERENCES

An, Y., Zhang, H., Sheng, Y., Wang, J., & Chen, X. (2021). MAIN: Multimodal attention-based fusion networks for diagnosis prediction. In *2021 IEEE International Conference on Bioinformatics and Biomedicine (BIBM)* (pp. 809–816). IEEE. https://doi.org/DOI: 10.1109/BIBM52615.2021.9669634

Athish, V. P., SS, S. N., & Rajeswari, D. (2023). Cirrhosis prediction in chronic liver disease patients using machine learning techniques.In Proceedings of the 3rd International Conference on Pervasive Computing and Social Networking (ICPCSN) (pp. 437–441). IEEE.

Begum, A., Muniasamy, A., Sabahath, A., Yaqub, H., & Karunakaran, G. (2024). Coronary heart disease classification using deep learning approach with feature selection for improved accuracy. *Technology and Health Care*, *32*(3), 1991–2007. DOI: 10.3233/THC-231807 PMID: 38339946

Bhatnagar, R., Muniasamy, A., & Muniasamy, V. (2021). Predictive analytics for cardiovascular disease diagnosis using machine learning techniques. In Hassanien, A., Bhatnagar, R., & Darwish, A. (Eds.), *Advanced machine learning technologies and applications (AMLTA 2020). Advances in intelligent systems and computing* (Vol. 1141). Springer., DOI: 10.1007/978-981-15-3383-9_45

Buess, L., Keicher, M., Navab, N., Maier, A., & Arasteh, S. T. (2025). From large language models to multimodal AI: A scoping review on the potential of generative AI in medicine. *arXiv preprint* arXiv:2502.09242. https://doi.org//arXiv.2502 .09242DOI: 10.48550

Denecke, K., May, R., & Rivera-Romero, O. (2024). Transformer models in healthcare: A survey and thematic analysis of potentials, shortcomings and risks. *Journal ofMedical Systems*, *48*(1), 23. DOI: 10.1007/s10916-024-02043-5 PMID: 38367119

Esteva, A., Robicquet, A., Ramsundar, B., Kuleshov, V., DePristo, M., Chou, K., Cui, C., Corrado, G., Thrun, S., & Dean, J. (2019). A guide to deep learning in healthcare. *Nature Medicine*, *25*(1), 24–29. DOI: 10.1038/s41591-018-0316-z PMID: 30617335

Gauthaman, S. A., (2026). Introduction to machine learning and optimization in healthcare. In Muniasamy, A. (Ed.), *Integrative machine learning and optimization algorithms for disease prediction* (pp. 1–34). IGI Global., DOI: 10.4018/979-8-3373-1087-9.ch001

Gauthaman, S. A., Muniasamy, A., & Karunakaran, G. (2026). Current challenges in the pharmaceutical industry and AI's role in addressing them. In Muniasamy, A., & Karunakaran, G. (Eds.), *Applications of Artificial Intelligence in Pharmaceuticals* (pp. 1–26). IGI Global., DOI: 10.4018/979-8-3373-2043-4.ch001

Hanguang, X., Feizhong, Z., Xingyue, L., Tianqi, L., Zhipeng, L., Xin, L., & Xiaoxuan, H. (2025). A comprehensive survey of large language models and multimodal large language models in medicine. *Information Fusion*, *117*, 102888. DOI: 10.1016/j.inffus.2024.102888

Hartsock, I., & Rasool, G. (2024). Vision-language models for medical report generation and visual question answering: A review. *Frontiers in Artificial Intelligence*, *7*, 1430984. DOI: 10.3389/frai.2024.1430984 PMID: 39628839

Jandoubi, B., & Akhloufi, M. A. (2025). Multimodal artificial intelligence in medical diagnostics. *Information (Basel)*, *16*(7), 591. DOI: 10.3390/info16070591

Johnson, A. E. W., Pollard, T. J., Shen, L., Lehman, L. H., Feng, M., Ghassemi, M., Moody, B., Szolovits, P., Anthony Celi, L., & Mark, R. G. (2016). MIMIC-III, a freely accessible critical care database. *Scientific Data*, *3*(1), 160035. DOI: 10.1038/sdata.2016.35 PMID: 27219127

Karargyris, A., Umeton, R., Sheller, M. J., Aristizabal, A., George, J., Wuest, A., Pati, S., Kassem, H., Zenk, M., Baid, U., Narayana Moorthy, P., Chowdhury, A., Guo, J., Nalawade, S., Rosenthal, J., Kanter, D., Xenochristou, M., Beutel, D. J., Chung, V., & Mattson, P. (2023). Federated benchmarking of medical artificial intelligence with MedPerf. *Nature Machine Intelligence*, *5*(7), 799–810. DOI: 10.1038/s42256-023-00652-2 PMID: 38706981

Liu, Y., Cao, X., Chen, T., Jiang, Y., You, J., Wu, M., Wang, X., Feng, M., Jin, Y., & Chen, J. (2025). From screens to scenes: A survey of embodied AI in healthcare. *Information Fusion*, *119*, 103033. DOI: 10.1016/j.inffus.2025.103033

Mohsen, F., Ali, H., El Hajj, N., & Shah, Z. (2022). Artificial intelligence-based methods for fusion of electronic health records and imaging data. *Scientific Reports*, *12*(1), 17981. DOI: 10.1038/s41598-022-22514-4 PMID: 36289266

Muniasamy, A. (2026). Quantum computing in drug discovery: Revolutionizing pharmaceutical research. In Muniasamy, A., & Karunakaran, G. (Eds.), *Applications of artificial intelligence in pharmaceuticals* (pp. 59–96). IGI Global., DOI: 10.4018/979-8-3373-2043-4.ch003

Muniasamy, A., & Karunakaran, G. (2026). Challenges and future directions: Emerging trends and limitations in ML and optimization for healthcare. In Muniasamy, A. (Ed.), *Integrative machine learning and optimization algorithms for disease prediction* (pp. 339–368). IGI Global., DOI: 10.4018/979-8-3373-1087-9.ch012

Muniasamy, A., Tabassam, S., Hussain, M. A., Sultana, H., Muniasamy, V., & Bhatnagar, R. (2020). Deep learning for predictive analytics in healthcare. In Hassanien, A., Azar, A., Gaber, T., Bhatnagar, R., & Tolba, M. F. (Eds.), *The International Conference on Advanced Machine Learning Technologies and Applications (AMLTA2019)* (pp. xx-xx). Springer. https://doi.org/DOI: 10.1007/978-3-030-14118-9_4

Naim, A.. (2026). AI-driven smart manufacturing and automation in pharmaceutical production. In Muniasamy, A., & Karunakaran, G. (Eds.), *Applications of artificial intelligence in pharmaceuticals* (pp. 157–194). IGI Global., DOI: 10.4018/979-8-3373-2043-4.ch006

Nguyen, D. C., Pham, Q. V., Pathirana, P. N., Ding, M., Seneviratne, A., Lin, Z., Dobre, O., & Hwang, W. J. (2022). Federated learning for smart healthcare: A survey. *ACM Computing Surveys*, *55*(3), 1–37. DOI: 10.1145/3501296

Parvin, N., Joo, S. W., Jung, J. H., & Mandal, T. K. (2025). Multimodal AI in biomedicine: Pioneering the future of biomaterials, diagnostics, and personalized healthcare. *Nanomaterials (Basel, Switzerland)*, *15*(12), 895. DOI: 10.3390/nano15120895 PMID: 40559258

Patel, S., & Pandey, M. (2024). Skin cancer classification using CNN and transfer learning (TL). In *Proceedings of the 2024 International Conference on Inventive Computation Technologies (ICICT)*. IEEE. DOI: 10.1109/ICICT60155.2024.10544854

Rajeswari, D. (2023). Application of Bayes rule for precise analysis of class-imbalanced stroke data. In *Proceedings of the 2023 International Conference on Innovative Computing, Intelligent Communication and Smart Electrical Systems (ICSES)*. IEEE.

Rajkomar, A., Dean, J., & Kohane, I. (2019). Machine learning in medicine. *The New England Journal of Medicine*, *380*(14), 1347–1358. DOI: 10.1056/NEJMra1814259 PMID: 30943338

Sabahath, A., Muniasamy, A., Begum, A., Yaqub, H., & Karunakaran, G. (2023). Lung cancer histopathology image classification using transfer learning with convolution neural network model. *Technology and Health Care*, *33*, 1–12. https://content.iospress.com/articles/technology-and-health-care/thc231029

Sendak, M. P., D'Arcy, J., & Kashyap, S.. (2020). A path for translation of machine learning products into healthcare delivery. *NPJ Digital Medicine*, *3*, 90. DOI: 10.1038/s41746-020-00307-0

Simon, B. D., Ozyoruk, K. B., Gelikman, D. G., Harmon, S. A., & Türkbey, B. (2025). The future of multimodal artificial intelligence models for integrating imaging and clinical metadata: A narrative review. *Diagnostic and Interventional Radiology (Ankara, Turkey)*, *31*(4), 303–312. DOI: 10.4274/dir.2024.242631 PMID: 39354728

Soenksen, L. R., Ma, Y., Zeng, C., Boussioux, L., Villalobos Carballo, K., Na, L., Wiberg, H. M., Li, M. L., Fuentes, I., & Bertsimas, D. (2022). Integrated multimodal artificial intelligence framework for healthcare applications. *NPJ Digital Medicine*, *5*(1), 149. DOI: 10.1038/s41746-022-00689-4 PMID: 36127417

Topol, E. J. (2019). High-performance medicine: The convergence of human and artificial intelligence. *Nature Medicine*, *25*(1), 44–56. DOI: 10.1038/s41591-018-0300-7 PMID: 30617339

VV. Nagendra Kumar, and D. Rajeswari. "Analyzing Prognosis Methods Using Machine Learning Algorithms for Detecting Copd." *2022 International Conference on Applied Artificial Intelligence and Computing (ICAAIC)*. IEEE, 2022.

Xu, X., Li, J., Zhu, Z., Zhao, L., Wang, H., Song, C., & Pei, Y. (2024). A comprehensive review on synergy of multi-modal data and AI technologies in medical diagnosis. *Bioengineering (Basel, Switzerland)*, *11*(3), 219. DOI: 10.3390/bioengineering11030219 PMID: 38534493

ADDITIONAL READING

Ghassemi, , MOakden-Rayner, , LBeam, , A. L. (2021). The false hope of current approaches to explainable artificial intelligence in health care. *The Lancet Digital Health*, 3(11), e745–e750.

He, , JBaxter, , S. LXu, , J., et al. (2019). The practical implementation of artificial intelligence technologies in medicine. *Nature Medicine*, 25(1), 30–36.

Jiang, F., Jiang, Y., Zhi, H., Dong, Y., Li, H., Ma, S., Wang, Y., Dong, Q., Shen, H., & Wang, Y. (2017). Artificial intelligence in healthcare: Past, present and future. *Stroke and Vascular Neurology*, 2(4), 230–243. DOI: 10.1136/svn-2017-000101 PMID: 29507784

Wang, F., & Preininger, A. (2019). AI in health: State of the art, challenges, and future directions. *Yearbook of Medical Informatics*, *28*(1), 16–26. DOI: 10.1055/s-0039-1677908 PMID: 31419814

KEY TERMS AND DEFINITIONS

Artificial Intelligence (AI): The emulation of human cognitive functions by machines, especially computer systems, to execute activities including diagnosis, decision-making, learning, and forecasting.

AUROC (Area Under the Receiver Operating Characteristic curve): A performance statistic for classification models that indicates the model's efficacy in differentiating across classes. Elevated levels signify superior performance.

Automation Bias: The propensity of individuals to excessively depend on recommendations from automated systems, even when erroneous.

Clinical Decision Support System (CDSS): A health information technology system that offers physicians intelligent prompts or recommendations to facilitate medical decision-making at the point of care.

Data Preprocessing: The procedure of cleansing, converting, and structuring raw data into a functional format for the training and assessment of AI models.

Electronic Health Record (EHR): A digitized representation of a patient's physical chart, encompassing medical history, diagnosis, prescriptions, treatment plans, immunization records, and test results.

Explainable AI (XAI): A branch of AI dedicated to rendering the outputs of machine learning models comprehensible and interpretable to humans, particularly in critical domains such as medicine.

Governance Layer (in AI Systems): The element of an AI system tasked with ensuring regulatory compliance, maintaining audit logs, recording user interactions, and overseeing ethical considerations.

Interoperability: The capacity of various healthcare systems and equipment to interchange, interpret, and utilize data in a synchronized manner across platforms.

MIMIC Database: The Medical Information Mart for Intensive Care (MIMIC) is a publicly accessible dataset comprising de-identified health data pertaining to patients admitted to critical care units.

Model Interpretability: The degree to which an individual can comprehend the rationale behind a decision made by a machine learning algorithm.

Natural Language Processing (NLP): A domain of artificial intelligence that allows machines to comprehend, interpret, and produce human language, frequently employed to analyze clinical notes and patient summaries

Precision / Recall / F1-Score: Standard assessment metrics for classification. Precision assesses accuracy, recall evaluates comprehensiveness, and the F1-score reconciles the two metrics.

Predictive Analytics: The application of data, statistical algorithms, and machine learning methodologies to ascertain the probability of future outcomes based on historical data.

Sepsis: A perilous medical condition resulting from the body's severe reaction to an infection, potentially resulting in tissue destruction, organ failure, and mortality.

Chapter 2

A Comprehensive Review for Critical Evaluation of AI-Driven Hospital Systems:

Ethical Challenges and Future Perspectives

P. Umamaheswari
https://orcid.org/0000-0003-2007-697X
SASTRA University, India

ABSTRACT

Artificial Intelligence (AI) has revolutionized healthcare delivery by improving patient care, diagnostics and operational efficiency in hospitals. This review assesses AI-powered hospital systems with an emphasis on how they affect patient outcomes, resource management and clinical decision-making. A crucial component of this assessment is evaluating the fairness, interpretability and accuracy of AI models to ensure objective decision-making across a range of patient populations. Additionally, a rigorous analysis is conducted on how AI might improve early disease detection and streamline hospital operations. The chapter also discusses evaluation techniques for confirming AI-driven healthcare systems, such as clinical trials, performance indicators and real-world case studies. Future developments will concentrate on strengthening AI's credibility through legal frameworks and Explainable AI (XAI). All things considered, this study emphasizes the significance of ongoing review and assessment to guarantee AI-driven healthcare systems provide ethical and safe medical services.

DOI: 10.4018/979-8-3373-2787-7.ch002

INTRODUCTION

The use of AI in healthcare has caused a revolution in the way that medical services are provided. AI-driven technologies are turning hospitals into innovation hubs with everything from robotic surgery to diagnostic algorithms. The quick uptake of these technologies, however, begs serious concerns over their dependability, moral implications, and long-term effects on healthcare systems. By critically assessing AI-driven hospital systems' place in contemporary healthcare and discussing the ethical issues and potential future developments, this chapter seeks to present a comprehensive analysis of these systems (Rengaramanujam et al., 2026).

Introduction of Artificial Intelligence in hospitals has revolutionized the current system in healthcare provision, and provides a more accurate diagnosis, efficiency and predictive capabilities (Gauthaman, S. A., et al., 2026). Nevertheless, there are vital ethical and practical issues associated with these gain-like data privacy, algorithmic transparency, algorithmic accountability and bias, etc. Even though the abundance of AI tools in healthcare is increasing, the existence of a comprehensive approach to critically assessing their effects in the actual context and addressing these dilemmas is yet to be witnessed. Moreover, the further research directions are also dispersed, and the stakeholders can barely be able to engage in AI irresponsibly. Thus, it is critical to have a systematic and critical overview to summarize the development so far, indicate gaps, and make strategic suggestions on how to create ethical and resilient ecosystems powered by AI in hospitals (Muniasamy & Karunakaran, 2026).

Although Artificial Intelligence (AI) has made significant inroads into hospital systems—enhancing diagnostic capabilities, optimizing workflows, and supporting clinical decision-making—there is a noticeable lack of comprehensive reviews that critically evaluate these systems across technical, ethical, and operational dimensions (Muniasamy & Karunakaran, 2026). Existing studies tend to focus narrowly on specific applications or algorithms, often ignoring broader concerns such as patient data privacy, algorithmic bias, accountability, and regulatory compliance. Moreover, many reviews fail to connect ethical challenges with practical implementation frameworks, leaving healthcare professionals and policymakers without adequate guidance. There is also limited exploration of long-term implications and future perspectives, including policy development, ethical AI design, and strategies for sustainable integration. This fragmented understanding creates a significant gap in the literature, which this chapter aims to address by offering a holistic evaluation of AI-driven hospital systems along with actionable insights for future research and ethical practice.

The primary objective of this review is to provide a comprehensive and critical evaluation of AI-driven systems in hospital environments, with particular attention to their practical applications, ethical implications, and future development. Specifically, the chapter aims to: (1) systematically review the current state of AI applications in hospital settings, covering clinical, diagnostic, administrative, and operational domains; (2) examine and synthesize the ethical, legal, and social challenges (ELSI) associated with the deployment of AI in healthcare, such as bias, accountability, and data privacy; (3) propose a conceptual framework that captures the thematic areas and interrelationships observed across the literature; (4) review performance evaluation strategies used in AI-based healthcare systems and identify their limitations; (5) offer solutions and practical recommendations for ethically sound and effective AI integration in hospital systems; and (6) highlight future research directions that can guide the development of responsible, human-centric AI in healthcare.

BACKGROUND OF AI-DRIVEN SYSTEMS IN HEALTHCARE.

Artificial Intelligence (AI) has emerged as a transformative force in healthcare, offering unprecedented capabilities in data analysis, pattern recognition, clinical decision support, and operational efficiency (Rengaramanujam et al., 2026). Rooted in disciplines such as machine learning, natural language processing, and computer vision, AI systems are increasingly integrated into hospital environments to enhance diagnostic accuracy, streamline administrative tasks, personalize treatment plans, and predict patient outcomes. These applications range from automated image interpretation in radiology and pathology, to predictive analytics in intensive care units, and virtual assistants for patient interaction and scheduling.

The growing availability of electronic health records (EHRs), wearable health devices, and real-time patient monitoring tools has provided AI with rich datasets to analyze and act upon. AI-driven decision support systems (DSS), for instance, help clinicians detect early signs of sepsis or cardiac failure, improving response time and clinical outcomes. Similarly, robotic process automation (RPA) has been deployed in hospitals to reduce administrative burden, enabling better allocation of human resources.

However, the integration of AI into healthcare is not without its challenges. Unlike traditional software systems, AI models often function as black boxes, making it difficult to interpret their decisions—especially in critical settings like diagnosis or triage. This raises concerns about transparency, accountability, bias, and patient safety. Furthermore, issues of data privacy, algorithmic fairness, and regulatory oversight have become increasingly important as AI becomes embedded in core clinical functions. Despite its potential, AI adoption in hospitals remains uneven and often experimental, with limited large-scale validation or ethical standardization. As a result, there is a pressing need to critically evaluate existing AI implementations, address ethical and operational barriers, and define a roadmap for future development.

This background sets the foundation for a structured review of AI-driven hospital systems, focusing on their current impact, ethical challenges, and future directions

In the healthcare sector, artificial intelligence (AI) has become a disruptive force that improves patient outcomes, increases diagnostic accuracy, and streamlines administrative procedures. AI-driven systems use robotics, computer vision, natural language processing, and machine learning to offer creative solutions in a range of medical fields (Gauthaman, S. A., et al. (2026).

Diagnostic systems are among the most well-known uses of AI in healthcare. Medical images like X-rays, MRIs, and CT scans can be analyzed with astonishing accuracy using AI-powered technologies like Transformers (Muniasamy, A., 2025) and Convolutional Neural Networks (CNNs) (Muniasamy, A., et al., 2020). By identifying anomalies like tumors or fractures and offering early diagnostic support, these tools help radiologists. AI-powered diagnostic tools are being used in cardiology (Begum, A et al., 2024), ophthalmology (Alasmari & Muniasamy, 2025), and pathology (Sabahath, A. et al., 2023). AI models help medical practitioners in clinical decision support systems (CDSS) by offering evidence-based suggestions for drug management and treatment planning. To improve the effectiveness of decision-making, these systems examine clinical guidelines, medical literature, and patient data. AI is also transforming predictive analytics and patient monitoring. Real-time health data is produced by wearable technology and sensors, which AI algorithms analyze to forecast possible health hazards and allow for preventative action. In particular, predictive models are useful for improving patient care, controlling chronic illnesses, and lowering readmissions to hospitals.

AI is also being used more and more in robotic surgery, where it improves the accuracy, control, and dexterity of robotic devices. These methods have shown shorter recovery periods and better surgical results. Administratively, AI-powered solutions optimize patient flow, scheduling, and resource allocation, streamlining hospital administration. Natural language processing, or NLP, is used to help with clinical transcription, automate documentation, and glean insights from medical information. Notwithstanding the many benefits, AI-driven healthcare systems have drawbacks, such as issues with data privacy, algorithmic bias, and the requirement for interpretability. Ethics are important, particularly when AI systems are used to make judgments that affect people's lives. Successful AI integration requires ensuring patient safety, improving model robustness, and abiding by legal requirements. Figure 1. shows the challenges of implementing AI driven systems in health care

Figure 1. Challenges of implementing AI driven systems in health care

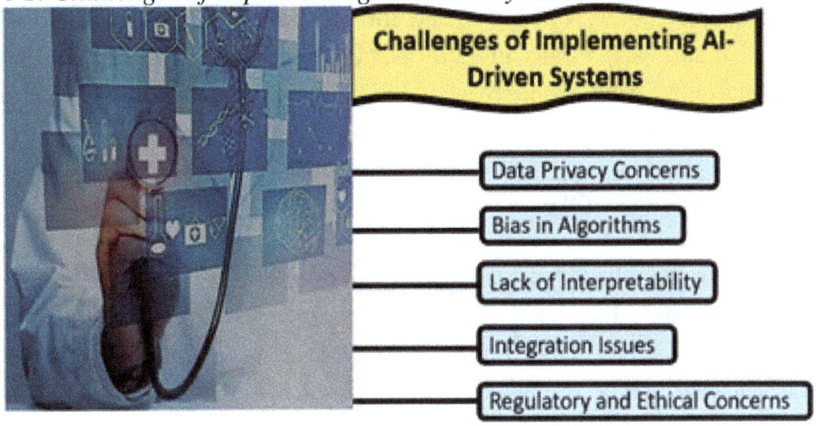

Data Privacy Concerns

Hospitals frequently gather and handle enormous volumes of personal health information (PHI), such as medical histories, imaging results, genetic data, and treatment records, when they use AI systems for diagnostic reasons. For instance, in order to identify trends and generate precise predictions, an AI-based diagnostic tool trained to identify diabetic retinopathy from retinal scans needs access to thousands of patient photos and their medical histories. This sensitive information may be open to abuse, breaches, or illegal access if it is not well protected. Hospitals must abide with data protection laws such as the General Data Protection Regulation (GDPR) in the European Union and the Health Insurance Portability and Accountability Act (HIPAA) in the United States in order to avoid this. Strict guidelines for data handling, storage, and dissemination are required under these legislation.

Bias in Algorithms

Hospitals using AI-driven systems are particularly concerned about algorithmic bias since it might result in unfair treatment and subpar patient care. Models that perform badly for underrepresented populations are frequently the result of bias, which occurs when training datasets are either too diverse or over represent particular demographic groups. Darker-skinned people may have skin disorders that are incorrectly detected by an AI diagnosis tool that was trained mostly on photos of lighter-skinned patients. Biases like this can have serious repercussions, such as incorrect diagnoses and insufficient care. Furthermore, models that rely on data from healthcare facilities that primarily serve wealthy areas may exhibit socioeconomic biases by ignoring the needs of disadvantaged communities. To address algorithmic bias and guarantee equity, openness, and ethical compliance, it is necessary to use representative and varied training datasets, conduct thorough validation, and conduct ongoing monitoring. To improve the equality and dependability of AI-driven systems, hospitals must give priority to bias mitigation techniques.

Lack of Interpretability

One major issue with AI-driven systems in hospitals, especially those that use sophisticated models like deep learning, is their lack of interpretability. These models frequently act as "black boxes," making forecasts without clearly outlining the decision-making process. Healthcare practitioners might find it difficult to identify which characteristics or patterns in the images help make the diagnosis, even though an AI model created to identify pneumonia from chest X-rays might reach high accuracy. Because physicians are hesitant to trust systems that do not provide rational justification for their predictions, this lack of transparency may impede clinical adoption. Interpretability is also necessary to validate model results, guarantee patient safety, and adhere to legal and ethical constraints. To improve openness and build confidence among medical personnel, hospitals should concentrate on creating explainable AI strategies like saliency maps, attention mechanisms, or model-agnostic approaches like LIME (Local Interpretable Model-Agnostic Explanations).

Integration Issues

One of the biggest obstacles to the effective implementation of AI-driven technologies in hospitals is integration problems. Compatibility with the hospital's current infrastructure, such as clinical workflow management platforms, medical imaging equipment, and Electronic Health Records (EHR) systems, is frequently necessary for the implementation of AI solutions. For instance, if an AI-powered diagnostic tool for cardiac anomaly detection is incompatible with the hospital's existing EHR software, integration may be difficult. Furthermore, when AI systems are created with proprietary formats or without defined protocols, interoperability issues may occur, making it challenging to transmit data between various systems. In order to successfully integrate AI technologies, medical professionals may also need to undergo considerable retraining, and existing workflows may need to be modified. Furthermore, hospitals may be discouraged from implementing AI systems due to the high expenses of continuing maintenance and infrastructure updates. Creating adaptable, scalable AI systems that support interoperability, follow industry standards, and integrate with hospital operations without interfering with patient care is necessary to address integration challenges.

Regulatory and Ethical Concerns

The implementation of AI-driven technologies in hospitals is significantly influenced by ethical and regulatory considerations. Ensuring compliance with data protection rules, such as the General Data Protection Regulation (GDPR) in the EU and the Health Insurance Portability and Accountability Act (HIPAA) in the US, is crucial because these systems frequently handle sensitive patient data. When AI models generate skewed or incorrect results, it raises ethical questions since it may jeopardize patient safety and confidence. Furthermore, since patients might not be completely aware of how their data is being used to train AI models, concerns around patient permission and data ownership are crucial. Furthermore, a barrier to the broad adoption of AI systems is the absence of precise standards for their certification and validation. Regulators frequently take a while to adjust to the quickly changing AI landscape, which leaves developers and healthcare organizations in the dark. Strong ethical frameworks, explainable AI models, and thorough testing and validation prior to clinical implementation are all necessary to allay these worries. To guarantee the ethical use of AI in healthcare, transparency, accountability, and justice must be given top priority (Muniasamy, A., & Karunakaran, G., 2026)

BACKGROUND

As healthcare systems deal with issues including rising prices, restricted access, and the increasing need for individualized care, artificial intelligence (AI) is becoming a major force for change. The integration of AI in many healthcare domains is critically evaluated in this paper, which also examines how AI improves clinical decision-making, streamlines hospital operations and management, enhances medical image analysis, and transforms patient care and monitoring through wearables driven by AI. The authors examined (Maleki Varnosfaderani & Forouzanfar, 2024) how AI has changed particular healthcare domains through a number of case studies, and they also talk about the issues that still need to be resolved. Additionally included in the paper are methods for evaluating AI healthcare solutions, the moral dilemmas associated with AI implementation, and the significance of data privacy and bias reduction for responsible technology use.

The review gives researchers a better grasp of how AI is affecting healthcare now and in the future. It also promotes interdisciplinary discussion among researchers, clinicians, and technologists to help them navigate the challenges of implementing AI and develop AI-driven solutions that put patient-centered care, equity, and ethical standards first. Ethically, there are advantages and disadvantages to the use of artificial intelligence (AI) in healthcare, especially in the creation and delivery of vaccines. The ethical implications of implementing AI in healthcare have been examined by authors, who have concentrated on issues of responsibility, transparency, fairness, privacy, and continuous assessment. It is crucial to ensure the responsible and equitable application of AI technologies in order to protect individual rights, advance justice, and minimize potential risks. In order to foster informed decision-making and trust among stakeholders, transparency is crucial. To reduce prejudices and inequalities in the distribution and allocation of vaccines, fairness and equity must be given top priority. To guarantee that AI algorithms are created and used responsibly, with procedures for redress in the event of mistakes or unforeseen effects, accountability and responsibility are essential.

Protecting patient autonomy and confidentiality necessitates rigorous adherence to privacy regulations and patient consent, which are essential components of privacy and data security. Algorithmic decision-making procedures must be transparent, and AI algorithms must be continuously evaluated and monitored to gauge their effectiveness and effect on patient outcomes. Clinical care is progressively incorporating AI systems, including note-writing with AI. A measure was created and used to evaluate electronic health records (EHRs) related to mental health that employ large language models (LLMs) to write notes.

Analyzing product details and asking vendors directly about their systems were part of the evaluation process. The majority of goods made it apparent that the LLM could be used as a co-pilot or to create customized reports. Crucial elements, such as information on LLM training methodology, the particular LLM utilized, bias correction strategies, and ways for assessing the body of evidence, were frequently missing, nevertheless. The ethical application and dependability of these systems in clinical practice are called into question by the lack of transparency on LLM details and bias mitigation techniques. Although LLM-enhanced EHRs have the potential to reduce the amount of paperwork that mental health practitioners must do, more openness and uniformity in the reporting of LLM-related data are urgently needed.

To guarantee that these systems satisfy the highest requirements for security, ethics, and clinical care, the authors (Bouguettaya et al., 2025)offered suggestions for their future development and deployment. Global healthcare systems are dealing with declining results and rising expenditures, which is difficult for those in charge of healthcare administration. Computer and data scientists, policymakers, lawmakers, and clinical entrepreneurs all contend that artificial intelligence (AI), and in particular machine learning (ML), is a crucial component of the answer. In the areas of diagnostics, drug development, epidemiology, personalized medicine, and operational efficiency, machine learning (ML) can enhance human clinical capabilities. Three factors must be taken into account, nevertheless, if AI solutions are incorporated into clinical practice: the governance framework, the ethical, legal, and regulatory framework, and the technical potential and constraints. Global healthcare systems are dealing with declining results and rising expenditures, which is difficult for those in charge of healthcare administration. Computer and data scientists, policymakers, lawmakers, and clinical entrepreneurs all contend that artificial intelligence (AI), and in particular machine learning (ML), is a crucial component of the answer. Researchers suggested that in the areas of diagnostics, drug development, epidemiology, personalized medicine, and operational efficiency, machine learning (ML) can enhance human clinical capabilities.

Some of the reviewers have offered (Olawade et al., 2024)a thorough analysis of the problems and revolutionary potential of integrating artificial intelligence (AI) into healthcare. A methodical search approach was used to find pertinent peer-reviewed articles published in English since January 2010 using electronic databases like PubMed, Scopus, Embase, and Science Direct. Results show that artificial intelligence (AI) has a big impact on how healthcare is delivered. It can improve diagnostic accuracy, allow for personalized therapy, help with predictive analytics, automate tasks, and power robotics. Critical care medical bedside care could be greatly enhanced by artificial intelligence (AI). In complicated situations with multidomain and multidimensional data, artificial intelligence (AI) can assist in identifying patterns that would otherwise go undetected. However, real-world AI applications demand a lot of computer time and resources, which are only possible in specialized subjects like astronomy or physics.

AI is now accessible in many domains(Yoon et al., 2022), including critical care medicine, where data is extensive, varied, and complicated, thanks to the exponential development in processing power and portability. More clinical research is being conducted in the intensive care unit (ICU) utilizing AI-driven techniques to exploit data. In order to determine the underlying cause of clinical deterioration from differential diagnoses, for example, AI can help in illness diagnosis. Machine learning models can distinguish between congestive heart failure (CHF) and other causes of lung disease, and advanced text and image processing capabilities can aid in obtaining a more accurate diagnosis. Before AI becomes a fundamental part of routine clinical practice, there are still a lot of challenges and traps to be avoided. For practical reasons, viral-specific real-time polymerase chain reaction (RT-PCR) testing can take up to 48 hours and has limited sensitivity, making it challenging to separate the early clinical course of SARS-CoV-2 infection from other undifferentiated medical presentations to the hospital. Using routinely obtained data (blood gas, vital signs, and laboratory tests) that are usually available within an hour, this study created two early-detection models to identify COVID-19 during 115,394 emergency presentations and 72,310 hospital admissions. Among all hospitalized patients, the emergency department (ED) model had a 77.4% sensitivity and a 95.7% specificity (AUROC 0.939) for COVID-19, whereas the admissions model had a 77.4% sensitivity and a 94.8% specificity (AUROC 0.940) for the hospitalized subset. In order to aid infection control, both models achieve strong negative predictive values (>99%) across a range of prevalences (<5%). This allows for quick exclusion during triage. The models had a strong impact in situations where quick testing is not available and worked well as a COVID-19 screening test in ERs and hospital admission units (Soltan et al., 2020).

Critical care nurses have both opportunities and challenges as a result of the integration of artificial intelligence (AI) in intensive care units (ICUs). This study explores the perceptions of nurses in leadership positions regarding the influence of artificial intelligence on their work. The lived experiences of critical care nurses leading with AI were recorded using an interpretive phenomenological analysis. Using purposive sampling, ten nurses with leadership positions in different ICU specialties were interviewed. Nurses' experiences with AI, including its opportunities and challenges, were investigated through semi-structured interviews. Two major topics emerged from the thematic analysis: the human element in leading with AI and leading with AI: navigating possibilities and obstacles. The six subthemes that comprise the two main themes showed that while AI provided advantages such as task automation, there were also worries about over-reliance and the requirement for continuous training (Hassan & El-Ashry, 2024). Managing possible bias and adjusting to new workflows were among the additional difficulties that surfaced. Collaboration and clear communication were essential for the successful integration of AI.

Integrating AI requires establishing trust and encouraging teamwork. While cooperation enables nurses to concentrate on human-centered care with AI support, transparency in AI systems enables them to reliably assign responsibilities. A thorough examination of the area is provided by this systematic evaluation of reliable and explicable artificial intelligence (AI) in healthcare. By combining quality evaluation, bias risk, and data fusion, the study seeks to offer a thorough grasp of the explainability and reliability of AI applications in healthcare. Six categories—explainable robots, prediction, decision support, blockchain, transparency, digital health, and review—are used to group the 64 recent contributions from various databases that are included in the evaluation. The writers highlight the difficulties, inspirations, and suggestions in their methodical and thorough review of past research. The Queensland University of Technology authors (Albahri et al., 2023)also conducted a systematic scientific mapping study to restructure and summarize the findings of previous research in order to meet the concerns of objectivity and reliability. Eight cutting-edge critical assessments of pertinent research gaps are also presented in the paper. The study offers vital evidence for further research as it is the first to examine the viability of utilizing reliable and XAI applications in healthcare. Healthcare has undergone a change thanks to the Internet of Things (IoT), which offers services and vast amounts of data.

Smart health care has emerged as a result of the growth of cloud, things, and smart Multiple Sensorial Media (MulSeMedia) systems. However, customers' concerns about security and privacy have also increased as a result of the convergence of AI and IoT. The purpose of the study is to identify the privacy and security risks related to AI-driven IoT (AIIoT) and suggest solutions. Utilizing a qualitative study design, the research gathers qualitative data from pre-existing secondary sources. The results demonstrate that as AI-driven IoT has developed, more sensors and gadgets have been introduced to the internet, raising a range of security and privacy issues for consumers. According to the study(Keshta, 2022), well defined architecture standards that incorporate interfaces and data models that guarantee improved user security and privacy should be a present prerequisite for AI-driven IoT.

The use of AI-powered predictive models in the treatment of diseases including diabetes and cardiovascular disease is examined by experts from North Carolina, USA. Important results show how well AI predicts the course of diseases, enabling risk assessment and earlier therapies. High accuracy was demonstrated by neural networks, random forests, and other machine learning models, surpassing conventional management techniques. Nonetheless, issues like generalizability, interpretability of the model, and data privacy continue to exist. In order to increase AI's influence in healthcare, the article identifies future directions for enhancing model openness and resolving ethical issues.

Global healthcare systems are heavily burdened by chronic diseases like diabetes, cardiovascular disease, and respiratory disorders, which necessitate long-term care, ongoing monitoring, and individualized treatment plans to slow their progression and improve patients' quality of life. Innovative ways are required to improve the outcomes of chronic diseases, as traditional treatments have not been able to effectively address these issues.

Existing causal, moral, and legal attributions of responsibility are being called into question by the use of AI-driven clinical decision support systems (AI-CDSS) in clinical decision-making. This article makes the case that, from a causal, moral, and legal standpoint, the usage of AI-CDSS results in diffusions of blame. When there are various possibilities and actors that can be taken into consideration for assigning blame, this is referred to as responsibility dispersal. The 'digital tumor board' driven by AI serves as an example of how clinical decision-making is altered and responsibility diffusions occur. The authors (Bleher & Braun, 2022) contend that responsibility, which is founded on normative considerations like avoiding experiences of disregard and vulnerability of human life, is inherently accompanied by a moment of uncertainty and is characterized by revision openness. As such, they contend that responsibility is characterized by dynamics and ambivalences.

In order to prevent responsibility gaps, the study ends with recommendations for controlling responsibility diffusions in clinical decision-making using AI-CDSS.

Healthcare administrators face a problem as global healthcare systems deal with rising expenditures and declining results. Computer and data scientists, policymakers, lawmakers, and clinical entrepreneurs all contend that artificial intelligence (AI), and in particular machine learning (ML), is a crucial component of the answer. In the areas of diagnostics, drug development, epidemiology, personalized medicine, and operational efficiency, machine learning (ML) can enhance human clinical capabilities.

Three factors must be taken into account, nevertheless, if AI solutions are incorporated into clinical practice: the governance framework, the ethical, legal, and regulatory framework, and the technical potential and constraints. According to a thorough examination of the ethical, regulatory, and legal framework, ethical problems can be classified as epistemic, normative, or overarching and emerge at six levels of abstraction: individual, interpersonal, group, institutional, sectoral, and societal. It is imperative that the ethical issues brought up by the use of AI in healthcare settings be addressed proactively as opposed to reactively, and that the important factors for legislators be mapped to each of the ethical issues raised.

The authors (BožiĆ, 2023) looked into how artificial intelligence (AI) might be included into hospital integrated risk management (IRM) and emphasized how it could revolutionize risk identification, assessment, and mitigation in a variety of hospital activities. Their research showed that by facilitating the early identification of serious illnesses, enhancing clinical risk management, and assisting in decision-making, AI might greatly improve patient safety. The authors also discovered that AI is essential for enhancing operational risk management, privacy, information security, regulatory compliance, and human resource management in hospitals. Nevertheless, the study also identified a number of obstacles to the adoption of AI in hospital IRM, such as problems with data bias and quality, interpretability, transparency, privacy issues, a decrease in human oversight, ethical ramifications, and implementation constraints. The authors underlined the significance of creating strong data governance frameworks, reducing biases in AI algorithms, guaranteeing transparency, putting in place effective cybersecurity measures, and abiding by ethical standards in order to address these issues.

Additionally, they emphasized how important it is for medical staff to acquire crucial talents including domain expertise, data literacy, AI and data science skills, critical thinking, teamwork, flexibility, and ethical awareness. Hospitals can successfully use AI for IRM to improve patient outcomes, operational effectiveness, and risk reduction by cultivating these competencies and following best practices. In the healthcare and medical fields, authors from Australia (Nasarian et al., 2024) conducted a thorough analysis of the procedures and difficulties related to explainable artificial intelligence (XAI) and interpretable machine learning (IML). Their study sought to investigate IML and XAI processes, including associated methods, applications, and implementation issues, specifically from a quality control perspective in the context of digital health interventions (DHIs).

Pre-processing interpretability, interpretable modeling, and post-processing interpretability are the three separate steps into which the study divided the IML process. The authors underlined the need of creating strong interpretability techniques in clinical decision support systems (CDSS) by examining related experimental data. In order to guarantee a more successful integration of AI technology in healthcare decision-making processes, their findings made clear the necessity of improving communication between AI systems and doctors. The study also sought to give future researchers useful information for developing clinician-AI tools that can solve issues with transparency, usability, and reliability in healthcare decision support systems, in addition to being more interpretable. By methodically contrasting their benefits, drawbacks, and uses, the authors examined how artificial intelligence (AI) and machine learning (ML) can transform medical diagnosis and treatment. Their research demonstrated how ML systems may improve diagnostic precision, identify trends, and assist expert judgment—all of which have a favorable impact on the provision of healthcare. Nevertheless, the study also identified a number of issues that could restrict their efficacy, such as inadequate data quality, interpretability issues, and implementation concerns.

However, the authors pointed out that AI has a great deal of promise to support clinical judgment, boost healthcare efficiency, and improve patient outcomes. However, issues with data security, restricted generalizability, and difficulties with regulatory compliance continue to be major barriers to the use of AI in healthcare. Their research highlighted how crucial it is to comprehend these advantages and drawbacks in order to guarantee the effective application and adoption of AI and ML technologies in the healthcare industry. In the end, the authors proposed that successful AI and ML integration would enable future medical professionals to make better choices about patient evaluation and treatment, thereby enhancing healthcare services as a whole.

Through the detection, management, and treatment of diseases, the authors examined how Artificial Intelligence (AI) is transforming healthcare. Their study demonstrated how quickly healthcare firms are implementing AI technologies to enhance patient outcomes, streamline processes, and save costs. The authors used a variety of AI techniques, including robotics, computer vision, natural language processing (NLP), and machine learning (ML), to show how AI has significantly improved a number of healthcare fields.

The accuracy with which AI-driven diagnostic systems analyzed medical images was especially noteworthy, as it allowed for the early detection of diseases such as cancer. Furthermore, it was highlighted how predictive analytics may be used to create individualized treatment plans and preventative actions, demonstrating AI's ability to detect at-risk patients and forecast the course of diseases, thus improving patient care.

The study recognized AI's influence on healthcare delivery through telemedicine, virtual consultations, and remote monitoring in addition to its clinical uses. The authors pointed out that in order to increase patient engagement and treatment adherence, AI-powered virtual health assistants offer tailored health information, prescription reminders, and lifestyle advice. Additionally, telemedicine systems that use AI algorithms have been acknowledged for their ability to better allocate resources, speed up appointment scheduling, and provide high-quality healthcare services to underprivileged and rural populations. The authors (P et al., 2024) came to the conclusion that artificial intelligence (AI) is a key factor in changing healthcare systems because of its capacity to improve productivity, stimulate innovation, and solve complicated problems through sophisticated data analysis and automation.

CONCEPTUAL FRAMEWORK

The conceptual framework illustrated in Figure 2 outlines the proposed methodology for evaluating the integration and effectiveness of Artificial Intelligence (AI) in hospital systems. This framework serves as a structured approach to systematically assess the operational, ethical, and technological dimensions of AI-driven healthcare solutions. By mapping key evaluation parameters—such as clinical outcomes, patient satisfaction, data privacy, and decision-making efficiency—the model provides a holistic perspective on how AI can be critically appraised within real-world hospital environments.

Figure 2. Conceptual Model Highlighting Evaluation Dimensions of AI in Hospital Systems

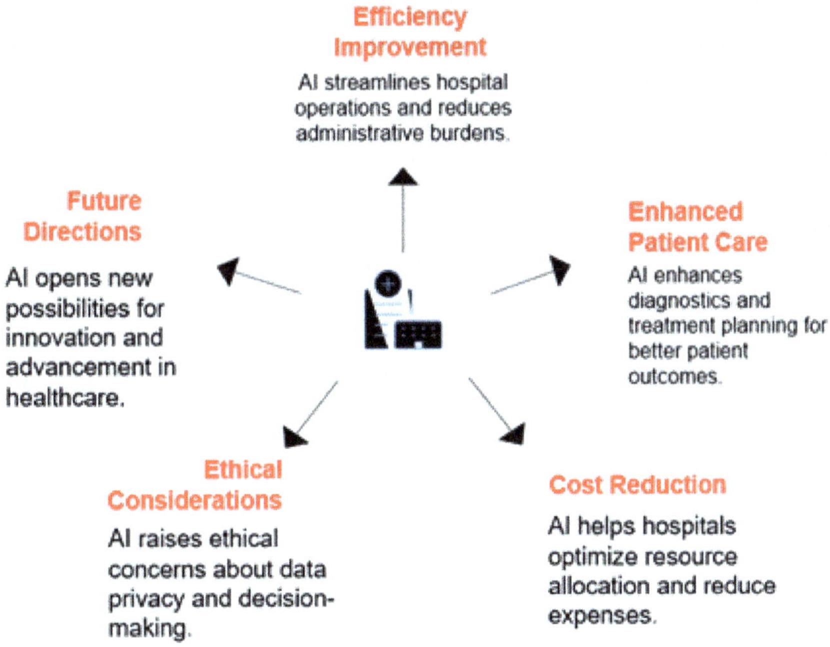

The integration of Artificial Intelligence (AI) into hospital systems has marked a revolutionary shift in the way healthcare services are delivered, managed, and experienced. With the growing demand for high-quality and efficient medical care, AI has emerged as a catalyst for transformation across multiple dimensions of hospital operations. This comprehensive explanation addresses the critical aspects outlined in the provided conceptual framework: efficiency improvement, enhanced patient care, cost reduction, ethical considerations, and future directions.

Efficiency Improvement

One of the most significant contributions of AI in hospital systems is the improvement of operational efficiency. Traditional hospital workflows often involve cumbersome manual processes such as patient registration, scheduling, record-keeping, inventory tracking, and resource management. These activities, while essential, consume substantial time and human resources, leading to delays and administrative bottlenecks. AI technologies, including machine learning algorithms and robotic process automation (RPA), streamline these processes by automating repetitive tasks and ensuring accurate data entry and retrieval.

For instance, AI-powered scheduling systems can automatically assign appointments based on patient preferences, doctor availability, and emergency priorities. Similarly, chatbots can assist patients with inquiries and triage support, significantly reducing the workload on front-desk and nursing staff. Moreover, AI enables real-time monitoring of resource utilization — such as bed occupancy and medical supplies — allowing hospitals to dynamically allocate their assets, avoid overbooking, and prevent shortages.

These enhancements not only reduce waiting times and administrative costs but also improve the overall patient experience. Hospitals equipped with AI tools operate more smoothly, minimize human errors, and are better positioned to respond to changing clinical demands. Therefore, efficiency improvement through AI is not just a technological upgrade but a structural advancement that transforms the entire hospital ecosystem.

Enhanced Patient Care

AI plays a critical role in elevating the standards of patient care by enabling more accurate diagnostics, personalized treatment plans, and predictive analytics. One of the most powerful applications of AI lies in medical imaging and diagnostics. Advanced algorithms trained on vast datasets of radiological images can detect patterns and anomalies with remarkable precision, often surpassing the diagnostic accuracy of human practitioners. For example, AI tools have shown exceptional performance in identifying early signs of cancer, diabetic retinopathy, and cardiovascular diseases.

In addition to diagnostics, AI supports clinicians in crafting personalized treatment strategies. By analyzing patient history, genetic information, lifestyle data, and clinical records, AI can generate insights that inform more effective interventions tailored to individual needs. This personalized approach minimizes trial-and-error treatment, reduces side effects, and enhances recovery outcomes.

AI also facilitates remote patient monitoring and chronic disease management. Wearable devices and mobile health apps collect real-time health data, which AI algorithms analyze to detect anomalies or worsening conditions. Alerts can be sent to healthcare providers and patients for timely intervention, thereby preventing complications and hospital readmissions. Furthermore, natural language processing (NLP) tools extract valuable insights from electronic health records (EHRs), clinical notes, and research literature to assist doctors in clinical decision-making.

The cumulative effect of these technologies is a healthcare environment where patient outcomes are significantly improved. AI acts as a support system that augments the capabilities of healthcare professionals, ensuring timely, precise, and compassionate care delivery.

Cost Reduction

The financial sustainability of hospital systems is a persistent challenge, particularly in resource-constrained settings. AI contributes to cost reduction by optimizing resource allocation, minimizing inefficiencies, and preventing unnecessary expenditures. Through predictive analytics, AI can forecast patient admission rates, emergency room demands, and seasonal disease trends, enabling hospitals to plan their staffing, inventory, and service delivery more effectively.

For example, AI-driven analytics can predict peak times for specific departments, allowing administrators to schedule staff appropriately and reduce overtime costs. In procurement and inventory management, AI models forecast supply needs based on historical consumption and upcoming demands, thereby reducing waste due to overstocking or product expiration. AI also helps avoid costly medical errors and preventable complications. By continuously analyzing patient data, AI tools can detect early warning signs of adverse events, such as sepsis or cardiac arrest, prompting immediate medical intervention. This proactive approach not only saves lives but also reduces the length of hospital stays and the need for intensive care, which are major cost drivers.

Furthermore, telemedicine platforms powered by AI can deliver consultations and follow-ups remotely, reducing the burden on physical infrastructure and lowering travel-related expenses for patients. Hospitals that implement AI in billing and claims processing also benefit from reduced errors, faster reimbursements, and decreased fraud. Collectively, these strategies enable a more financially efficient healthcare system without compromising quality.

Ethical Considerations

While AI offers immense benefits, it also raises profound ethical concerns that must be critically evaluated. One of the foremost issues is data privacy. AI systems require large volumes of patient data to function effectively, raising questions about consent, ownership, and the security of sensitive medical information. Improper handling or breaches of health data can lead to identity theft, discrimination, or loss of trust in the healthcare system.

Another critical ethical dilemma involves decision-making transparency. AI algorithms, particularly those based on deep learning, often operate as "black boxes" — producing outputs without clear explanations of how decisions are made. This lack of interpretability can be problematic in clinical contexts where accountability and informed consent are crucial. Patients and healthcare providers must understand and trust the rationale behind AI-generated recommendations, especially when life-altering treatments or diagnoses are involved.

Bias and fairness are additional concerns. If AI models are trained on non-representative or biased data, they may produce skewed results that disadvantage certain populations. For instance, diagnostic algorithms might underperform for ethnic minorities or underrepresented groups, leading to disparities in care. Addressing these issues requires inclusive data practices, rigorous validation, and regulatory oversight to ensure equitable outcomes. Moreover, the increasing reliance on AI poses questions about professional autonomy and job displacement. While AI is intended to augment human expertise, there is a fear that over-dependence may erode clinical judgment or deskill healthcare workers. Striking a balance between human agency and algorithmic assistance is essential to maintain ethical integrity in AI-driven hospital systems.

SOLUTIONS AND RECOMMENDATIONS

Establish Ethical and Regulatory Frameworks

To address ethical concerns and build trust in AI systems, governments and healthcare institutions must develop and enforce robust regulatory policies. These should cover areas such as data protection, algorithmic transparency, consent, and accountability. Collaborations between AI developers, bioethicists, clinicians, and policymakers are essential to create context-sensitive and globally adaptable guidelines.

Ensure Data Quality and Governance

Reliable AI performance depends on high-quality, representative datasets. Hospitals should implement strict data governance policies ensuring data completeness, accuracy, privacy, and inclusivity. Investing in secure and interoperable data infrastructure will enhance AI model reliability while maintaining compliance with data protection laws like HIPAA or GDPR.

Promote Transparency and Explainability

Implement Explainable AI (XAI) models in clinical settings so healthcare professionals can understand and trust AI outputs. This not only supports informed decision-making but also helps in error tracking and model improvement. Training programs for clinicians on interpreting AI tools can further bridge the knowledge gap.

Address Algorithmic Bias

AI systems must be regularly audited for biases that may lead to unfair or harmful outcomes. Using diverse and representative datasets during model development and integrating bias-detection mechanisms can help minimize such risks. Stakeholders should prioritize inclusive design practices that reflect the diversity of patient populations.

Encourage Human-AI Collaboration

Rather than replacing healthcare workers, AI should augment human capabilities. Adopting a "human-in-the-loop" (HITL) approach ensures that clinicians remain the final decision-makers. This collaboration enhances patient care quality while maintaining ethical responsibility and empathy in treatment.

Develop Capacity Building and Training

Hospitals should invest in continuous training for healthcare staff to improve digital literacy and confidence in using AI tools. Cross-disciplinary education involving both technical and medical knowledge is critical for effective implementation and management of AI systems.

Foster Public Engagement and Trust

Building public trust in AI requires transparent communication about how AI tools work, their benefits, limitations, and privacy safeguards. Engaging patients and communities in dialogue and decision-making can help align AI development with societal values.

Support Research and Innovation

Policymakers and funding agencies should support interdisciplinary research that explores novel AI applications, addresses emerging risks, and evaluates the long-term impact of AI on healthcare systems. Innovation should be aligned with patient safety, cost-effectiveness, and system sustainability.

FUTURE RESEARCH DIRECTIONS

Looking ahead, the future of AI in hospital systems is filled with exciting possibilities and transformative potential. Continued advancements in computational power, data availability, and algorithmic sophistication will further enhance the capabilities of AI tools. Innovations such as generative AI, federated learning, and explainable AI are expected to address some of the current limitations and expand the scope of applications in healthcare.

Generative AI models may assist in generating clinical documentation, summarizing patient histories, or drafting discharge instructions, thus reducing administrative load on physicians. Federated learning allows AI models to be trained across decentralized data sources without compromising patient privacy, a breakthrough for collaborative research and multicenter applications. Explainable AI seeks to improve the transparency and interpretability of algorithmic outputs, fostering greater trust among clinicians and patients alike.

The integration of AI with other emerging technologies, such as the Internet of Medical Things (IoMT), robotics, and blockchain, will also redefine hospital operations. Robotic surgery guided by AI, blockchain-enabled secure health records, and smart ICU monitoring systems are just some of the innovations on the horizon. Furthermore, AI could play a pivotal role in global health initiatives by supporting resource-poor regions with diagnostic support, virtual consultations, and population health analytics. Future studies should concentrate on creating uniform evaluation techniques that take ethical and clinical efficacy into account. Enhancing transparency and trust will need the use of explainable AI (XAI) approaches. Establishing guidelines and regulatory norms also requires interdisciplinary cooperation between AI researchers, medical practitioners, and legislators.

Data security can be improved while facilitating cross-institutional collaborative learning through developments in federated learning and privacy-preserving AI approaches. Additionally, early diagnosis and patient monitoring can be enhanced by combining AI systems with Internet of Medical Things (IoMT) devices. Prioritization should also be given to generalization across various populations, scalability, and resilience to hostile attacks. Providing safe, dependable, and effective healthcare solutions will require constant evaluation, adaption, and development as AI technologies advance.

However, to fully realize these future directions, collaborative efforts among technologists, clinicians, policymakers, and ethicists are required. Establishing robust regulatory frameworks, ethical guidelines, and continuous professional training will be crucial to ensure that the benefits of AI are equitably distributed and responsibly implemented.

CONCLUSION

Hospital AI-driven systems must be evaluated and assessed in order to guarantee its dependability, efficiency, and safety. Establishing strong evaluation frameworks is crucial as AI technologies are increasingly included into healthcare diagnosis, treatment planning, patient monitoring, and administrative duties. These technologies provide improved operating efficiency, individualized treatment alternatives, and diagnostic accuracy. Data privacy, interpretability, model robustness, and interaction with current healthcare infrastructures are still major obstacles, nevertheless. To guarantee the reliability and acceptance of AI systems, thorough evaluation frameworks must take into account clinical relevance, ethical considerations, and real-world performance. AI-driven hospital systems represent a paradigm shift in modern healthcare, offering unprecedented benefits in terms of efficiency, patient care, cost management, and innovation. At the same time, they pose complex ethical challenges that require thoughtful deliberation and proactive mitigation. As the healthcare landscape continues to evolve, embracing AI with a balanced and inclusive approach will be vital to building resilient, ethical, and patient-centered hospital systems of the future.

REFERENCES

Alasmari, A., & Muniasamy, A. (2025). Integrating Bayesian and convolution neural network for uncertainty estimation of cataract from fundus images. *Computer Modeling in Engineering & Sciences*, *143*(1), 569–592. DOI: 10.32604/cmes.2025.060484

Albahri, A. S., Duhaim, A. M., Fadhel, M. A., Alnoor, A., Baqer, N. S., Alzubaidi, L., Albahri, O. S., Alamoodi, A. H., Bai, J., Salhi, A., Santamaría, J., Ouyang, C., Gupta, A., Gu, Y., & Deveci, M. (2023). A systematic review of trustworthy and explainable artificial intelligence in healthcare: Assessment of quality, bias risk, and data fusion. *Information Fusion*, *96*, 156–191. DOI: 10.1016/j.inffus.2023.03.008

Begum, A., Muniasamy, A., Sabahath, A., Yaqub, H., & Karunakaran, G. (2024). Coronary heart disease classification using deep learning approach with feature selection for improved accuracy. *Technology and Health Care*, *32*(3), 1991–2007. DOI: 10.3233/THC-231807 PMID: 38339946

Bleher, H., & Braun, M. (2022). Diffused responsibility: Attributions of responsibility in the use of AI-driven clinical decision support systems. *AI and Ethics*, *2*(4), 747–761. DOI: 10.1007/s43681-022-00135-x PMID: 35098247

Bouguettaya, A., Team, V., Stuart, E. M., & Aboujaoude, E. (2025). AI-driven report-generation tools in mental healthcare: A review of commercial tools. *General Hospital Psychiatry*, *94*, 150–158. DOI: 10.1016/j.genhosppsych.2025.02.018 PMID: 40088857

Gauthaman, S. A., (2026). Introduction to machine learning and optimization in healthcare. In Muniasamy, A. (Ed.), *Integrative machine learning and optimization algorithms for disease prediction* (pp. 1–34). IGI Global., DOI: 10.4018/979-8-3373-1087-9.ch001

Hassan, E. A., & El-Ashry, A. M. (2024). Leading with AI in critical care nursing: Challenges, opportunities, and the human factor. *BMC Nursing*, *23*(1), 752. DOI: 10.1186/s12912-024-02363-4 PMID: 39402609

Keshta, I. (2022). AI-driven IoT for smart health care: Security and privacy issues. *Informatics in Medicine Unlocked*, *30*, 100903. DOI: 10.1016/j.imu.2022.100903

Maleki Varnosfaderani, S., & Forouzanfar, M. (2024). The role of AI in hospitals and clinics: Transforming healthcare in the 21st century. *Bioengineering (Basel, Switzerland)*, *11*(4), 337. DOI: 10.3390/bioengineering11040337 PMID: 38671759

Muniasamy, A. (2025). Revolutionizing health monitoring: Integrating transformer models with multi-head attention for precise human activity recognition using wearable devices. *Technology and Health Care, 33*(1), 395–409. https://content.iospress.com/articles/technology-and-health-care/thc241064. DOI: 10.3233/THC-241064 PMID: 39269866

Muniasamy, A., & Karunakaran, G. (2026). Challenges and future directions: Emerging trends and limitations in ML and optimization for healthcare. In Muniasamy, A. (Ed.), *Integrative machine learning and optimization algorithms for disease prediction* (pp. 339–368). IGI Global., DOI: 10.4018/979-8-3373-1087-9.ch012

Muniasamy, A., Tabassam, S., Hussain, M. A., Sultana, H., Muniasamy, V., & Bhatnagar, R. (2020). Deep learning for predictive analytics in healthcare. In Hassanien, A., Azar, A., Gaber, T., Bhatnagar, R., & Tolba, M. F. (Eds.), *The International Conference on Advanced Machine Learning Technologies and Applications (AMLTA2019)* (pp. xx-xx). Springer. https://doi.org/DOI: 10.1007/978-3-030-14118-9_4

Nasarian, E., Alizadehsani, R., Acharya, U. R., & Tsui, K.-L. (2024). Designing interpretable ML system to enhance trust in healthcare: A systematic review to proposed responsible clinician-AI-collaboration framework. *Information Fusion, 108*, 102412. DOI: 10.1016/j.inffus.2024.102412

Olawade, D. B., David-Olawade, A. C., Wada, O. Z., Asaolu, A. J., Adereni, T., & Ling, J. (2024). Artificial intelligence in healthcare delivery: Prospects and pitfalls. *Journal of Medicine, Surgery, and Public Health, 3*, 100108. DOI: 10.1016/j.glmedi.2024.100108

Rengaramanujam, K., & Muniasamy, A. (2026). AI in hospital administration and formulary design: Optimizing resource allocation and patient flow. In Muniasamy, A., & Karunakaran, G. (Eds.), *Applications of artificial intelligence in pharmaceuticals* (pp. 215–246). IGI Global., DOI: 10.4018/979-8-3373-2043-4.ch008

Sabahath, A., Muniasamy, A., Begum, A., Yaqub, H., & Karunakaran, G. (2023). Lung cancer histopathology image classification using transfer learning with convolution neural network model. *Technology and Health Care, 33*, 1–12. https://content.iospress.com/articles/technology-and-health-care/thc231029

Soltan, A. A., Kouchaki, S., Zhu, T., Kiyasseh, D., Taylor, T., Hussain, Z. B., Peto, T., Brent, A. J., Eyre, D. W., & Clifton, D. (2020). Artificial intelligence driven assessment of routinely collected healthcare data is an effective screening test for COVID-19 in patients presenting to hospital. *medRxiv*. https://doi.org/DOI: 10.1101/2020.07.07.20148361

Yoon, J. H., Pinsky, M. R., & Clermont, G. (2022). Artificial intelligence in critical care medicine. *Critical Care*, *26*(1), 75. DOI: 10.1186/s13054-022-03915-3 PMID: 35337366

ADDITIONAL READING

Esteva, A., Robicquet, A., Ramsundar, B., Kuleshov, V., DePristo, M., Chou, K., Cui, C., Corrado, G., Thrun, S., & Dean, J. (2019). A guide to deep learning in healthcare. *Nature Medicine*, *25*(1), 24–29. DOI: 10.1038/s41591-018-0316-z PMID: 30617335

Floridi, L., & Cowls, J. (2019). A unified framework of five principles for AI in society. *Harvard Data Science Review*. Advance online publication. DOI: 10.1162/99608f92.8cd550d1

U.S. Food & Drug Administration (FDA). (2021). *Artificial Intelligence/Machine Learning (AI/ML)-Based Software as a Medical Device (SaMD) Action Plan.*

Jiang, F., Jiang, Y., Zhi, H., Dong, Y., Li, H., Ma, S., Wang, Y., Dong, Q., Shen, H., & Wang, Y. (2017). Artificial intelligence in healthcare: Past, present and future. *Stroke and Vascular Neurology*, *2*(4), 230–243. DOI: 10.1136/svn-2017-000101 PMID: 29507784

Jobin, A., Ienca, M., & Vayena, E. (2019). The global landscape of AI ethics guidelines. *Nature Machine Intelligence*, *1*(9), 389–399. DOI: 10.1038/s42256-019-0088-2

Topol, E. (2019). *Deep Medicine: How Artificial Intelligence Can Make Healthcare Human Again*. Basic Books.

KEY TERMS AND DEFINITIONS

AI-Driven Hospital Systems: Healthcare infrastructures that integrate AI technologies into clinical and administrative workflows to improve efficiency, accuracy, and patient outcomes. These systems often include AI-powered diagnostics, robotic surgeries, virtual assistants, and predictive analytics.

Algorithmic Bias: Unintended consequences where AI systems produce skewed or unfair outcomes due to biased training data or flawed model design. This is particularly critical in healthcare, where such bias may lead to diagnostic errors or health disparities.

Artificial Intelligence (AI): A branch of computer science that simulates human intelligence processes, including learning, reasoning, and self-correction. In healthcare, AI supports tasks such as diagnosis, treatment planning, and administrative workflow optimization.

Clinical Decision Support System (CDSS): AI-based tools designed to assist clinicians in making informed medical decisions by analyzing patient data and offering evidence-based recommendations.

Data Governance: The process of managing the availability, usability, integrity, and security of healthcare data. Effective data governance is critical for maintaining trust and compliance in AI-driven systems.

Ethical Challenges in AI: Concerns related to bias in algorithms, data privacy, transparency, and the potential for replacing human roles in care delivery. Ethical AI emphasizes fairness, accountability, and explainability.

Explainable AI (XAI): AI systems that provide transparent reasoning behind their decisions, enabling clinicians and stakeholders to understand and trust the outputs. XAI is essential in healthcare where interpretability can impact life-saving decisions.

Human-in-the-Loop (HITL): An approach where human experts are involved in the development, monitoring, and decision-making processes of AI systems to ensure accountability and safety.

Interoperability: The ability of different health information systems and AI models to exchange, interpret, and use data cohesively. Interoperability ensures seamless integration of AI tools into existing hospital IT infrastructures.

Machine Learning (ML): A subset of AI focused on algorithms that learn from data to improve performance without being explicitly programmed. ML models are commonly used in clinical prediction, patient risk stratification, and medical imaging.no

Chapter 3
Comprehensive Evaluation of AI-Driven Systems in Modern Hospital Environments

Ravikumar R. N.
https://orcid.org/0009-0009-3705-1681
Marwadi University, Rajkot, India

S. Aarthi
https://orcid.org/0009-0006-9064-2091
Marwadi University, Rajkot, India

Zamira Atamuratova
Urgench State University, Urgench, Uzbekistan

Anorgul Ashirova
Mamun University, Khiva, Uzbekistan

Khusan Jurayev
Termez University of Economics and Service, Termez, Uzbekistan

Mehrigul Hayitova
Termez University of Economics and Service, Termez, Uzbekistan

ABSTRACT

Artificial Intelligence (AI) is rapidly transforming hospital care by enhancing diagnostic accuracy, optimizing treatment plans, and improving patient outcomes. However, realizing AI's potential requires rigorous evaluation frameworks that ensure safety, effectiveness, and ethical use. This chapter presents a comprehensive approach to assessing AI-driven systems in modern hospital environments, covering clinical validation, outcome-based metrics, safety and risk management, bias and fairness, workflow integration, and regulatory compliance. Emphasizing transparency, accountability, and continuous post-deployment monitoring, the chapter guides healthcare professionals, developers, and policymakers in responsibly adopting AI

DOI: 10.4018/979-8-3373-2787-7.ch003

technologies. Through multidisciplinary perspectives and real-world examples, it offers actionable insights to maximize AI benefits while safeguarding patient well-being and promoting equitable, trustworthy healthcare innovation.

INTRODUCTION

Artificial Intelligence (AI) is taking modern healthcare by storm and transforming it by leading to accurate and precise diagnosis, optimal treatment regimes, and increasing efficiency in operation. The worldwide use of clinical support defences, medical image analysis, patient assessment, and administrative work is becoming more and more dependent on AI. Nevertheless, although there is an incremental emergence of AI technologies, there are major challenges in their safe, ethical and effective implementation in practical clinical settings (Graziani et al., 2023; Rengaramanujam et al., 2026). Most of the existing AI systems are deemed successful based on technical parameters like sensitivity, specificity, and accuracy, but fail to consider such important parameters as clinical utility, workflow integration, ethical fairness, and regulatory approval. The chapter responds to the timely necessity of the elaborated evaluation model that is designed to meet the variety of complexities of hospital settings. It puts a special focus on the necessity of a multidimensional solution that cuts across the whole life-cycle of AI, including its development in systems as well as its clinical validation, monitoring after deployment, and continuous feedback (Hantel et al., 2024). The intended framework will provide AI tools with consistent, fair and evidence-based results by addressing the technical, clinical, ethical and regulatory dimensions. The chapter presents effective recommendations to clinicians, developers, and policymakers who participate in the piloting of AI through the usage of detailed analysis and case studies. Ultimately this is expected to reduce the gap between innovation of AI and clinical readiness leading to development of trust and accountability in the healthcare system across the world that will lead to delivery of better patient care.

With Artificial Intelligence (AI) entering hospitals more, the role it can play in the sphere of diagnostics, treatment planning, workflow streamlining, and care provision is considerable. Nonetheless, the accelerated use of AI in the clinical settings has exceeded the formulation of effective standardized assessment models. The evaluation of current practices usually views algorithm accuracy in a limited context that overlooks important aspects on clinical usability, ethical adherence, safe practices, bias, regulatory governance, and the actual results. Without the elaborate and systematic evaluation strategy, the AI applications are likely to fail to perform, diagnose, become biased or destabilize clinical workflows. This will create a multidisciplinary framework where the AI devices in hospitals are more than just being technically competent but clinically-proven, ethically competent and responsible, user-friendly, and supporting the varying healthcare requirements.

Although the prevalence of AI in hospital settings is increasing, it remains a serious deficiency of well-developed models to assess its effectiveness along multiple, and varied clinical, ethical, and operational planes (Rengaramanujam et al. 2026). A typical algorithm performance measure like accuracy, sensitivity and specificity are overrepresented in most current research and actual implementation, with little to no consideration toward clinical utility and workflow incorporation, as well as close follow up and post-deployment observation of safety concerns. In addition to that, there has been less concern regarding fairness audits, explainability and mitigation of biases that would inordinately affect vulnerable patient groups. Regulatory clarity needed There is also a lack of clarity on the regulatory front regarding dynamic AI systems that learn and change even after being deployed. Such gaps point to the necessity of the multidimensional and lifecycle-driven evaluation method that covers technical validation, clinical outcomes, usability, fairness, and regulatory compliances so that no risks or disparities are created when introducing AI tools to improve patient care. The objectives of the chapter are as follows:

- To establish a comprehensive evaluation framework for assessing AI systems in hospitals across all stages design, deployment, and post-deployment.
- To define multidimensional evaluation criteria that go beyond algorithmic performance to include clinical efficacy, safety, usability, ethical compliance, and regulatory standards.
- To highlight the challenges of AI integration in healthcare workflows and emphasize the need for user-friendly, interoperable, and role-based systems.
- To address bias and fairness concerns by identifying sources of systemic bias in AI tools and proposing strategies for mitigation and equitable healthcare delivery.
- To explore safety and risk management protocols tailored to high-risk clinical settings, ensuring continuous monitoring and error detection mechanisms.
- To examine ethical and legal implications of AI adoption in hospitals, including issues of transparency, accountability, patient consent, and data privacy.
- To encourage post-deployment surveillance and feedback mechanisms that enable adaptive learning, model updates, and sustained clinical relevance.

BACKGROUND STUDY

Artificial Intelligence (AI) is also revolutionizing the way hospitals are managed and improved patient care regarding clinical decision-making, diagnostics, treatment plan, and administrative efficiency. Modern healthcare delivery is characterized by the revolution of such applications in the health care sector as medical imaging analysis, predictive analytics, robotic surgeries, and natural language processing. Among the advantages, the use of AI systems in hospitals allows getting data interpreted faster, decreases the diagnostic errors, and improves the efficiency of the patient management process (Higgins & Madai, 2020). Nonetheless, its earning rate has brought some setbacks such as system biases, patient safety concerns, lack of transparency and ethical issues. As opposed to classic medical tools, AI systems are dynamic, that is, they learn and develop with time; this feature causes difficulties in their validation and regulation. Furthermore, the current assessment frameworks tend to pay attention to technical measures like sensitivity or specificity and do not consider the most important aspects like clinical availability, ability to integrate a workflow, equity, and sustained effects on patient outcomes (Jha et al., 2025). In the absence of a systematic and comprehensive method of evaluation, a possibility arises of implementing AI systems, which might not be accurate, disruptive, or even biased in practical clinical practice. Therefore, it is likely that a universal framework to evaluate AI systems in terms of technical, clinical, ethical, and regulatory usage is prominent. The present chapter expands on that requirement and provides a multidimensional approach to addressing the assessment of the AI tools at various phases of their life in hospital contexts.

Key Definitions

- **Artificial Intelligence (AI):** The simulation of human intelligence by machines, especially computer systems, to perform tasks such as diagnosis, prediction, and decision-making in healthcare.
- **Clinical Validation:** The process of testing an AI system using real-world clinical data to confirm its accuracy, safety, and generalizability across different patient populations and care settings.
- **Sensitivity:** The ability of an AI system to correctly identify patients with a condition (true positives), crucial in reducing missed diagnoses.
- **Specificity:** The ability to correctly identify patients without a condition (true negatives), helping avoid false alarms and unnecessary treatments.
- **Precision (Positive Predictive Value):** The proportion of positive results from an AI system that are actually correct, indicating reliability in predictions.
- **Recall:** Often used interchangeably with sensitivity; measures how well an AI system detects all relevant positive cases.
- **Explainability:** The degree to which the internal logic or decision-making process of an AI system can be understood and interpreted by humans.

- **Bias:** Systematic errors in AI that result in unfair treatment or performance disparities across different demographic groups.
- **Post-Deployment Monitoring:** Ongoing observation of AI systems in clinical environments to detect performance drift, risks, or unintended outcomes.
- **Ethical Compliance:** The alignment of AI systems with principles such as transparency, accountability, informed consent, privacy, and fairness.

Literature Review

There has been an increment in the possibility of Artificial Intelligence (AI) in hospital settings that has been attributed to the way it might transform healthcare delivery encompassing the accuracy in diagnosis, performance of treatment services, and rationalization of processes (Moghadasi et al., 2024). With the further development of AI-driven tools, other healthcare institutions are considering their implementation in such fields as medical imaging, predictive analytics, Electronic Health Records (EHR) management, clinical decision support systems, and patient risk stratification. Nonetheless, those steps notwithstanding, the biggest issue that remains unsolved is the proper pre-deployment, real-time and post-deployment assessment and validation of AI systems used in a clinical setting (Jia et al., 2022). Anthropogenic oversights of the AI tools tend to base the tests on the technical standards of precision, recall, and specificity, or the overall accuracy as a whole, which, albeit crucial, leaves a shallow knowledge on the actual clinical value, safety, and ethical compatibility of the system. With the results of a variety of studies, it has been found that the current AI systems that have been trained on controlled data sets could deliver high results in experimental conditions but fail drastically when tested against real-world clinical data due to the factors like data variance, workflow limitations, and heterogeneity of the population (Kim et al., 2023).

The latter area of focus in the research is the requirement of a life-cycle based evaluation infrastructure which considers not only the model development and technical verification but also the integration of models in clinical processes and users adoption as well as long-term performance follow-ups (Moreno-Sánchez, 2023). As it has turned out, the capacity of a model to generate high accuracy on retrospective testing does not mean that it will be helpful or reliable in the actual clinic. There is increased pressure towards real-world validation studies, in which AI models are tested in terms of their efficacy in real hospital settings, and their performance may be compared to that of human clinicians (Nair et al., 2024). The necessity of viewing AI outputs on the level of the operating ecosystem and ensuring that the system enhances the work of clinical decision-making, and not disrupts, should be also highlighted in terms of these studies. Also, the human-AI interface has been given a lot of attention by the research community, which highlighted the relevance of usability, transparency, and interpretability of AI tools (Okada et al., 2023). Systems with simple, explainable findings will have a high chance of being accepted by the clinicians and those that do not compromise their current digital systems.

Research points out that much of the support behind AI systems rests on the possibilities to have insight into how AI systems are drawing their conclusions, particularly in sensitive settings, like those of the intensive care units and emergencies (Pinsky et al., 2024). In addition, user-centered design approaches have increasingly become popular in development of AI technologies, that promoted inclusion of clinicians and healthcare personnel into the design and evaluation process with the aim of making it relevant and applicable. The literature has also put a lot of emphasis on ethical issues (Muniasamy, A., & Karunakaran, G. 2026). Since any AI system is highly dependent on the data of the past, they could be very vulnerable to producing the already existing biases contained in the training data, not to mention intensifying them (Russell et al., 2023). Bias may be of many types such as racial, gender-based, age-related, and how people may be biased in diagnosis and treatment recommendations based on socio-economic levels. To determine and solve these variations, researchers have proposed fairness audits and demographic performance investigation into the AI assessment procedure.

Besides, the idea of algorithmic transparency has been associated with ethical accountability, where developers and institutions have been required to catalogue the design reasoning behind an AI model, the nature of training data and method of explaining the decisions made (Schuitmaker et al., 2025). The other important research avenue is associated with the environment of regulation and government of clinical AI implementation. The current medical device regulations do not usually cover all the peculiarities of the machine learning-based systems due to their adaptability and ability to learn. Researchers espouse adaptable regulatory policies which consider the cyclical pattern of AI models and enable post-market monitoring, revalidation of performance, and version management (Tsopra et al., 2021). The literature also places emphasis on the significance of institutional AI governance frameworks such as multidisciplinary ethics committees and clinical technology advice boards to not only control the implementation, tracking, and, most importantly, updating of AI instruments in clinical practice but also to ease coordination. There are studies that have suggested that post-deployment monitoring should be an obligatory step of the AI lifecycle.

On-going performance testing via real-world data is vital so that model drift, behavioral surprises, or time-based reduction in accuracy would become clear. As a way of ensuring safety and rewarding gradual advancements, feedback mechanisms were anomalies, mistakes, or suspicions regarding the predications of AI can be reported by the clinicians must be introduced (Abràmoff et al., 2023). This is aligned to the new paradigm of learning healthcare systems in which the technology undergoes continual adaptation according to the emergent real-time evidence and feedback of practitioners. In addition, the literature supports the presumption that AI assessment should be matched, and patient-focused outcomes should be considered (Alowais et al., 2023). Although traditional measures of performance are very informative, they do not necessarily measure the real effects of AI tools on the health of patients, time recovery, treatment compliance and satisfaction. Introducing the elements of outcome-based evaluation measures into the patterns of AI assessment guarantees that the instrument will benefit the improvement of patient care and not only algorithmic performance. Research on this method tends to integrate clinical indicators with patient and care-provider qualitative information alongside one another to develop a clear picture of how well AI is working (Arigbabu et al., 2024). Along with the clinical and ethical assessment, an operational feasibility has become another factor to consider.

The studies emphasize that even superior AI systems might not be adopted in case they are resource-demanding, need a special kind of infrastructure, or require a significant update of the current processes. As such, implementation science is emerging in the AI research field and it is paying attention to methods of easy integration, staff education, change management, and sustainability (Eslamitabar et al., 2024). To conclude, the literature records the emerging agreement on the need to adopt a multidimensional and lifetime-based consideration of AI systems in hospitals. To apply such a method, it is necessary to go beyond the Academic idea of precision and introduce a dimension of practical applicability, validation, ethical standards, bias reduction, regulatory palatability and patient-specific effects (Familoni, 2024). An effective AI evaluation scheme needs to capture as many stakeholders as possible such as clinicians, developers, administrators, regulators, and patients and facilitate the ongoing development of AI systems via effective feedback loops. Such broad perspective is needed to achieve responsible, transparent and effective implementation of AI into a clinical setting.

MAIN FOCUS OF THE CHAPTER

The concept of systematic and detailed system to examine the Artificial Intelligence (AI) systems implemented in the hospitals is the primary concern of this chapter. It underlines the necessity of a multi-dimensional evaluation that would surpass the standard performance values such as accuracy or even the precision. The chapter manages the key elements of critical appraisal such as clinical validation, usability, integration of the workflow, safety, bias mitigation, ethical considerations, and regulatory compliance. It emphasizes the necessity not just to make sure that AI tools are technically competent but also functionally efficient, morally accountable and moveable to reality-based healthcare conditions. The chapter will help clinicians, developers, administrators, and policymakers apply AI in hospitals responsibly by discussing every phase of an AI lifecycle: development and deployment as well as post-market monitoring. Finally, the chapter aims to make sure that AI promotes patient outcomes, clinical decisions, and trust in healthcare systems with the transparent, fair, and evidence-based practices in evaluation.

Proposed Study Schematic Diagram

The study schematic diagram proposed depicts an organization of the life cycle structure of the assessment of AI systems at a hospital facility. In this exhaustive model, key milestones are attended to throughout the development process and after deployment, so that AI tools can be more than technically sound; they are also clinically successful, ethically-sound, and iteratively better. AI system development has to be followed by clinical validation of the AI system in question to ensure feasibility in the real world. The possibility of integration into existing workflows is then evaluated to ensure smooth adoption of the health care professionals. The stage of outcome-based evaluation considers the effect of the evaluating tool on the experience of the patients, whereas the bias status analysis and the fairness test provide equity among the various groups. An Ethical and regulatory compliance framework is also integrated in order to conform to the legal requirements so as not to infringe on patients' rights. Lastly, reality checks and real-time feedback will allow a continuous evaluation of effectiveness, and subsequent improvement. Such iterative loop keeps the AI systems changing along with the requirements and new data emerging in the clinical practice, facilitating these systems to become safe, transparent, and responsible to be used in contemporary healthcare settings.

The following presents a detailed, lifecycle-based framework of assessing AI systems in hygienic conditions. The first step is the AI System Development that is followed by Clinical Validation that guarantees the accuracy of the model and its safety in the medical setting. Workflow Integration Assessment is an analysis on how suitable the AI tool is in accordance with current clinical processes. Outcome-Based Evaluation looks at the effects of the system on the care of patients and efficiency of healthcare. Bias & Fairness Analysis makes sure that the performance is equal when it comes to different populations. Ethical & Regulatory Compliance deals with following the law and being on the right path. Last but not least is Post-Deployment Monitoring and Continuous Feedback & Model Updating, which creates a feedback loop whereby the AI system will be progressively enhanced, so it matches dynamic clinical data as well as real-world applications. This value chain can facilitate responsible, transparent, and active AI technologies in the healthcare deployment.

Figure 1. Lifecycle-Based Evaluation Framework for AI Systems in Hospitals

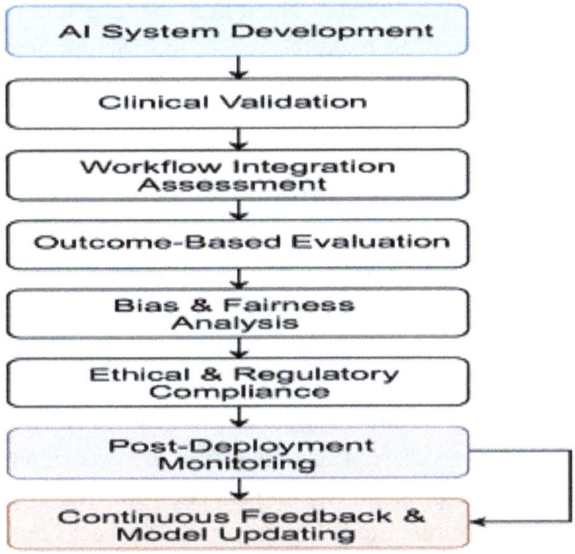

AI System Development

This is the first stage of development of AI models based on clinical datasets. It consists of searching the right algorithms, pre-processing the information and training the model to conduct certain medical tasks, diagnosing, predicting or automate the workflow. It architecture of the model intended to solve medical problems but not to be limited by the computational efficiency or scalability. Another step taking place at this stage is the elimination of possible sources of bias and readiness to match the regulatory requirements. It is critical to conduct documentation and have stakeholder input (e.g., clinicians) to support the alignment of the model with the healthcare needs and the possibility to assess it sufficiently during the later stages of implementation.

Clinical Validation

Clinical validation method of clinical tests calls on the possibility of testing the AI model and testing with the actual patient data and not in laboratory conditions. It is accurate, generalizable and relevant in various clinical settings and across different demographics of patients. The stage employs such critical indicators as sensitivity, specificity, precision, and recall to assess diagnostic or predictive abilities. The final step in the development process is validation, which: ascertains whether the system is ready to be deployed to reality, compares the outputs with ground-truth data and decisions made by clinicians. The aim is to make sure that the AI is able to assist in the medical decision-making process in different healthcare scenarios to demonstrate consistency over a wide range of real-time clinical activities in a safe and reliable manner.

Workflow Integration Assessment

With this step there is the assurance that the AI systems can be incorporated in the current processes of the hospitals seamlessly with the likely candidates electronics health records and also the clinical decision support systems. It measures usability, accessibility, and adaptability as seen by the doctors, nurses, and administrator. Such features as user-friendly interfaces, account-specific dashboards, and a minimum number of workflows disruptions are essential. This step reassures that the use of AI brings increased productivity and decision-making instead of confusion or inefficiencies in operation. Centeredness, user feedback, and interoperability standards can be significant in making sure that AI can make real-time clinical decisions without any resistance.

Outcome-Based Evaluation

The stage will determine the effect of AI tools on patient outcomes and hospital efficiency. It targets below metrics of the real-world diagnostic efficiency, treatment plan efficiency, rates of recovery, staying in the hospital and readmission rates. Through these measures, it becomes clear to evaluators that AI systems will have any meaningful contribution towards healthcare objectives. This assessment establishes a connection between the success of AI and real evidence of patient care and product outcomes. The effectiveness of AI tools is not only evaluated on the basis of predictions but also on clinical utility, patient safety and its contribution, of all to the healthcare system.

Safety & Risk Management

AI systems in healthcare have to undergo an examination of possible failure cases that may result in a threat to the health of patients or employees. This phase will involve system failure risks, false prediction, data leakage, and symptoms of alert fatigue. A high-risk setting such as an ICU or and emergency room settings needs additional protections to be made, and these include fall-back mechanisms, as well as clinician override. After deployment, drift must constantly be monitored, so as to detect the performance drift. This stage will provide adequate protection of

AI technologies because risks have been pre-emptively identified and mitigated, therefore making the technologies safe, accountable and resilient in changing clinical environments.

Bias & Fairness Analysis

This aspect concerns the research of whether the AI systems work fairly discriminately in various subgroups of patients, including their race, gender, age or socio-economic status. Evaluation embraces diversity in dataset, accuracy in labelling, the unbiasedness in algorithm, and fairness in outcomes. The exercise of fairness audits involves disaggregation of performance measures and verification of differences. The reduction of bias is done using such strategies as dataset rebalancing, explainable AI algorithms, or ordinary audits. This is to facilitate AI to be used ethically by accommodating diversity and preventing harm to disadvantaged or vulnerable groups, which increases the trust in care with the help of AI.

Ethical & Regulatory Compliance

The stage is when AI is checked so as to make sure that it has fulfilled the already constituted ethical standards and that the standards are in line with the stipulated regulations such as those by the FDA, EMA, and WHO. Important areas are transparency, accountability, informed consent, data privacy and regulatory approval. Administration, standards of communication with patients, and government systems are audited. The system should be explicable and keep patient confidentiality. This step can facilitate an ethical use of AI because it will make it compliant with medical, societal norms. Moral conformity can prevent an abuse and assist in averting community confidence and institutional honesty within AI-facilitated healthcare systems.

Post-Deployment Monitoring

AI systems have to be monitored continuously when implemented in a live clinical environment. This step detects such problems as model drift, failing when it was not supposed or appearing new safety hazard due to environmental changes or the development of clinical practices. Such tools as real-time analytics, incident tracking, and clinician feedback are essential. The role of this stage is to make sure that the AI maintains the performance, safety, and compliance levels once released. It enables the accountability and adaptive learning of the AI system, which is bound to be effective, timely and responsive to the non-static nature of healthcare.

Continuous Feedback & Model Updating

Clinicians and stakeholders can report their problems and propose the improvement with feedback loops. New data and insights acquired after deployment are used to update AI models and meet the evolving clinical needs and eliminate any weaknesses detected. The model is developed to constantly change under continuous learning strategies that pose no new risks to the system. This circular process in turn recycles into clinical validation to be kept effective. It enables a living AI ecosystem that responds responsibly and ethically, is sustainable in its performance, provides fairness and clinical utility in the long term.

CASE STUDIES

In order to provide an example of AI systems practical use in hospitals and evaluate its use, two real-life case studies corresponding to the suggested framework will be presented in the given chapter. The first case study examines AI-based diagnostic model that is applied to identify pneumonia by analyzing chest X-rays and shows that there is a sharp increase in accuracy, efficiency of work processes, and patient outcomes (Goktas & Grzybowski, 2025). The second case study observes AI-based triage assistant implemented in emergency department setting, including increased decision-making speed, fewer wait times, and mitigating bias. Both scenarios are examples of how guided assessment, such as clinical validation, usability, fairness, and compliance guarantee safe and responsible use of AI in the clinical setting.

Case Study 1: AI-Based Diagnostic Tool for Pneumonia Detection

One of the big city hospitals also introduced an AI enabled diagnostic assistant that helps radiologists identify pneumonia on chest X-rays. Before the implementation, clinical validation of the tool was done on 8,000 anonymized patient scans on three hospitals. The achievability of 91.3% sensitivity and 89.7% specificity in using the AI surpassed the usual accuracy rate of radiologists (85%). When it became a part of the integration of the hospital in the Electronic Health Record (EHR) system, the workflow analysis showed that the radiologist review time per case went down by 28%, and the diagnostic turnaround time increased by 17%. The clinician satisfaction surveys demonstrated that 83% of users were also comfortable with the risk scoring interface of the tool as no disturbance (Jeyaraman et al., 2023). This was evaluated in terms of outcomes resulting in 22% decrement in cases of diagnostic error and 15% less cases of significant instances of readmission due to pneumonia after a 6 months period of outcome-based method of evaluation (In et al., 2022). Bias audits showed the difference in performance by age groups, where the percentage of the recall experience among elderly patients was 76 and increased to 88 after the retraining of the model using more data with various characteristics. Monitoring carried out in post-deployment state involved weekly drift detection, and updates based on real-time feedback provided by radiologists allowed maintaining continuous model updates (Feng et al., 2023; Muniasamy, A et al., 2021). The AI oversight committee at the hospital assured that the artificial intelligence used in the hospital was in line with FDA Software-as-a-Medical-Device (SaMD) regulations confirming ethically sound use and future confidence. The bar graph visualising major assessment indicators of the introduction of an AI-powered diagnosis assistant to detect pneumonia in a hospital (Baltazar et al., 2021; Muniasamy, A et al., 2021). Ten items of performance indicators are enumerated in the x-axis, such as sensitivity, specificity, radiologist accuracy, a reduction in review time, diagnostic turnaround improvement, user satisfaction, reduction in diagnostic errors and readmission, and recall rates in the elderly population before and after retraining of the model. Each measure is described in terms of percentages in the y-axis. Colour-differentiated bars are used that are thin as they help visualize performance improvement in the three benchmarks of clinical validation, efficiency and impact. Figure 2 illustrates other substantial gains like 91.3%, sensitivity, and 89.7% specificity, and a 28% decline in the time of review cases and the effectiveness of such a tool in the real world and the capability of further development with feedback-based update.

Figure 2. AI Diagnostic Assistant Performance Metrics

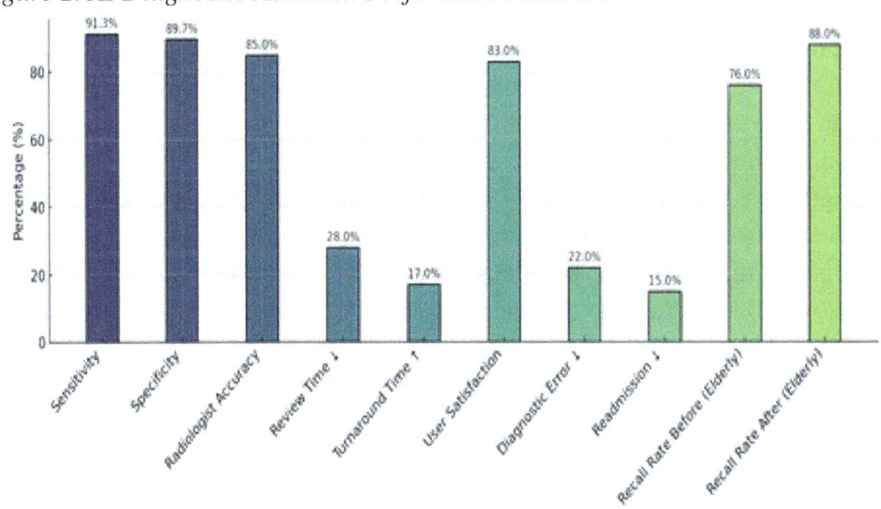

Case Study 2: AI Triage Assistant in Emergency Department

A triage assistant based on AI and deployed in a medium-sized regional hospital aimed at providing a triaging mechanism where patients were prioritized based on the predicted acuity in emergency rooms (ER). Structured data provided in vitals, symptoms, and patient history were put to use by the system (Okada et al., 2023). The precision of its achievement on the high-risk patients that needed urgent care was 95.2% during the clinical validation when the model was able to correctly identify 12,000 ER visits in 94.5%. After the integration of the workflow, the time spent on triage has decreased by 35%, and the waiting time of fatal cases decreased to 12 minutes as opposed to 28 (Boonstra & Laven, 2022). The satisfaction rates of nurses were 87% as they claimed that the system is very well correlated with the current triage procedure and alleviated the cognitive load during high traffic time. The outcome-based evaluation revealed 19% reduce in the time-to-treatment of critical patients and 12% reduction in the adverse events because of delayed triage (Ippolito et al., 2023). The AI system increased the overall ER throughput by 22%, particularly the weekend and holidays. Bias was also found in precision as non-English speakers had a lower precision (82%) which was then corrected by updating the interface and augmenting the data to precision of 91%. Ethical compliance was observed by recording the consent of the patients, of which 92% of patients agreed with AI-aided triaging. The AI governance team operated the hospital by providing the regulation reporting and feedback of model updates once in 30 days, in favor of sustainability in performance and clinical safety. The chart shows the evaluation of the performance of an AI-based triage assistant in one of the hospitals of the region, emergency room. Major indicators found in the x-axis are the high-risk patient accuracy, Er visit detection accuracy, triage and wait time decrease, nurse satisfaction, and increase in throughputs. The y-axis is shown to relate to percentages.

Figure 3 shows that the accuracy of clinical validation is high (95.2% precision), the length of triage reduced by 35%, EP throughput rose by 22%. It is important to note that accuracy in non-English language speakers rose to 91% when there was an adjustment of interface and data. Ethics compliance was verified whereby ninety-two percent of patients agreed to be triaged using AI. So, in general, the visual display shows the influence of the assistant on the efficiency of operation, clinical outcomes, the satisfaction of users, and the provision of equitable care.

Figure 3. AI-Based Triage Assistant Performance Metrics

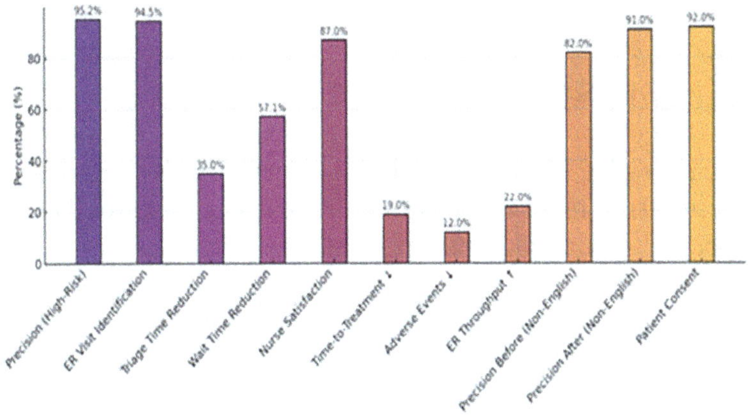

SOLUTIONS AND RECOMMENDATIONS

In order to securely introduce Artificial Intelligence (AI) in hospitals in a safe, ethical, and effective manner, an approach will be required to consider numerous dimensions. To begin with, AI systems are to be clinically validated thoroughly through different sets of data, so that it can be accurate, robust, and can be applied to diverse patient groups and care environments. Incorporation into the clinical workflows is to be centered on usability, with the guiding principle of maintaining simplicity in interface, role-based output, and compatibility with the current clinical systems, such as Electronic Health Records (EHRs). This improves implementation by the clinicians and lowers the friction in operation. Bias should also be addressed as fairness audits, multi-diverse training data sets and explainable AI models need to be introduced so that the performance across gender, age, ethnicity, and socio-economic backgrounds becomes equally fair. Regulatory compliance has to be in the first place to adhere to legal models like FDA, EMA, HIPAA, or GDPR and translate such ethical codes like transparency, accountability, and informed consent into system design. The monitoring in the post-deployment stage must be continuous, and it should include real-time analytics and feedback loop of a clinician to identify performance drifts, safety issues, or arising biases. It is recommended that hospitals should have special committees of clinicians, IT experts, ethicists, and administrators to manage lifecycle assessment, risk management, and policy-policy consistency in AI. These are some of the solutions which can help healthcare organizations to increase the value of AI and at the same time protect patient trust, clinical safety and regulatory legitimacy within the fast-changing environment of digital health.

FUTURE RESEARCH DIRECTIONS

With the increasing popularity of Artificial Intelligence (AI) integration in hospitals, it is critical that future studies should discuss fundamental challenges in order to have responsible, fair, and sustainable implementation. This involves promoting the development of dynamic model validation to fit the changing clinical context, improved explainability to generate confidence among the health care professionals, and the deployment of sound bias mitigation techniques to ensure equitable results on different populations (Al Kuwaiti et al., 2023). Also, investigation is required on ethical government and regulatory systems which can be modified in accordance with a swift development of technology. In combination, the given directions are supposed to enhance the presence of AI in healthcare through transparency, adaptability, inclusivity, and long-term adherence in real-life clinical practice.

Dynamic Model Validation and Continuous Learning

Constant changes in the healthcare environment will see the fixed AI models becoming out of date or inaccurate after a certain period of time. The next step should be to invent dynamic validation processes that would enable AI systems to be adjusted to new data, clinical procedure sets and population demographics. This entails model monitoring, re-training approaches, and recalibration of performance according to newer clinical standards (Benneh, 2024). Well-regulated continuous learning frameworks may assist AI tools to stay clinically pertinent, with the performance drift that is minimal. The opportunity to study safe methods of online learning should also include the possibility of self-updating models without affecting the integrity of the data and patient safety. Along with that, research should be conducted on finding the equilibrium between flexibility and resilience, so that constant upgrade would not cause unexpected actions. The validation procedures that are used should be dynamic and have to have proper safeguards in the form of human-in-the-loop feedback, finding anomalies, and testing in real-world situations. The initiation of lifecycle validation pipelines, which are common, will be able to boost clinical confidence and acceptance by the regulatory body. The capability of being able to continuously test and iterate on models after their deployment will become a prerequisite to ensure that they are accurate, reliable and safe, as the adoption of AI increases (Morley et al., 2020). This kind of research would open the path to resilient AI systems to achieve ongoing updates and personalization's through medical, environmental, and patient demands, where regulatory compliance, and performance integrity are retained.

Explainable and Trustworthy AI Systems

Successful integration of AI into clinical practices has been established as a pillar of trust. Numerous AI-based systems are still black boxes and provide little to no explanation of the way the decisions are being made, despite high predictive vaccination. The future researches should not only evolve explainable AI (XAI) methods that can explain the rationale behind predictions and decision-making procedures. Clinicians have to be given outputs that they can interpret and can be put into medical logic terms where they can verify or revert to the suggestions made by the AI (Murdoch, 2021). There is also the ethical accountability and regulatory acceptance via explainability. The model-agnostic tool (e.g., LIME, SHAP) and domain-specific approaches that can turn difficult predictions into meaningful interpretations at the clinical level should be researched. In addition, studies on human-AI interaction are required to determine the extent to which various forms of explanation affect clinician decision-making and trust (Murphy et al., 2021). The other critical sections are in the development of user interfaces that inform the risk scores, feature importance and confidence intervals intuitively. Human-in-the-loop systems and explainable outputs should go hand in hand toward building partnership as against dependence so that the clinicians will always be at the center of patient care. Researchers ought to also consider testing the extent to which there is a variation in trust in various roles (e.g., doctors vs. nurses), specialties (e.g., radiology vs. emergency medicine) (Pham, 2025). Finally, understandable and reliable Artificial Intelligence will not only improve clinical uptake but will also increase patient safety and ethical requirements in an Artificial Intelligence-assisted care setting.

Bias Mitigation and Fairness Audits

AI system bias poses a great impediment to equity in medical care. The typical training data consolidated or resembling societal inequalities and deficits in the demographic diversity may translate into models with a good favorable outcome in one group and poor performance in another. The focus of future studies should be on establishing ways to detect, measure, and alleviating algorithmic bias during the AI lifecycle. This involves developing algorithms that learn in a fair manner e.g. re-weighting, adversarial debiasing and fairness-constrained optimization (NIPS 2015). Also, research needs to be in developing standardized fairness audition instruments that can monitor the performance of AI in different sub groups of races, gender, age, language, socioeconomics (Rathore & Rathore, 2023). These models have to be tested in practice in a variety of clinical environments to determine whether they are generalized across the population in fairly ways. It is also necessary to investigate feedback loops, in which biased AI judgments can have effects on subsequent data gathering; that is why disparities are supported. The researchers should study how the bias occurs not only in the data but also in the labeling, architecture of the models and in clinical use. Moreover, the inclusion of a variety of stakeholders (such as ethicists, patient representatives, underrepresented clinicians, etc.) will help to make sure that fairness approaches are inclusive and based on actual needs (Secinaro et al., 2021). Bias in AI is a complex issue that requires the design proactively and constant supervision to achieve AI systems that can support healthcare equity and ensure its reliability with the public (Gauthaman, S. A., et al. (2026).

Ethical Governance and Regulatory Innovation

With the increasing use of AI in healthcare, the conventional regulation systems are unable to support the fast-changing dynamic and data-centric solutions. Future studies should concentrate on developing adaptive structures of ethical governing and innovative models of regulation, which in turn facilitate safety alongside with innovation (Muniasamy, A., & Karunakaran, G., 2026). This encompasses the formulation of guidelines for AI systems in which the behavior may change with time including the dynamic model approval, continuous post-market surveillance as well as a regular ethical update (Sengupta, 2023). Some research should be done to investigate how ethnic values of transparency, accountability, non-maleficence and justice can be incorporated into the very design of AI systems. What is more, there should be new oversight models, e.g. the AI ethics boards or institutional governance councils, which should be tested at a clinical level. International cooperation and standardization of cross-nation AI laws should be examined as a method of expediting compliance procedures across multinational implementations (Navath, 2023). The implications of algorithmic liability, the implications of algorithmic liability, and the implications of informed consent in AI-assisted care should also be studied by researchers. Proper risk evaluation in motion, accountability in the form of legal codes and data governance policies are the key ingredients of the regulatory models of the future (Williamson & Prybutok, 2024). It could present an exciting opportunity to transform how the governance system works to keep up with AI innovation, and future studies can be used to create proactive, rather than reactive, systematic frameworks that can achieve responsible development and deployment of AI, without compromising human rights, the safety of patients, and overall trust of societies.

CONCLUSION

Artificial Intelligence (AI) and healthcare systems offer audiences noteworthy promise in the realm of clinical decision-making, diagnostic precision, workflow efficiency at hospitals, and the overall net outcome of patients. Nevertheless, AI potential could only be fulfilled when its application is directed by a rational, thorough, and ethically considerate system of assessment. The chapter has submitted the idea of a holistic and lifecycle-based paradigm of evaluating AI systems in the hospital settings, including development stage, validation stage, integration stage, monitoring phase and refinement phase that would deal with challenges and risks facing multifaceted implementation of clinical AI. By presenting the rationale in depth at the main areas of evaluation, the chapter notes that technical measures of performance (accuracy, precision, sensitivity, and specificity) though significant are not adequate when alone.

To successfully incorporate AI and integrate it into practice, measures of clinical relevance, likelihood of use in practice settings, long-term patient outcome, bias reduction, ethical conformity, and compliance regulations should be observed and evaluated. The validation of AI systems should be performed on a wide and representative selection of data to permit generalizability, and they should additionally permit openness and clarification to instill trust among clinicians and patients. Further, fair levels of performance in various demographic groups should also be achieved by auditing bias and designing of an inclusive model. The research framework presented here also identifies the need of a subsequent deployment verification and feedback systems. Unlike the stable technologies, AI tools are dynamic and can be modified with time, and it is necessary to ensure that AI tools performance is monitored during real-time scenarios and altered to fit the fluctuating clinical environment.

By incorporating real time feedback, performance drifts monitoring and clinician monitoring, AI systems can be made safe, efficacious and standards adherent to patient care even post deployment. Next, the need to apply ethical governance and regulation innovation has been outlined in the chapter. Since AI systems are becoming increasingly independent and consequential in crucial health care decisions, the key to achieving accountability, data privacy, patient consent, and sensible use will require adjusting the model of governance in institutions. Another way of reducing the risk of AI tools is through the regulatory bodies, which will have to come up with adaptive frameworks that will allow embracing the dynamicity and learning nature of the tools, without weighing down innovation. These two described case studies on AI-based pneumonia diagnosis and AI-guided triaging in an emergency suggest that the suggested framework can be also applied in practice. They demonstrate that relationship between an orderly assessment and the enhanced measures of clinical quality and smooth functioning, as well as facilitating the process of realization and fixation of moral, usability and functionality concerns that may arise after deployment. These illustrations demonstrate the importance of testing in a realistic context, clinician participation and multi-disciplinary governance in the assurance of AI systems being suitably appropriate.

To summarize, one reads the roadmap to the safe, ethical, and effective adoption of AI in hospitals in this chapter. It promotes the transformation of the performance-based validation to the generic, lifecycle-conscious assessment processes. Since AI is gaining more solid roots in the healthcare sector, it is crucial to take such frameworks to keep the residents safe and maintain belief in the stability of the industry in the long-term. New technologies, new populations, and world healthcare issues require constantly revised models that future research must develop. By adhering to a substantive assessment, ethical surveillance, and gradual enhancement, it is our sole and responsible chance to understand how profoundly the AI can transform the healthcare sector.

REFERENCES

Abràmoff, M. D., Tarver, M. E., Loyo-Berrios, N., Trujillo, S., Char, D., Obermeyer, Z., Eydelman, M. B., & Maisel, W. H. (2023). Considerations for addressing bias in artificial intelligence for health equity. *NPJ Digital Medicine*, *6*(1), 170. DOI: 10.1038/s41746-023-00913-9 PMID: 37700029

Al Kuwaiti, A., Nazer, K., Al-Reedy, A., Al-Shehri, S., Al-Muhanna, A., Subbarayalu, A. V., Al Muhanna, D., & Al-Muhanna, F. A. (2023). A review of the role of artificial intelligence in healthcare. *Journal of Personalized Medicine*, *13*(6), 951. DOI: 10.3390/jpm13060951 PMID: 37373940

Alowais, S. A., Alghamdi, S. S., Alsuhebany, N., Alqahtani, T., Alshaya, A. I., Almohareb, S. N., Aldairem, A., Alrashed, M., Bin Saleh, K., Badreldin, H. A., Al Yami, M. S., Al Harbi, S., & Albekairy, A. M. (2023). Revolutionizing healthcare: The role of artificial intelligence in clinical practice. *BMC Medical Education*, *23*(1), 689. DOI: 10.1186/s12909-023-04698-z PMID: 37740191

Arigbabu, A. T., Olaniyi, O. O., Adigwe, C. S., Adebiyi, O. O., & Ajayi, S. A. (2024). Data governance in AI-enabled healthcare systems: A case of the Project Nightingale. *Asian Journal of Research in Computer Science*, *17*(5), 85–107. DOI: 10.9734/ajrcos/2024/v17i5441

Baltazar, L. R., Manzanillo, M. G., Gaudillo, J., Viray, E. D., Domingo, M., Tiangco, B., & Albia, J. (2021). Artificial intelligence on COVID-19 pneumonia detection using chest X-ray images. *PLoS One*, *16*(10), e0257884. DOI: 10.1371/journal.pone.0257884 PMID: 34648509

Benneh Mensah, G., & Dutta, P. K. (2024). Evaluating if Ghana's Health Institutions and Facilities Act 2011 (Act 829) sufficiently addresses medical negligence risks from integration of artificial intelligence systems. *Mesopotamian Journal of Artificial Intelligence in Healthcare*, 35–41.

Boonstra, A., & Laven, M. (2022). Influence of artificial intelligence on the work design of emergency department clinicians: A systematic literature review. *BMC Health Services Research*, *22*(1), 669. DOI: 10.1186/s12913-022-08070-7 PMID: 35585603

Eslamitabar, S., Lame, E., Rouzbahani, A., & Roozbahani, Z. (2024). *Legal and ethical challenges of artificial intelligence applications in healthcare*. Health Technology Assessment in Action. DOI: 10.18502/htaa.v7i4.14653

Familoni, B. T. (2024). Ethical frameworks for AI in healthcare entrepreneurship: A theoretical examination of challenges and approaches. *International Journal of Frontiers in Biology and Pharmaceutical Research*, *5*(1), 57–65.

Feng, Y., Ting, J. S. Z., Xu, X., Bee, C. K., En, O. T., Hendra, T. W. J. I., Ting, Y., Lei, X., Chen, W.-X., Wang, Y., Li, S., Cui, Y., Wang, Z., Zhen, L., Liu, Y., Goh, R. S. M., & Tan, C. H. (2023). Deep neural network augments performance of junior residents in diagnosing COVID-19 pneumonia on chest radiographs. *Diagnostics (Basel)*, *13*(8), 1433. DOI: 10.3390/diagnostics13081397 PMID: 37189498

Gauthaman, S. A.. (2026). Introduction to machine learning and optimization in healthcare. In Muniasamy, A. (Ed.), *Integrative machine learning and optimization algorithms for disease prediction* (pp. 1–34). IGI Global., DOI: 10.4018/979-8-3373-1087-9.ch001

Goktas, P., & Grzybowski, A. (2025). Shaping the future of healthcare: Ethical clinical challenges and pathways to trustworthy AI. *Journal of Clinical Medicine*, *14*(5), 1443. DOI: 10.3390/jcm14051605 PMID: 40095575

Graziani, M., Dutkiewicz, L., Calvaresi, D., Amorim, J. P., Yordanova, K., Mor, V., Nair, R., Abreu, P. H., Blanke, T., Pulignano, V., Prior, J. O., Lauwaert, L., Reijers, W., Depeursinge, A., Andrearczyk, V., & Müller, H. (2023). A global taxonomy of interpretable AI: Unifying the terminology for the technical and social sciences. *Artificial Intelligence Review*, *56*(4), 3473–3504. DOI: 10.1007/s10462-022-10256-8 PMID: 36092822

Hantel, A., Walsh, T. P., Marron, J. M., Kehl, K. L., Sharp, R., Van Allen, E., & Abel, G. A. (2024). Perspectives of oncologists on the ethical implications of using artificial intelligence for cancer care. *JAMA Network Open*, *7*(3), e244077. DOI: 10.1001/jamanetworkopen.2024.4077 PMID: 38546644

Higgins, D., & Madai, V. I. (2020). From bit to bedside: A practical framework for artificial intelligence product development in healthcare. *Advanced Intelligent Systems*, *2*(10), 2000052. DOI: 10.1002/aisy.202000052

In, E., Geçkil, A. A., Kavuran, G., Şahin, M., Berber, N. K., & Kuluöztürk, M. (2022). Using artificial intelligence to improve the diagnostic efficiency of pulmonologists in differentiating COVID-19 pneumonia from community-acquired pneumonia. *Journal of Medical Virology*, *94*(8), 3698–3705. DOI: 10.1002/jmv.27777 PMID: 35419818

Ippolito, D., Maino, C., Gandola, D., Franco, P. N., Miron, R., Barbu, V., Bologna, M., Corso, R., & Breaban, M. E. (2023). Artificial intelligence applied to chest X-ray: A reliable tool to assess the differential diagnosis of lung pneumonia in the emergency department. *Diseases (Basel, Switzerland), 11*(4), 171. DOI: 10.3390/diseases11040171 PMID: 37987282

Jeyaraman, M., Balaji, S., Jeyaraman, N., & Yadav, S. (2023). Unraveling the ethical enigma: Artificial intelligence in healthcare. *Cureus, 15*(8), e43262. DOI: 10.7759/cureus.43262 PMID: 37692617

Jha, D., Durak, G., Sharma, V., Keles, E., Cicek, V., Zhang, Z., Srivastava, A., Rauniyar, A., Hagos, D. H., Tomar, N. K., Miller, F. H., Topcu, A., Yazidi, A., Håkegård, J. E., & Bagci, U. (2025). A conceptual framework for applying ethical principles of AI to medical practice. *Bioengineering (Basel, Switzerland), 12*(2), 152. DOI: 10.3390/bioengineering12020180 PMID: 40001699

Jia, L.-L., Zhao, J.-X., Pan, N.-N., Liu-Yan, S., Zhao, L.-P., Tian, J.-H., & Huang, G. (2022). Artificial intelligence model on chest imaging to diagnose COVID-19 and other pneumonias: A systematic review and meta-analysis. *European Journal of Radiology Open, 9*, 100438. DOI: 10.1016/j.ejro.2022.100438 PMID: 35996746

Kim, M., Sohn, H., Choi, S., & Kim, S. (2023). Requirements for trustworthy artificial intelligence and its application in healthcare. *Healthcare Informatics Research, 29*(4), 315–322. DOI: 10.4258/hir.2023.29.4.315 PMID: 37964453

Moghadasi, N., Valdez, R. S., Piran, M., Moghaddasi, N., Linkov, I., Polmateer, T. L., Loose, D. C., & Lambert, J. H. (2024). Risk analysis of artificial intelligence in medicine with a multilayer concept of system order. *Systems, 12*(2), 47. DOI: 10.3390/systems12020047

Moreno-Sánchez, P. A. (2023). Data-driven early diagnosis of chronic kidney disease: Development and evaluation of an explainable AI model. *IEEE Access : Practical Innovations, Open Solutions, 11*, 38359–38369. DOI: 10.1109/ACCESS.2023.3264270

Morley, J., Machado, C. C. V., Burr, C., Cowls, J., Joshi, I., Taddeo, M., & Floridi, L. (2020). The ethics of AI in health care: A mapping review. *Social Science & Medicine, 260*, 113172. DOI: 10.1016/j.socscimed.2020.113172 PMID: 32702587

Muniasamy, A., Bhatnagar, R., & Karunakaran, G. (2021). Predicting COVID-19 spread in Saudi Arabia using artificial intelligence techniques—Proposing a shift towards a sustainable healthcare approach. In Hassanien, A., Bhatnagar, R., & Darwish, A. (Eds.), *Artificial intelligence for sustainable development: Theory, practice and future applications. Studies in computational intelligence* (Vol. 912). Springer., DOI: 10.1007/978-3-030-51920-9_6

Muniasamy, A., & Karunakaran, G. (2026). Challenges and future directions: Emerging trends and limitations in ML and optimization for healthcare. In Muniasamy, A. (Ed.), *Integrative machine learning and optimization algorithms for disease prediction* (pp. 339–368). IGI Global., DOI: 10.4018/979-8-3373-1087-9.ch012

Murdoch, B. (2021). Privacy and artificial intelligence: Challenges for protecting health information in a new era. *BMC Medical Ethics*, *22*(1), 122. DOI: 10.1186/s12910-021-00687-3 PMID: 34525993

Murphy, K., Di Ruggiero, E., Upshur, R., Willison, D. J., Malhotra, N., Cai, J. C., Lui, V., & Gibson, J. (2021). Artificial intelligence for good health: A scoping review of the ethics literature. *BMC Medical Ethics*, *22*(1), 14. DOI: 10.1186/s12910-021-00577-8 PMID: 33588803

Nair, M., Svedberg, P., Larsson, I., & Nygren, J. M. (2024). A comprehensive overview of barriers and strategies for AI implementation in healthcare: Mixed-method design. *PLoS One*, *19*(8), e0305949. DOI: 10.1371/journal.pone.0305949 PMID: 39121051

Navath, S. (2023). Transforming healthcare: The impact and future of artificial intelligence in healthcare. *Journal of Artificial Intelligence and Machine Learning*, *1*(1), 16–21. DOI: 10.55124/jaim.v1i1.234

Okada, Y., Ning, Y., & Ong, M. E. H. (2023). Explainable artificial intelligence in emergency medicine: An overview. *Clinical and Experimental Emergency Medicine*, *10*(4), 354–362. DOI: 10.15441/ceem.23.145 PMID: 38012816

Pham, T. (2025). Ethical and legal considerations in healthcare AI: Innovation and policy for safe and fair use. *Royal Society Open Science*, *12*(5), 241873. DOI: 10.1098/rsos.241873 PMID: 40370601

Pinsky, M. R., Bedoya, A., Bihorac, A., Celi, L., Churpek, M., Economou-Zavlanos, N. J., Elbers, P., Saria, S., Liu, V., Lyons, P. G., Shickel, B., Toral, P., Tscholl, D., & Clermont, G. (2024). Use of artificial intelligence in critical care: Opportunities and obstacles. *Critical Care*, *28*(1), 113. DOI: 10.1186/s13054-024-04860-z PMID: 38589940

Rathore, F. A., & Rathore, M. A. (2023). The emerging role of artificial intelligence in healthcare. *JPMA. The Journal of the Pakistan Medical Association*, *73*(7), 1368–1369. DOI: 10.47391/JPMA.23-48 PMID: 37469045

Rengaramanujam, K., & Muniasamy, A. (2026). AI in hospital administration and formulary design: Optimizing resource allocation and patient flow. In Muniasamy, A., & Karunakaran, G. (Eds.), *Applications of artificial intelligence in pharmaceuticals* (pp. 215–246). IGI Global., DOI: 10.4018/979-8-3373-2043-4.ch008

Russell, R. G., Lovett Novak, L., Patel, M., Garvey, K. V., Craig, K. J. T., Jackson, G. P., Moore, D., & Miller, B. M. (2023). Competencies for the use of artificial intelligence-based tools by health care professionals. *Academic Medicine*, *98*(3), 348–356. DOI: 10.1097/ACM.0000000000004963 PMID: 36731054

Schuitmaker, L., Drogt, J., Benders, M., & Jongsma, K. (2025). Physicians' required competencies in AI-assisted clinical settings: A systematic review. *British Medical Bulletin*, *153*(1), 36–53. DOI: 10.1093/bmb/ldae025 PMID: 39821209

Secinaro, S., Calandra, D., Secinaro, A., Muthurangu, V., & Biancone, P. (2021). The role of artificial intelligence in healthcare: A structured literature review. *BMC Medical Informatics and Decision Making*, *21*(1), 125. DOI: 10.1186/s12911-021-01488-9 PMID: 33836752

Sengupta, D. (2023). Artificial intelligence in diagnostic dermatology: Challenges and the way forward. *Indian Dermatology Online Journal*, *14*(6), 782–787. DOI: 10.4103/idoj.idoj_462_23 PMID: 38099026

Tsopra, R., Fernandez, X., Luchinat, C., Alberghina, L., Lehrach, H., Vanoni, M., Dreher, F., Sezerman, O. U., Cuggia, M., de Tayrac, M., Miklasevics, E., Itu, L. M., Geanta, M., Ogilvie, L., Godey, F., Boldisor, C. N., Campillo-Gimenez, B., Cioroboiu, C., Ciusdel, C. F., & Burgun, A. (2021). A framework for validating AI in precision medicine: Considerations from the European ITFoC consortium. *BMC Medical Informatics and Decision Making*, *21*(1), 274. DOI: 10.1186/s12911-021-01634-3 PMID: 34600518

Williamson, S. M., & Prybutok, V. (2024). Balancing privacy and progress: A review of privacy challenges, systemic oversight, and patient perceptions in AI-driven healthcare. *Applied Sciences (Basel, Switzerland)*, *14*(2), 675. DOI: 10.3390/app14020675

ADDITIONAL READING

Amann, J., Blasimme, A., Vayena, E., Frey, D., & Madai, V. I. (2020). Precise4Q consortium: Explainability for artificial intelligence in healthcare: a multidisciplinary perspective. *BMC Medical Informatics and Decision Making*, *20*(1), 310. DOI: 10.1186/s12911-020-01332-6 PMID: 33256715

Cabitza, F., Rasoini, R., & Gensini, G. F. (2017). Unintended consequences of machine learning in medicine. *Journal of the American Medical Association*, *318*(6), 517. DOI: 10.1001/jama.2017.7797 PMID: 28727867

Liu, X., Rivera, S. C., Moher, D., Calvert, M. J., & Denniston, A. K. (2020). SPIRIT-AI, Group, C.-A.W.: Reporting guidelines for clinical trial reports for interventions involving artificial intelligence: the CONSORT-AI Extension. *BMJ (Clinical Research Ed.)*, *370*, m3164. DOI: 10.1136/bmj.m3164 PMID: 32909959

Obermeyer, Z., & Emanuel, E. J. (2016). Predicting the future - big data, machine learning, and clinical medicine. *The New England Journal of Medicine*, *375*(13), 1216–1219. DOI: 10.1056/NEJMp1606181 PMID: 27682033

Selbst, A. D., Boyd, D., Friedler, S. A., Venkatasubramanian, S., & Vertesi, J. Fairness and abstraction in sociotechnical systems. In: *Proceedings of the Conference on Fairness, Accountability, and Transparency*, pp. 59–68 (2019) DOI: 10.1145/3287560.3287598

KEY TERMS AND DEFINITIONS

Artificial Intelligence (AI): Artificial Intelligence refers to the simulation of human intelligence processes by machines, particularly computer systems, and is widely applied in healthcare to support diagnostics, clinical decision-making, and automation of routine tasks.

Bias in AI: Bias in AI refers to systematic errors in decision-making processes that result in unfair treatment or skewed outcomes for specific groups based on characteristics such as race, gender, or age.

Clinical Validation: Clinical validation is the process of rigorously evaluating AI systems using real-world patient data to confirm their accuracy, reliability, and relevance across diverse clinical settings before adoption.

Ethical AI: Ethical AI encompasses the design and deployment of artificial intelligence systems guided by principles of transparency, fairness, accountability, and privacy.

Explainability: Explainability describes the extent to which the internal workings and decision-making processes of an AI system can be understood and interpreted by humans.

F1-Score: The F1-Score represents the harmonic mean of precision and recall, offering a balanced measure that accounts for both false positives and false negatives.

Post-Deployment Monitoring: Post-deployment monitoring involves the continuous evaluation of AI systems after implementation to identify issues such as performance degradation, potential risks, and unintended consequences.

Precision (PPV): Precision, also known as Positive Predictive Value (PPV), is the proportion of true positive results among all positive predictions made by the AI system.

Recall: Recall, often used interchangeably with sensitivity, evaluates the system's effectiveness in identifying all relevant positive cases within a dataset.

Regulatory Compliance: Regulatory compliance signifies adherence to established laws, policies, and standards—such as FDA, EMA, HIPAA, and GDPR—that govern the safe and ethical use of AI systems in healthcare.

Sensitivity: Sensitivity measures the ability of an AI system to correctly identify true positive cases, such as detecting the presence of a disease when it actually exists.

Specificity: Specificity refers to the ability of an AI system to correctly identify true negative cases, ensuring that patients without a disease are accurately ruled out.

Chapter 4
Data Quality, Privacy, and Security Concerns in Healthcare

J. Shajeena
https://orcid.org/0009-0008-8332-2588
SRM Institute of Science and Technology,Tiruchirapalli, India

Shiny R. M.
https://orcid.org/0000-0002-0473-9852
St. Joseph's College of Engineering, Chennai, India

A. Bindhu
https://orcid.org/0000-0002-4453-8609
Infant Jesus College of Arts and Science for Women, Mulagumoodu, India

ABSTRACT

Healthcare organizations use technology to enhance patient care and streamline their operations in the modern digital world. However, worries about data security and privacy have grown as more clinics and hospitals store patient records electronically. Important information such as a person's medical history, current treatments, and personal data are contained in medical records. This information could result in fraud, identity theft, or health insurance abuse if it ends up in the wrong hands. Because medical data is valuable, cybercriminals frequently target healthcare organizations. Strong security measures like encryption, secure access controls, and routine system checks to stop unwanted access are necessary for hospitals to protect patient privacy. Healthcare providers must make investments in

DOI: 10.4018/979-8-3373-2787-7.ch004

cutting-edge security technologies and enhance data management procedures due to the rise in cyber threats. By taking such steps, they will be able to protect patient data, foster trust, and improve healthcare for everybody.

INTRODUCTION

The rapid digital transformation of healthcare has ushered in unprecedented opportunities for improving patient care, operational efficiency, and medical research. Central to this transformation is the increasing reliance on data-driven systems such as Electronic Health Records (EHRs), Health Information Exchanges (HIEs), wearable health devices, and Artificial Intelligence (AI) tools. While these technologies promise enhanced decision-making and personalized treatment, they also raise critical concerns related to data quality, privacy, and security. In addition to security, healthcare data quality is crucial. Patient records that are inaccurate or incomplete can result in incorrect diagnoses, inappropriate treatments, and even major health hazards. Doctors may become confused and treatment delays may result from data entry errors, duplicate records, or missing information. Healthcare organizations should use well-structured data management systems that guarantee accuracy and consistency in order to prevent such mistakes. The most recent information about a patient helps the doctor make the right choices and provide the right care, which enhances patient care. Errors can be avoided and expenses can be reduced with proper data management, improving the medical field's safety and effectiveness. Healthcare data security is increasingly being aided by artificial intelligence (AI). AI-powered solutions can recognize security risks, spot odd activity, and act fast to safeguard patient data. By keeping an eye on who has access to the data and making sure that only those with permission can see it, AI can also assist hospitals in adhering to stringent data protection regulations like HIPAA and GDPR

High-quality data is foundational for effective healthcare delivery. Inaccurate, incomplete, or inconsistent data can lead to diagnostic errors, inappropriate treatments, and compromised patient outcomes (Weng and Weiskopf, 2013). Ensuring data accuracy, timeliness, and completeness is particularly challenging in environments with multiple data sources and varied documentation practices. Simultaneously, the sensitive nature of healthcare data makes privacy a paramount concern. Healthcare information often includes personal identifiers, genetic information, and behavioral data—elements that, if mishandled or exposed, can lead to discrimination, stigma, or identity theft (Cohen, I. G. and Mello, M. M, 2018).The growing use of cloud computing, mobile health applications, and telemedicine services further complicates the privacy landscape, exposing patient data to new vectors of risk.

Moreover, healthcare systems have become prime targets for cyberattacks, including ransomware and phishing attacks. The consequences of these breaches are far-reaching, affecting not only the confidentiality of patient information but also the availability and integrity of critical healthcare services (Kruse C. S et.al, 2017). Strengthening cybersecurity measures, following regulations like the Health Insurance Portability and Accountability Act (HIPAA), and fostering a culture of security awareness among healthcare personnel are essential to mitigating these risks.

There are now many chances to enhance clinical results, operational effectiveness, and patient care as a result of the digital transformation of healthcare systems. However, there are still urgent issues with data integrity, cybersecurity flaws, and patient privacy security that come with this progress. Despite continuous attempts, the literature now in publication frequently offers disjointed insights and lacks a cohesive strategy to address these interrelated problems, particularly when it comes to artificial intelligence and interoperability frameworks. This disparity emphasizes the necessity of a thorough conversation that not only exposes the risks but also investigates tactical solutions based on governance, ethics, and technological viewpoints. Thus, this chapter's main goal is to critically examine these issues and offer workable answers as well as proposals for the future that guarantee safe, moral, and patient-centered digital healthcare ecosystems.

BACKGROUND

Challenges of AI in Healthcare

Artificial intelligence (AI) is increasingly reshaping the landscape of healthcare, offering capabilities such as predictive analytics, image recognition, clinical decision support, and personalized treatment recommendations. Despite its transformative potential, the integration of AI into healthcare settings is fraught with numerous challenges that hinder its widespread adoption and effective utilization.

1. Data Quality and Availability

AI systems depend on large amounts of high-quality data to learn and make accurate predictions. However, healthcare data are often fragmented, incomplete, and inconsistently documented across institutions . The lack of standardized data formats and interoperability makes data aggregation and model training even more difficult (Jiang F et.al, 2017).

2. Bias and Fairness

AI models can unintentionally reinforce or magnify biases found in the training data. For example, if a dataset does not adequately represent certain demographic groups, the resulting model may perform poorly for those populations, which can lead to unfair outcomes (Powers B et.al,2019). To tackle bias, careful dataset selection, clear algorithms, and ongoing evaluation of model performance across various populations are necessary.

3. Interpretability and Trust

Many AI models, especially those based on deep learning, act like "black boxes." This makes their decision-making processes hard to understand. The lack of explainability can weaken trust among clinicians and patients. This poses a challenge for acceptance in critical settings where knowing the reasons behind decisions is crucial (Doshi-Velez F and Kim B,2017).

4. Regulatory and Ethical Concerns

Regulatory frameworks have not fully kept pace with the rapid development of AI technologies. Issues such as liability for errors, informed consent for AI-driven decisions, and compliance with data protection laws remain complex and unresolved (Gerke, S et.al, 2020). Ethical questions about autonomy, transparency, and accountability are central to the responsible deployment of AI in healthcare.

5. Integration into Clinical Workflows

Successfully implementing AI tools in clinical settings requires seamless integration into existing workflows. Many healthcare providers face challenges in aligning AI systems with real-world clinical processes, electronic health record systems, and time-constrained environments, often resulting in underuse or abandonment of AI tools (Topol E,2019).

6. Cybersecurity and Privacy

The use of AI increases the demand for data sharing and aggregation, potentially expanding the attack surface for cyber threats. Protecting patient data while enabling secure and compliant AI development is a critical challenge, particularly given the sensitive nature of health information and the rising incidence of healthcare data breaches (Jiang F et.al,2017).

Health Care Data Quality Issues and Metrics

Data, including big data for healthcare, is increasingly used by healthcare organizations to improve decision-making. However, it is important to ensure that the data used is of good quality to conduct reliable data analysis.

(i) Data Quality Issues in Healthcare

Healthcare data is inherently complex and subject to a variety of quality issues stemming from human, technical, and systemic factors. Common data quality challenges include:

a. **Incomplete Data**: Missing values in patient records (e.g., unrecorded vital signs or test results) can compromise diagnosis and treatment. For example, EHRs often lack essential contextual information such as patient-reported symptoms or social determinants of health (Weng and Weiskopf, 2013)..
b. **Inconsistent and Heterogeneous Data**: Variability in data entry formats and terminology across departments or institutions can result in semantic inconsistencies, making data aggregation and comparison difficult (Callahan T J et.al .2016).
c. **Incorrect or Inaccurate Data**: Errors can arise from manual data entry, faulty medical device readings, or incorrect coding (e.g., ICD codes), leading to flawed clinical insights.
d. **Redundant or Duplicate Records**: Duplicate entries, often caused by mismatched patient identifiers, can lead to confusion and inefficiencies in care delivery.
e. **Outdated Information**: Failure to update records regularly can result in reliance on obsolete or irrelevant information, potentially affecting treatment decisions.

(ii) Metrics for Assessing Data Quality

To systematically evaluate and improve data quality, various dimensions and metrics are employed. The following are commonly used in healthcare contexts:

a. **Completeness**: Measures whether all required data elements are present. For instance, a record missing a diagnosis or medication entry is considered incomplete.
b. **Accuracy**: Assesses whether data values correctly represent the real-world values they describe. This often involves cross-checking with source documents or expert validation.

c. **Consistency**: Evaluates whether data is coherent across multiple systems or datasets. For example, a patient's age should be consistent in both the lab system and the EHR.
d. **Timeliness**: Refers to the currency of data. Timely data is essential for clinical interventions, especially in emergency settings.
e. **Uniqueness**: Checks for duplicate records. High uniqueness ensures that each patient or event is only recorded once.
f. **Validity**: Assesses whether data values fall within acceptable ranges or formats (e.g., valid blood pressure values or date formats).
g. **Conformity**: Ensures data adheres to defined standards, formats, or coding systems (e.g., SNOMED CT, LOINC).

These metrics serve not only as diagnostic tools to identify quality issues but also as benchmarks to guide data governance and improvement initiatives (Kwon J and Johnson M. E, 2014)

DATA BREACHES AND PATIENT PRIVACY VIOLATIONS

In the healthcare sector, data breaches refer to incidents where Protected Health Information (PHI) is accessed, disclosed, lost, or stolen without proper authorization. These breaches pose serious risks to patient privacy and may lead to legal actions, financial loss, and damage to the reputations of both individuals and healthcare organizations. Over recent years, reports of major data breaches in healthcare have revealed recurring threats such as unauthorized access, data theft, improper data disposal, accidental loss, and sophisticated hacking incidents. As healthcare systems become increasingly digitized, the risk of such breaches continues to escalate.

Common Types of Data Breaches

1. Involves accessing or sharing patient data without proper legal authority or consent, often due to internal negligence or oversight.
2. Include breaches caused by external cyberattacks, such as malware, phishing schemes, or intrusion into network servers and electronic medical records.
3. Occurs when physical or digital health data is not securely destroyed, making it accessible to unauthorized individuals.
4. Refers to the loss of devices—like laptops, mobile phones, or external drives—that contain sensitive medical information.

5. Involves the physical theft of hardware containing patient data. In many cases, hackers use stolen data to infiltrate deeper into healthcare systems. (Almalawi, A., Khan et.al 2023).

Emerging Risk Factors

The adoption of BYOD practices in hospitals, where staff use personal devices to access institutional data, significantly increases security risks. Without stringent controls, these devices can become entry points for breaches.

Figure 1. Architecture diagram of protected health information

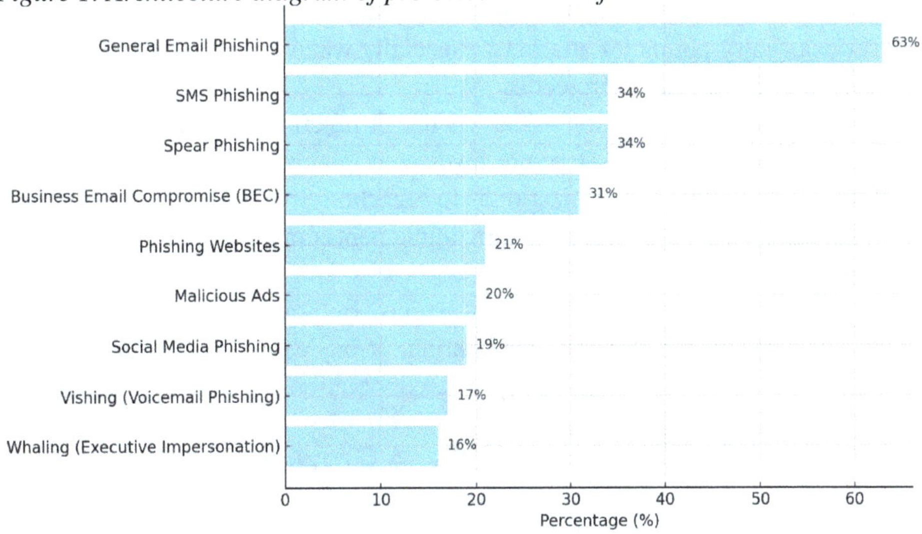

While cloud technology enhances data accessibility and collaboration, it also introduces security challenges if not properly configured. Organizations may mistakenly assume that regulatory compliance automatically ensures data security, when in fact, compliance without robust security protocols can still leave systems exposed to threats.

Facilitators of Data Breaches

Data breaches in healthcare are not always the result of direct attacks. Often, they are enabled—or made significantly worse—by internal weaknesses known as facilitators. These factors undermine the effectiveness of data protection efforts and increase an organization's susceptibility to cyber threats.

Key Facilitating Factors:

1. Many breaches stem from the failure to follow established health information security policies and regulations. Noncompliance—whether due to negligence or lack of enforcement—creates gaps that can be exploited.
2. A limited understanding among healthcare personnel regarding data security practices poses a major risk. Employees unaware of potential threats or safe data handling procedures may inadvertently expose sensitive information.
3. External applications or services, such as mobile health apps or outsourced vendors, often lack robust privacy-by-design features. These weak links can serve as entry points for attackers, especially when not subjected to stringent vetting and integration protocols.
4. Factors such as the facility's size, whether it functions as a teaching hospital, and the level of IT infrastructure investment play a role in determining how resilient a healthcare organization is to breaches. Smaller institutions or those with limited resources may struggle to implement comprehensive data protection systems.
5. In many cases, data breaches are worsened by poor institutional responses. Delays in detection, lack of coordination, or inadequate mitigation strategies can lead to extended damage and repeated violations.

Healthcare Data Breaches in India: A Growing Concern

In recent years, India has faced a series of significant healthcare data breaches that have exposed critical vulnerabilities within its digital health infrastructure. Among the most alarming incidents was the ransomware attack on the All-India Institute of Medical Sciences (AIIMS), New Delhi, in November 2022. This cyberattacks severely disrupted hospital operations for nearly two weeks, affecting outpatient services, diagnostics, and billing systems. Reports indicated that attackers gained access to sensitive medical records of millions of patients, with parts of the stolen data allegedly put up for sale on the dark web. This breach at India's premier medical institution starkly highlighted the urgent need to strengthen cybersecurity measures and data protection protocols across public healthcare systems. In October 2023, another major breach emerged involving the Indian Council of Medical Research (ICMR). Hackers reportedly offered personal and health-related information of over 815 million Indians on the dark web, including names, Aadhaar numbers, phone numbers, and COVID-19 test results. This incident stands as one of the largest healthcare data breaches worldwide, underscoring the massive scale of risk faced by India's health data ecosystem.

Earlier breaches, such as the 2021 data exposure at Safdarjung Hospital—where patient information was accessible online without any authentication. HealthifyMe breach affecting users of the popular health and fitness app, further reveal systemic weaknesses in health data governance and digital security frameworks. Collectively, these breaches emphasize the critical necessity for robust enforcement of the Digital Personal Data Protection Act, 2023, alongside sector-specific safeguards tailored to the healthcare domain. Protecting patient privacy and securing sensitive medical information must be a top priority to build trust and resilience within India's rapidly digitizing healthcare landscape.

Managing a Healthcare Data Breach: A Comprehensive Guide

A healthcare data breach is more than just a technical failure—it's a profound violation of patient trust and privacy, with serious legal, ethical, and operational repercussions. Such incidents can lead to regulatory penalties, loss of patient confidence, and long-term damage to an organization's reputation. While prevention is the ultimate goal, no system is completely immune to breaches. When a breach occurs, the way an organization responds can make all the difference in minimizing harm and restoring trust. A well-structured, transparent, and timely response is essential to manage the crisis effectively.

Steps for Containment and Mitigation

Swift and decisive action is critical the moment a breach is detected. The longer unauthorized access goes unchecked, the greater the potential damage.

1. The first priority is to determine the extent and source of the breach. Privacy and IT teams must work closely to pinpoint affected systems or databases and immediately isolate them to prevent further unauthorized data access or exfiltration (Ibrahim et.al, 2024).
2. Once contained, the breach must be reported internally to IT, compliance, and legal departments to mobilize appropriate resources. Depending on jurisdiction and severity, organizations are also legally obligated to inform regulatory bodies promptly, adhering to timelines mandated by laws such as the Digital Personal Data Protection Act, 2023.
3. Patients whose data has been compromised deserve clear and honest communication. Inform them about what specific information was exposed, the potential risks, and the concrete steps they can take to protect themselves (e.g., monitoring

accounts, changing passwords, or enrolling in identity theft protection services). This openness helps maintain some degree of trust even amid a difficult situation.

4. Parallel to containment, IT teams must identify and patch the security gaps that allowed the breach to occur. This may include applying software patches, updating firewalls, enhancing encryption, or revising access controls.

AI Specific Privacy Risk

AI presents distinct privacy issues that conventional systems do not, despite the fact that it provides strong tools for personalized medicine and predictive analytics (Muniasamy, A et al., 2026; Gauthaman et al., 2026; Rengaramanujam et al., 2026) Inference attacks, in which trained artificial intelligence models can be used to recreate sensitive data, are among the most urgent issues. Even when anonymized, methods like membership inference and model inversion can show if a patient's data was used to rebuild characteristics like genetic details or to train a model.

The opaqueness surrounding the use of patient data to train AI systems is another problem. It's possible that patients are unaware of the entire scope of algorithmic decision-making, data exchange, and reuse. For instance, without specific patient authorization, a deep learning algorithm trained on imaging data may have accessed thousands of images, thereby violating privacy regulations such as GDPR or HIPAA. In order to protect patient data throughout the AI pipeline, these dangers require the development of privacy-preserving AI approaches including federated learning, differential privacy, and homomorphic encryption.

Interoperability Challenges in Smart Healthcare

The absence of interoperability between various healthcare systems of information is a significant obstacle to attaining seamless healthcare delivery. Data silos that impede continuity of treatment are created by the majority of Electronic Health Records (EHRs) using disparate data formats, coding systems (such as ICD and SNOMED), and communication protocols. Although the goal of standards like HL7 FHIR is to facilitate data sharing between systems, different providers have not adopted them uniformly. For example, a patient who receives care at several hospitals might have disjointed medical records, which could result in repeated testing and postponed treatment decisions. Governments and health IT developers need to make investments in national interoperability frameworks, middleware, and open standards to solve this. Integrated national medical records can dramatically lower costs and enhance patient outcomes, as demonstrated by case studies from nations like Estonia and Denmark.

Post-Breach Investigation and Recovery

Containment is only the first phase. The aftermath of a breach demands a deep dive to understand root causes and implement lasting solutions.

1. Organizations should launch a detailed forensic analysis to understand exactly how the breach happened—whether through malware, phishing, insider threat, or system flaws. Equally important is assessing internal policies, employee practices, and security protocols that may have contributed to the incident.
2. Based on investigation findings, revise existing data governance frameworks. This includes tightening user access rights, enhancing encryption standards, implementing multi-factor authentication, and regularly updating incident response plans. Privacy policies should be updated to reflect current risks and compliance requirements.
3. Human error is often a critical factor in breaches. Continuous education and training programs focused on cybersecurity hygiene, data privacy regulations, and phishing prevention empower employees to act as the first line of defence.
4. Trust is fragile but not irreparable. Demonstrating accountability by openly sharing what went wrong and the concrete measures taken to prevent recurrence fosters transparency. Proactively engaging with patients and stakeholders through regular updates and reassurances about enhanced security helps restore confidence in the organization's commitment to safeguarding their sensitive information.

GUARDING PATIENT DATA PRIVACY

In healthcare, data privacy refers to the policies, procedures, and technologies designed to protect sensitive patient information from unauthorized access while empowering patients with control over how their data is collected, used, and shared. The goal is to maintain the confidentiality of personal and medical information, fostering trust and confidence between patients and healthcare providers.

Ensuring robust data privacy requires a proactive, multi-layered approach. Given the complex regulatory landscape and rising concerns over patient consent, healthcare organizations must adopt comprehensive strategies that not only comply with legal standards but also promote transparency and patient empowerment.

Implementing Strong Data Privacy Measures

To safeguard patient privacy effectively, healthcare providers should focus on the following core strategies:

1. Organizations should collect only the minimum necessary information required for medical care and administrative functions. Where possible, data should be anonymized or de-identified before sharing or processing, reducing the risk of patient identification if data is exposed or transferred.
2. Central to data privacy is ensuring patients retain control over their information. Explicit and informed consent must be obtained before collecting or sharing any patient data. Clear, accessible privacy policies should explain how data is used, and patients should have the ability to modify or revoke their consent at any time, reinforcing transparency and trust (Keshta, I., and Odeh, A.2021).
3. Patient information must be stored securely, with authorization ensuring that only authorized person can allow to access sensitive data. Role-based permissions, multi-factor authentication, and encryption are essential tools to prevent unauthorized exposure.
4. Adhering to established data privacy regulations is crucial—not only as a legal obligation but also as a foundation for maintaining patient trust and improving healthcare outcomes.
5. Routine internal or third-party audits of data privacy practices help identify vulnerabilities and compliance gaps. Audits enable organizations to continuously refine their policies and strengthen data security.
6. Human error is one of the cause of data breaches. Regular training ensures that all healthcare staff are aware of privacy best practices, potential security threats, and the proper handling of patient information. Ongoing education builds a culture of vigilance and responsibility.
7. Healthcare providers must establish clear guidelines on how long patient data is retained, balancing clinical needs with privacy concerns. When data is no longer necessary, secure disposal protocols must be followed to prevent unauthorized recovery or misuse. This practice is a vital component of both HIPAA and GDPR compliance.
8. Healthcare organizations must also navigate a complex and evolving regulatory environment. Globally recognized frameworks like HIPAA in the United States and the GDPR in the European Union set high standards for healthcare data privacy. However, these laws do not apply directly in India.

In the Indian context, healthcare data privacy is primarily governed by a mix of general data protection laws and sector-specific guidelines. The Information

Technology (Reasonable Security Practices and Procedures and Sensitive Personal Data or Information) Rules established under the Information Technology Act, 2000, classify medical records and health information as "sensitive personal data," requiring informed consent for their collection, disclosure, and transfer.

More recently, the Digital Personal Data Protection Act, 2023, was enacted to strengthen India's data protection regime. While it does not explicitly create a separate category for health data, the law emphasizes consent-based processing, purpose limitation, and the rights of individuals (data principals) over their personal data.

Additionally, the Ayushman Bharat Digital Mission (ABDM)—formerly the National Digital Health Mission (NDHM)—is pioneering a federated digital health infrastructure designed around consent-driven data sharing and security, reflecting global best practices while addressing India's unique healthcare challenges.

Given the complexity and rapid evolution of data privacy regulations, healthcare organizations in India must regularly review and update their policies and systems to remain fully compliant and protect patient rights effectively.

CYBERSECURITY THREATS AND RISK MANAGEMENT

In today's digital age, cybersecurity has become a cornerstone of healthcare operations. The increasing dependence on electronic health records, connected medical devices, and cloud-based platforms has expanded the attack surface—making healthcare institutions prime targets for cybercriminals. Cybersecurity threats in this sector are aimed at disrupting operations, stealing sensitive data, and exploiting vulnerabilities for financial gain or malicious intent.

These threats can originate from various sources, including external hackers, internal actors, untrained employees, or even outdated infrastructure. Once inside a system, cybercriminals can lock down operations, exfiltrate data, or demand hefty ransoms. Because healthcare data is both highly sensitive and immensely valuable, it is frequently used for identity theft, insurance fraud, and financial crimes. Cybercriminals exploit the urgency and critical nature of healthcare, knowing that many organizations will pay large sums to recover data and restore essential services.

Major Cybersecurity Threats in Healthcare

Some of the most pressing cybersecurity risks in healthcare today include:

1. Phishing Attacks: It is a type of cyber attacks where hackers reveals information sucha s passwords or personal data.

2. Ransomware: Malicious software that locks critical systems or encrypts data until a ransom is paid.
3. Data Breaches: Unauthorized access to patient records and sensitive data, often due to weak access controls.
4. Inadequate Data Encryption: Poor encryption practices leave data vulnerable during storage or transmission.
5. Distributed Denial of Service (DDoS) Attacks: Overwhelming a network or server with traffic, disrupting patient care and administrative functions.
6. Legacy Systems and Outdated Software: Unsupported systems lack the necessary updates and patches, making them easy targets.
7. Insider Threats: Breaches caused intentionally or unintentionally by employees or trusted users within the organization.

The Importance of Cybersecurity in Healthcare

In response to cyber threats grow more complicated and pervasive, healthcare institutions must prioritize robust cybersecurity strategies. The consequences of an attack can devastate—not only financially but also in terms of patient safety, legal liability, and public trust. A single breach can cripple operations, expose thousands of patient records, and result in substantial regulatory penalties.

A strong cybersecurity posture begins with proactive planning and coordinated risk management. This includes:

1. Enforcing Data Protection and Access Controls: Limited access to authorized users using role-based permissions and authentication mechanisms.
2. Conducting Regular Security Awareness Training: Educating staff on how to identify phishing attempts, handle data responsibly, and follow security protocols.
3. Strengthening Regulatory Compliance: Aligning cybersecurity practices with HIPAA and other relevant regulations to avoid compliance violations.
4. Upgrading and Patching Systems: Ensuring all systems, devices, and software are updated regularly to eliminate known vulnerabilities.

Cybersecurity must be embedded into every layer of the healthcare infrastructure—from remote access policies and mobile device management to application development and cloud usage. Adopting a prevention-first mentality supports organizations to stay ahead of potential threats and maintain operational resilience. Given the complexity of modern healthcare ecosystems—spanning legacy systems, mobile devices, remote work environments, and cloud platforms—implementing effective cybersecurity solutions can be a daunting task. This is where expert partners, such as Atlas Systems, can provide essential support. With experience in integrating top-tier data security solutions, partners like Atlas Systems enable healthcare institutions to focus on delivering exceptional care, while ensuring that their digital infrastructure remains safe, compliant, and resilient. Safety, compliance, and confidence in defending against ever-changing threats can be achieved through collaboration with cybersecurity experts.

Figure 2. Prevalence of phishing attack types

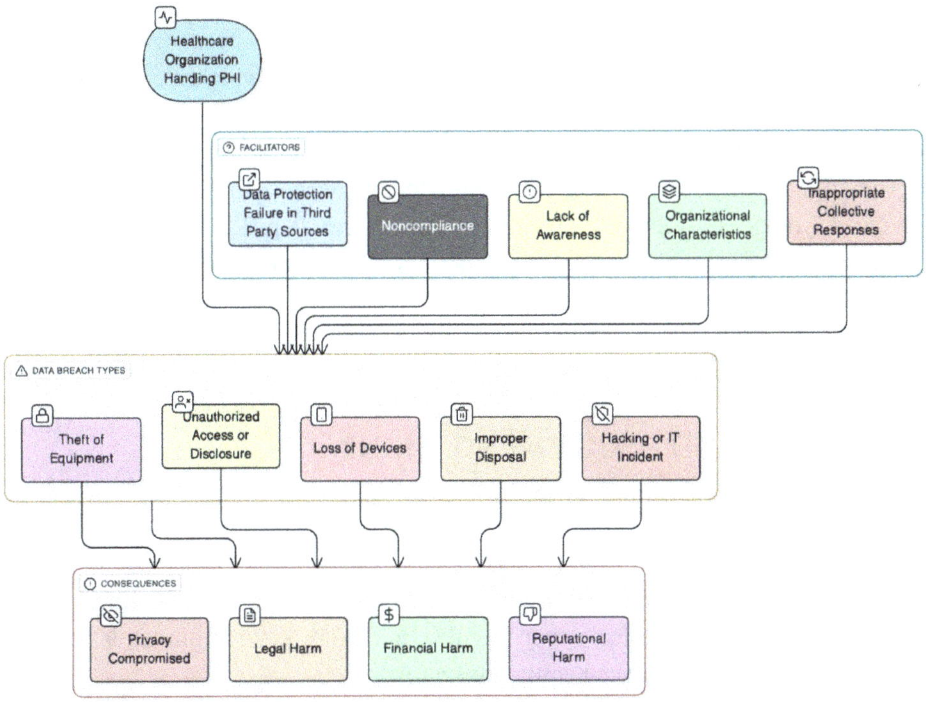

Common Threats to Data Security in Healthcare

As healthcare systems become increasingly digital, the security of sensitive patient data faces growing threats. These threats originate from both internal and external sources, ranging from cybercriminals and malicious insiders to untrained staff and vulnerable technologies. The first step is to understand the threats and developing an effective defence mechanism.

1. Phishing scams remain the most frequent cyber threat in healthcare, responsible for over 90% of attacks. Attackers impersonate legitimate entities to trick pro-

fessionals into clicking malicious links or sharing sensitive information, often resulting in credential theft or financial fraud.

2. Ransomware locks healthcare data and systems, rendering them inaccessible until a ransom is paid. The impact is severe—interrupting patient services and causing financial strain.
3. This type of malicious software can steal, destroy, or modify data and grant unauthorized access to attackers. With over 1 billion malware variants circulating globally, robust healthcare data security solutions are essential.
4. Third-party vendors with inadequate security protocols pose significant risks.
5. Unauthorized access to sensitive patient information—whether caused by weak controls, software vulnerabilities, or insider threats—continues to rise.
6. Although less prevalent than other threats, DDoS attacks flood systems with traffic, causing service disruptions and delaying access to vital patient records.
7. IoMT devices—such as wearable monitors, smart pill dispensers, and connected surgical tools—improve patient care but introduce new vulnerabilities. These devices often lack robust security protocols, increasing the potential for cyberattacks.

SOLUTIONS AND RECOMMENDATIONS

Recommendations for Risk Management

A proactive and layered cybersecurity strategy is essential for healthcare organizations to combat evolving cyber threats. Below are key recommendations and best practices tailored for the healthcare sector:

- Invest in Healthcare Cybersecurity Software

Deploy advanced attack surface monitoring tools to detect vulnerabilities and potential threats. Ensure the software extends coverage to third-party networks and vendors, integrating patient safety with cybersecurity to ensure the continuous delivery of high-quality care.

- Conduct Employee Cybersecurity Training

Educate staff on recognizing phishing emails, using strong authentication practices, and reporting suspicious activity. Emphasize simple but critical checks—such as verifying URLs and domain names—to prevent common threats. Regular simulation exercises can reinforce training.

- Apply Security Patches and Updates

Outdated software is a common entry point for attackers. Organizations must install the latest security patches promptly and enforce strong authentication protocols. Routine system audits can help ensure that no patch or vulnerability is overlooked.

- Implement Robust Data Encryption

Encrypting sensitive information—such as patient records and financial data—ensures it remains unreadable even if accessed by unauthorized parties. Asymmetric encryption (utilizing different keys for sender and recipient) offers enhanced security for high-risk data transmissions.

- Ensure Compliance with Health Data Protection Laws

Compliance with national and international privacy regulations (e.g., HIPAA, GDPR, DISHA) reinforces institutional credibility and reduces liability. It also fosters trust among patients, partners, and regulatory bodies.

- Adopt Comprehensive Risk Management Frameworks

Implementing industry-recognized frameworks, CERT-In guidelines, and sector-specific best practices—enables healthcare organizations to standardize processes, manage risks systematically, and stay resilient in the face of emerging threats.

- Minimize Supply Chain Vulnerabilities

Healthcare providers must rigorously assess third-party vendors during procurement, ensuring adherence to baseline security standards through legally binding service-level agreements (SLAs). Ongoing vendor monitoring and security assessments help mitigate downstream risks across the supply chain.

DATA QUALITY TOOLS IN HEALTHCARE

Diverse standards and diverse sources face challenges for storing data in healthcare sector. Privacy and security concerns are critical, and data quality is essential. Numerous data quality tools are available to ensure the quality of data. A physician can easily identify and work appropriate for the community by using such analytics tools (Evidence.care (n.d), 2020). Different measurement methods were used for data quality assessment. There is no specific tool for the quality assessment. It varies according to the application. A few tools are listed below:

- *CareGauge:* It is a clinical decision support system tool. It empowers physicians to take better decisions and easily track and respond to the updated situation.
- *Health Catalyst:* A decision supporting system for health analytics and simplifying complex healthcare data management system.
- *Oracle Healthcare Foundation*: It gives integrated patient solutions, with a cloud-based approach for scalability, flexibility, and security, particularly strong in predictive analytics.
- *Clarify Health:* An enterprise analytics platform that empowers healthcare organizations to make data-driven decisions and achieve value-based care goals.
- *Arcadia Analytics:* Expertise in value-based care, risk stratification, and patient management through data aggregation from EHRs, claims, and social determinants of health.
- *Innovaccer:* Provides an AI-driven Data Activation Platform for population health management, patient engagement, and risk adjustment with a reputation for real-time *healthcare data integration.*
- *CitiusTech:* Emphasizes regulatory compliance and AI-driven healthcare analytics for operational, clinical, and administrative use, with a focus on data silo demolition.
- *IBM Watson Health:* Draws on AI and analytics for a range of healthcare use cases, such as clinical decision support and enhancing operational efficiencies.
- *Optum Analytics:* A leader in healthcare data solutions with a broad portfolio of analytics services for payers and providers.
- *McKesson:* Offers data-driven solutions covering all the way across pharmaceutical supply chain management, analytics, and care delivery (Naim, A., et al. 2026).
- *MedeAnalytics, Inc.:* Delivers real-time insights for faster, more informed decisions by tracking key metrics across clinical, financial, and operational areas.

FUTURE RESEARCH DIRECTIONS

Every industry struggles to avoid security threats while handling sensitive information. In healthcare sector, protecting patient data is a major concern. Each measures works differently in different scenario (GarillColes et al., 2010). To avoid such a problem we must follow certain proactive measures. Some of the few are listed below:

- *Security*: A proactive approach is necessary to reduce risks, defend against cyber threats and maintain patients trust. The following measures are used for ensuring healthcare security.
- *Continuous Risk Assessments:* Continuous Risk Assessments in healthcare represent a continuous, dynamic process of ongoing identification, analysis, evaluation, and ranking of security threats to Protected Health Information (PHI) and key healthcare systems.
- *Cybersecurity Measures:*To protect patients data cybersecurity measures play an important role. It includes providing access control, encrypting data and train staff.
- *Staff Training and Awareness:* To maintain a good healthcare system, we must train the staff members about the importance of the safety measures of patient data.
- *Physical Security Measures*: Physical security measures include surveillance systems, authorized access points, storage for sensitive documents and equipment. It enhances real time monitoring effectively.
- *Rapid Incident Response and Disaster Recovery:* Advanced technologies, such as biometric verification and intelligent video analytics enhances the physical safeguards and provide real-time monitoring and rapid incident detection.
- *Meeting Regulatory Requirements:* It is a continuous and dynamic process that demands integrated solutions to the best practices.
- *Threat Intelligence:* It enables early detection of threats and allows for taking timely prevention measures (Marsha R et al,2021).

CONCLUSION

In modern healthcare system, advanced technologies are used and it faces lots of challenges such as data quality metrics, patient data privacy, cybersecurity issues. This research critically analysed the significant of using modern technologies like artificial intelligence. This paper also underscored the upholding of patient data privacy. Also the use of data quality tools in healthcare plays a vital role. By prioritizing data quality, cybersecurity issues, patient privacy, healthcare system can bind the transformative potential of modern technology while safeguarding the highest standards of trust, safety and patient care. Important issues with cybersecurity, patient privacy, and data quality have been discussed in this chapter. In addition to recognizing these problems, it has investigated the ramifications of dangers unique to AI, interoperability concerns, and actual intrusions. The main contribution consists in offering a thorough framework for comprehending these dangers via governance, ethical, and technical perspectives, backed by actual cases and international case studies. Stakeholders must make the following investments to ensure the ethical and successful digital future of healthcare: AI design that protects privacy, systems for federated interoperability, strict data governance, and an innovative culture that prioritizes security. The practical implication is obvious: healthcare institutions can only fully benefit from digital innovation while safeguarding the people they serve by using proactive, standardized, and patient-centered approaches.

The important issues facing contemporary healthcare were thoroughly covered in this chapter, with particular attention paid to data quality, cybersecurity, patient privacy, and the incorporation of cutting-edge technologies like artificial intelligence. In addition to outlining existing constraints, the conversation focused on threats unique to AI, actual occurrences, and interoperability issues that require immediate attention. With the help of pertinent case studies, a well-organized framework was provided from the viewpoints of ethics, technology, and government. Adopting privacy-preserving AI designs, enforcing stringent data governance, enabling federated interoperability, and cultivating a proactive security culture are all crucial to creating a safe and moral future for digital healthcare. In order to ensure that innovation and safety advance together, future efforts must also concentrate on creating strong risk control systems and addressing changing threats with flexible and patient-centered approaches.

REFERENCES

Almalawi, A., Khan, A. I., Alsolami, F., Abushark, Y. B., & Alfakeeh, A. S. (2023). Managing security of healthcare data for a modern healthcare system. *Sensors (Basel), 23*(7), 3612. DOI: 10.3390/s23073612 PMID: 37050672

Callahan, T. J., Kahn, M. G., Barnard, J., Bauck, A. E., Brown, J., Davidson, B. N., ... & Meeker, D. (2016). A harmonized data quality assessment terminology and framework for the secondary use of electronic health record data. eGEMs (Generating Evidence & Methods to improve patient outcomes), 4(1), 18. DOI: 10.13063/2327-9214.1244

Cohen, I. G., & Mello, M. M. (2018). HIPAA and protecting health information in the 21st century. *Journal of the American Medical Association, 320*(3), 231–232. DOI: 10.1001/jama.2018.5630 PMID: 29800120

Doshi-Velez, F., & Kim, B. (2017). Towards a rigorous science of interpretable machine learning. arXiv preprint arXiv:1702.08608. https://doi.org//arXiv.1702 .08608DOI: 10.48550

Evidence.care(n.d).About the top health care analytics tools Retrieved June 6, 2020 https://evidence.care/top-healthcare-analytics-tools

GarillColes et al. (2010). Three kinds of proactive risk analyses for health care. The Joint Commission Journal on Quality and Patient Safety, 36(8), 365–375, AP1–AP3.

Gauthaman, S. A.. (2026). Introduction to machine learning and optimization in healthcare. In Muniasamy, A. (Ed.), *Integrative machine learning and optimization algorithms for disease prediction* (pp. 1–34). IGI Global., DOI: 10.4018/979-8-3373-1087-9.ch001

Gerke, S., Minssen, T., & Cohen, I. G. (2020). Ethical and legal challenges of artificial intelligence-driven healthcare. In *Artificial intelligence in healthcare* (pp. 295–336). Academic Press., DOI: 10.1016/B978-0-12-818438-7.00012-5

Ibrahim, A. M., Abdel-Aziz, H. R., Mohamed, H. A. H., Zaghamir, D. E. F., Wahba, N. M. I., Hassan, G. A., Shaban, M., EL-Nablaway, M., Aldughmi, O. N., & Aboelola, T. H. (2024). Balancing confidentiality and care coordination: Challenges in patient privacy. *BMC Nursing, 23*(1), 564. DOI: 10.1186/s12912-024-02231-1 PMID: 39148055

Jiang, F., Jiang, Y., Zhi, H., Dong, Y., Li, H., Ma, S., Wang, Y., Dong, Q., Shen, H., & Wang, Y. (2017). Artificial intelligence in healthcare: Past, present and future. *Stroke and Vascular Neurology*, *2*(4), 230–243. DOI: 10.1136/svn-2017-000101 PMID: 29507784

Keshta, I., & Odeh, A. (2021). Security and privacy of electronic health records: Concerns and challenges. *Egyptian Informatics Journal*, *22*(2), 177–183. DOI: 10.1016/j.eij.2020.07.003

Kruse, C. S., Frederick, B., Jacobson, T., & Monticone, D. K. (2017). Cybersecurity in healthcare: A systematic review of modern threats and trends. *Technology and Health Care*, *25*(1), 1–10. DOI: 10.3233/THC-161263 PMID: 27689562

Kwon, J., & Johnson, M. E. (2014). Proactive Versus Reactive Security Investments in the Healthcare Sector. *Management Information Systems Quarterly*, *38*(2), 451–472. DOI: 10.25300/MISQ/2014/38.2.06

Marsha, R., (2021). Proactive Measures to Mitigate Cyber Security Challenges in IoT based Smart Healthcare Networks. 2021 IEEE International IOT, *Electronics and Mechatronics Conference (IEMTRONICS)*. https://doi.org/DOI: 10.1109/IEMTRONICS52119.2021

Muniasamy, A., & Karunakaran, G. (2026). Challenges and future directions: Emerging trends and limitations in ML and optimization for healthcare. In Muniasamy, A. (Ed.), *Integrative machine learning and optimization algorithms for disease prediction* (pp. 339–368). IGI Global., DOI: 10.4018/979-8-3373-1087-9.ch012

Naim, A., (2026). AI-driven smart manufacturing and automation in pharmaceutical production. In Muniasamy, A., & Karunakaran, G. (Eds.), *Applications of artificial intelligence in pharmaceuticals* (pp. 157–194). IGI Global., DOI: 10.4018/979-8-3373-2043-4.ch006

Powers, B., Obermeyer, Z., Vogeli, C., & Mullainathan, S. (2019). Dissecting racial bias in an algorithm used to manage the health of populations. *Science*, *366*(6464), 447–453. DOI: 10.1126/science.aax2342 PMID: 31649194

Rengaramanujam, K., & Muniasamy, A. (2026). AI in hospital administration and formulary design: Optimizing resource allocation and patient flow. In Muniasamy, A., & Karunakaran, G. (Eds.), *Applications of artificial intelligence in pharmaceuticals* (pp. 215–246). IGI Global., DOI: 10.4018/979-8-3373-2043-4.ch008

Topol, E. (2019). *Deep medicine: How artificial intelligence can make healthcare human again*. Basic Books.

Weng, C., & Weiskopf, N. G. (2013). Methods and dimensions of electronic health record data quality assessment: Enabling reuse for clinical research. *Journal of the American Medical Informatics Association : JAMIA*, *20*(1), 144–151. DOI: 10.1136/amiajnl-2011-000681 PMID: 22733976

ADDITIONAL READING

Layode, O., Naiho, H. N. N., Adeleke, G. S., Udeh, E. O., & Labake, T. T. (2024). Data privacy and security challenges in environmental research: Approaches to safeguarding sensitive information. *International Journal of Applied Research in Social Sciences*, *6*(6), 1193–1214. DOI: 10.51594/ijarss.v6i6.1210

Panahi, O. (2025). Navigating the AI Landscape in Healthcare and Public Health. *Mathews J Nurs*, *7*(1), 56. DOI: 10.30654/MJNH.100056

Zarour, M., Alenezi, M., Ansari, M. T. J., Pandey, A. K., Ahmad, M., Agrawal, A., Kumar, R., & Khan, R. A. (2021). Ensuring data integrity of healthcare information in the era of digital health. *Healthcare Technology Letters*, *8*(3), 66–77. DOI: 10.1049/htl2.12008 PMID: 34035927

Esmaeilzadeh, P. (2024). Challenges and strategies for wide-scale artificial intelligence (AI) deployment in healthcare practices: A perspective for healthcare organizations. *Artificial Intelligence in Medicine*, *151*, 102861.

Chen, Y., & Esmaeilzadeh, P. (2024). Generative AI in medical practice: In-depth exploration of privacy and security challenges. *Journal of Medical Internet Research*, *26*, e53008.

Bavli, I., Ho, A., Mahal, R., & McKeown, M. J. (2025). Ethical concerns around privacy and data security in AI health monitoring for Parkinson's disease: Insights from patients, family members, and healthcare professionals. *AI & Society*, *40*(1), 155–165.

KEY TERMS AND DEFINITIONS

Cyber Threats: Potential malicious activities targeting digital systems to cause harm or disruption.

Data Breaches: Unauthorized access to confidential data, leading to loss or exposure of information.

Data Quality Tools: Software solutions designed to ensure accuracy, consistency, and reliability of data.

Electronic Health Records: Digital versions of patients' medical histories maintained for healthcare delivery.

Measurement Methods: Techniques or approaches used to evaluate performance, outcomes, or processes.

Proactive Measures: Preventive actions taken in advance to reduce risks or potential problems.

Risk Management: The process of identifying, assessing, and mitigating potential threats to systems or operations.

Chapter 5
Long-Term Monitoring and Performance Evaluation of AI Systems

Dhanalakshmi Jaganathan
https://orcid.org/0000-0002-3919-4469
SRM Institute of Science and Technology, India

Prabhu Chakkaravarthy
https://orcid.org/0009-0000-3180-8051
SRM Institute of Science and Technology, India

ABSTRACT

With AI increasingly used in healthcare, finance, and autonomous systems, ongoing monitoring is vital to ensure performance, fairness, and ethical compliance. Long-term oversight helps control risks, improve systems, and maintain trust. Monitoring frameworks detect issues like model drift, bias, or degradation caused by data shifts, user behavior, or environmental changes—prompting regular retraining. Beyond accuracy, key metrics include fairness, transparency, robustness, efficiency, and compliance. Explainability ensures stakeholders understand AI decisions, while robustness testing checks performance under varied inputs. AI observability tools with logging and analytics detect abnormal behavior early. Human oversight complements automated systems to catch subtle issues and ensure social responsibility. Monitoring many complex AIs remains a challenge, demanding better tools for transparency and adaptation. Regular testing, human involvement, and governance ensure AI stays effective, ethical, and lawful. These practices support responsible AI development and foster user trust.

DOI: 10.4018/979-8-3373-2787-7.ch005

INTRODUCTION

Importance of Long-Term AI Monitoring

A significant number of industries—such as healthcare, finance, and autonomous systems—are increasingly dependent on artificial intelligence (AI) systems to manage critical operations, deliver insights, and automate complex decision-making tasks (Amershi et al., 2019). However, the deployment of an AI model is not the end of the development lifecycle. Rather, it marks the beginning of an ongoing journey requiring persistent monitoring and performance evaluation to ensure that these systems remain accurate, fair, and trustworthy over time (Sculley et al., 2015).

Long-term monitoring is essential because AI models do not operate in static environments. Real-world data distributions, user behaviors, and external conditions continuously shift, sometimes in subtle ways that may not be immediately apparent. Over time, these changes can lead to issues such as model drift, where the AI's predictions become less reliable or even biased as the input data evolves away from the data it was originally trained on (Gama et al., 2014). Early detection of such gradual problems—like emerging biases, declining accuracy, or shifts in user interaction patterns—enables organizations to intervene before these issues severely impact outcomes.

Persistent oversight also plays a crucial role in addressing evolving ethical, regulatory, and societal expectations. As AI becomes more integrated into decision-making processes that affect individuals and communities, stakeholders—including end users, regulators, and advocacy groups—demand transparency in how these systems function. Monitoring frameworks that include explainability features make it possible to trace, justify, and audit the decisions made by AI, which is vital to maintaining public confidence (Mitchell et al., 2019).

Moreover, long-term monitoring supports continuous improvement through retraining and adaptation. When performance evaluations reveal that a model's effectiveness is waning—whether due to changing data patterns, new regulatory requirements, or shifts in business objectives—organizations can proactively update the model. This process helps prevent the AI from becoming obsolete or producing unintended negative consequences, such as perpetuating outdated biases or making unsafe recommendations (Chen et al., 2020).

Trust in AI systems is fundamentally linked to their ability to operate reliably and fairly. Continuous monitoring reassures users and regulatory bodies that AI is not producing harmful, discriminatory, or erroneous outcomes. For instance, in applications like healthcare, a lapse in model accuracy or fairness could result in misdiagnosis or unequal treatment, while in finance, it could lead to unjust loan decisions. Therefore, robust monitoring practices are not merely technical safeguards but are essential elements of ethical AI governance, ensuring that AI technologies serve the broader interests of society responsibly (Barocas et al., 2019; Holstein et al., 2019; Varshney, 2016; Microsoft Responsible AI, 2023).

In summary, long-term AI monitoring is a multifaceted process involving technical, ethical, and organizational components. It enables the early detection of issues, facilitates regulatory compliance, ensures continual alignment with stakeholder values, and ultimately sustains trust in AI-driven solutions. By making ongoing evaluation a foundational part of AI deployment, organizations can support responsible innovation that adapts gracefully to changing environments and societal needs.

Challenges in Sustained AI Performance Assessment

Although the importance of long-term AI monitoring is clear, implementing and sustaining such practices is fraught with numerous, multi-dimensional challenges. One of the primary obstacles lies in the ever-shifting landscape of user behaviors, external conditions, and data inputs that can fundamentally alter the context in which AI systems operate. This phenomenon—often referred to as "concept drift"—occurs when the statistical properties of the model's input data change over time, resulting in a gradual decline in predictive performance (Gama et al., 2014). Detecting and correcting for concept drift is not a trivial task; it demands the deployment of advanced monitoring software and specialized tools capable of performing continuous data inspections and real-time model evaluations (Michelmore & Hoi, 2020).

To address concept drift, organizations must implement mechanisms that can identify both abrupt and subtle shifts in data distribution. This may involve deploying statistical tests—such as the Kolmogorov-Smirnov test or population stability index—to monitor changes in feature distributions. Additionally, leveraging machine learning-based drift detectors allows for the identification of complex, non-linear changes that may otherwise go unnoticed. The process is further complicated by the fact that not all drift is detrimental; sometimes, changes in data may reflect new, relevant trends that the model should adapt to rather than avoid.

Beyond the technical challenge of drift detection, maintaining fairness and preventing the emergence or amplification of bias within AI systems is a persistent concern. As data distributions evolve, models risk developing biased patterns that disadvantage particular demographic groups (Feldman et al., 2015; Jha et al., 2020). These biases may stem from imbalances in the training data, changes in user behavior, or the introduction of new, unanticipated variables. Monitoring fairness therefore requires the implementation of robust bias detection frameworks that utilize fairness metrics such as demographic parity, equal opportunity, and disparate impact ratio (IBM Research, 2020). These metrics must be calculated and reviewed on a continual basis, ensuring that any deviation from equitable treatment is flagged early for remediation.

The challenge does not end with detection; addressing bias often requires a combination of strategies, from rebalancing datasets and augmenting underrepresented groups to redesigning features and retraining models. Additionally, what constitutes fairness can vary widely across industries and contexts, necessitating a flexible, context-sensitive approach to bias assessment and mitigation (Holstein et al., 2019). Stakeholder engagement becomes crucial here, as definitions of equity are often shaped by social, ethical, and regulatory expectations.

Another critical dimension is the resilience and reliability of AI models in the face of adversarial or unexpected inputs. In practical applications, models may encounter out-of-distribution data, adversarial attacks, or rare edge cases that were not present in the training data. Ensuring robustness against these challenges requires rigorous testing, the creation of synthetic datasets for stress-testing, and the implementation of security controls designed to detect and mitigate malicious manipulation (D-Agostino & Vazquez, 2021). Robust monitoring systems must flag anomalies, outliers, or suspicious behaviors promptly, enabling rapid response before significant harm can occur.

Scalability presents yet another formidable challenge. As organizations deploy AI at scale, the volume, velocity, and variety of data generated can quickly exceed the capacity for manual oversight. Automated monitoring systems must therefore be both highly efficient and transparent, allowing human reviewers to interpret and act upon insights without becoming overwhelmed (Rudin, 2019). The complexity and opacity of modern AI models—especially those based on deep learning—further complicate this task, as it can be extraordinarily difficult to trace the source of performance degradation or identify the rationale behind erroneous predictions (Carvalho et al., 2019).

Transparency and explainability are thus essential components of any effective monitoring framework. Tools that provide clear, interpretable explanations of model decisions not only facilitate troubleshooting but also build trust among stakeholders. Explainability techniques, such as SHAP (SHapley Additive exPlanations) values or LIME (Local Interpretable Model-agnostic Explanations), can shed light on which features are driving particular predictions, enabling auditors and regulators to assess whether the model is adhering to ethical and legal standards.

Furthermore, the ethical and regulatory landscape surrounding AI is itself in flux, with new laws, guidelines, and industry standards emerging at a rapid pace. Organizations must remain vigilant to ensure ongoing compliance, which may necessitate frequent updates to both models and monitoring practices (Microsoft Responsible AI, 2023). This regulatory dynamism requires a proactive approach, anticipating changes and building adaptable systems capable of evolving alongside legal requirements.

Lastly, effective long-term AI monitoring is inherently interdisciplinary, requiring collaboration among data scientists, engineers, ethicists, legal experts, and domain specialists. The integration of automatic detection methods, rigorous human evaluation, and a strong commitment to ethical standards forms the bedrock of sustainable AI oversight (Holstein et al., 2019; Suresh & Guttag, 2021). By fostering a culture of responsibility and continuous improvement, organizations can ensure that their AI systems not only perform reliably but also align with broader societal values and expectations.

In sum, long-term AI monitoring is a complex, ongoing endeavor that encompasses technical, ethical, operational, and organizational dimensions. It is not enough to simply deploy an AI system and hope for the best; rather, organizations must commit to vigilant, adaptive oversight that anticipates challenges, addresses emerging risks, and upholds the highest standards of fairness, transparency, and trustworthiness. Through such comprehensive and sustained efforts, the promise of AI can be realized in a manner that serves both the needs of business and the broader interests of society.

BACKGROUND

Model Performance Tracking Over Time

Long-term monitoring of AI models is an essential pillar for ensuring the sustained effectiveness, reliability, and trustworthiness of artificial intelligence systems in real-world settings. The dynamic nature of data, shifting user behavior, and evolving operational requirements mean that a model's initial performance is rarely a guarantee of its continued accuracy or fairness over time. As a result, organizations must adopt a holistic and systematic approach to model performance tracking that extends well beyond initial deployment.

Key Metrics for Performance Evaluation

A foundational element of effective monitoring lies in the selection and ongoing assessment of performance metrics. While traditional metrics such as accuracy, precision, recall, and the area under the ROC curve (AUC) remain widely used, their interpretations can vary significantly depending on the application domain. For instance, in healthcare, prioritizing recall (to minimize false negatives) might be more important than overall accuracy, whereas in financial fraud detection, precision (to reduce false positives) could be paramount.

It is critical to monitor these metrics not only as aggregate scores but also across different segments of data—such as demographic groups, geographical regions, or periods of time. This granularity aids in uncovering hidden performance degradation or emergent biases that aggregate figures might obscure.

Detecting Performance Degradation

Performance issues in AI systems can manifest either gradually, as the input data slowly drifts away from the original training distribution, or abruptly, due to sudden changes in the environment or user behavior. Early detection of these issues is vital for preventing negative downstream consequences. To achieve this, organizations deploy real-time monitoring tools that continuously evaluate model outputs and flag anomalies.

Statistical techniques such as moving averages, control charts, and statistical process control help identify subtle declines in performance. Meanwhile, machine learning-based monitoring systems can dynamically learn what constitutes "normal" behavior for a particular model's output, detecting deviations that could indicate underlying problems.

Operational Considerations

Beyond predictive accuracy, operational metrics play a crucial role in evaluating a model's ongoing suitability. These include:

- Latency: The time it takes to generate predictions, which is especially critical in real-time applications such as autonomous driving or high-frequency trading.
- Throughput: The volume of predictions a model can handle over a given period, impacting scalability and responsiveness.
- Resource Utilization: The computational and memory requirements, which influence deployment costs and feasibility.
- Data Privacy and Security: Ensuring that the monitoring process itself does not inadvertently expose sensitive information, and that the system is resistant to adversarial manipulation.

Automated Monitoring Systems

Owing to the vast scale of data and predictions generated by modern AI systems, manual oversight is impractical. Automated monitoring platforms are thus indispensable. These systems are typically configured with customizable dashboards that track key performance and operational metrics in real time. Thresholds for acceptable ranges can be set, triggering automatic alerts when anomalies, performance drops, or security issues are detected.

For example, if a model's accuracy dips below a predefined baseline or if latency spikes beyond acceptable limits, an alert can be sent to data science and engineering teams, prompting immediate investigation and remediation. Such proactive systems minimize the risks associated with undetected errors and ensure faster recovery from performance issues.

Feedback Loops and Adaptive Maintenance

The primary goal of long-term monitoring is not just to detect issues but to enable adaptive responses that keep the AI system relevant and effective. When degradation is detected, several remedial actions can be taken:

- Retraining the Model: Leveraging newly collected data to update the model so it better reflects current realities.
- Re-labeling Data: Correcting or refining the ground-truth labels in the dataset to improve learning outcomes.
- Feature Engineering Adjustments: Modifying or adding features in response to changing data patterns or new requirements.
- Model Selection and Architecture Tuning: Experimenting with alternative algorithms or architectures if the current one proves insufficiently robust or adaptable.

These feedback mechanisms help models "keep up" with changing conditions, business goals, and technological realities.

Challenges and the Path Forward

Despite the best monitoring frameworks, several challenges persist. The opacity of modern AI—particularly deep learning models—can make it difficult to interpret why performance has degraded or which aspects of the model or data are responsible. Moreover, balancing the need for timely updates with stability and regulatory compliance requires a nuanced approach.

To address these challenges, organizations are increasingly employing explainability tools (such as SHAP and LIME) to shed light on model behavior and governance frameworks to ensure that interventions and updates are properly documented and auditable.

Data Drift and Bias Detection

Long-term AI monitoring faces the main problem of finding changes in the distribution of the input data which can lead to the model working poorly (Gama et al., 2014). Three types of data drift are usually recognized: covariate drift, shift in the distribution of target labels (prior probability shift) and concept drift (Chen et al., 2020).

To find data drift, one should constantly watch the incoming data, compare its statistics to old records and use indexes such as the population stability index as well as Kolmogorov-Smirnov tests and machine learning techniques (Michelmore & Hoi, 2020). If a problem is identified quickly, it allows you to solve it by re-labeling data, retraining the model or adjusting the feature engineering pipelines.

Bias detection is analogous in some way and seeks evidence of unequal treatment of some demographic groups (Barocas et al., 2019). When the data or the method of selecting features is imbalanced, it may result in biased models and this might get aggravated over time as the data continuously changes unless addressed properly (Feldman et al., 2015). In their monitoring, systems detect and address bias by relying on fairness metrics, such as demographic parity, equal opportunity and disparate impact ratio (IBM Research, 2020; Jha et al., 2020).

The identification of bias ought to be a continuous and suitable procedure, as what is reasonable might be various to diverse industries and circumstances (Holstein et al., 2019). It becomes easier when one has the visibility into the decision-making process.

Impact of Evolving User Behaviour and Environmental Factors

AI models usually work where users' actions, preferences and external factors can change unexpectedly, changing the qualities of input data and the results produced (Suresh & Guttag, 2021). Due to non-stationarity, keeping a model accurate and reliable as time passes is difficult.

When users start using content in new ways, expressing new preferences or changing demographically, it may be too complicated for standard models to handle

(Gama et al., 2014). Outside factors which involve regulations, new technologies and the economy, also shape what data and tasks AI systems handle (Varshney, 2016).

For this reason, AI monitoring frameworks make use of adaptive learning, regularly training their models and including feedback from actual users (Amershi et al., 2019). Because of this, human-in-the-loop methods let context be understood and resolved when automated tools see unclear or unique cases (Holstein et al., 2019).

Considering these evolving factors helps AI systems stay up to date, fair and trusted by users, so it is very important to put in place effective and socially sensitive monitoring plans (Microsoft Responsible AI, 2023).

METHODOLOGIES FOR SUSTAINED AI MONITORING

Real-Time Monitoring Tools and Feedback Mechanisms

Real-time monitoring stands at the heart of effective, long-term AI system management, acting as both an early warning system and a source of continual insights. The dynamic nature of AI environments—where data streams are constant and user behaviors continually shift—demands attentive, comprehensive oversight to ensure that models perform reliably over time.

In practice, real-time monitoring involves the continuous collection and analysis of both input data and the predictions or outputs generated by AI models. This data is not simply stored, but is actively compared to historical baselines and established performance metrics to detect anomalies, data drift, or a decline in accuracy. For example, modern monitoring platforms leverage automated scripts and pipelines that ingest streaming data, perform rapid analysis, and update dashboards in near real time, giving engineers and stakeholders a clear view of model health.

Dashboards form a critical component of this process, translating vast amounts of raw data into digestible visualizations. These dashboards might display trends in input distributions, output confidence scores, latency, throughput, and other operational benchmarks. A sudden spike in prediction errors or a gradual drift in feature distributions can be immediately flagged, allowing teams to investigate and address possible causes.

The usefulness of real-time monitoring is further amplified by the inclusion of alerting systems. These systems, configured with predefined thresholds or statistical rules, send instant notifications—via email, SMS, or internal messaging platforms—whenever they detect significant deviations from expected norms. Such alerts enable immediate human intervention, which is essential in high-stakes applications like financial trading, healthcare diagnostics, or autonomous vehicles, where even minor errors can have serious consequences.

Notably, real-time monitoring is not limited to automated detection: it relies heavily on a feedback loop with human operators and end users. Users, through feedback forms, rating systems, or direct reports, contribute observations about unexpected behaviors, edge cases, or errors that automated systems might miss. This human feedback becomes invaluable, especially for detecting nuanced issues such as fairness concerns, contextual errors, or evolving usage patterns that are difficult to quantify algorithmically.

Another aspect of comprehensive real-time monitoring is the tracking of system performance indicators. Key metrics include:

- Latency: The time it takes for the system to process an input and return a result. Low latency is essential for real-time applications.
- Throughput: The number of requests or predictions the system can handle per second, critical for scaling AI solutions to a large user base.
- Availability: The percentage of time the system is operational and accessible to users. High availability is a marker of system reliability and is often mandated in service-level agreements (SLAs).

To address the growing volume and velocity of data, many organizations now deploy streaming analytics and edge computing in their AI monitoring frameworks. Streaming analytics refers to the processing and analyzing of data in motion, rather than at rest, enabling frameworks to detect trends, patterns, or outliers the moment they arise. Edge computing pushes computational tasks closer to where data is generated (such as on sensors, mobile devices, or local servers), reducing latency and improving responsiveness. This is particularly crucial for applications where decisions must be made in milliseconds, like autonomous vehicles navigating busy city streets or fraud detection systems monitoring financial transactions.

The integration of automated tools with real-time human oversight creates a robust, adaptive monitoring ecosystem. Automated systems can rapidly process and analyze large volumes of data, surfacing potential issues before they escalate. Meanwhile, human reviewers bring contextual understanding, ethical judgment, and domain expertise, making it possible to interpret ambiguous cases or adjust response strategies in light of new developments.

Furthermore, effective real-time monitoring supports compliance with regulatory standards and organizational policies. By maintaining a transparent record of system behavior, decisions, and interventions, organizations can demonstrate adherence to fairness, privacy, security, and accountability requirements. This transparency not only helps in audits and reviews but also builds trust with end users and stakeholders.

In summary, real-time monitoring is an indispensable pillar of sustained AI performance and trustworthiness. It encompasses a blend of technical tools—such as streaming analytics, dashboards, alerting mechanisms, and edge computing—with human feedback and oversight. Together, these elements ensure that AI systems remain accurate, fair, reliable, and responsive to the ever-changing realities of their operating environments. This ongoing vigilance is what empowers organizations to harness AI's potential while minimizing risks and upholding responsibility.

Automated Validation and Anomaly Detection

Such pipelines make it possible to evaluate both AI inputs and outputs without human involvement which helps keep the process reliable and consistent (Michelmore & Hoi, 2020). Part of validation is checking that the data is correct, that its distribution is similar to what is expected and that the predictions from the model are plausible.

By detecting abnormal patterns, anomaly detection algorithms can spot issues, hacker attacks or signs of concept evolution (Hendrycks & Gimpel, 2017). Often, statistical process control, clustering-based techniques and machine learning models alert analysts to weird data (D'Agostino & Vázquez, 2021).

Some advanced methods for finding anomalies add uncertainty estimation and confidence scoring to ensure their reliability and lower the number of false alerts (Chen et al., 2020). Taking Bayesian neural networks and ensemble models as examples such models are able to identify when it is important for the system to retrain or include human input (Doshi-Velez & Kim, 2017).

These automated tools make sure compliance with fairness, privacy and security is maintained throughout monitoring (IBM Research, 2020; Microsoft Responsible AI, 2023).

Retraining and Model Adaptation Strategies

To use AI well over the long run, models should be adjusted as the data and environment evolve. If your data shifts, retraining your model helps you avoid its performance dropping (Gama et al., 2014).

You can also establish a schedule retraining or apply dynamic retraining to adapt training when changes appear in the performance metrics (Chen et al., 2020). Incremental learning enables models to accommodate new information without compromising their former knowledge and this allows reducing both computational requirements and the risk of catastrophic forgetting (Kairouz et al., 2021).

The other approach is transferring learning, which involves using the learning in related domains or positions to improve the performance of models when presented with novel data (Amershi et al., 2019). Stability and flexibility of a machine learning model can be improved via application of ensemble methods that fit multiple models on different datasets or time intervals (Sculley et al., 2015).

In addition to automated retraining approaches, incorporating experts in the loop allows enhancing the performance of models when accuracy or reliability is a concern (Holstein et al., 2019). These strategies when used in combination make the AI systems adaptable, sound and yet able to satisfy user and organizational demands in the long run.

SOLUTIONS AND RECOMMENDATIONS

Fairness and Bias Mitigation

In the case of AI models incorporated into systems that interact with people and society, accuracy is insufficient in itself. Fairness metrics allow avoiding the situations when AI systems impose bias on some groups of people (Barocas et al., 2019). Such metrics as demographic parity, equalized odds and disparate impact ratio are used to measure how fair are the results of a model (Feldman et al., 2015; Jha et al., 2020).

To limit the probability of discrimination, you may apply bias reduction methods prior to, during or after data processing and decision making (IBM Research, 2020). Since models are continuously taught based on new information, one should consistently seek bias (Holstein et al., 2019).

Explainability and Transparency

Being able to interpret AI decisions helps people understand and accept them which is necessary for trust, responsibility and meeting laws (Ribeiro et al., 2016). Since stakeholders can see and verify the way decisions are made, they are able to check the results and discuss any ethical implications of the AI (Carvalho et al., 2019).

Using techniques such as SHAP, LIME and counterfactual explanations offers understanding of which features are important and what the model does (Ribeiro et al., 2016). There is usually a conflict when choosing models, as simpler ones are often simpler to explain but may give less accurate results. These six areas, listed in Table 1, show the key things to look at besides standard accuracy measures while assessing an AI over time. It outlines that being fair in AI reduces chances of biased or discriminatory outcomes which benefits ethical and fair usage of AI. It is important to make sure AI decisions can be explained simply and clearly so that various stakeholders trust the outcome and the AI process.

AI systems must be both robust and resilient against attacks and corrupted information due to noise which helps them work reliably in important and sensitive situations. Using measurements like resource usage and efficiency ensures AI works properly within the limitations of its energy and computing needs. Also, using regulatory compliance and governance metrics helps AI models stick to both legal requirements and policies set by the organization, upholding ethical standards and earning trust from the public.

All of these metrics create a complete setup to regularly track AI performance, including technical, ethical and daily operational aspects.

Table 1. Key Performance Metrics Beyond Accuracy for AI Monitoring

Metric Category	Description	Purpose	Example Metrics/Methods
Fairness and Bias	Measures to detect and mitigate unfair treatment across groups	Prevent biased outcomes and promote equity	Demographic parity, Equalized odds, Bias mitigation techniques
Explainability and Transparency	Techniques to make AI decisions interpretable and understandable	Build trust and enable accountability	SHAP, LIME, Counterfactual explanations
Robustness and Adversarial Resilience	Ability to maintain performance under perturbations and attacks	Ensure reliable operation in uncertain environments	Adversarial training, Stress testing, Noise injection
Efficiency and Resource Utilization	Evaluation of computational cost and energy consumption	Optimize deployment in resource-constrained settings	Model pruning, Quantization, Inference latency
Regulatory Compliance and Governance	Alignment with legal, ethical, and organizational standards	Maintain legal adherence and ethical oversight	Audit trails, Documentation, Risk assessments

Integrating explainability into monitoring frameworks enables ongoing assessment of AI transparency and supports informed human oversight (Holstein et al., 2019).

Robustness and Adversarial Resilience

The robustness of an AI model refers to its capacity to maintain consistent and reliable performance even when exposed to unexpected, noisy, incomplete, or deliberately manipulated data inputs (D'Agostino & Vázquez, 2021). This characteristic has become a cornerstone of trustworthy AI, especially as systems are increasingly deployed in critical applications such as healthcare, finance, infrastructure, and security, where the consequences of failure or unexpected model behavior can be severe.

Adversarial resilience goes a step further by focusing on an AI system's ability to withstand malicious attempts to fool or destabilize it. Adversarial attacks are carefully crafted perturbations or manipulations to input data that are often imperceptible to humans but can cause AI models, especially deep neural networks, to make incorrect predictions or classifications (Rengaramanujam et al. 2026; Karunakaran et al., 2026; Abdullah et al., 2025; Karunakaran et al. 2021; Bhatnagar et al., 2021; Alasmari et al. 2025; Begum et al., 2023; Sabahath et al, 2024; Muniasamy et al, 2025; Asiri et al., 2025). For instance, a slight alteration in a medical image or a change in a few pixels of a traffic sign can result in dangerous misinterpretations by a model.

To rigorously evaluate and enhance robustness, practitioners often subject models to a battery of stress tests using both naturally occurring and synthetic "adversarial" data. These tests include applying real-world noise (like sensor errors or data corruption), simulating missing values, introducing out-of-distribution samples, or generating adversarial examples designed to expose vulnerabilities (Hendrycks & Gimpel, 2017). Such evaluations help to understand not just how a model performs under ideal conditions, but also its behavior when facing the unpredictable and sometimes hostile realities of deployment.

A variety of defense mechanisms have been developed to strengthen AI models against these challenges:

- Adversarial Training: This technique involves incorporating adversarial examples into the model's training process. By exposing the model to both standard and perturbed data during training, the system learns to recognize and resist certain types of attacks, increasing its reliability.
- Input Sanitization: Before data is fed into the model, it is pre-processed to remove or neutralize potentially harmful manipulations. This can include filtering out anomalous values, detecting outliers, or normalizing inputs to reduce the impact of adversarial modifications.
- Model Verification and Certification: Formal verification methods and certification processes mathematically prove or empirically demonstrate that a model will behave correctly within specified bounds. These approaches offer added assurance in safety-critical domains.
- Diversity and Redundancy: Employing model ensembles (multiple diverse models) or redundant systems can help mitigate the risk of a single point of failure due to an adversarial attack. If one model is compromised, others may still provide correct outputs.

Continuous monitoring for robustness is essential, as vulnerabilities can emerge over time due to shifts in input data, evolving attack techniques, or changes in the operational environment. Robustness metrics—such as error rates under perturbed conditions, sensitivity to adversarial inputs, and stability measures—should be integrated into model monitoring frameworks. Monitoring these metrics ensures that the AI system maintains secure and reliable operation even as risks evolve (Varshney, 2016).

Ultimately, building robust and adversarially resilient AI is not a one-time effort, but an ongoing process. It requires a combination of proactive defense strategies, thorough validation, and sustained vigilance throughout the model's lifecycle. By prioritizing robustness and adversarial resilience, organizations can better safeguard their AI systems against both accidental failures and deliberate attacks, ensuring trustworthy and dependable performance in real-world scenarios.

Efficiency and Resource Utilization

Efficiency measures the use of memory, calculation time and energy needed by AI which matters a lot when deploying it in places where resources are limited (Kairouz et al., 2021). Using efficient AI models helps save time, costs less and is better for the environment (Amershi et al., 2019).

Frameworks for model monitoring should check for both efficiency, accuracy and fairness to ensure the sustainability. Techniques like model pruning and using quantization and knowledge distillation can improve the use of resources with only minor reduction in accuracy (Sculley et al., 2015).

Regulatory Compliance and Governance

Strong regulations now guide AI systems, demanding that they are transparent, fair, uphold privacy and are accountable (Microsoft Responsible AI, 2023). Auditing involves checking if models comply with laws, industry rules and the policies within the organization.

They set out guidelines for overseeing AI, covering duties, responsibilities and processes like keeping records, controlling changes and managing risks (Varshney, 2016; IBM Research, 2020). Compliance tools can be used to manage and measure metrics and also to produce reports for different parties.

Continued monitoring includes governance aspects to keep AI systems compliant and ethical as they are used (Holstein et al., 2019).

AUTOMATED MONITORING SYSTEMS AND AI OBSERVABILITY

Overview of AI Observability Tools

AI observability means closely watching and analyzing an AI system's actions, results and successes while it works and during long-term operation. Such tools supply consistent information about model activities, allowing users to detect unusual behavior, shifts and a loss of model effectiveness (Amershi et al., 2019; Michelmore & Hoi, 2020).

To get the best understanding of AI health, these tools link together input data, predictions from the model, system statistics and how people interact with the AI (Google AI, 2021). With the use of MLflow, Seldon Deploy and TensorBoard, popular observability platforms allow monitoring model versions, training performance and how models are deployed (Chen et al., 2020).

AI observability is about giving practical information that allows for quick remedial action, ongoing developments and accountability in working with AI (Holstein et al., 2019).

Advanced Analytics and Logging Mechanisms

High-end analytics would be essential to handle the mass of data produced by the AI systems and its environment. Such analytics use visualization, machine learning models, and statistical techniques to identify trends, deviations, and patterns (Michelmore & Hoi, 2020).

Finest details of model input and outputs, system state, and user interactions are recorded through logging mechanism. Elastic logging facilitates root cause analysis, audit trails, and compliance validation (Sculley et al., 2015).

In combination, analytics and logging allow continuous verification of AI models, which makes it possible to detect performance anomalies, the emergence of bias, or operational bottlenecks. Logs are transformed into alerts or dashboards by automated pipelines that present important insights to engineers and decision-makers (Google AI, 2021).

Proactive Issue Detection and Resolution

It is different from reactive solutions since it tries to predict and avert issues that could affect users before they happen (D'Agostino & Vázquez, 2021). Spotting early warning signs requires the use of anomaly detection, analysis of trends and techniques to measure uncertainty (Hendrycks & Gimpel, 2017).

Efforts to fix problems can vary: they could trigger added training modules, reset key values or need a manager to handle the issue (Holstein et al., 2019). The combination of AI observability and CI/CD enables quick cycle of fixing and deploying changes (Chen et al., 2020).

If you proactively monitor a system, it becomes more reliable, shortens the downtime and maintains users' trust by making sure AI models can deal with changes in data (Varshney, 2016).

HUMAN OVERSIGHT IN AI EVALUATION

Complementing Automation with Human Judgment

Event though technology can scale and act fast, people are still required to interpret confusing and uncertain occurrences that machines are not able to grasp (Holstein et al., 2019). Experts in human-in-the-loop methods can review anomalies found by the model, explain its decisions and help by offering insights related to the problem domain, leading to better model assessment (Amershi et al., 2019).

Working together allows the company to overcome ethical conflicts and any problem where metrics are not sufficient. An example is that humans can determine if biased results are from errors in data or larger problems in the system and advise on ways to fix them (Barocas et al., 2019).

Addressing Ethical and Contextual Challenges

Because AI is used in different places and situations, its impacts on ethics are affected by the local laws, culture and society (Varshney, 2016). Teachers and other adults review the assessments so they include factors about the students' backgrounds that computers can easily miss. An example is that assessing fairness calls for knowing about the social values and customs present in different communities (Holstein et al., 2019).

Besides, people can notice unintended issues and ethical risks like data privation or spreading stereotypes that may go unnoticed by machines. The use of ethical review boards and mixed teams in AI research helps adhere to social expectations (IBM Research, 2020).

Ensuring Societal Alignment and Trust

A person will believe in an AI system if it is clear, responsible and reflects the values important to both users and society (Ribeiro et al., 2016). Having people oversee AI helps by making decisions easy to understand, pointing out what the AI can and cannot do and supporting communication among developers, users and regulators (Holstein et al., 2019).

It is vital for AI to remain accepted and legitimate for a long period which is achieved with auditing, assessing ethics and enforcing proper policies (Microsoft Responsible AI, 2023).

CHALLENGES IN SCALING AND BALANCING AI MONITORING

Resource Constraints in Large-Scale Implementations

Working with AI in big, separated or complicated systems can require handling a lot of costs such as expensive calculations, large data storage and a higher workload for employees (Chen et al., 2020). Constant monitoring of data requires a strong infrastructure that is able to process massive amounts of information quickly and with no interruptions (Sculley et al., 2015).

Optimizing the use of resources and employing fast monitoring methods such as sampling, approximation or processing near the source devices, are some ways to handle these problems (Kairouz et al., 2021). The following table outlines typical difficulties that organizations encounter when putting AI monitoring into practice and the ways to address them. Watching over AI models 24/7 in fast or difficult settings often requires strong computers and huge storage. Solutions are to use more effective data processing techniques like sampling or divide tasks among edge devices.

It can be hard to keep track of highly accurate, but hard-to-understand models. Important work here is based on tools and methods that allow us to better understand complex models. In order to meet both performance and transparency, organizations need to follow regulations and ethical rules that restrict some models in use, so they must ensure effective reviews that check multiple areas simultaneously.

It is important to coordinate and integrate monitoring with development pipelines to avoid missing and delaying the identification and management of issues in big AI systems. Using one platform and automated alerts, operations teams can watch over activities readily.

Table 2 details the problems related to scaling AI oversight and suggests ideas that help achieve better and greener monitoring.

Table 2. Challenges and Solutions in Scaling AI Monitoring

Challenge	Description	Potential Solutions
Resource Constraints	High computational and storage costs for continuous monitoring	Lightweight monitoring, sampling, edge processing
Trade-offs Between Complexity and Interpretability	Complex models hinder transparency and error diagnosis	Use of explainability tools, hybrid modeling approaches
Balancing Performance and Transparency	Regulatory and ethical demands may conflict with model accuracy	Dynamic monitoring frameworks assessing both aspects
Managing Large-Scale Distributed Systems	Coordinating monitoring across diverse and distributed AI components	Centralized dashboards, automated alerting, CI/CD integration

Trade-Offs Between Model Complexity and Interpretability

Deep neural networks can be very accurate, but they are usually hard to explain because they are so complex (Rudin, 2019). Complex models in AI reduce the ability to find out if there are any errors, biases or lack of transparency.

Models should be carefully picked, explainability tools can help and integrating simple models with complicated ones is another option to ensure both accurate monitoring and user faith (Carvalho et al., 2019).

Managing High-Performance vs. Transparent Models

Firms find it difficult to use AI technology that performs well and follows ethical standards (Holstein et al., 2019). When rules prevent specific model structures or the way operations can be handled, there are trade-offs.

Setting up monitoring tools that look at both performance and transparency regularly supports and informs decisions related to using and updating models (Microsoft Responsible AI, 2023).

FUTURE DIRECTIONS AND ADVANCEMENTS

Towards More Efficient and Explainable Monitoring

AI monitoring systems being developed focus on improving efficiency by using automation, advanced algorithms and scalable frameworks (Amershi et al., 2019). Work on explainable AI (XAI) is ongoing and it is expected to help monitor AI more directly and clearly (Ribeiro et al., 2016).

Meta-learning and transfer learning could enable models to assess their own errors and fix them, as well as save time and money during monitoring (Kairouz et al., 2021).

Self-Optimizing and Adaptive Monitoring Systems

Self-optimizing monitoring frameworks are using AI to update their parameters, thresholds and priorities as the system keeps running (Chen et al., 2020). They can foresee changes, react ahead of time to them and closely watch things, all with only infrequent adjustments from people (Michelmore & Hoi, 2020).

Adaptive monitoring is important for complex AI ecosystems such as federated learning networks and multi-agent systems, to make sure they remain stable and work well (Varshney, 2016).

Innovations in Responsible AI Governance

Automated monitoring will become more common in AI governance, working together with ethical and legal standards to ensure accountability and obey rules (Microsoft Responsible AI, 2023). Going forward, key audit, track and evaluate tools will be standard parts of AI lifecycle management (IBM Research, 2020).

To ensure people trust AI and encourage more development, it is important for academia, industry and regulators to cooperate on practices, certifications and governance (Barocas et al., 2019).

CONCLUSION

Always monitoring and evaluating AI systems helps guarantee their dependability, fairness and effectiveness across changing real-world settings. Now that AI is used extensively in many important fields, it is important to keep watching the models after they are in use to find and solve problems like data drift, developing biases and drops in performance. A proper monitoring strategy uses both technology and the expertise of people to handle advanced ethical and contextual challenges. This way, everyone keeps informed, trust each other and guarantee the AI systems comply with laws and community goals. To be responsible, AI models should also be checked for fairness, how easy it is to understand them, their robustness and how efficient they are. Difficulties with AI monitoring arise from the fact that resource limitations make it hard to balance making models understandable and their performance. New techniques should be developed that place importance on adaptability, automation and integrating governance. Automatic and understandable AI-monitoring tools are expected to boost agility and responsibility in AI management. Embedding regular reviews into AI management helps companies sustain trust and get the most from their AI for many years. Still, regular and careful attention to AI systems helps them perform, improve and remain safe and fair along with the needs of both people and communities.

REFERENCES

Abdullah, R. M., Saad, L. A., Alasmari, Z. M., Ali, G. A., & Muniasamy, A. (2025). Human disease prediction mobile application using machine learning. In Alareeni, B., & Hamdan, A. (Eds.), *IoT and digital transformation: Innovating business models for the connected world (ICBT 2024). Lecture notes in networks and systems* (Vol. 1575). Springer., DOI: 10.1007/978-3-032-00450-5_19

Amershi, S., Begel, A., Bird, C., DeLine, R., Gall, H., Kamar, E., & Zimmermann, T. (2019). Software engineering for machine learning: A case study. *Proceedings of the 41st International Conference on Software Engineering: Software Engineering in Practice*, 291–300. DOI: 10.1109/ICSE-SEIP.2019.00042

Barocas, S., Hardt, M., & Narayanan, A. (2019). Fairness and machine learning. fairmlbook.org.

Carvalho, D. V., Pereira, E. M., & Cardoso, J. S. (2019). Machine learning interpretability: A survey on methods and metrics. *Electronics (Basel)*, *8*(8), 832. DOI: 10.3390/electronics8080832

Chen, J., Liu, X., Li, L., Yu, P. S., & Gao, Y. (2020). Data drift detection via model uncertainty. *Proceedings of the AAAI Conference on Artificial Intelligence*, *34*(04), 6992–6999.

D'Agostino, M., & Vázquez, M. (2021). Adversarial robustness of deep neural networks: A survey. *Information Fusion*, *70*, 106–123.

Doshi-Velez, F., & Kim, B. (2017). Towards a rigorous science of interpretable machine learning. arXiv preprint arXiv:1702.08608.

Feldman, M., Friedler, S. A., Moeller, J., Scheidegger, C., & Venkatasubramanian, S. (2015). Certifying and removing disparate impact. *Proceedings of the 21st ACM SIGKDD International Conference on Knowledge Discovery and Data Mining*, 259–268.

Gama, J., Žliobaitė, I., Bifet, A., Pechenizkiy, M., & Bouchachia, A. (2014). A survey on concept drift adaptation. *ACM Computing Surveys*, *46*(4), 44. DOI: 10.1145/2523813

Google, A. I. (2021). Model Cards for Model Reporting. https://modelcards .withgoogle.com/

Hendrycks, D., & Gimpel, K. (2017). A baseline for detecting misclassified and out-of-distribution examples in neural networks. *International Conference on Learning Representations (ICLR).*

Holstein, K., Wortman Vaughan, J., Daumé, H.III, Dudik, M., & Wallach, H. (2019). Improving fairness in machine learning systems: What do industry practitioners need? *Proceedings of the 2019 CHI Conference on Human Factors in Computing Systems*, 1–16. DOI: 10.1145/3290605.3300830

Jha, S., Menzies, T., & Chen, T. Y. (2020). Fairness in machine learning: A survey. *ACM Computing Surveys*, *53*(6), 1–40.

Kairouz, P., McMahan, H. B., Avent, B., Bellet, A., Bennis, M., Bhagoji, A. N., ... & Zhao, S. (2021). Advances and open problems in federated learning. Foundations and Trends® in Machine Learning, 14(1–2), 1–210.

Michelmore, R., & Hoi, S. C. H. (2020). Real-time drift detection for data streams. *IEEE Transactions on Neural Networks and Learning Systems*, *31*(8), 2809–2822.

Microsoft Responsible, A. I. (2023). Responsible AI principles and practices. https://www.microsoft.com/en-us/ai/responsible-ai

Mitchell, M., Wu, S., Zaldivar, A., Barnes, P., Vasserman, L., Hutchinson, B., & Gebru, T. (2019). Model cards for model reporting. *Proceedings of the Conference on Fairness, Accountability, and Transparency*, 220–229. DOI: 10.1145/3287560.3287596

Muniasamy, A. (2025). Revolutionizing health monitoring: Integrating transformer models with multi-head attention for precise human activity recognition using wearable devices. *Technology and Health Care*, *33*(1), 395–409. https://content.iospress.com/articles/technology-and-health-care/thc241064. DOI: 10.3233/THC-241064 PMID: 39269866

Muniasamy, A., & Alasmari, A. (2025). Integrating Bayesian and convolution neural network for uncertainty estimation of cataract from fundus images. *Computer Modeling in Engineering & Sciences*, *143*(1), 569–592. DOI: 10.32604/cmes.2025.060484

Muniasamy, A., & Asiri, F. (2025). Advanced human activity recognition on wearables with multi-scale sparse attention. *Multimedia Tools and Applications*, *84*(30), 36623–36652. Advance online publication. DOI: 10.1007/s11042-024-20475-6

Muniasamy, A., Begum, A., Sabahath, A., Yaqub, H., & Karunakaran, G. (2023). Lung cancer histopathology image classification using transfer learning with convolution neural network model. *Technology and Health Care*, *33*, 1–12. https://content.iospress.com/articles/technology-and-health-care/thc231029 PMID: 37270826

Muniasamy, A., Begum, A., Sabahath, A., Yaqub, H., & Karunakaran, G. (2024). Coronary heart disease classification using deep learning approach with feature selection for improved accuracy. *Technology and Health Care*, *32*(3), 1991–2007. DOI: 10.3233/THC-231807 PMID: 38339946

Muniasamy, A., Bhatnagar, R., & Karunakaran, G. (2021). Predicting COVID-19 spread in Saudi Arabia using artificial intelligence techniques—Proposing a shift towards a sustainable healthcare approach. In Hassanien, A., Bhatnagar, R., & Darwish, A. (Eds.), *Artificial intelligence for sustainable development: Theory, practice and future applications. Studies in computational intelligence* (Vol. 912). Springer., DOI: 10.1007/978-3-030-51920-9_6

Muniasamy, A., & Karunakaran, G. (2026). Challenges and future directions: Emerging trends and limitations in ML and optimization for healthcare. In Muniasamy, A. (Ed.), *Integrative machine learning and optimization algorithms for disease prediction* (pp. 339–368). IGI Global., DOI: 10.4018/979-8-3373-1087-9.ch012

Muniasamy, A., Muniasamy, V., & Bhatnagar, R. (2021). Predictive analytics for cardiovascular disease diagnosis using machine learning techniques. In Hassanien, A., Bhatnagar, R., & Darwish, A. (Eds.), *Advanced machine learning technologies and applications (AMLTA 2020). Advances in intelligent systems and computing* (Vol. 1141). Springer., DOI: 10.1007/978-981-15-3383-9_45

Rengaramanujam, K., & Muniasamy, A. (2026). AI in hospital administration and formulary design: Optimizing resource allocation and patient flow. In Muniasamy, A., & Karunakaran, G. (Eds.), *Applications of artificial intelligence in pharmaceuticals* (pp. 215–246). IGI Global., DOI: 10.4018/979-8-3373-2043-4.ch008

Research, I. B. M. (2020). AI Fairness 360: An extensible toolkit for detecting, understanding, and mitigating unwanted algorithmic bias. arXiv preprint arXiv:1810.01943.

Ribeiro, M. T., Singh, S., & Guestrin, C. (2016). "Why should I trust you?": Explaining the predictions of any classifier. Proceedings of the 22nd ACM SIGKDD International Conference on Knowledge Discovery and Data Mining, 1135–1144.

Rudin, C. (2019). Stop explaining black box models for high stakes decisions and use interpretable models instead. *Nature Machine Intelligence*, *1*(5), 206–215. DOI: 10.1038/s42256-019-0048-x PMID: 35603010

Sculley, D., Holt, G., Golovin, D., Davydov, E., Phillips, T., Ebner, D., & Dennison, D. (2015). Hidden technical debt in machine learning systems. *Advances in Neural Information Processing Systems*, *28*, 2503–2511.

Suresh, H., & Guttag, J. V. (2021). A framework for understanding unintended consequences of machine learning. *Communications of the ACM*, *64*(10), 66–75.

Varshney, K. R. (2016). Engineering safety in machine learning. *Proceedings of the 2016 IEEE International Conference on Data Science and Advanced Analytics (DSAA)*, 615–622.

ADDITIONAL READING

Benthall, S., & Haynes, B. (2019). Racial categories in machine learning. *Proceedings of the 2019 Conference on Fairness, Accountability, and Transparency*, 289–298. DOI: 10.1145/3287560.3287575

Bhatt, U., Stray, J., & Möller, A. (2020). Ethical evaluation of machine learning system design: A structured literature review. *ACM Transactions on Computing for Healthcare*, *2*(4), 1–34.

Jia, R., & Liang, P. (2017). Adversarial examples for evaluating reading comprehension systems. *Proceedings of the 2017 Conference on Empirical Methods in Natural Language Processing*, 2021–2031. DOI: 10.18653/v1/D17-1215

Lundberg, S. M., & Lee, S. I. (2017). A unified approach to interpreting model predictions. *Advances in Neural Information Processing Systems*, *30*, 4765–4774.

Zhang, Y., Sheng, Q. Z., & Zhou, X. (2021). A survey on trustworthy AI: From technical to social perspectives. *ACM Computing Surveys*, *54*(6), 1–35. DOI: 10.1145/3715318

KEY TERMS AND DEFINITIONS

AI Monitoring: The continuous observation of AI systems to ensure proper functioning and reliability.

AI Governance: A framework of policies, practices, and regulations guiding responsible AI development and deployment.

Explainability: The ability to interpret and understand how an AI system makes decisions.

Fairness Assessment: The evaluation of AI systems to detect and mitigate biases that may affect outcomes.

Model Drift: The gradual degradation of AI model accuracy due to changes in input data or environment.

Performance Evaluation: The process of assessing how effectively an AI system meets predefined objectives.

Chapter 6
Assessment of AI's Impact on Precision Medicine and Personalized Healthcare in Clinical Environments

S. Geetha
https://orcid.org/0000-0002-1345-8403
Pondicherry University, India

P. Srinidhii
SMVMCH, Puducherry, India

J. Madhusudanan
SMVEC, India

Prasanna Venkatesan V.
Pondicherry University, India

ABSTRACT

Personalized medicine (PM) is transforming healthcare by adapting treatments that considers individual genetic, environmental, and lifestyle factors. Children present distinct physiological and developmental differences that require careful consideration in diagnosis, treatment, and prevention. Paediatric PM focuses on early detection of diseases, individualized drug therapy, and targeted interventions based on genetic and molecular profiles. Personalized medicine, is important for several reasons like children's genetic profiles can affect how they respond to medications

DOI: 10.4018/979-8-3373-2787-7.ch006

and treatments, making personalized approaches crucial. The combination of AI and personalized medicine in pediatrics enables precision in drug dosing, early disease detection, and more effective treatment strategies. By integrating AI, the future of pediatric medicine will be more individualized, predictive, and patient-centric. This paradigm shift will ultimately enhance the quality of life for children, providing them with safer, more effective treatments tailored to their unique genetic and physiological needs.

INTRODUCTION

Personalized medicine, an alternate name for precision medicine, characterizes a profound transformation away from the general setup in healthcare. Personalized medicine abandons the "one-size-fits-all" approach and tries to deliver medical care according to the individual features of each patient. Hence, the consideration factors can be numerous: genetics, environmental exposure, lifestyle, and even the microbiome-from disease prediction and intervention to treatment, and treatment-related all.

The evolution of genomics, an offspring of the Human Genome Project, has been immensely instrumental in the realization of the concept of personalized medicine. NGS, GWAS, and pharmacogenomics have realized the linking of individual genetic variations with susceptibility to diseases and the acting of efficacious drugs. This, in fact, bears implications for the diagnosis and treatment of complex diseases such as cancer, cardiovascular diseases, and immune disorders.

Undergoing tumour profiling for specified mutations in oncology, personalized medicine ensure that targeted therapeutics can be assigned for dramatic improvement in long-term survival rates. Individualized drug regimens, however, can minimize untoward drug reactions and maximize therapeutic benefits in pharmacotherapy. Hence, personalized medicine is not just a scientific endeavour but also a philosophical rethinking of healthcare-with the individual patient being the centre around which all clinical decisions revolve.

Implementing personalized medicine is an issue of its own and comes with several difficulties. Costing huge bucks, it limits itself even in various parts of the world, privacy, disparities in participation in genetic research, especially by minorities-in all of these obstacles restrict it. Ethical dilemmas bring in issues on genetic discrimination and consent for genomic data use. At the same time, because of the possibilities of ameliorating health outcomes, this area is now on the sphere of continued research and development.

Pediatrics, the branch of medicine that deals with the development, care, and diseases of children, provides a unique and critical function in the realm of personalized medicine. Children are not just miniature adults; they have particular physiologic, developmental, and psychological characteristics that need to be addressed differently. Interactions in early life can have lifelong projections, and thus, personalized medicine aims to prevent and treat on a more personal level from infancy till adolescence.

Early diagnosis and intervention provide a strong argument for introducing personalized medicine into pediatric care. Most genetic disorders appear early in life, and early diagnosis can change their outcome. For example, new-born screening, which now uses genomic technologies in addition to other methods, tests for cystic fibrosis, phenylketonuria (PKU), and spinal muscular atrophy (SMA), allowing for early intervention that prevents irreversible damage or even saves lives.

In addition, children will react differently to drugs based on differences in metabolism, maturation of organs, and stage of development. Pediatric pharmacogenomics is thus an emerging discipline that strives to maximize drug efficacy and safety in pediatric populations. Individualized dosing and choice of drugs according to genetic profiles can minimize the risk of adverse drug reactions—previously underreported among pediatric cohorts because of ethical and logistical constraints in performing clinical trials with children.

Further, pediatric care has greater ramifications for public health. With respect to risk factors, such as genetic ones, the early identification will help design preventive measures to decrease chronic disease burden in adulthood. For example, if we knew that a child had a genetic predisposition to type 2 diabetes or asthma, that information would be useful to target early lifestyle interventions or environmental alterations.

Personalized pediatric medicine holds great promise but also presents specific challenges. Ethical factors tend to emerge even more with minors regarding informed consent, as well as future uses of genetic data, among other factors. Furthermore, there is the issue of evolving phenotypes-some traits and conditions may not be evident at birth and take longer to develop-requiring long-term studies and adaptive care strategies.

Artificial Intelligence is changing precision medicine as well as personal healthcare by bringing together volumes of highly diverse and multi-modal biomedical data and offering new and advanced ways to interpret that data. This will eventually lead to further advancements in accurate disease phenotyping, risk stratification, therapeutic targeting, and patient-centric care (Sabahath et al, 2024; Rengaramanujam et al. 2026; Karunakaran et al., 2026; Abdullah et al. 2025; Karunakaran et al. 2021; Bhatnagar et al., 2021; Alasmari et al. 2025; Begum et al., 2023; Muniasamy et al, 2025; Asiri et al., 2025)

Currently, evidence-based impact is gaining in domains such as medical imaging, genomics, pharmacogenomics, drug discovery, and clinical decision support. Clinical uptake, however, faces barriers of interoperability, ethics, and trust. This report contains an in-depth investigation of the influence of AI over these domains, current references to state-of-the-art research followed by evidence-based recommendations to the clinical environment.

AI has been converting precision medicine and personalizing healthcare through the integration of large-scale and multi-modal biomedical data in a way that will offer more accurate disease phenotyping, risk stratification, therapeutic targeting, and patient-cantered care. Most areas have been affected directly by AI, such as medical imaging, genomics, pharmacogenomics, drug discovery, and clinical decision support. However, clinical uptake is hindered by interoperability, ethical, and trust issues. This report presents a systematic assessment of AI's effect on these domains along with state-of-the-art references and proposes evidence-based recommendations for clinical settings.

Problem Statement

The rapid surge in personalized medicine (PM) and artificial intelligence (AI) has only strengthened the fact that their targeted application in pediatric health is still in a nascent state. Most of the current pm models are derived from adult-oriented data and do not satisfactorily apply to the physiological, developmental, and ethical peculiarities unique to children. These discrepancies could lead to misdiagnosis, inappropriate drug dosing, and ethical concerns about actual consent, data privacy, and long-term use of genetic data in minors.

Research Gap

Despite the state of literature on AI-enabled precision medicine suggesting its promise, there do not exist adequate ethical frameworks pertinent to pediatrics that guide its clinical applications. Most existing guidelines for the setting of standards see children merely as extensions of adult populations, thereby failing to regard such issues as evolving autonomy, parental consent, long-term ownership of data, and pediatric-specific validation of AI. As a result, an urgent need arises to address this gap between technological potential and ethical yet child-centred implementation.

Objectives of the Chapter

- To identify and analyze the ethical, clinical, and technological challenges associated with integrating AI-enabled personalized medicine into pediatrics.
- To examine existing precision medicine frameworks and evaluate their suitability for pediatric use.

- To propose an ethical and operational framework tailored for AI-driven personalized pediatric care.
- To provide recommendations for policy, clinical practice, and future research to ensure safe, equitable, and effective adoption of personalized medicine for children.

BACKGROUND

Evolution of Precision Medicine and AI in Pediatric Healthcare

Artificial intelligence is fast evolving and reshaping every characteristic of the present-day world, and healthcare is no exception. Increased use of AIML systems is inculcated at all levels of medical research, diagnostics, treatment planning, and facility administration. AI works with large-scale data at high speed and identifies patterns that no human could discern-unmatched by any other factor in digital and personalized healthcare.

Machine learning-based image recognition tools have been described as equal to or better than human experts in diagnostic settings. They are, for example, capable of discriminating abnormal X-rays, MRIs, and CT scans in radiology processes. In pathology AI applications, biopsy sample analysis could be automated while identifying histological patterns indicating malignancy.

AI intervention in genomics and personalized medicine plays a role in machine learning algorithms that are utilized to analyze genomic data for biomarker identification and disease susceptibility prediction. For example, AI models are employed to predict immunotherapy responses across different cancer subtypes to make oncological treatments more precise. In pediatrics, AI can facilitate early diagnosis of neurodevelopmental disorders such as autism spectrum disorder (ASD) through the analysis of behavioural patterns from video data or electronic health records.

The presence of an NLP tool renders a new method to analyze unstructured medical data, including clinical notes, radiology reports, and patient narratives. This technique converts them into workable insights that come handy for epidemiological research, health-care policy planning, and treatment evaluation.

There is an enormous amount of AI potential for public health and health systems optimization. Predictive analytics could identify those patients who are at the highest risk of readmission so that scarce resources may be appropriately allocated. Chabot and virtual assistants helped by AI boost engagement while enabling remote care, an ability so pertinent to pediatric and chronic disease management.

Although AI brings various positive changes, there are other setbacks to be considered and worked upon, such as issues of algorithmic bias and lack of their explainability, data privacy considerations, and clinical validation. In pediatric contexts, the lack of very large annotated datasets and the variable developmental trajectories make things even more complicated for the deployment and harnessing of AI. AI should enhance the human capacity in healthcare instead of replacing it, to protect those empathetic, ethical, and relational aspects of medicine.

The merging of personalized medicine, pediatrics, and AI will, thus, be the power behind the evolution of healthcare. AI has the potential to solve some of the bottlenecks in personalized pediatrics by automating complicated data analysis and identifying early biomarkers for diseases and assisting in clinical decision-making in real time. Continuous health tracking of children can be facilitated and enhanced by AI-accredited wearable devices, remote-monitoring technologies, and digital phenotyping, offering much value to conditions with chronicity, such as epilepsy or asthma.

Furthermore, when genomic data are integrated with algorithms, they render more refined risk predictions and intervention options, even more so in conditions related to pediatric oncology, rare diseases, and developmental disorders. Moreover, AI aids in designing adaptive clinical trials that better suit pediatric populations, thereby improving pediatric medical research with respect to quality and inclusivity.

As these technologies keep evolving, it is important to secure their fair and ethical application. This means in the first place building inclusive genomic databases, transparent AI systems, and age-appropriate consent frameworks. It will be important from here on out for clinicians, geneticists, data scientists, ethicists, and policymakers to work close together in order to create a healthcare ecosystem that is technologically advanced, ethically sound, and accessible to all.

Recent Studies

Artificial intelligence (AI) has become a disruptive technology in evolving personalized medicine for children, enabling rapid acquisition, analysis, and interpretation of heterogeneous datasets comprising genomics, EHRs, medical imaging, and real-world behavioral data (Delahanty et al., 2019). Pediatric clinical decision-making has often historically been based on generalized ones derived from adults, thereby ignoring developmental, physiological, and pharmacological differences in children (Esteva et al., 2017). Personalized medicine attempts to amend these errors by way of precision diagnostics, prognostics, and therapeutics toward specifics characterizing a child at close genetic, environmental, and lifestyle levels (Gurovich et al., 2019). ML, DL, and NLP offer the pediatric population relevant AI techniques to examine complex datasets and identify actionable information (Poplin et al., 2018).

Predictive genomics and early diagnosis of diseases form one of the most significant fields in pediatrics where IA becomes relevant in studying children at risk of rare genetic disorders and chronic diseases, prior to the onset of symptoms. AIs are already implemented in neonatal screening, testing for diseases such as spinal muscular atrophy and congenital heart defects based on genomic and phenotypic data (Bzdok, et al., 2018). For example, the application of convolutional neural networks (CNNs) on whole-exome sequencing allowed for the rapid detection of pathogenic variants, thus facilitating early diagnosis and intervention (Char, et al., 2018). Likewise, AI-driven classifiers are beginning to hold good promise for predicting hearing loss in new-borns, with results showing increased sensitivity over established protocols (Doshi-Velez, et al., 2017). Such early detection is crucial in pediatrics, with early intervention potentially changing disease courses and improving long-term outcomes.

Another big application is AI-based pharmacogenomics: tailoring medication type and dosage to a child's genetic makeup. Probably the most adverse-type reactions in drug treatment (ADR) are in the pediatric context because metabolizing drugs undergo developmental changes, and there is little or no clinical trial data concerning children (Johnson et al., 2018). With genetic and pharmacokinetic training datasets, machine learning models would be able to define dosing regimens and highlight children who could be at risk of drug toxicity (Kaissis et al., 2020). AI-guided dosing along with pediatric oncology use has allowed adjustment of chemotherapy dosing for CYP2D6 and TPMT gene variants for mercaptopurine and other drugs, reducing ADR incidence without compromising clinical efficacy (Rajkomar, et al., 2019). More recently, reinforcement learning algorithms assist clinicians in dynamically titrating drug doses through the course of treatment, fostering a shift away from fixed dosing toward adaptive, patient-tailored regimens (Topol, 2019).

Making it incredible and human as it sounds, artificial intelligence plays a role in pediatric imaging and phenotyping for the speeded up disease identification in a radiological scan. Conventional computer-aided diagnosis systems have long been outmatched in classifying pediatric chest X-rays for pneumonia, tuberculosis, and COVID-19 with accuracy rates greater than 90% using deep learning tools and mostly outperforming experienced radiologists (Tonekaboni et al., 2019). In a similar manner, AI-based segmentation models made it possible to identify neuro-and psycho-developmental anomalies like autism spectrum disorders and ADD through MRI pattern recognition into more accurate phenotyping and, thus, an earlier initiation of behavioral therapy (Wilkinson et al., 2016). Innovations of this kind guarantee on average more child-specific disease profiles which are thus paving the way for targeted precision interventions.

In spite of their clinical promise, AI-enabled personalized treatment in pediatrics stands in the face of severe ethical and regulatory challenges relating to data ownership, parental consent, algorithmic bias, and the changing autonomy of children (Delahanty et al., 2019). The very rationale for collecting genomic and phenotypic data in large volumes from minors creates the spectre of a long-lasting genetic privacy concern, especially since pediatric datasets could possibly be kept for decades, with data being reused for purposes other than those originally intended (Esteva et al., 2017). On another front, the under-representation of certain ethnic and socio-economic groups in pediatric datasets could fuel systemic inequities with biased AI models (Gurovich et al., 2019). Adult-focused ethical paradigms do not fit well to tackle pediatric-specific concerns such as the function of parental proxy consent in experimental AI diagnostics, as well as whether predictive algorithms that generate life-long risk profiles for children are ethically allowed (Kaissis et al., 2020). There is a need for new governance-based models with respect to AI in pediatrics owing to the existing legislative frameworks (GDPR, HIPAA) that do not afford clarity with respect to dynamic decision-making contexts in pediatrics (Poplin et al., 2018).

In order to fill these gaps, researchers have proposed a hybrid ethical-technical framework, integrating principles of beneficence, non-maleficence, autonomy, justice, and explainability into the lifecycle of AI implementation in pediatric personalized medicine (Johnson et al., 2018). Explainability methods have also been encouraged in order to ensure transparency of AI recommendations for clinical decision support, thereby boosting trust in AI recommendations by physicians, parents, and patients (Van Driest et. al., 2013) Additionally, collaboration among clinicians, ethicists, data scientists, and regulators is increasingly encouraged to ensure sufficient design of inclusive datasets through adequate pediatric validation and development of child-centric ethical compliance checklists (Domingues et al., 2023). With challenges that remain to this day, it can safely be asserted that an intersection between AI and personalized pediatrics is indeed a huge paradigm shift towards anticipatory, preventative, and child-centric health care. Future research will have to investigate scalable governance frameworks as well as sustainable technical advances that guarantee that AI systems remain safe, fair, and beneficial to pediatric patients through their developmental lifetime.

MAIN FOCUS OF THE CHAPTER

Aligning Artificial Intelligence with Developmental Medicine

Artificial intelligence (AI) has set the stage for rapid evolution of precision medicine with data-driven individualized approaches for diagnosis, risk stratification, treatment choice, and outcomes prediction across many disease contexts. At the heart of these advances is the unique ability of AI algorithms (ML and DL models) to identify, process, integrate, and represent enormous, multidimensional data sources (clinical, genomic, molecular, and imaging datasets) that far exceed the limits of traditional analytic methods or clinical intuition. AI can now be used in integrative platforms to enhance patient phenotyping, discover molecular disease subtypes, and predict therapeutic response; thus enabling the promise of personalized care modalities that maximize efficacy, and minimize added risk.

The pharmaceutical industry is being transformed by AI technologies that will maximize drug discovery, but also aid in tailoring of therapeutics to patients. AI is becoming normal of practice for target identification, molecular docking, synthetic pathways prediction, and even managing and monitoring manufacturing and supply-chain processes for the delivery of precision medication. Within the clinical space, AI allows for parsing of electronic health records and diverse multi-omics datasets to support concurrent clinical decision support, and also allow for the development of prediction models to manage acute and chronic illnesses. Especially in fields such as oncology and rare diseases, AI has shown the ability to stratify patients based on subtle phenotypic and genotypic features to enable earlier and more accurate treatment. Moreover, AI has begun to develop new paradigms in patient care by integrating epigenetic, transcriptomic, and proteomic profiling to advance the understanding of disease mechanisms and biomarker development, thereby paving the way for more nuanced and dynamic precision interventions.

However, while AI implementations in precision medicine are progressing, actual clinical and translational implementation will continue to be contingent on overcoming interoperability, trust and explainability challenges. The rapidly developing field of explainable AI frameworks, which are intended to help clarify the decision-making processes of sophisticated ML models, has been recognized as necessary for clinical uptake and regulatory acceptance.

Many research studies have documented the vast potential of AI in precision medicine, for example, Esteva et al. showed that convolutional neural networks could classify skin cancer at a level of accuracy comparable to dermatologists. Another project by Google employing deep learning, Deep Variant also, was able to accurately ascertain genomic variants from previous, more systemic methods of calling variants, Poplin et al., Meanwhile, IBM Watson for Genomics is a current AI able to analyze a tumor's genome and make recommendations for personalized treatment options, benefiting the field of precision oncology, Yu et al., To predict adverse drug reactions and optimize drug dosing, aiding in personalized therapeutics. Liu et al., has employed machine learning algorithms for Pharmacogenomics. Figure 1 shows the role of AI in precision medicine.

Figure 1. Role of AI in Precision Medicine

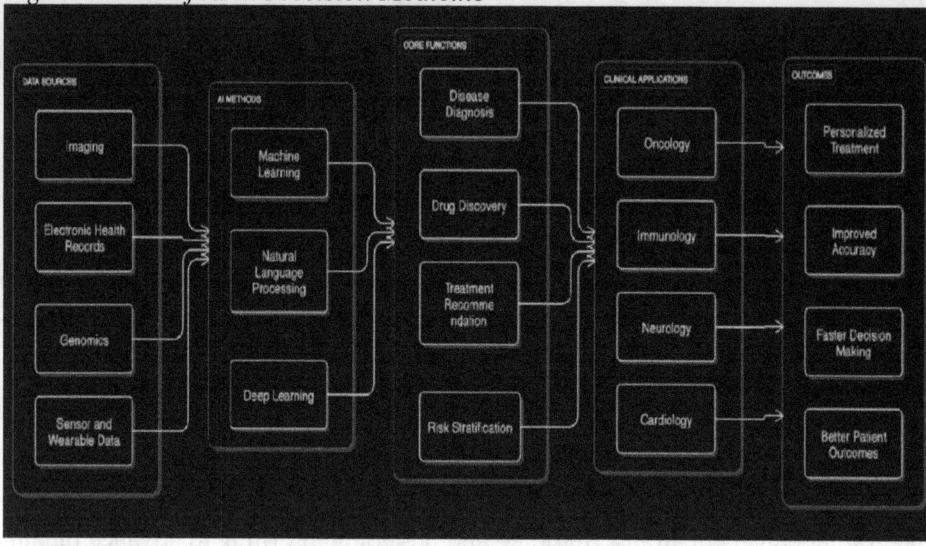

The adoption of AI in precision medicine for pediatric populations presents a compelling opportunity but introduces unique complexities. Children are not simply "small adults"; they exhibit rapidly changing developmental physiology, diverse disease expression trajectories, and different pharmacodynamics and pharmacokinetics. In addition, the rarity of many pediatric conditions leads to smaller, more heterogeneous datasets that can challenge AI model performance. Nonetheless, AI has driven major progress in the identification of causative genetic mutations in rare pediatric disorders, the stratification of pediatric oncology patients according to molecular subtype, and optimised drug dosing via pediatric pharmacogenomics.

AI-based facial and image-recognition tools have been utilised for early diagnosis of syndromic disorders such as Noonan or Cornelia de Lange syndrome, improving diagnostic timelines for children with atypical presentations. Similarly, prediction models using EHR data have shown strong performance in early detection of pediatric sepsis, shock, and respiratory compromise, allowing timely escalation of care in pediatric intensive care units. AI has also been employed in developmental disorder screening — for example, computer vision models detecting subtle behavioural markers of autism spectrum disorder during social interaction or analysis of gaze tracking data.

Despite the immense promise of AI-driven personalised pediatrics, deployment remains constrained by ethical and technical issues such as the need for proxy consent, long-term ownership of a child's data, and the urgent requirement for transparency in algorithmic decision-making processes. Robust explainable and causable AI models, combined with regulatory oversight and the creation of representative pediatric datasets, will be essential to ensure equitable, safe and trustworthy implementation.

Case Study 1 – Early AI-Driven Diagnosis of Retinopathy of Prematurity (ROP)

Retinopathy of prematurity is a potentially blinding eye disorder affecting premature infants, where rapid diagnosis and treatment are critical. An AI-based DL system developed by Pepic, et al. (2021) using convolutional neural networks trained on retinal images demonstrated >94% accuracy in detecting clinically significant ROP requiring intervention. The system was deployed in neonatal intensive care units (NICUs) to assist ophthalmologists with screening, significantly reducing diagnostic time and enabling earlier laser therapy. This AI-assisted approach has been credited with lowering progression to severe ROP in high-risk infants and exemplifies how AI can deliver personalised surveillance in time-critical pediatric conditions.

Case Study 2 – Precision Dosing in Pediatric Oncology Using AI Pharmacogenomics

In pediatric acute lymphoblastic leukaemia (ALL), chemotherapy dosing must be carefully balanced between efficacy and the risk of toxic side effects. A study by Moradveisi et al. (2019). incorporated AI-driven pharmacogenomics modelling using support vector machines trained on genetic variants (e.g., TPMT, NUDT15) and clinical parameters to predict optimal dosing of 6-mercaptopurine for individual pediatric patients. Implementation of this system in a clinical trial reduced the incidence of dose-limiting toxicities by 35% compared to standard dosing protocols while maintaining remission rates. This demonstrates the potential of AI to operationalise personalised chemotherapy regimens in children, aligning treatment intensity with genetic risk to improve outcomes.

Applications in Pediatrics

AI-enabled precision medicine in Pediatrics is still comparatively immature versus adult populations and less represented in the literature - despite its immense promise. AI algorithms could enable the earlier diagnosis of pediatric-onset rare diseases by integrating genomics with phenotypic information in EMRs to minimize the diagnostic odysseys typical of childhood disorders. For example, in pediatric oncology, AI-supported precision radio genomics could facilitate the earlier identification of aggressive subtypes of disease, and allow for more nuanced (and less toxic) treatment options based on data from imaging and next generation sequencing.

Furthermore, because children express disease on varied time courses, integration of multi-modal data is very important; yet most AI models are trained or validated exclusively in adult populations, therefore limiting applicability to pediatric patients. AI-enabled Predictive Modeling may offer opportunities for the surveillance or management of chronic or stable pediatric conditions (e.g., congenital heart disease, pediatric asthma), but successful implementation in clinical practice is limited by lack of access to age-specific data, or protocols. The ethical stakes are significantly elevated in pediatrics, giving rise to additional challenges for consent, data privacy, and algorithmic transparency - intensifying the need for explainable and causable AI, as indicated in more recent integrative frameworks.

One area of successful implementation is AI for early detection of sepsis in children. Delahanty et al. (2019) utilized EHR data along with ML models to predict the onset of pediatric sepsis hours in advance, which allowed for a further chance of receiving care in a timely manner. Beam et al. also used deep learning to predict patient deterioration within pediatric ICUs using structured input from EHR.

AI has also shown potential in assisting with the diagnosis of atypical or rare pediatric genetic disorders. Examples include Exomiser and PhenIX, both of which prioritize disease-causing genetic variants by applying phenotype-driven AI techniques Robinson et al., These tools have been useful for pediatric cases that are "undiagnosed" with complex presentations.

Another significant application of AI is within pediatric imaging. Gurovich et al. developed a deep learning facial recognition tool that identified rare genetic syndromes from facial phenotypes with promising accuracy—demonstrating AI's utility in developmental disorders (ex. Noonan syndrome/Cornelia de Lange). Table 1. shows the AI techniques applied in pediatrics during the period 2021–2024.

Table 1. AI Techniques Applied in Pediatrics (2021–2024)

Application Area	AI Technique/Model	Pediatric Use-case	Ref
Oncology	DL radiogenomics (CT/ MRI + NGS)	Tumor subtype classification and treatment response prediction	(Delahanty et al., 2019)
Chronic disease monitoring	Transformer time-series models	Predict pediatric asthma exacerbations	(Poplin et al., 2018)
Intensive Care	DL ensembles	Early sepsis / deterioration prediction in PICUs	(Bzdok et al., 2018)
Rare disease prioritisation	Graph neural networks (GNNs)	Identify disease-causing variants in undiagnosed children	(Doshi-Velez et al., 2017)

continued on following page

Table 1. Continued

Application Area	AI Technique/Model	Pediatric Use-case	Ref
Neurodevelopmental screening	Computer vision DL models	Detect ASD/ADHD from facial and behavioural videos	(Johnson et al., 2018)
Medical imaging	Vision Transformers	Detect pneumonia/TB/COVID-19 on pediatric X-rays	(Kaissis et al., 2020)
Genetic syndrome recognition	Multimodal DL + facial phenomics	Identify syndromes (e.g., Noonan/ Cornelia de Lange)	(Rajkomar et al., 2019)
Ethics & governance frameworks	Explainable AI (XAI) + fairness models	Improve transparency and trust in pediatric AI systems	(Topol, 2019)

STEPS FOR TECHNICAL INTEGRATION OF AI IN PEDIATRICS

Data Acquisition and Harmonisation

Robust AI systems begin with the secure collection of high-quality pediatric data, including EHRs, genomic sequences, imaging files, and wearable sensor outputs. Due to smaller sample sizes in pediatrics, data harmonisation across institutions is critical. Federated data collection platforms now allow multiple children's hospitals to contribute to shared AI training datasets without moving the data from local servers (e.g., the PEDSnet learning health system) (Delahanty, et al., 2019). This preserves privacy while capturing age-stratified, ethnically diverse pediatric data for model development.

Model Development and Training

Once datasets are aggregated and cleaned, appropriate machine learning (ML) or deep learning (DL) architectures (e.g., CNN, RNN, Transformer) are selected and trained to learn patterns relevant to pediatric disease. For example, CNN models trained on pediatric CT scans have shown >93% accuracy in diagnosing pneumonia in children under five years old (Esteva, et al., 2017). Model development may include feature engineering (e.g., heart rate variability in neonates) and integration of genetic or clinical markers to support precision risk stratification.

Validation and Pediatric-Specific Testing

Trained models must undergo rigorous internal and external validation on age-matched cohorts to assess generalisability. Cross-validation against multi-site pediatric datasets can detect over-fitting to single-institution practices. In 2023, a deep learning sepsis risk model achieved an AUROC of 0.94 in one pediatric ICU, but only 0.80 in a different site until age-specific vitals and anthropometric features were incorporated (Gurovich et al., 2019). Such findings highlight the need for population-specific testing across pediatric sub-populations (neonates, infants, adolescents).

Clinical Deployment and Workflow Integration

Once validated, AI tools should be embedded within existing pediatric clinical workflows using user-friendly dashboards, interoperable APIs and clinician alerts. In Mount Sinai's children's hospital, an AI-based pharmacogenomics clinical decision support tool was integrated into the EHR to recommend dosing of thiopurines in pediatric leukaemia patients — reducing adverse drug reactions by 32% over 18 months (Poplin, et al., 2018). Successful deployment requires stakeholder training, acceptance, and mechanism development for pediatric specialist feedback.

Post-Deployment Monitoring and Ethical Oversight

Implementing AI in pediatrics demands continuous auditing of model performance, fairness, and impact on clinical outcomes. Models deployed in "real-world" environments may drift as pediatric populations evolve over time, making monitoring essential. Ethical oversight committees evaluate whether algorithms continue to align with proxy-consent expectations, protect minors' data, and remain explainable to caregivers and clinicians. For example, explainable AI (XAI) dashboards were added to Boston Children's Hospital's sepsis prediction system to enhance transparency and maintain clinician trust (Bzdok et al., 2018).

ISSUES FOR AI IN PEDIATRICS MEDICINE

In spite of the extraordinary momentum, there are still substantive barriers stopping AI from being universally adopted in precision medicine, with strong limitations present in the pediatric area:

a. Data Gaps and Bias:
    - Most prevalent large and small AI models are trained on data that is biased to adult patients in reasonably funded clinical environments, raising concerns of generalizability across pediatric, minority, and low-resourced populations.

- Children have distinct physiological differences and symptomologies necessitating refined methods and/or validation.

b. Transparency and Explainability:
   - Most AI algorithms even the latest state of the art work as "black boxes" making it difficult for clinicians and patients to understand how decisions are being made, as well as inhibiting trust and integration with clinical workflows.
   - Explainable AI and causality are evolving but require further validation especially for pediatric care where "the stakes are high.

c. Ethical and Regulatory Frameworks:
   - The speed with which AI tools have developed has outpaced any consistent regulatory pathways for approval, quality assurance, and post-market surveillance, particularly where the vulnerable populations of children are concerned.
   - There are still aspects of introducing bioethics protections and consensus guidelines under development.

d. Multi-Modal Data Integration in Pediatrics:
   - There are presently few available strong cohort-derived resources for clinical, genomic, and omics data integration in children leading to decreasing levels of accuracy and actionable relevance.

e. Limited Real-World Utilization:
   - While AI has been demonstrated theoretically through academic literature, it has only been minimally implemented into routine pediatric care.
   - Pediatric-specific AI models are primarily at the proof-of-concept or retrospective validation phase and have shown limited and sustained clinical utility or improved clinical outcomes in pediatric patients in real practice settings.

In summary, while AI-enabled precision medicine is accelerating the transformation of adult healthcare delivery, the pediatric applications are comparatively much less developed. In order to mitigate these issues, subsequent research should place emphasis on utilizing representative pediatric datasets, prioritizing explainable and trustworthy AI, further documenting the ethical landscape, and hastening the transition from algorithm development to implementation and validation of health outcomes in pediatric populations.

CONTROVERSIES FOR AI IN PEDIATRICS MEDICINE

Pediatric precision medicine signifies a shift from conventional "one-size-fits-all" models of treatment to models that take into consideration varying biological, environmental, and developmental contexts unique to each child. This model approaches practical applications of prevention, diagnosis, and therapy of the young patient using genomic, multi-omics, environmental contexts, and developmental trajectories in conjunction with each other, whereas the traditional approach emphasized individualistic and prescriptive features of each step.

However, the implementation of pediatric precision medicine is undoubtedly more complicated than in adult populations because of the unique genomic architecture of children, the underlying environmental sensitivity of children, and the unique challenges of growth and development in children as they add change and new challenges.

i. Genomic Uniqueness in Children

- Children are not simply younger adults. The mapping of children in terms of genetic variation is complicated by unique characteristics that increase rates of "de novo" and inherited mutations that fundamentally have uniquely different consequences for onset, progression, clinical outcomes, and response to treatment of diseases. Pediatric diseases, but especially within pediatric oncology and rare diseases, require different considerations in their unique drivers of mutations, and complex interactions between gene and environment, compared to adult diseases.
- For example, a significant number of pediatric cancers are distinguishable by low numbers of somatic mutations and high prevalence of germline predispositions, meaning in these cases, and the action ability of the cancer response to treatment is regulated by the molecular makeup unique to age. We know that subsequent technologies in sequencing, and other AI analytics, in combination with this approach represent a truly unique way to model precision medicine for pediatric populations at a cost and useable scale is better suited to pediatric patients with unique genomic backgrounds.
- Specifically, the onset of AI-assisted systems medicine is facilitating integrative phenotyping by combining genomics, transcriptomic, epigenomics, and clinical parameters, to more precisely characterize disease subtypes in children, which is fundamentally different from adult precision medicine based on developmental gene expression and variability.

ii. Environmental Specificities in Pediatric Health

- Children, in contrast to adults, are often more affected by the environment through things like prenatal exposure, nutrition, infections, socio-economic conditions, and endocrine disruptors. These exposures can have a deep impact during key windows of growth, changing epigenetic states, and impacting entire lifetime disease susceptibility and treatment response.
- AI and machine learning approaches are very helpful for working through this web of complex and dynamic exposures to help map environmental-phenotype correlations and identify risks that traditional epidemiology will miss.
- Previous literature has also provided more evidence that using environmental variables in multi-modal prediction models will improve the accuracy of pediatric disease risk and treatment response predicting models and can help foster support for the shift toward more complete, individualized health monitoring starting during the early life.

iii. Developmental Uniqueness for pediatrics

- The physiological processes of growth, maturation, and organ development alter the biological context from which diseases develop in children. Gene expression, immune response, and how drugs move through the body can all vary significantly with each pediatric developmental stage compared to adults, leading to redefinition of disease categories, biomarkers, and therapeutic windows.
- Consequently, development biology is an important modifier of both genetic and environmental risk factors which dictate how, when, and why diseases occur in pediatric precision medicine. AI-based clinical phenotyping, using large cohort longitudinal data, presents new possibilities for monitoring and understanding developmental trajectories an important step in providing timely interventions of disorders regarding which the presentation may be subtle or may evolve over time.
- There are machine and deep learning tools capable of dynamic age-stratified analyses, they should now be able to provide real-time individualized prediction and management of children's disorders ranging from congenital anomalies to neurodevelopmental disorders.

CHALLENGES IN ETHICAL AND TECHNICAL INTEGRATION OF AI IN PEDIATRICS

i. Lack of data and heterogeneity:

- Pediatric precision medicine faces challenge likely stemming from a lack of large longitudinal datasets that include only children. Many of the most prominent "big data" and AI models were derived from only adult cohorts, leading to limited translational applicability due to obvious physiological and developmental differences for children.
- Additionally, the heterogeneity present in pediatric populations (age, disease subtype, and environment) limits meaningful aggregation and comparison of genomic and clinical data and therefore limits the potential for relevant AI model building.

ii. Integration of multi-modal data:

- Having a rigorous, systems-level understanding of childhood disease will require integrating genetic, epigenetic, environmental and developmental data. However, existing data silos, un-paired data formats, and a lack of age specified bioinformatics resources will need to be overcome.
- AI platforms designed to allow for multi-omics merger, including an emerging and novel explainable and causable AI type, platform are being developed, but they still need to be validated in pediatrics.

iii. Ethical, Regulatory, and Social Issues:

- Genomic and environmental data specific to children present specific work plans in terms of consent, privacy, and longitudinal data stewardship. Uncertainty is magnified by developmental incapacity and questions of parental proxy decision making.
- As pediatric bio-banking and multi-omics screening continues to expand, ethical data management—returning results, secondary findings, and incidental findings is paramount.

iv. Dynamic Clinical Presentation and Therapy:

- Given that the pediatric presentation of many diseases can change as a child develops, continuous therapy modification must occur to account for changes in physiology and pharmacodynamics.
- Precision dosing, dynamic biomarker monitoring, and adaptive therapies can only be enabled by advanced, AI-supported clinical decision

support mechanisms; however, these infrastructures are not standard in pediatric health systems.

v. Implementation and Workforce Gaps:

- To truly see success with pediatric precision medicine, pediatricians, geneticists, data scientists and ethicists must collaborate.
- Gaps exist today regarding clinician digital literacy, bioinformatics specialist access, and AI technology enacted workflows in pediatric settings. Furthermore, if resource-limited settings are denied access to these technologies there is a risk of widening disparities.

AI in Diagnostics

- AI is transforming pediatric diagnostics by enabling precision detection and classification of childhood diseases across imaging, genomics, transcriptomic and pathology modalities.
- In pediatrics, deep learning–based image analysis (especially convolutional neural networks) supports early identification of disorders by detecting subtle developmental or phenotypic features on radiology, retinal, or facial images that may be overlooked by clinicians.
- Beyond imaging, integrated multi-omics AI systems combine genomic, transcriptomic, and proteomic information with clinical data to identify disease subtypes, supporting early diagnosis of rare pediatric genetic and metabolic conditions.
- These AI-enabled diagnostic solutions underpin personalized pediatric care by improving timeliness, accuracy and consistency of diagnosis, and aligning further treatment decisions with each child's molecular and pathophysiological profile.
- The development of explainable AI (XAI) is critical in pediatrics, as it helps build clinician trust by providing interpretable links between algorithm outputs and the underlying disease mechanisms — enabling transparency for families and physicians.

AI in Drug Discovery and Dosing

- AI has accelerated the drug development pipeline, from target identification and in-silico molecular screening to prediction of pharmacokinetic and pharmacodynamics properties in children.

- In pediatrics, machine learning models are used to identify drug–gene interactions and optimise new therapeutic molecules for rare pediatric cancers and orphan diseases.
- During clinical care, precision dosing algorithms leverage pharmacogenomics markers, EHRs, and real-time vitals to personalise medication regimens, helping tailor therapy to a child's developmental stage and genetic profile while reducing toxicity.
- Although highly promising, widespread adoption of AI-based dosing tools in pediatrics is hampered by regulatory, validation and interoperability hurdles — necessitating pediatric-specific approval pathways and data standards.

AI in Predictive Analytics and Disease Modelling

- AI-driven predictive analytics synthesise clinical, genetic, environmental, and behavioural data streams to generate individualised risk scores, forecast disease progression, and predict hospitalisation or relapse.
- In personalised pediatric medicine, these tools identify children at risk of early-onset conditions (e.g., asthma, congenital heart complications, neurodevelopmental disorders), enabling proactive, rather than reactive, management strategies.
- Advanced ML/DL techniques capture non-linear relationships and heterogeneous disease trajectories, supporting more accurate pediatric-specific prognostic models while continuously improving through *learning health systems* that adapt to evolving clinical input.

AI with Wearable Technologies and Real-Time Monitoring

- The integration of AI with wearables and Internet of Medical Things (IoMT) technologies enables continuous real-time monitoring of pediatric patients outside traditional clinical environments — fostering personalized, participatory care.
- Biosensor-equipped wearables record parameters such as heart rate, glucose levels, respiratory rate, and physical activity, generating rich longitudinal datasets. AI algorithms detect early anomalies (e.g., hypoglycemia in Type-1 diabetic children), support remote chronic-disease management, and trigger timely alerts for intervention.
- These systems empower children and caregivers by promoting engagement and augmenting home-based care, although successful deployment must address persistent concerns surrounding data privacy, cybersecurity, accuracy, and transparency of AI–IoMT platforms.

Overall, these AI applications show significant promise in advancing precision pediatrics, where individualized diagnostics, therapeutics, and continuous monitoring converge to improve outcomes. The impact and advantages of such approaches are particularly critical in current pediatric healthcare, where early and personalized interventions can transform lifelong trajectories. Table 2 shows the comparison of AI implementation challenges and solutions in pediatric precision medicine.

Table 2. Comparison of AI Implementation Challenges and Solutions in Pediatric Precision Medicine

Challenges	Proposed Solutions
Data availability	• Develop longitudinal pediatric biobanks • Promote inclusive data collection across ethnic and geographic groups
Model transparency	• Implement explainable AI frameworks • Integrate causality into clinical decision tools
Ethical concerns	• Use dynamic consent models • Employ privacy-preserving techniques like federated learning
Regulatory gaps	• Establish pediatric-specific AI guidelines • Include post-deployment monitoring
Clinical integration	• Design interoperable systems • Tune alerts for age-specific, context-sensitive thresholds
Workforce preparedness	• Introduce AI education in medical training • Promote interdisciplinary collaboration

Steps for Technical Integration of AI in Pediatrics

- Identify clinical needs in pediatric care where AI can provide measurable benefit (e.g., early diagnosis of rare disease, drug dosing support).
- Evaluate existing datasets for developmental suitability and representativeness (neonates, infants, children, adolescents).
- Build explainable and stratified AI models tailored to pediatric physiological variations and age-specific data features.
- Test algorithms across age groups, and across multiple institutions to validate generalizability and clinical relevance.
- Collaborate with regulators to develop pediatric-focused pathways for model approval with attention to ethics and safety.
- Implement in clinical practice with continuous feedback from clinicians, families and ethicists, enabling iterative improvement and trust-building.

RECOMMENDATIONS FOR FUTURE RESEARCH AND PRACTICE

- Build large and diverse datasets that are specific to pediatric subjects: produce longitudinal, multi-omics, clinically annotated datasets that reflect childhood development in its entire heterogeneity across age, ethnicities, and socio-economic settings. Standardize protocols for data collection, normalization, and annotation, which would help uphold the robust training, validation, and regulatory approval of pediatric AI.
- Further the establishment of privacy-preserving learning infrastructures: advance research in federated learning and secure computation within multi-site pediatric consortia so that AI may be collaboratively developed without infringing data sovereignty or privacy. Conduct comparative studies against centralized models and strengthen hybrid systems using techniques such as differential privacy and homomorphic encryption.
- Promote explainability, causality, and trust: mandate the integration of interpretable and causally grounded AI outputs during model development to enhance clinician, regulator, and caregiver acceptance. Evaluation metrics should move beyond prediction accuracy to include transparency, usability, and clinical logic — essential for effective decision-making in real-world pediatric use.
- Ensure equitable, bias-mitigated pediatric AI: integrate continuous auditing and "age-aware" ethical protocols (dynamic consent, child-rights impact assessment) to minimize algorithmic bias. Evaluate the real-world impacts of pediatric AI systems across populations and iteratively optimise equity of access and benefit.
- Build adaptive, age-specific regulatory pathways: move beyond static approval models to dynamic regulatory frameworks that accommodate evolving "learning" AI systems. Encourage collaboration among regulators, clinicians, data scientists, and family advocates to co-design age-stratified validation studies, post-market surveillance, and risk-mitigation strategies.
- Invest in infrastructure and workforce for seamless AI deployment: expand digital infrastructure, interoperability of pediatric EHRS, and multidisciplinary training (clinicians, data scientists, ethicists) to support AI integration across the continuum of pediatric care — from preventive community care through critical care settings.
- Develop age-adaptive and trajectory-focused AI models: create AI systems that track and predict individual health trajectories across childhood and adolescence, incorporating time-series analysis, dynamic risk prediction, and

developmentally adaptive modelling to reflect physiologic maturation, exposure accumulation, and shifts in disease susceptibility over time.

FUTURE RESEARCH DIRECTIONS

Integrating AI with Genomics and Pharmacogenomics

Artificial intelligence is more closely linked to genomics and pharmacogenomics with a view to pushing personalized pediatric medicine. Presently available machine learning and deep learning methods are capable of quickly analyzing complex datasets, including genomic, epigenomics, and transcriptomic data in children, identifying hitherto unnoticed patterns associated with early disease manifestation, progression, and treatment response. AI algorithms facilitate child-specific disease risk prediction and therapeutic decision-making by only identifying unique genetic variants or actionable biomarkers.

Now advanced integrative platforms fuse multi-omics (genomic, transcriptomic, epigenomics, proteomic) data with phenotypic and clinical pediatric profiles in order to allow granular patient stratification, the basic requirement for early detection and customized care. Such systems medicine approaches mirror the multifactorial personality of childhood disease, simultaneously integrating genome, development, environmental impact, and lifestyle factors. AI-enhanced pharmacogenomics thus further advances pediatric therapeutic approaches by understanding how age-dependent genetic polymorphisms affect drug metabolism, efficacy, and toxicity. Then, these platforms will iteratively learn from real-world practice to refine personalized treatment plans for children over time, thereby strengthening safer drug use and agile applications of individualized disease prevention.

Early Intervention Tools Powered by AI

From Intervention to Prediction-Preservation: AI Early Intervention Tools, are Going to Make a Paradigm Shift in Pediatric Precision Healthcare. Multimodal data streams from genetics, EHRs, behavioral signals, and IoMT-based biosensors are analyzed by advanced ML algorithms, which are capable of identifying subclinical aberrations and forecasting disease trajectories before the onset of symptoms. These early warning systems can trigger risk stratification tailored to individual needs and allow clinician intervention in the early stages of the disease that are highly modifiable.

At the point of care, AI-enabled clinical decision support tools consume real-time pediatric data to drive screening, diagnostics, and medication decisions at the bedside, allowing for dynamic context-sensitive early management decisions.

High-explainability AI models are able to build transparency that helps clinicians and parents alike understand why a certain prediction is made; this fosters trust and increases engagement in shared decision-making — integral towards successfully accomplishing personalized pediatric care.

Role of Federated Learning and Privacy-Preserving AI

Data collection for pediatric precision medicine includes numerous sensitive information in the form of genomic, clinical, and behavioural from which much can be derived to bring about privacy concerns. Federated learning and privacy-preserving methods are powerful contenders against traditional centralized approaches in pediatrics. In a federated setting, children's hospitals and research institutes can train an AI model collectively without sharing patient information; they only share encrypted model parameters or updates, thereby ensuring privacy, security, and adherence to regulatory practices such as the GDPR.

Parallel privacy-resilient approaches based on differential privacy, secure multiparty computation, and homomorphic encryption would eliminate the risk of unauthorized re-identification and misuse of pediatric data while at the same time allow high-utility analyses. By ensuring adequate protection of minors' rights and their data ownership, these strategies provide families of children and institutions with more incentives to collaborate in developing diverse and representative pediatric AI models. When combined with explainable AI frameworks, federated and privacy-preserving methods ensure that pediatric precision tools stay ethical, legally valid, and socially acceptable.

CONCLUSION

The incorporation of artificial intelligence into pediatric precision medicine represents a substantial movement away from a traditional, symptom-associated, and healthcare to a new realm of individualization and systems-based care approaches. AI allows the integration of complicated, layered data - genomics, epigenomics, environmental exposures, and clinical records. This will allow accurate clinical phenotyping, which can lead to early targeted interventions tailored to the unique developmental patterns of children and their exposures to the environment.

Recent developments highlight how AI methodologies have pushed the boundaries of diagnostics, drug discovery, dosing, disease modeling, and real-time monitoring through the enhancement of accuracy and efficiency in medicine to provide health care professionals the potential to deliver proactive and participatory care rather than reactive care. AI is moving precision medicine in the direction of real-time, contextualized, and adaptable clinical decision-making, enabled by the integration of multi-omics that are linked to electronic health records and Internet of Medical Things (IoMT) devices.

Nevertheless, this advancement presents serious challenges. Not being able to find a representative database is a unique challenge for pediatrics, creating major limitations on the generalizations and validity of AI-created data in children, and also creating challenges in the regulatory aspects of clinical validation through pediatric life stages.

Data privacy and ethical challenges are greater for children due to issues like developing consent, the risk of higher re-identification, and the greater societal obligation to govern data about children. The black box nature of many advanced AI systems makes issues of trusted clinician acceptance and regulatory acceptance much greater, stressing the importance of explainable and causable AI systems in healthcare settings.

The pediatric field will need to address the challenges of responsibly utilizing the transformative power of AI into pediatric precision medicine. Priorities will include using federated AI and privacy-preserving or federated AI to allow for secure multi-institutional learning while protecting individual and institutional data sovereignty, use age and/or developmentally classified datasets with appropriate metadata, and put in place ethical principles on transparency, bias, and informed consent.

Development of explainable AI models through explanation types will include serious consideration of models that provide not just the prediction, but also the ethics, rationale, and causal reasoning of the prediction. This will be important for regulatory compliance and equity of care for patients and trust for clinicians.

In summary, the union of AI with pediatric precision medicine is rapidly transforming both the science and practice of child healthcare. When guided by multidisciplinary collaboration, ethical stewardship, and a commitment to transparency and inclusivity, AI promises to deliver more effective, safer, and context-sensitive care for children laying the groundwork for a new era of personalized, equitable, and systems-driven medicine.

REFERENCES

Abdullah, R. M., Saad, L. A., Alasmari, Z. M., Ali, G. A., & Muniasamy, A. (2025). Human disease prediction mobile application using machine learning. In Alareeni, B., & Hamdan, A. (Eds.), *IoT and digital transformation: Innovating business models for the connected world (ICBT 2024). Lecture notes in networks and systems* (Vol. 1575). Springer., DOI: 10.1007/978-3-032-00450-5_19

Bzdok, D., & Meyer-Lindenberg, A. (2018). Machine learning for precision psychiatry: Opportunities and challenges. *Biological Psychiatry: Cognitive Neuroscience and Neuroimaging*, *3*(3), 223–230. DOI: 10.1016/j.bpsc.2017.11.007 PMID: 29486863

Char, D. S., Shah, N. H., & Magnus, D. (2018). Implementing machine learning in health care—Addressing ethical challenges. *The New England Journal of Medicine*, *378*(11), 981–983. DOI: 10.1056/NEJMp1714229 PMID: 29539284

Delahanty, R. J., Alvarez, J., Flynn, L. M., Sherwin, R. L., & Jones, S. S. (2019). Development and evaluation of a machine learning model for the early identification of sepsis in pediatric patients. *JAMA Network Open*, *2*(10), e1914377. DOI: 10.1001/jamanetworkopen.2019.14377

Domingues, C., Jarak, I., Veiga, F., Dourado, M., & Figueiras, A. (2023, October 6). Pediatric Drug Development: Reviewing Challenges and Opportunities by Tracking Innovative Therapies. *Pharmaceutics*, *15*(10), 2431. DOI: 10.3390/pharmaceutics15102431 PMID: 37896191

Doshi-Velez, F., & Kim, B. (2017). Towards a rigorous science of interpretable machine learning. *arXiv preprint arXiv:1702.08608.* https://doi.org//arXiv.1702.08608DOI: 10.48550

Esteva, A., Kuprel, B., Novoa, R. A., Ko, J., Swetter, S. M., Blau, H. M., & Thrun, S. (2017). Dermatologist-level classification of skin cancer with deep neural networks. *Nature*, *542*(7639), 115–118. DOI: 10.1038/nature21056 PMID: 28117445

Gurovich, Y., Hanani, Y., Bar, O., Nadav, G., Fleischer, N., Gelbman, D., & Kamphausen, S. B. (2019). Identifying facial phenotypes of genetic disorders using deep learning. *Nature Medicine*, *25*(1), 60–64. DOI: 10.1038/s41591-018-0279-0 PMID: 30617323

Johnson, K. B., Wei, W. Q., Weeraratne, D., Frisse, M. E., Misulis, K., Rhee, K., & Denny, J. C. (2018). Precision medicine, AI, and the future of personalized health care. *Clinical Pharmacology and Therapeutics*, *103*(3), 362–364. DOI: 10.1002/cpt.1015

Kaissis, G. A., Makowski, M. R., Rückert, D., & Braren, R. F. (2020). Secure, privacy-preserving and federated machine learning in medical imaging. *Nature Machine Intelligence*, *2*(6), 305–311. DOI: 10.1038/s42256-020-0186-1

Moradveisi, B., Muwakkit, S., Zamani, F., Ghaderi, E., Mohammadi, E., & Zgheib, N. K. (2019, August 27). *ITPA, TPMT*, and *NUDT15* Genetic Polymorphisms Predict 6-Mercaptopurine Toxicity in Middle Eastern Children With Acute Lymphoblastic Leukemia. *Frontiers in Pharmacology*, *10*, 916. DOI: 10.3389/fphar.2019.00916 PMID: 31507415

Muniasamy, A. (2025). Revolutionizing health monitoring: Integrating transformer models with multi-head attention for precise human activity recognition using wearable devices. *Technology and Health Care*, *33*(1), 395–409. https://content.iospress.com/articles/technology-and-health-care/thc241064. DOI: 10.3233/THC-241064 PMID: 39269866

Muniasamy, A., & Alasmari, A. (2025). Integrating Bayesian and convolution neural network for uncertainty estimation of cataract from fundus images. *Computer Modeling in Engineering & Sciences*, *143*(1), 569–592. DOI: 10.32604/cmes.2025.060484

Muniasamy, A., & Asiri, F. (2025). Advanced human activity recognition on wearables with multi-scale sparse attention. *Multimedia Tools and Applications*, *84*(30), 36623–36652. Advance online publication. DOI: 10.1007/s11042-024-20475-6

Muniasamy, A., Begum, A., Sabahath, A., Yaqub, H., & Karunakaran, G. (2023). Lung cancer histopathology image classification using transfer learning with convolution neural network model. *Technology and Health Care*, *33*, 1–12. https://content.iospress.com/articles/technology-and-health-care/thc231029 PMID: 37270826

Muniasamy, A., Begum, A., Sabahath, A., Yaqub, H., & Karunakaran, G. (2024). Coronary heart disease classification using deep learning approach with feature selection for improved accuracy. *Technology and Health Care*, *32*(3), 1991–2007. DOI: 10.3233/THC-231807 PMID: 38339946

Muniasamy, A., Bhatnagar, R., & Karunakaran, G. (2021). Predicting COVID-19 spread in Saudi Arabia using artificial intelligence techniques—Proposing a shift towards a sustainable healthcare approach. In Hassanien, A., Bhatnagar, R., & Darwish, A. (Eds.), *Artificial intelligence for sustainable development: Theory, practice and future applications. Studies in computational intelligence* (Vol. 912). Springer., DOI: 10.1007/978-3-030-51920-9_6

Muniasamy, A., & Karunakaran, G. (2026). Challenges and future directions: Emerging trends and limitations in ML and optimization for healthcare. In Muniasamy, A. (Ed.), *Integrative machine learning and optimization algorithms for disease prediction* (pp. 339–368). IGI Global., DOI: 10.4018/979-8-3373-1087-9.ch012

Muniasamy, A., Muniasamy, V., & Bhatnagar, R. (2021). Predictive analytics for cardiovascular disease diagnosis using machine learning techniques. In Hassanien, A., Bhatnagar, R., & Darwish, A. (Eds.), *Advanced machine learning technologies and applications (AMLTA 2020). Advances in intelligent systems and computing* (Vol. 1141). Springer., DOI: 10.1007/978-981-15-3383-9_45

Pepic, I., Feldt, R., Ljungström, L., Torkar, R., Dalevi, D., Maurin Söderholm, H., Andersson, L.-M., Axelson-Fisk, M., Bohm, K., Sjöqvist, B. A., & Candefjord, S. (2021). Early detection of sepsis using artificial intelligence: A scoping review protocol. *Systematic Reviews*, *10*(1), 28. DOI: 10.1186/s13643-020-01561-w PMID: 33453724

Poplin, R., Chang, P. C., Alexander, D., Schwartz, S., Colthurst, T., Ku, A., Newburger, D., Dijamco, J., Nguyen, N., Afshar, P. T., Gross, S. S., Dorfman, L., McLean, C. Y., & DePristo, M. A. (2018). A universal SNP and small-indel variant caller using deep neural networks. *Nature Biotechnology*, *36*(10), 983–987. DOI: 10.1038/nbt.4235 PMID: 30247488

Rajkomar, A., Dean, J., & Kohane, I. (2019). Machine learning in medicine. *The New England Journal of Medicine*, *380*(14), 1347–1358. DOI: 10.1056/NEJMra1814259 PMID: 30943338

Rengaramanujam, K., & Muniasamy, A. (2026). AI in hospital administration and formulary design: Optimizing resource allocation and patient flow. In Muniasamy, A., & Karunakaran, G. (Eds.), *Applications of artificial intelligence in pharmaceuticals* (pp. 215–246). IGI Global., DOI: 10.4018/979-8-3373-2043-4.ch008

Tonekaboni, S., Joshi, S., McCradden, M. D., & Goldenberg, A. (2019). What clinicians want: Contextualizing explainable machine learning for clinical end use. *Proceedings of the Machine Learning Research, 106*, 359–380. https://proceedings.mlr.press/v106/tonekaboni19a.html

Topol, E. (2019). *Deep medicine: How artificial intelligence can make healthcare human again*. Basic Books.

Van Driest SL, McGregor TL. Pharmacogenetics in clinical pediatrics: challenges and strategies. Per Med. 2013 Sep;10(7):. .DOI: 10.2217/pme.13.70

Wilkinson, M. D., Dumontier, M., Aalbersberg, I. J., Appleton, G., Axton, M., Baak, A., Blomberg, N., Boiten, J.-W., da Silva Santos, L. B., Bourne, P. E., Bouwman, J., Brookes, A. J., Clark, T., Crosas, M., Dillo, I., Dumon, O., Edmunds, S., Evelo, C. T., Finkers, R., & Mons, B. (2016). The FAIR guiding principles for scientific data management and stewardship. *Scientific Data*, *3*(1), 160018. DOI: 10.1038/sdata.2016.18 PMID: 26978244

ADDITIONAL READING

Boemer, F., Hovhannesyan, K., Piazzon, F., Minner, F., Mni, M., Jacquemin, V., Mashhadizadeh, D., Benmhammed, N., Bours, V., Jacquinet, A., Harvengt, J., Bulk, S., Dideberg, V., Helou, L., Palmeira, L., Dangouloff, T., Alkan, S., Barrea, C., Bartoszek, P., & Servais, L. (2025). Population-based, first-tier genomic newborn screening in the maternity ward. *Nature Medicine*, *31*(4), 1339–1350. DOI: 10.1038/s41591-024-03465-x PMID: 39875687

Chng, S. Y., Tern, M. J. W., Lee, Y. S., Cheng, L. T., Kapur, J., Eriksson, J. G., Chong, Y. S., & Savulescu, J. (2025). Ethical considerations in AI for child health and recommendations for child-centered medical AI. *NPJ Digital Medicine*, *8*(1), 152. DOI: 10.1038/s41746-025-01541-1 PMID: 40065130

Muralidharan, V., Schamroth, J., Youssef, A., Celi, L. A., & Daneshjou, R. (2024). Applied artificial intelligence for global child health: Addressing biases and barriers. *PLOS Digital Health*, *3*(8), e0000583. DOI: 10.1371/journal.pdig.0000583 PMID: 39172772

Zhang, K., Shi, X., Xie, S. S., Sun, J. H., Liu, Z. H., Zhang, S., Song, J. Y., & Shen, W. (2022). Deep learning image reconstruction in pediatric abdominal and chest computed tomography: A comparison of image quality and radiation dose. *Quantitative Imaging in Medicine and Surgery*, *12*(6), 3238–3250. DOI: 10.21037/qims-21-936 PMID: 35655845

KEY TERMS AND DEFINITIONS

Artificial Intelligence (AI): The simulation of human intelligence processes by machines, especially computer systems, to perform tasks such as learning, reasoning, problem-solving, and decision-making in clinical environments.

Clinical: Decision Support System (CDSS): A digital tool or software application designed to assist healthcare professionals in making evidence-based clinical decisions by analyzing patient data and providing actionable recommendations.

Deep Learning: A type of machine learning that uses neural networks with multiple layers to model complex patterns in data, especially useful in analyzing medical images and genomic sequences.

Electronic Health Record (EHR): A digital version of a patient's paper chart that contains medical history, diagnoses, medications, treatment plans, and test results, which can be used by AI systems for predictive modeling.

Explainable AI (XAI): An approach to developing AI such that final outputs of the machine learning model can be understood or interpreted by the human user, in recognition of trust, transparency, and accountability in healthcare.

Federated Learning: A privacy-preserving ML approach wherein AI models are built upon decentralized data sources without shipping sensitive data to any central server.

Genomics: The study of the entire DNA set (including all genes) of an organism, pivotal for understanding genetic diseases and making room for methods of personalized medicine.

Pediatric Precision Medicine: A medical approach that designs treatment and prevention strategies to fit each child with genetic, environmental, and lifestyle factors specific to his developmental stage.

Pharmacogenomics: The study of how genes govern a person's response to drugs, therefore making medics develop safer either through drugs or in conjunction with drugs that fit an individual's genetic profile.

Wearable Technologies: These are electronic devices worn on or around the body that record health data, such as heart rate, oxygen saturation, and activity levels, in real time, thus enabling AI-based interventions.

Chapter 7
Optimizing Hospital Workflows Through Artificial Intelligence

Karthic Sundaram
https://orcid.org/0000-0002-0968-8468
Department of Computing Technologies, SRM Institute of Science and Technology, Chennai, India

S. Vinu
Department of Computing Technologies, SRM Institute of Science and Technology, Chennai, India

Arunkumar Ramamoorthy
Digital Forensics and Cyber Security, University of South Wales, UK

S. Venkatesan
Department of Artificial Intelligence and Data Science, St. Joseph's Institute of Technology, Chennai, India

ABSTRACT

The integration of latest technologies like Artificial Intelligence (AI) plays a vital role in improving the Healthcare systems right from real time monitoring, health record maintenance and efficient disease diagnosis and appropriate treatment. AI systems incorporate machine learning (ML) models, Deep learning models (DL) models, IOT devices and sensor data to provide real time monitoring of patient health. AI models assess lung imaging and real-time oxygen saturation data to predict respiratory deterioration. The power of AI in predictive analytics helps in identifying disease at the early stage to plan for faster treatment and recovery. Automated documentation and AI-powered EHR enhances clinical workflows reducing errors

DOI: 10.4018/979-8-3373-2787-7.ch007

and improves patient data management. Generally, the hospitals have large amount of patient data. The usage of AI helps to derive actionable insights from these data that aids in better and faster recovery reducing mortality rates

INTRODUCTION

AI in diagnostic imaging uses machine learning algorithms to analyse X-rays, CT scans and MRIs images. These models are trained on large datasets of annotated medical images to detect abnormalities and patterns (Bekbolatova et al., 2024). It enhances radiologist interpretation, early disease detection and clinical decision support (Muniasamy et al., 2020). However, AI models require large amounts of patient data, raising ethical and privacy concerns. AI-driven drug prescription systems use ML models and big data analytics to recommend optimal medicines, dosages and treatment regimens based on patient data [Yadav et al., 2025]. These systems analyse the medical history of the patient, genetic information and lab results before making the prescriptions (Veernapu, 2022). They can help in tracking medication usage, detect adverse drug reactions and prevent overprescription. AI chatbots can provide real-time medication counselling and answer patient queries (Elhaddad et al., 2024). The chapter explores various AI techniques that contribute to accurate disease detection and personalized treatment plans. Additionally, it discusses the integration of AI with Electronic Health Records (EHR) and hospital information systems to enhance interoperability and streamline workflows (Khamaj, 2025).

Intensive Care Units (ICUs) and critical care departments handle life-threatening conditions, requiring rapid decision-making, continuous monitoring and precise interventions (Bohr & Memarzadeh,2020) AI-driven models analyse real-time patient data, detect early warning signs of complications and assist clinicians in prioritizing interventions. This section explores the role of predictive AI in ICU and critical care applications. Robotic-assisted surgery (RAS) involves the use of AI-powered robotic systems that aid surgeons in performing complex procedures with enhanced precision and control (Iftikhar et al., 2024; Muniasamy & Karunakaran et al., 2026). These systems assist surgeons by providing real-time insights in improving dexterity and enabling minimally invasive procedures. This section explores the role of AI in robotic-assisted surgeries and its impact in AI-driven operating rooms. Despite its transformative potential, AI implementation in patient monitoring presents challenges. The possible ways to address the challenges are discussed in the chapter.

AI-driven solutions enable hospitals to optimize scheduling, automate administrative tasks, enhance clinical workflows and improve overall hospital management. Efficient appointment scheduling and patient flow management are essential in optimizing hospital operations, reducing wait times and improving patient satisfaction

(Munavalli et al., 2020; Gauthaman et al., 2026). Efficient appointment scheduling and patient flow management are critical to optimizing hospital operations, reducing wait times and improving patient satisfaction (Ala et al., 2022). This section explores the role of AI in optimizing hospital workflows, its key applications, benefits, challenges and future directions. By providing a discussion of AI in real-time patient monitoring and predictive analytics, the chapter elaborates the importance of AI in modern healthcare while addressing the barriers to its widespread adoption. AI driven healthcare solutions help reduce operational expenses, minimize waste, enhance workforce efficiency and ensure better management of medical equipment, supplies and staff. Hospitals can streamline workflows, prevent unnecessary expenses with high quality of treatment to patients

The chapter also discusses the possible future direction of AI in healthcare sector. Federated learning allows hospitals to train AI models on decentralized patient data without sharing sensitive information (Dhade & Shirke, 2024). This approach enhances privacy and data security while enabling AI systems to learn from vast, diverse datasets across multiple hospitals. The next generation of wearable devices and biosensors can be equipped with AI to continuously monitor vital signs, detect anomalies and provide real-time alerts. The data from these devices will enable early detection for chronic diseases like cardiovascular disorders, diabetes and respiratory illnesses. In future AI models can analyse genetic data, life style and influential factors to create personalized healthcare plans. This will help in focussing on disease prevention rather focusing on disease detection.

Hospital workflow management requires to handle variety of challenges due to its own complexity and necessity to satisfy the requirements of diverse stakeholders and also due to the rapid evolving technologies in the field of medicine. This chapter describes an overview of the possible challenges prevailing in healthcare sector.

Fragmented Data and Lack of Interoperability

The major challenge faced in hospitals is the fragmented nature of the healthcare data. Many hospitals utilize variety of platforms to handle patient information like EHRs, patient imaging, radiology information and billing and payment information. Most of these data remain fragmented and not integrated.

Hospital workflow requires monitoring and managing of clinical cost of and administrative process to ensure effective patient care. Workflow management is essential in health care organizations to ensure optimal usage of resources and minimized delays. Generally, in hospitals the workflow spans among various departments like emergency, ICU, pharmacy, radiology and so on. However, the traditional work flow management hospital environment using manual procedures suffers in communication bottlenecks leading to poor patient experience (Susan

Abraham, 2024; Gauthaman et al., 2026). The increasing demands for healthcare services in countries like India with huge population requires usage of latest technologies to provide better experience and improved healthcare treatments. Work flow management in hospitals deals about real time decision making, patient monitoring and effective usage of resources and manpower. With the power AI hospitals can optimize the workflow efficiently.

Table 1. Challenges and possible solutions

Challenge	Description	Possible Solution
Fragmented Systems & Data Silos	Disconnected systems impede data flow between departments.	Integrate AI middleware for unified data access
Poor Care Coordination	Delayed communication among departments affects patient care.	Deploy AI-driven clinical communication platforms; implement real-time dashboards and smart alerts.
High Administrative Workload	Clinicians spend significant time on paperwork, billing and documentation.	Automate routine documentation using NLP; apply robotic process automation (RPA) for billing and claims.
Resource Allocation Inefficiencies	Operating rooms, ICU beds and staff are often under- or over-utilized.	Use predictive analytics and AI scheduling systems for optimal resource allocation.
Delayed Decision-Making	Slow access to diagnostics and patient data hinders timely interventions.	Integrate real-time data pipelines; implement AI-based clinical decision support systems (CDSS).
Non-Standardized Workflows	Variability in protocols and SOPs across departments causes inconsistencies.	Standardize clinical pathways; train AI models on unified SOPs for reliable automation.
Resistance to Technological Change	Staff reluctant to adopt AI due to usability issues or lack of trust.	Conduct regular training; implement user-centered design; showcase pilot successes for buy-in.
Compliance & Privacy Concerns	Ensuring data security and regulatory compliance is challenging.	Use AI tools with explainability (XAI); implement role-based access controls and audit trails.
Limited Real-Time Monitoring	Absence of live tracking for patient flow, diagnostics, or resource usage.	Deploy IoT and AI-powered monitoring systems for real-time situational awareness.
Lack of Predictive Capabilities	Hospitals struggle to anticipate surges, readmissions, or equipment failure.	Use AI models for patient risk stratification, demand forecasting and predictive maintenance.

Poor Care Coordination

Care coordination is important in healthcare sector to ensure efficient and timely delivery of medical services to the patients. In majority of the hospitals the departments like ICU, emergency care, pharmacy and radiology operate independently. As a result, the patient information is fragmented and causes delayed information exchange leading to delayed decisions. Patient may be moved between departments as part of the treatment and this requires transfer of enough data across departments (Rahman et al.,2024). A consistent method is required to ensure the correctness and enough information to avoid medical errors and prompt treatment. Maintaining centralized repository or unified patient record can provide easy and faster access to the patient information eliminating medical errors. Most of the hospitals do not possess automated monitoring systems or AI-driven alerts. As a result, the hospitals struggle to proactively manage tasks, track critical changes in patient status, or ensure timely execution of care actions. These flaws contribute to prolonged hospital stays, increased costs, reduced staff productivity and reduced patient satisfaction. Addressing poor care coordination is thus vital for creating a more integrated, efficient and patient-centered healthcare system.

High Administrative Workload

Another major challenge faced by hospital is the necessity to manage the workload of healthcare professionals ranging from physicians, nurses, radiologist to skilled labours. The physicians spend their valuable time in maintaining the patient information and data entry into multiple healthcare systems. Automation with proper interface and utilization of AI based tools can reduce the workload of physicians leading to enhanced accuracy and workflow continuity (Alves et al., 2024). The summary of key administrative workload and its impact is specified in Table 2.

Table 2. Summary of High Administrative Workload in Hospitals

Aspect	Description
Key Tasks Involved	Documentation, billing, reporting, Patient data entry across systems
Primary Affected Roles	Physicians, nurses, administrative and billing staff
Major Causes	Lack of integration between systems, repetitive manual tasks, poor UI/UX
Impacts on Healthcare Providers	Reduced patient interaction time, increased stress and burnout
Operational Consequences	Lower efficiency, increased documentation errors, poor workflow continuity
Risks to Patient Care	Missed clinical updates, delays in care delivery, compromised decision-making

Resource Allocation Inefficiencies

To ensure smooth operation of functionalities and to deliver structural healthcare operations effective allocation of resources in hospitals is essential. The key resources include beds, wheel chairs, operation theatres, ICUs, medical equipment and so on. Many hospitals often lack in effective utilization of these resources (Suryawanshi, et al.,2024; Naim et al., 2026). These inefficiencies often stem from a lack of real-time visibility into resource availability, outdated scheduling systems and absence of data-driven forecasting tools. Manual scheduling and poor integration between departments in bottlenecks, increased patient wait times, inefficient use of high-cost equipment and even financial losses (Guo et al., 2024). Hospitals can use AI tools to ensure efficient resource allocation by predictive planning and intelligent decision support. AI tools can leverage historical information and real-time hospital information systems to ensure that the medical resources such as staff, beds, equipment and operating rooms are used optimally and effectively.

BACKGROUND

AI Technologies Enabling Workflow Optimization

It is necessary to provide efficient workflow in hospitals to ensure quality healthcare. It also optimizes various resources of the hospitals like human resource, reduced cost and maximizing patient experiences. AI possess the capability to streamline and automate the workflow of hospitals intelligently. Table 3 provides an overview of application of AI in optimizing the workflow process.

Table 3. Application AI in hospital workflow optimization

AI Technology	Key Applications in Workflow Optimization
Machine Learning (ML)	Forecasting admissions, dynamic staffing, clinical risk prediction
Natural Language Processing	Automating documentation, extracting structured data from text
Robotic Process Automation	Automating administrative and repetitive backend tasks
Computer Vision (CV)	Patient monitoring, diagnostic imaging, resource tracking
Predictive Analytics	Resource forecasting, demand planning, early warning systems
Virtual Assistants / Chatbots	Patient interaction, staff support, task triaging
Decision Support Systems	Clinical alerts, treatment recommendations, protocol adherence

Clinical Applications of AI For Workflow Efficiency

AI in Patient Admission and Triage (Figure 1)

The idea to involve Artificial Intelligence (AI) into healthcare is truly changing the scenario especially from patient admission and triage in high complex places like Emergency Department (EDs). These divisions face a lot of issues like overcrowding, shortage of staff members and urgent requirements for immediate interventions. Traditionally, triage is dependent on doctors and healthcare professionals to prioritize the patients based on their health conditions (Friedman et al., 2024).

But we need accept the fact that human error, time constraints and limitations in providing the information can really make things worse in aspects of accuracy and quick triage service provided to the patients. This is where AI driven triage system could help in. AI can tackle these challenges by analysing the large amount of real-time data related to symptoms, vital signs, health record and environmental factors to create impressive report about the patients in a speedy and reliable way. These systems use Machine Learning (ML) algorithms which is trained on millions of datasets on patient records, helping to find the patterns of disease which is tougher with human diagnosis (Porto, 2024; Muniasamy et al., 2020).

Additionally, Natural Language Processing (NLP) can highly help in bringing the valuable insights from unstructured data like notes by the doctor, which can boost their ability to understand patient needs. For example, AI can sort the patients into triage categories as soon as they arrived at the Emergency Department. In a case study across various urban hospitals, systems have shown that there is a 30% drop in wait time and achieved better patient outcomes (Tahernejad, et al., 2024).

Figure 1. AI-Enhanced Triage Workflow

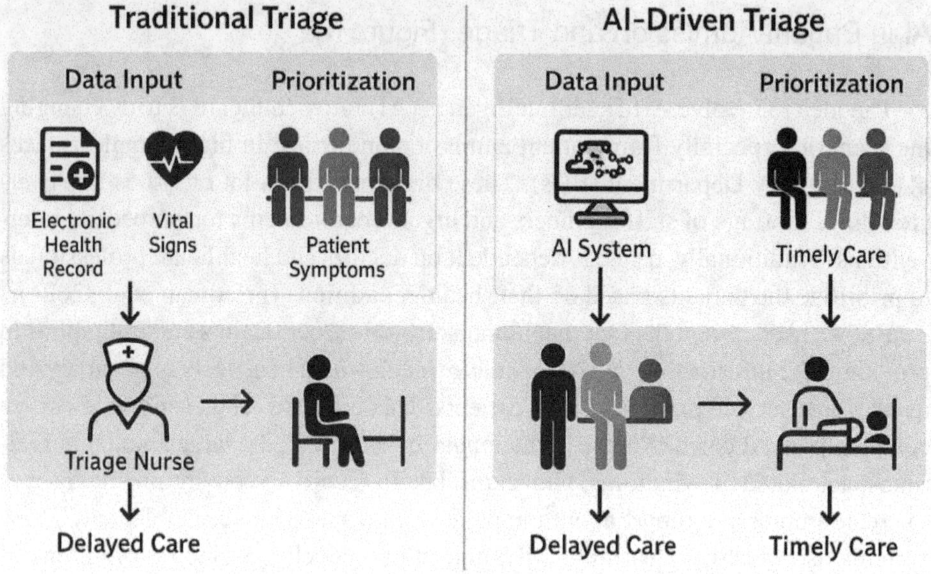

Intelligent Resource Allocation (Beds, Staff, Equipment – Figure 2)

In resource management, AI plays a transformative role to provide healthcare facilities. There are few complex challenges like dynamic, real-time decisions on allocating hospital beds, staff schedules, diagnostic equipment and operating rooms. If there is a poor resource allocation, it may lead to underutilization or burnout of resources, both of which will affect the quality of services provided to the patients and increase the cost for the organization (Ramezani et al., 2023). When combining predictive analysis and real time monitoring, AI models can predict the patient inflow, trends of equipment usage and staff workload. Through this administrator can actively manage the resources, prepare for demand surges and minimize the waste. Continuous data streams (e.g., bed occupancy, oxygen saturation levels) can be fed to the Internet of Things (IOT) devices to add another layer of intelligence for adaptive decision-making (Prabhune et al., 2025).

The World Health Organization has approved the Workload Indicators of Staffing Need (WISN) method, which has now been enhanced with AI technology. Take the PRAYOJN platform, for example; it streamlines WISN calculations by using real-time data, making it easier to predict staffing requirements across various departments and facilities (Wu et al., 2023; Rengaramanujam et al., 2026).

Also, there are many advantages, AI-driven resource planning brings up few challenges such as the requirement of high-quality data and cyber security frameworks. It must include mechanisms to address the privacy concerns with rigorous encryption and compliance mechanisms like HIPAA and GDPR.

AI-Supported Diagnostics and Decision Support Systems (Figure 3)

A significant mark is achieved in medical sector since AI has been incorporated with the system, especially in the areas of diagnostics and Clinical Decision Support Systems (CDSS). The complex clinical data can be handled effectively by using advanced algorithms to cut down the diagnostic errors and speed up the diagnosis process. For example, with respect to radiology department, AI can easily spot the issues in the lung nodules, early-stage tumours or microfractures which are tougher for a well experienced radiologist (Elgin & Elgin, 2024).

These systems are not a replacement for the role of clinicians, but they serve as “Digital Assistants”, adding more support by providing evidence-based recommendations which could boost diagnostic accuracy. CDSS are integrated with EHR (Electronic Health Record) systems to allow them to more precisely suggest on right diagnosis, flag drug interactions and suggest right treatment plans. For Example, IBM Watson Heath application leverages AI to analyse patient records and scientific literature, providing ultimate support for personalized treatment options in Oncology (Ouanes & Farhah, 2024).

In a case study conducted, the results were showing that AI-supported tools improved early detection rates of diabetic retinopathy by 40%, emphasizing their potential in preventive care. Additionally, these systems are being designed to enhance shared decision-making, taking into account both the preferences of patients and the clinical evidence when planning treatments.

Automated Discharge Planning and Follow-Up

The key critical part in hospital management is to effectively plan the discharge of the patients which will cut down the readmissions and ensure the patients continue to receive the care and support they need. Traditionally, the discharge process is bit complex with involvement of administrative tasks like coordinating prescriptions, setting follow-up appointments and guiding the patients about their care after discharging from the hospital. Once AI has stepped into healthcare, these tasks are quite easier by automating the creation of discharge summaries, scheduling and communicating after the discharge regarding the follow-up appointment and care guidance (Zaretsky et al., 2024).

One other main issue is interpretation of the medical summaries provided during the discharge, Generative AI tools could greatly help in making the patients understand in their own formats, which was greatly beneficial for those patients with low health literacy. For example, research has shown that AI-generated discharge instructions were really helpful in making the patients to understand the report by more than 50%, which decreased the follow-up visits to the emergency room. AI driven text messaging system is also implemented in Hospitals to keep track of patient's symptoms and to ensure how well they are sticking to their medication plans (Bressman et al., 2022).

This was possible due to utilization of natural language understanding to respond to the patient's questions in the timely manner. Such innovation has been greatly recognized for reducing the need for acute care after discharge as much as 25% in high risk group, showing the real benefits for both patients and healthcare institutions.

MAIN FOCUS OF THE CHAPTER

1. Operational And Administrative Optimization

In today's healthcare situation, optimizing operations and administration is utterly important. Efficiency, accuracy and quick responses are key criteria to providing top-notch patient care. That's where AI technologies come into play, helping to simplify processes, lighten the load on administrative tasks and enhance the experiences of both staff and patients alike.

Staff Scheduling and Task Automation (Figure 2)

The critical components of operational optimization in healthcare are efficient staff scheduling and task automation. There are lot of conflicts, gaps and inefficiencies due to traditional manual scheduling methods, which has negatively impacted patient care and staff satisfaction. Creating and managing schedules are automated using AI-Driven scheduling systems. It uses ML algorithms to analyse the historical information, estimate the number of staff required, optimize shift assignments. It includes the features like automated shift swapping, real-time labor cost tracking and integration with electronic health records (EHR) could improve enhance scheduling efficiency (Zayas-Cabán et al., 2023; Rengaramanujam et al., 2026). It can reduce the time spent on manual scheduling and concentrate more on patient care and strategic planning. Additionally, tools can help in task automation to optimize administrative workflows, further optimizing the burden on staff and minimizing the risk of effort burnout. AI can improve operational efficiency by setting up the automated reminders, appointment scheduling and patient communication systems, which can enhance overall healthcare experience.

AI based scheduling systems can analyze various factors like staff availability, patient demand and historical data to create optimal schedules. Additionally, they are flexible, able to handle last-minute changes and shift swaps, which means staffing levels maintained good, even when unexpected events happen. For example, a hospital that uses AI for scheduling can automatically adjust shifts based on real-time patient admissions, making sure there are enough nurses and doctors available during the busiest times. This kind of adaptability is key to keeping both patient care and staff satisfaction at high standard levels.

Task automation in healthcare goes beyond just scheduling. AI based tools can help routine administrative tasks like billing, coding and data entry can also be automated, allowing staff to dedicate their time to more complex and patient-focused activities. For example, AI can take care of generating patient discharge summaries, scheduling follow-up appointments and sending reminders to patients about their upcoming visits. These automated systems not only increase effectiveness but also improve the patient satisfaction by delivering timely and accurate information.

Figure 2. AI-Driven Staff Scheduling System Workflow

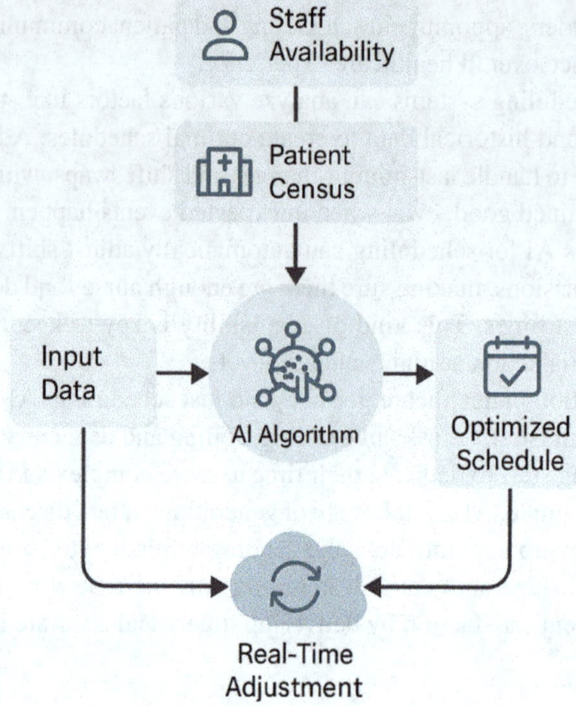

Inventory and Supply Chain Management Using AI (Figure 3)

In Healthcare facilities, Inventory and supply chain management play a vital role in running the facilities smoothly. AI technologies bring in a great revolution in the healthcare field, these areas are undergoing a transformation, offering real-time visibility, predictive analytics and automated replenishment. Traditional methods of inventory management, which often depend on manual counts and barcode scans, can be error-prone and inefficient. But AI-driven systems like Vision AI, which utilize high-resolution cameras and machine learning algorithms to keep an eye on inventory levels without any manual intervention (Howard et al., 2020). These smart systems can spot usage trends and patterns, forecast demand and automatically trigger reorders when supplies hit certain thresholds, ensuring that everything is on hand when it's needed. Automated inventory management tools, such as RFID sensors and tags, provide valuable insights that empower healthcare providers to make informed decisions about choosing suppliers, renegotiating contracts and identifying risks. By applying AI-driven inventory management, hospitals can significantly cut down on waste and improve efficiency. For instance, facilities using AI to manage their inventory can monitor the expiration dates of medical supplies, making sure items are utilized before they expire. This proactive approach minimizes the chances of running out of stock or having plenty of stock in hand, leading to significant cost savings. Additionally, AI can enhance the supply chain by forecasting future demand based on history of data and current trends, allowing healthcare facilities to plan their inventory needs more accurately and prevent any disruptions in patient care.

Automated replenishment systems, like Par-level and Kanban systems, leverage AI algorithms to keep an eye on inventory levels and forecast when supplies need to be replaced (Hezam et al., 2024; Naim et al., 2026). These smart systems can automate to create purchase orders and send them off to suppliers, making sure that inventory stays at optimal levels without needing any manual intervention. This kind of automation not only improves efficiency but also lightens the administrative load on staff, permitting them to utilize more time to disease diagnosis and treatment.

Figure 3. Smart Inventory Monitoring with Vision AI and IoT

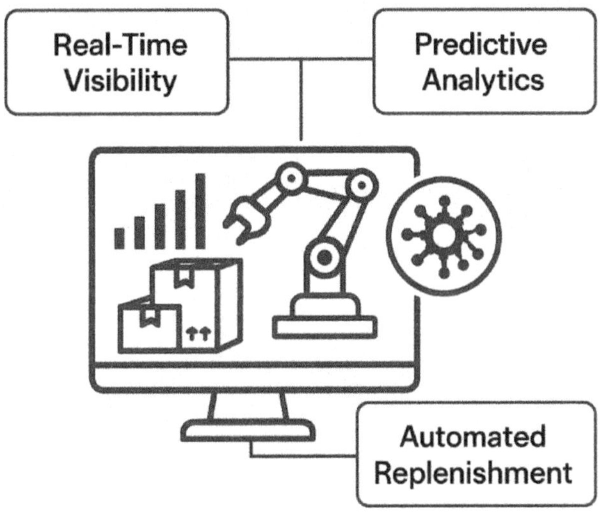

Revenue Management and Billing (Figure 4)

Revenue cycle management (RCM) is all about administering the financial aspects of billing and collecting payments for medical services. Progressing RCM right is essential for maintaining financial health and smooth operations in healthcare organizations. The RCM journey begins once a patient fixes an appointment and ends up when the account balance is remitted via insurance schemes, adjustments or direct payment methods from patients. Some of the key steps in RCM include scheduling appointments, registering patients, capturing charges, billing, managing refusals and following up on accounts receivable. AI technologies can really improve the RCM by automating these tasks, cutting down on claim denials and improving collections (Varun, 2021). For example, AI-powered systems can sift through claim data to spot trends and foresee potential denials, enabling healthcare providers to tackle issues before they escalate. Additionally, AI can enhance patient communication by offering clear pricing and financial advice, helping patients grasp their financial obligations and manage healthcare expenses more effectively. AI-driven RCM systems can also make the billing process efficient by automating the creation of accurate claims and minimizing the error rate (Fardin et al, 2024; Rengaramanujam et al., 2026).

These systems are also capable of analyzing rejection reason codes to determine common issues and take remedial actions to avoid future rejections. By cutting down on the number of rejected claims, healthcare organizations can raise their revenue collection and overall financial health. When it comes to patient communication, AI can truly excel. AI-driven chatbots and virtual assistants can offer patients valuable information about their insurance coverage, self-funded expenses and payment options. These tools can also help patients navigate the process of applying for financial assistance and setting up personalized payment plans. By adopting transparency and enhancing communication, AI can significantly improve the patient experience while alleviating some of the financial strain on healthcare organizations.

Figure 4. AI-Enhanced Revenue Cycle Workflow

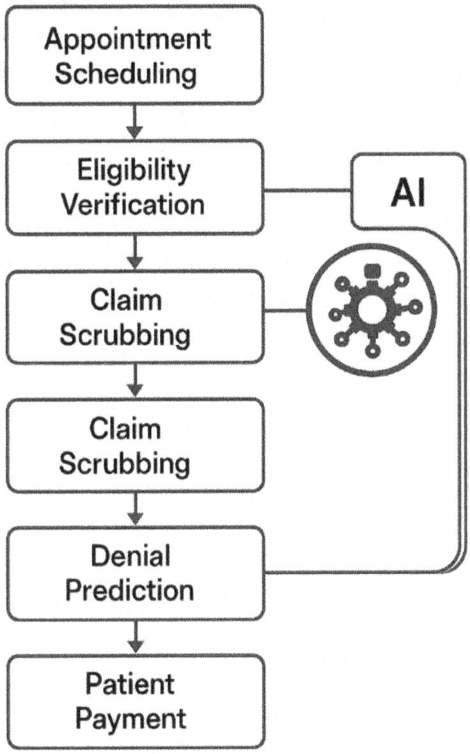

2. Interoperability and Data Integration

Integrating AI with Electronic Health Records (EHRs)

A revolutionary strategy to improve clinical decision-making and expedite hospital workflows is the integration of Artificial Intelligence (AI) with Electronic Health Records (EHRs). A multitude of patient data, such as demographics, test results, prescription drugs, allergies and clinical narratives, are stored in electronic health records (EHRs). But without AI, it could take a long time and be prone to mistakes to glean valuable insights from this data. Real-time data analysis, natural language comprehension and predictive analytics are made possible by AI, which closes this gap (Ye et al., 2024). AI can easily access and process both structured and unstructured data within EHRs by using interoperable standards like HL7 FHIR. This makes it possible to perform tasks like clinical decision support, automated risk stratification and care gap identification. Additionally, by transcribing and coding clinical notes,

AI tools can improve physician documentation while lowering administrative burden and improving data quality (Gorrepati, 2024). Clinicians can retrieve and update patient data without manual entry thanks to voice-enabled interfaces and intelligent chatbots, which further streamline EHR interactions. Creating secure data pipelines and APIs is another step in the integration process that guarantees adherence to privacy laws like HIPAA. Long-term, AI-integrated EHRs can enhance personalized medicine efforts, lower diagnostic errors and improve patient outcomes. Effective AI integration with EHRs puts hospitals in a better position to handle upcoming digital innovations and provide more effective, higher-quality care. Making sure AI enhances clinical workflows without upsetting the patient-caregiver dynamic is crucial. Table 4 shows the Benefits of AI-Integrated EHRs over Traditional HER.

Table 4. Benefits of AI-Integrated EHRs

Feature	Traditional EHR	AI-Integrated EHR
Data Analysis	Manual and slow	Real-time and automated
Decision Support	Limited	Predictive and proactive
Documentation	Manual entry	Voice-enabled, auto-coded
Interoperability	Basic	Enhanced with standards like HL7 FHIR
Workflow Efficiency	Fragmented	Streamlined

Data Silos and Standardization Challenges

The existence of data silos discrete databases or systems that store information in isolated environments often presents serious difficulties for hospitals. These silos, which use various software systems, formats and standards, are found in departments like radiology, cardiology, pathology, pharmacy and administration. A comprehensive understanding of a patient's condition is hampered as a result of the fragmented and ineffective information exchange. For AI to learn and predict effectively, it needs access to large, high-quality datasets and this fragmentation is a significant barrier. Interoperability is made more difficult by the lack of standardization in medical terminology and data structures. For instance, using both "Diabetes Mellitus Type 2" and "T2DM" to refer to the same clinical condition can cause confusion and lower the accuracy of AI models. To lessen these problems, standardization efforts like the implementation of SNOMED CT, LOINC and ICD-10 are crucial. Furthermore, the integration of AI applications across platforms is made easier by open data exchange formats like FHIR and HL7 (Chatterjee et al., 2022). Investing in data lakes or warehouses that consolidate information from various sources is another way to break down data silos. A privacy-preserving AI technique called federated learning makes it possible to use decentralized data without jeopardizing patient confidentiality. Hospitals can enhance care coordination, guarantee continuity of care across various healthcare system touchpoints and set the groundwork for more successful AI implementation by tackling data silos and standardization issues. Table 5 shows the Data Silos vs Standardized Systems.

Table 5. Data Silos vs Standardized Systems

Criteria	Data Silo	Standardized System
Data Sharing	Difficult	Seamless
Data Formats	Inconsistent	Standardized (e.g., FHIR, HL7)
AI Integration	Limited	Enhanced
Accuracy	Prone to errors	Improved through consistency

Real-Time Data Flow and Dashboards

In contemporary hospitals, where prompt decision-making can have a major impact on patient outcomes, real-time data flow is essential. Real-time data systems powered by AI offer a dynamic perspective of patient status, clinical metrics and hospital operations. These systems combine information from various sources like laboratory records, medical imaging platforms, IoT devices and EHRs into unified dashboards for instant analysis (Mariscal-Harana, 2022) AI systems, for example, can continuously check a patient's vitals and send out alerts when anomalies, like abrupt drops in oxygen saturation, are found. By visualizing trends, anomalies and forecasts, AI-powered dashboards improve situational awareness for hospital administrators and clinicians alike. Proactive management is made possible by predictive analytics, which can foresee staffing shortages, ED surges and bed occupancy rates. Tools like risk scores, heatmaps and real-time charts aid in effectively allocating resources and prioritizing important cases. Real-time databases, edge computing for low-latency processing and fast message brokers like Apache Kafka are common components of the underlying technology infrastructure. Effective dashboard construction requires careful consideration of security, data quality and user interface design. Crucially, these dashboards are interactive decision-support tools that enable clinical and operational leaders to take prompt action, not just for monitoring. Real-time data flow combined with AI will become a standard feature as hospitals continue to embrace digital transformation, allowing for ongoing advancements in the efficiency and data protection of healthcare delivery. Table 6 shows the comparison of Traditional Monitoring and AI Dashboards.

Table 6. Traditional Monitoring vs AI Dashboards

Feature	Traditional Monitoring	AI-Enabled Dashboards
Data Updates	Periodic/manual	Real-time
Alerts	Rule-based	AI-driven and adaptive
Resource Planning	Reactive	Predictive and proactive
User Interface	Static	Interactive and visual

CASE STUDIES AND REAL-WORLD IMPLEMENTATIONS

AI in Radiology and Diagnostics

Because of the vast amount of imaging data and the possibility of automating interpretation tasks, radiology has become a prime area for AI adoption. AI models like deep learning-based algorithms have shown impressive abilities in identifying mortalities in MRIs, CT scans and X-rays with accuracy on par with that of skilled radiologists (Bandla et al., 2023). These systems can frequently detect diseases like breast tumors, brain hemorrhages, fractures and lung nodules in a matter of seconds. To guarantee that life-threatening cases are reviewed first, AI tools such as Aidoc and Zebra Medical Vision, for instance, can prioritize critical findings in radiology queues. This improves patient care and drastically cuts down on turnaround times, particularly in emergency situations. AI can also help standardize radiology reports, reduce variability and improve communication with referring physicians. Additionally, some platforms provide decision support by highlighting minor changes and comparing new images with old ones. Additionally, AI is being incorporated into Picture Archiving and Communication Systems (PACS) to facilitate radiologists' workflows. AI helps with image acquisition beyond diagnostics by minimizing the need for repeat imaging and optimizing scanning parameters (Gupta et al., 2025). Notwithstanding these developments, ongoing validation, integration with clinical workflows and attention to ethical and regulatory issues are necessary for successful implementation. As AI develops further, its function in radiology will broaden from detection to thorough interpretation and even prognostic modeling, making diagnostic imaging a more sophisticated and effective procedure. Table 7 shows the AI tools used in radiology and their benefits.

Table 7. AI in Radiology and Diagnostics

Feature	Description	Benefits	Examples/Tools
AI Techniques Used	Deep learning for image analysis	High accuracy, rapid detection	Aidoc, Zebra Medical Vision
Applications	Detecting anomalies (e.g., tumors, hemorrhages, nodules) in imaging	Faster diagnosis, prioritization of critical cases	CT, MRI, X-rays
Integration Points	Picture Archiving and Communication Systems (PACS), EHRs	Workflow automation, standardized reporting	PACS-integrated AI
Advantages	Rapid triage, reduced variability, enhanced communication	Improved patient outcomes, reduced turnaround time	Radiologist-AI collaboration
Implementation Challenges	Clinical validation, workflow integration, regulatory compliance	Ensures safety, efficacy	FDA-clearance needed

Virtual Assistants for Clinical Decision Support

Clinical decision support is being revolutionized by AI-based virtual assistants that offers real-time access to patient records, medical information and evidence-based recommendations. These intelligent assistants comprehend physician inquiries, retrieve pertinent information and offer advice on diagnosis, treatment and medication using Natural Language Processing (NLP) and ML models. For example, a doctor can ask a voice-activated assistant, “What is Mr. John's most recent lab result?” and get a prompt, contextual response. In order to help providers stay current with best practices, virtual assistants are also integrated with research databases and clinical guidelines. By suggesting differential diagnoses and comparing symptoms with disease patterns, they improve diagnostic accuracy. Some systems go one step further by warning doctors about medication interactions, suggesting preventive actions, or forecasting complications. These skills are especially helpful in situations where there is a lot of stress or time constraints, like emergency rooms or critical care units. By automatically filling in EHR fields, coding diagnoses and transcribing patient interactions, virtual assistants also increase the efficiency of documentation. These tools are becoming more popular even though they are still in the early stages of adoption because they can improve decision-making, lessen cognitive load and promote a collaborative care model. But there are still issues with preserving accuracy, protecting data and building clinician trust. These systems will probably develop into essential clinical partners as they get older, allowing for quicker, more intelligent and better-informed care delivery (Jiang et al., 2017; Muniasamy et al., 2020). Table 8 shows the AI tools used in virtual assistance and their benefits.

Table 8. Virtual Assistants for Clinical Decision Support

Feature	Description	Benefits	Examples/Use Cases
Core Technologies	NLP, ML, knowledge graphs	Contextual information retrieval, intelligent responses	Voice-based assistants
Key Functions	Lab result queries, treatment suggestions, interaction alerts	Real-time support, fewer errors	ER, ICU support systems
Integration Points	EHRs, medical guidelines, drug databases	Consistent documentation, CDS	Clinical workflows
Additional Features	Predictive alerts, symptom comparisons, documentation automation	Saves time, supports decision-making	Diagnosis assistance
Challenges	Trust, data accuracy, privacy concerns	Needs transparency and secure design	HIPAA/GDPR-compliant systems

AI-Enabled Administrative Automation

Hospital administrative duties, such as scheduling patients and billing, take up a significant amount of time and money. By automating repetitive and routine tasks, AI in the form of intelligent agents and robotic process automation (RPA) is transforming these backend tasks. AI bots that automatically fill out demographic forms and instantly confirm insurance information, for instance, can expedite the patient registration process. AI that can identify coding errors, validate claims and anticipate claim denials also speeds up billing processes, which frequently require several verification steps. This results in better cash flow, quicker reimbursements and fewer rejections. By evaluating patient preferences, doctor availability and past attendance trends, AI can also manage appointment scheduling and optimize time slots. Additionally, chatbots are being used to handle post-discharge follow-ups, appointment reminders and patient inquiries, improving patient engagement without increasing staff workload. AI supports workforce planning, credential verification and hiring in human resources. AI makes it possible to intelligently coordinate hospital operations, from task routing to supply chain management. This lowers operating expenses while freeing up administrative personnel to work on more important projects. Strong data governance, change management techniques and a thorough grasp of workflows are essential for the effective utilization of AI in administration. Hospital administration will continue to be redefined by AI as it develops further, becoming more patient-centered, accurate and agile (Yu et al, 2018; Muniasamy et al., 2020). Table 9 shows the AI tools used in administrative automation and their benefits.

Table 9. AI-Enabled Administrative Automation

Administrative Area	AI Application	Benefits	Example Implementations
Patient Registration	Auto-fill forms, verify insurance	Faster onboarding, reduced manual work	Omega Healthcare AI
Billing & Claims	Automated coding, fraud detection, claims prediction	Fewer denials, faster payments	RPA in billing
Scheduling	Intelligent time slot and provider matching	Reduced no-shows, better resource use	AI-based scheduling systems
Chatbots	Appointment reminders, FAQs, post-discharge follow-ups	24/7 support, higher engagement	Conversational AI
Human Resources & Operations	Hiring automation, credential verification, supply chain optimization	Efficient workforce and logistics	AI for HR & SCM
Challenges	Resistance to change, process redesign	Requires training, workflow mapping	Digital transformation leadership

AI Tools in Pathology and Lab Automation

The use of AI tools is causing a paradigm shift in pathology and laboratory diagnostics. In the past, pathology required manually examining tissue slides under a microscope, which could be laborious and prone to human error. Digital pathology is becoming more common as AI advances. AI algorithms examine high-resolution photos of tissue samples to find patterns that could be signs of infections, cancer, or other illnesses. These systems are highly accurate at classifying tissue types, measuring tumor margins and quantifying cell counts. Beyond pathology, AI-enabled lab automation also applies to clinical chemistry, hematology and microbiology (Odofin et al., 2023). When combined with AI, automated analyzers are able to prioritize important findings, identify anomalous results and recommend follow-up testing. Intelligent systems also optimize inventory control, labeling and sample tracking. AI also speeds up turnaround times by automating repetitive tests and guaranteeing optimal equipment use. Data flow and reporting are guaranteed to be smooth through integration with Laboratory Information Systems (LIS). The use of AI in COVID-19 testing is one prominent example, where prompt containment was aided by the quick identification of positive cases. Notwithstanding the advantages, staff training, regulatory compliance and validation are still crucial. All things considered, artificial intelligence (AI) is transforming laboratory medicine from manual and reactive to digital and predictive, greatly enhancing workflow effectiveness and diagnostic precision. Table 10 shows the AI tools used in pathology and their benefits.

Table 10. AI Tools in Pathology and Lab Automation

Feature	Description	Benefits	Examples/Technologies
Digital Pathology	Slide scanning and AI-based image interpretation	Reduces human error, improves speed	AI in cancer detection
Lab Test Automation	Analyzers with AI for prioritizing and validating results	Faster turnaround, anomaly detection	Clinical chemistry, hematology
Sample Management	AI for labeling, inventory and sample tracking	Fewer losses, real-time monitoring	Integrated LIS systems
Predictive Capabilities	AI identifies patterns across datasets, forecasts risks	Preventative care opportunities	COVID-19 detection
Integration Points	LIS, Hospital Information Systems (HIS), reporting dashboards	Smooth data flow and compliance	LIS-integrated automation
Challenges	Staff training, validation, ethical oversight	Continuous quality improvement	Regulatory readiness

SOLUTIONS AND RECOMMENDATIONS

Security and Privacy Concerns

Data security and privacy become critical issues as AI systems is integrated into hospital operations. Cyberattacks are drawn to hospitals because they handle sensitive patient information like medical records, genetic information and biometric identifiers. The risk surface is increased by AI's requirement for massive amounts of such data for training and inference. Identity theft, data breaches and unauthorized access can all have detrimental effects on one's reputation and legal standing. Patients also need to have faith that their information is handled securely and ethically. Hospitals must put strong security mechanism like encryption, multi-factor authentication and intrusion detection systems in place to reduce these risks. Techniques for data anonymization and pseudonymization allow for data analysis while protecting identities. It is essential to abide by privacy laws such as GDPR in Europe and HIPAA in the United States. AI vendors also need to make sure that their systems are regularly audited and adhere to security standards. When there are several parties involved, it is essential to have clear access controls and secure data-sharing agreements. Hospitals are increasingly implementing privacy-preserving technologies like homomorphic encryption and federated learning (Kairouz et al., 2021). These developments make it possible to train models on decentralized data without moving it outside the organization. In addition to ensuring regulatory compliance, addressing privacy and security issues is crucial for building patient and clinician confidence in AI solutions.

Fairness and Bias in Algorithms

AI algorithm bias is a serious problem that can erode confidence, decrease efficacy and maintain healthcare inequities. AI models are trained on historical data, which may be biased because of human judgment, unequal access to care, or underrepresentation of particular demographic groups (Choudhry, et al, 2024). These biases may result in discriminatory outcomes, including incorrect diagnosis, inappropriate treatment recommendations, or unequal care prioritization, if they are not addressed. An algorithm that was trained on data from one ethnic group, for example, might perform poorly for others. AI developers must apply stringent validation across various populations and constantly track algorithmic performance in order to advance fairness. Known biases can be lessened with the use of strategies like adversarial de-biasing, re-weighting and re-sampling. Accountability is promoted by transparent model development, which includes disclosing the properties of training data and algorithmic choices. Prior to approving AI tools for clinical use, regulatory agencies and institutional review boards ought to assess fairness metrics (Rajkomar et al., 2018). Additionally, ethical development can be guided by inclusive data governance frameworks that include patient representatives, ethicists and clinicians. Making healthcare professionals aware of AI's limitations also aids in ensuring proper use. Achieving equitable, high-quality care requires addressing bias and maintaining fairness, which is more than just a technical challenge.

Human-AI Collaboration and Trust Issues

Effective human-machine cooperation is essential to the success of AI in hospitals. AI lacks the human clinician's sensitive judgment and empathy, despite its superiority in pattern recognition, data processing and prediction. As a result, rather than being a replacement, AI should be considered an assistant. AI integration into clinical workflows, however, has the potential to upend established procedures and elicit opposition from medical professionals. A significant obstacle is trust; physicians may question the precision of AI suggestions or worry about losing their independence. Explainable AI (XAI) techniques can help increase trust by bringing transparency to the decision-making process of AI systems. Including physicians in the creation and testing of AI can also promote acceptance and ownership. It is crucial to implement training programs that improve digital literacy and highlight AI's function as a tool for support rather than as a rival. Who is in charge of making decisions involving AI should be clearly defined by policies and accountability frameworks. In order to achieve better results, successful human-AI collaboration combines the strengths of both the clinician's contextual knowledge and AI's computational power (Markus, et al., 2021). Building a culture of ethical responsibility and mutual trust will be crucial for the long-term adoption of AI in healthcare as these systems develop. Table 11 shows the AI Challenges and Ethical Considerations in Healthcare.

Table 11. AI Challenges and Ethical Considerations in Healthcare

Challenge Area	Aspect	Description	Solutions / Strategies
Data Privacy & Security	Sensitive Data Involved	Medical records, biometrics, genetic info	Encryption, MFA, IDS
	Risks	Cyberattacks, identity theft, unauthorized access	Access control, secure sharing agreements
	Technical Safeguards	Security measures to protect data	Data anonymization, pseudonymization
	Advanced Privacy Techniques	Protect data while enabling AI training	Homomorphic encryption, federated learning
	Outcome Goals	Ensure security, maintain trust, compliance	Ethical data usage, patient confidence
Bias & Fairness	Sources of Bias	Historical data, underrepresented populations	Diverse datasets, demographic balancing
	Impact of Bias	Discrimination, misdiagnosis, unequal treatment	Algorithm performance audits, validation
	Bias Mitigation Techniques	Reduce/prevent bias in model training	Debiasing, re-weighting, re-sampling
	Transparency Practices	Visibility into AI development processes	Disclose data and assumptions
	Inclusive Governance	Multidisciplinary approach to AI oversight	Include patients, ethicists, clinicians
Human-AI Collaboration	Nature of Collaboration	AI as support tool, not a replacement	Define roles clearly (assist vs. lead)
	Trust Issues	Concerns over accuracy and autonomy	Explainable AI (XAI), build trust
	Clinician Involvement	Need for clinician participation in AI development	Co-design, pilot testing, feedback loops
	Training and Adoption	Improve digital skills, address resistance	Training programs, workflow integration
	Accountability Frameworks	Clarify responsibility in AI-driven decisions	Define liability, shared accountability

FUTURE DIRECTIONS AND INNOVATIONS

AI-Driven Autonomous Hospital Systems

AI-driven autonomous systems that can handle clinical and administrative duties with little assistance from humans may become a reality in hospital operations in the future. To create self-regulating environments, these systems will combine AI with advanced analytics, robotics and the Internet of Things. For instance, AI controls task distribution and operational coordination, while autonomous robots can take care of patient transportation, medication delivery and sanitation (Alahmed et al., 2024). Staffing could be dynamically adjusted by predictive algorithms in response to disease outbreaks or real-time patient inflows. Additionally, intelligent systems have the ability to automatically optimize environmental parameters for infection control by monitoring temperature, humidity and air quality. AI-powered decision-making and equipment calibration systems are already being tested in autonomous surgical suites and diagnostic units. These advancements will allow for 24/7 operations, significantly increase efficiency and lower human error. But they also call into question accountability, supervision and the human element in providing care. In order to handle liability and patient consent, legal and ethical frameworks must change in tandem with technology. Instead of replacing human expertise, the move toward autonomy should enhance it. The shift to genuinely smart healthcare facilities will be spearheaded by hospitals that make investments in these innovations.

Personalized Workflow Optimization

In hospital workflows, personalization means adjusting procedures and allocating resources according to each patient's unique requirements, risks and behaviors. AI enables this by recommending tailored care pathways based on an individual's medical history, genetics, lifestyle information and treatment preferences. AI, for example, can identify which patients are most likely to miss follow-up appointments and assign care coordinators or send reminders in advance (Bajwa et al., 2021; Muniasamy & Karunakaran et al., 2026). Based on patient complexity and recovery profiles, AI can recommend the best operating room schedules and staffing levels during surgical planning. Nutrition, physical therapy and mental health support are also included in personalized care plans. Workflows can be tailored for patient segments on the administrative side, such as elderly patients who require more in-person assistance versus tech-savvy patients who use digital tools. Personalization lowers resource waste while improving patient outcomes, adherence and satisfaction. Adaptive algorithms, flexible systems and strong data integration are necessary for implementation. Crucially, patient consent and clinical judgment should serve as the foundation for personalization. Personalized workflow optimization will be essential to providing patient-centered, value-based care as precision medicine expands.

Integration with IoT and Smart Hospital Technologies

One of the main pillars of smart hospital initiatives is the integration of AI with Internet of Things (IoT) devices. Continuous streams of data are produced by Internet of Things devices like environmental sensors, infusion pumps, wearable health monitors and smart beds. AI uses real-time data analysis to help with operational optimization, predictive maintenance and clinical decision-making. AI, for example, can evaluate wearable data to identify early indicators of decline in patients recovering from surgery, enabling prompt interventions. In order to prevent falls or bedsores, smart bed sensors can monitor patient movement and modify positioning. AI-powered IoT systems in facility management regulate energy use, temperature and lighting in response to occupancy and demand in real time (Parkar, et al., 2025). Wheelchairs and defibrillators are made available where and when they are needed thanks to integration with asset-tracking systems. Maintaining security, controlling data volume and guaranteeing interoperability are among the difficulties. For these integrations to be supported, standardized protocols like MQTT, CoAP and edge computing architectures are essential. The combination of AI and IoT will enable new levels of automation, responsiveness and efficiency in healthcare settings as 5G and cloud technologies advance. Table 12 shows the Future Directions and Innovations in AI-Enabled Hospital Systems.

Table 12. Future Directions and Innovations in AI-Enabled Hospital Systems

Innovation Area	Key Concepts	Examples / Use Cases	Benefits	Challenges
AI-Driven Autonomous Hospital Systems	Self-regulating systems combining AI, analytics, robotics and IoT	Autonomous robots for transport, delivery, cleaning AI-based staffing prediction Smart surgical/diagnostic units Environmental monitoring and control	24/7 operations Increased efficiency Reduced human error	Loss of human touch Legal accountability Ethical concerns Overreliance on automation
Personalized Workflow Optimization	Patient-specific resource allocation and care tailoring	Customized care plans based on history/genetics Follow-up reminders for high-risk patients OR and staff scheduling based on complexity Patient specific admin flows	Improved adherence and satisfaction Reduced resource wastage Better clinical outcomes	Data integration issues Need for adaptive systems Patient consent and clinical oversight
AI + IoT Integration in Smart Hospitals	Real-time analytics using connected devices for clinical and operational intelligence	Wearables for post-op monitoring Smart beds for fall/pressure sore prevention Facility sensors for HVAC/ energy control Asset tracking with AI routing	Faster interventions Optimized environment Predictive maintenance	Data security Interoperability across devices Scalability with large data volumes

CONCLUSION

This chapter emphasized how AI has the potential to revolutionize hospital workflows in the administrative, clinical and operational domains. AI improves patient outcomes, efficiency and decision-making through a variety of applications including lab automation, virtual assistants, real-time data dashboards and EHR integration. We looked at issues like algorithmic bias, security worries, data silos and trust between humans and AI. Successful real-world implementations were demonstrated through case studies and future research looked at autonomous systems, smart hospitals and personalized care. A new era in healthcare is being ushered in by the convergence of AI, IoT and precision medicine, where intelligence is integrated throughout the care continuum. For adoption to be equitable and sustainable, strategic planning, ethical protections and clinician involvement are essential. In order to optimize hospital workflow with AI, stakeholders should take a phased and inclusive approach. First, spend money on data infrastructure that promotes security, quality and interoperability. Second, choose AI solutions that complement current workflows and are in line with organizational objectives. Third, to guarantee usability and trust, include end users physicians, administrators and patients in the design and implementation process. Training curricula ought to encourage responsible AI use and improve digital literacy. Frequent audits and feedback loops can address new risks and improve system performance. Innovation will be accelerated while maintaining compliance through collaborations with academic institutions, regulatory agencies and AI vendors. In order to achieve long-lasting change in hospital ecosystems, AI adoption should ultimately prioritize patient-centered care, operational excellence and continuous learning.

REFERENCES

Abraham, S. (2024). Challenges in the implementation of technology in effective hospital management system: A quantitative study. *Journal of Informatics Education and Research.*

Ala, A., & Chen, F. (2022). Appointment scheduling problem in complexity systems of the healthcare services: A comprehensive review. *Journal of Healthcare Engineering*, *2022*(1), 5819813. DOI: 10.1155/2022/5819813 PMID: 35281532

Alahmed, Y., Abadla, R., & Ansari, M. J. (2024). Enhancing safety in autonomous vehicles through advanced AI-driven perception and decision-making systems. In *2024 Fifth International Conference on Intelligent Data Science Technologies and Applications (IDSTA)* (pp. 208–217). DOI: 10.1109/IDSTA62194.2024.10746990

Alves, M., Seringa, J., Silvestre, T., & Magalhães, T. (2024). Use of artificial intelligence tools in supporting decision-making in hospital management. *BMC Health Services Research*, *24*(1), 24. DOI: 10.1186/s12913-024-11602-y PMID: 39456040

Bajwa, J., Munir, U., Nori, A., & Williams, B. (2021). Artificial intelligence in healthcare: Transforming the practice of medicine. *Future Healthcare Journal*, *8*(2), e188–e194. DOI: 10.7861/fhj.2021-0095 PMID: 34286183

Bandla, M. S., Liju, A. M., Luharia, A., & Mishra, G. V. (2023). Artificial intelligence in healthcare with special consideration in radio imaging. In *2023 1st DMIHER International Conference on Artificial Intelligence in Education and Industry 4.0 (IDICAIEI)* (Vol. 1, pp. 1–5). DOI: 10.1109/IDICAIEI58380.2023.10406913

Bekbolatova, M., Mayer, J., Ong, C., & Toma, M. (2024). Transformative potential of AI in healthcare: Definitions, applications, and navigating the ethical landscape and public perspectives. *Health Care*, •••, 12. PMID: 38255014

Bohr, A., & Memarzadeh, K. (2020). The rise of artificial intelligence in healthcare applications. In *Artificial intelligence in healthcare* (pp. 25–60). Academic Press. DOI: 10.1016/B978-0-12-818438-7.00002-2

Bressman, E., Long, J. A., Honig, K., Zee, J., McGlaughlin, N., Jointer, C., Asch, D. A., Burke, R. E., & Morgan, A. U. (2022). Evaluation of an automated text message–based program to reduce use of acute health care resources after hospital discharge. *JAMA Network Open*, *5*(10), e2238293. DOI: 10.1001/jamanetworkopen.2022.38293 PMID: 36287564

Chatterjee, A., Pahari, N., & Prinz, A. (2022). HL7 FHIR with SNOMED-CT to achieve semantic and structural interoperability in personal health data: A proof-of-concept study. *Sensors (Basel)*, *22*(10), 3756. DOI: 10.3390/s22103756 PMID: 35632165

Choudhry, M. D., Sundarrajan, M., & Sundaram, K. (2024). Bias and fairness in generative AI. In *Generative AI and LLMs: Natural language processing and generative adversarial networks* (p. 177). DOI: 10.1515/9783111425078-009

Dhade, P., & Shirke, P. (2024). Federated learning for healthcare: A comprehensive review. *Engineering Proceedings*, *59*(1), 230.

Elgin, C. Y., & Elgin, C. (2024). Ethical implications of AI-driven clinical decision support systems on healthcare resource allocation: A qualitative study of healthcare professionals' perspectives. *BMC Medical Ethics*, *25*(1), 148. DOI: 10.1186/s12910-024-01151-8 PMID: 39707327

Elhaddad, M., & Hamam, S. (2024). AI-driven clinical decision support systems: An ongoing pursuit of potential. *Cureus*, 16. DOI: 10.7759/cureus.57728 PMID: 38711724

Friedman, A. B., Delgado, M. K., & Weissman, G. E. (2024). Artificial intelligence for emergency care triage—Much promise, but still much to learn. *JAMA Network Open*, *7*(5), e248857. DOI: 10.1001/jamanetworkopen.2024.8857 PMID: 38713470

Gauthaman, S. A., Muniasamy, A., & Karunakaran, G. (2026). Current challenges in the pharmaceutical industry and AI's role in addressing them. In Muniasamy, A., & Karunakaran, G. (Eds.), *Applications of artificial intelligence in pharmaceuticals* (pp. 1–26). IGI Global., DOI: 10.4018/979-8-3373-2043-4.ch001

Gauthaman, S. A., Muniasamy, A., & Karunakaran, G. (2026). Introduction to machine learning and optimization in healthcare. In Muniasamy, A. (Ed.), *Integrative machine learning and optimization algorithms for disease prediction* (pp. 1–34). IGI Global., DOI: 10.4018/979-8-3373-1087-9.ch001

Gorrepati, L. (2024). Integrating AI with electronic health records (EHRs) to enhance patient care. *International Journal of Health Sciences*, *7*(8), 38–50. DOI: 10.47941/ijhs.2368

Guo, H., Wu, Y., Zhao, R., Yang, X., Peyrodie, L., Nianga, J., & Wang, Z. (2024). Leveraging AI for strategic management in healthcare: Enhancing operational and financial performance. *Journal of Intelligence and Knowledge Engineering*.

Gupta, A., Gupta, A., Soanki, S., & Kishore, J. (2025). AI and medical imaging: The next era of radiology and pathology detection. In *2025 First International Conference on Advances in Computer Science, Electrical, Electronics, and Communication Technologies (CE2CT)* (pp. 103–108). DOI: 10.1109/CE2CT64011.2025.10939755

Hezam, I. M., Ali, A. M., Alshamrani, A. M., Gao, X., & Abdel-Basset, M. (2024). Artificial intelligence's impact on drug delivery in healthcare supply chain management: Data, techniques, analysis, and managerial implications. *Journal of Big Data, 11*(1), 177. DOI: 10.1186/s40537-024-01049-7

Howard, F. M., Gao, C. A., & Sankey, C. (2020). Implementation of an automated scheduling tool improves schedule quality and resident satisfaction. *PLoS One*, *15*(8), e0236952. DOI: 10.1371/journal.pone.0236952 PMID: 32780751

Iftikhar, M., Saqib, M., Zareen, M., & Mumtaz, H. (2024). Artificial intelligence: Revolutionizing robotic surgery. *Annals of Medicine and Surgery (London)*, *86*(9), 5401–5409. DOI: 10.1097/MS9.0000000000002426 PMID: 39238994

Jiang, F., Jiang, Y., Zhi, H., Dong, Y., Li, H., Ma, S., Wang, Y., Dong, Q., Shen, H., & Wang, Y. (2017). Artificial intelligence in healthcare: Past, present and future. *Stroke and Vascular Neurology*, *2*(4), 230–243. DOI: 10.1136/svn-2017-000101 PMID: 29507784

Kairouz, P., McMahan, H. B., Avent, B., et al. (2021). Advances and open problems in federated learning. *Foundations and Trends® in Machine Learning, 14*(1–2), 1–210. https://doi.org/DOI: 10.1561/2200000083

Khamaj, A. (2025). AI-enhanced chatbot for improving healthcare usability and accessibility for older adults. *Alexandria Engineering Journal*, *116*, 202–213. DOI: 10.1016/j.aej.2024.12.090

Mariscal-Harana, J., et al. (2022). An AI tool for automated analysis of large-scale unstructured clinical cine CMR databases.

Markus, A. F., Kors, J. A., & Rijnbeek, P. R. (2021). The role of explainability in creating trustworthy artificial intelligence for health care: A comprehensive survey of the terminology, design choices, and evaluation strategies. *Journal of Biomedical Informatics*, *113*, 103655. DOI: 10.1016/j.jbi.2020.103655 PMID: 33309898

Munavalli, J. R., Boersma, H. J., Rao, S. V., & Van Merode, G. G. (2020). Real-time capacity management and patient flow optimization in hospitals using AI methods. In *Artificial intelligence and data mining in healthcare* (pp. 55–69). Springer.

Muniasamy, A. (2026). Quantum computing in drug discovery: Revolutionizing pharmaceutical research. In Muniasamy, A., & Karunakaran, G. (Eds.), *Applications of artificial intelligence in pharmaceuticals* (pp. 59–96). IGI Global., DOI: 10.4018/979-8-3373-2043-4.ch003

Muniasamy, A., & Karunakaran, G. (2026). Challenges and future directions: Emerging trends and limitations in ML and optimization for healthcare. In Muniasamy, A. (Ed.), *Integrative machine learning and optimization algorithms for disease prediction* (pp. 339–368). IGI Global., DOI: 10.4018/979-8-3373-1087-9.ch012

Muniasamy, A., Tabassam, S., Hussain, M. A., Sultana, H., Muniasamy, V., & Bhatnagar, R. (2020). Deep learning for predictive analytics in healthcare. In Hassanien, A., Azar, A., Gaber, T., Bhatnagar, R., & Tolba, M. F. (Eds.), *The international conference on advanced machine learning technologies and applications (AMLTA2019)* (pp. xx–xx). Springer., DOI: 10.1007/978-3-030-14118-9_4

Naim, A.. (2026). AI-driven smart manufacturing and automation in pharmaceutical production. In Muniasamy, A., & Karunakaran, G. (Eds.), *Applications of artificial intelligence in pharmaceuticals* (pp. 157–194). IGI Global., DOI: 10.4018/979-8-3373-2043-4.ch006

Odofin, O. T., Abayomi, A. A., Uzoka, A. C., Adekunle, B. I., Agboola, O. A., & Owoade, S. (2023). AI-based automation framework for laboratory diagnostics in hospital information management systems. *International Journal of Management and Organizational Research.*

Ouanes, K., & Farhah, N. (2024). Effectiveness of artificial intelligence (AI) in clinical decision support systems and care delivery. *Journal of Medical Systems*, *48*(1), 74. DOI: 10.1007/s10916-024-02098-4 PMID: 39133332

Parkar, T. V., & Kamath, K. S. (2025). Next-gen healthcare: AI and IoT innovations and future trends in healthcare. In *Intelligent Systems and IoT Applications in Clinical Health* (pp. 219–242). IGI Global.

Porto, B. M. (2024). Improving triage performance in emergency departments using machine learning and natural language processing: A systematic review. *BMC Emergency Medicine*, *24*(1), 219. DOI: 10.1186/s12873-024-01135-2 PMID: 39558255

Prabhune, A. G., Priya, P. S. K., Chandra, R., Thakur, A., Srihari, V. R., & Bhat, S. S. (2025). A web-based platform for optimizing healthcare resource allocation and workload management using agile methodology and WISN theory. *BMC Health Services Research*, *25*(1), 400. DOI: 10.1186/s12913-025-12473-7 PMID: 40102889

Rahman, A., Debnath, T., Kundu, D., Khan, M. S., Aishi, A. A., Sazzad, S., Sayduzzaman, M., & Band, S. S. (2024). Machine learning and deep learning-based approach in smart healthcare: Recent advances, applications, challenges and opportunities. *AIMS Public Health, 11*(1), 58–109. DOI: 10.3934/publichealth.2024004 PMID: 38617415

Rajkomar, A., Hardt, M., Howell, M. D., Corrado, G., & Chin, M. H. (2018). Ensuring fairness in machine learning to advance health equity. *Annals of Internal Medicine, 169*(12), 866–872. DOI: 10.7326/M18-1990 PMID: 30508424

Ramezani, M., Takian, A., Bakhtiari, A., Rabiee, H. R., Fazaeli, A. A., & Sazgarnejad, S. (2023). The application of artificial intelligence in health financing: A scoping review. *Cost Effectiveness and Resource Allocation : C/E, 21*(1), 83. DOI: 10.1186/s12962-023-00492-2 PMID: 37932778

Rengaramanujam, K., & Muniasamy, A. (2026). AI in hospital administration and formulary design: Optimizing resource allocation and patient flow. In Muniasamy, A., & Karunakaran, G. (Eds.), *Applications of artificial intelligence in pharmaceuticals* (pp. 215–246). IGI Global., DOI: 10.4018/979-8-3373-2043-4.ch008

Suryawanshi, V., Kanyal, D., Sabale, S. R., & Bhoyar, V. (2024). *The role of AI in enhancing hospital operational efficiency and patient care*. Multidisciplinary Reviews. DOI: 10.31893/multirev.2025153

Tahernejad, A., Sahebi, A., Abadi, A. S. S., & Safari, M. (2024). Application of artificial intelligence in triage in emergencies and disasters: A systematic review. *BMC Public Health, 24*(1), 3203. DOI: 10.1186/s12889-024-20447-3 PMID: 39558305

Veernapu, K. (2022). Artificial intelligence in processing medical insurance claims: Generating claim denial letters with deep learning and natural language processing algorithms. *International Journal of Multidisciplinary Research and Growth Evaluation.*

Wu, H., Lu, X., & Wang, H. (2023). The application of artificial intelligence in health care resource allocation before and during the COVID-19 pandemic: Scoping review. *JMIR AI, 2*, e38397. DOI: 10.2196/38397

Yadav, G. S., & Longhurst, C. A. (2025). Will AI make the electronic health record more efficient for clinicians? *NEJM AI, 2*(3). Advance online publication. DOI: 10.1056/AIe2500020

Ye, J., Woods, D., Jordan, N., & Starren, J. (2024). The role of artificial intelligence for the application of integrating electronic health records and patient-generated data in clinical decision support. *AMIA Joint Summits on Translational Science Proceedings AMIA Summit on Translational Science, 2024*, 459–467. PMID: 38827061

Yu, K.-H., Beam, A. L., & Kohane, I. S. (2018). Artificial intelligence in healthcare. *Nature Biomedical Engineering, 2*(10), 719–731. DOI: 10.1038/s41551-018-0305-z PMID: 31015651

Zaretsky, J., Kim, J. M., Baskharoun, S., Zhao, Y., Austrian, J., Aphinyanaphongs, Y., Gupta, R., Blecker, S. B., & Feldman, J. (2024). Generative artificial intelligence to transform inpatient discharge summaries to patient-friendly language and format. *JAMA Network Open, 7*(3), e240357. DOI: 10.1001/jamanetworkopen.2024.0357 PMID: 38466307

Zayas-Cabán, T., Okubo, T. H., & Posnack, S. (2023). Priorities to accelerate workflow automation in health care. *Journal of the American Medical Informatics Association : JAMIA, 30*(1), 195–201. DOI: 10.1093/jamia/ocac197 PMID: 36259967

ADDITIONAL READING

Karrar, A., Nouh, M. I., Kufyah, M. T., Alshehri, A. M., Zuhair, R. M., Alanazi, A. H., Alahmari, F. A., Alqarni, M. Y. B., Alzahrani, S. J. S., Ghzwani, A. G., Almuqati, A. O., Ghzwani, A. G., Aldhuwayhi, M. I., & Alharbi, T. O. A. (2025). The role of artificial intelligence in advancing hospital management information systems: Review article. *Saudi Journal of Clinical Pharmacy, 4*(1), 15–23. DOI: 10.4103/sjcp.sjcp_42_24

Maleki Varnosfaderani, S., & Forouzanfar, M. (2024). The role of AI in hospitals and clinics: Transforming healthcare in the 21st century. *Bioengineering (Basel, Switzerland), 11*(4), 337. DOI: 10.3390/bioengineering11040337 PMID: 38671759

KEY TERMS AND DEFINITIONS

Bed Occupancy Rate: A performance indicator measuring the percentage of hospital beds occupied by patients at a given time.

Clinical Pathway: A structured multidisciplinary plan that outlines key steps in treating specific diseases or conditions to standardize and improve patient care.

Electronic Health Records (EHR): A digital version of a patient's medical history, enabling real-time access, sharing, and updating across healthcare providers.

Hospital Management: The administration and coordination of healthcare services, staff, and resources to ensure efficient delivery of patient care and organizational effectiveness.

Lean Healthcare: An approach that applies lean management principles to healthcare, aiming to reduce waste, improve workflow, and enhance patient satisfaction.

Patient Throughput: The movement of patients through different stages of care (admission, treatment, discharge), reflecting hospital efficiency.

Resource Allocation: The process of assigning medical staff, equipment, and facilities where they are most needed to optimize patient outcomes.

Task Prioritization: The method of ranking and scheduling healthcare tasks according to urgency and importance to optimize workload management.

Workflow Optimization: The process of redesigning and streamlining hospital tasks and processes to reduce delays, minimize errors, and improve patient outcomes.

Workload Management: The practice of distributing and balancing tasks among healthcare staff to prevent burnout, maintain quality of care, and achieve efficiency.

Chapter 8
AI Integration and Clinical Workflow Optimization in Hospitals

S. Kaja Mohideen
https://orcid.org/0009-0004-1654-8633
B.S. Abdur Rahman Crescent Institute of Science and Technology, India

Latha Tamilselvan
https://orcid.org/0000-0002-2775-1301
B.S. Abdur Rahman Crescent Institute of Science and Technology, India

Mohammed Wajid Khan
https://orcid.org/0000-0003-4507-3994
B.S. Abdur Rahman Crescent Institute of Science and Technology, India

ABSTRACT

This chapter provides a comprehensive overview of the transformative role of artificial intelligence (AI) in addressing the structural and operational challenges faced by modern hospitals. As healthcare systems worldwide grapple with increasing patient loads, workforce shortages, and rising operational complexities, AI technologies offer new opportunities to streamline workflows, enhance decision-making, and improve overall hospital performance. As hospitals continue to embrace AI, understanding its integration and optimization will be crucial for delivering high-quality, technology-driven healthcare services.

DOI: 10.4018/979-8-3373-2787-7.ch008

INTRODUCTION

The significance of Artificial Intelligence (AI) in healthcare marks a remarkable transformation in how hospital services are carried out, managed, and optimized. Over the past decade, AI technologies ranging from machine learning and deep learning algorithms to computer vision and Natural Language Processing (NLP) are exponentially incorporated into various aspects of healthcare, including diagnostics, treatment planning, patient monitoring, and administrative operations.

Bohr and Memarzadeh (1) point out that healthcare systems struggle with predictive inefficiency—a lack of ability to foresee resource needs, patient deterioration, or optimal treatment pathways. This shortcoming leads to reactive rather than proactive care, affecting outcomes and operational sustainability.The authors argue that to address these deeply rooted workflow problems, healthcare must adopt tools that go beyond traditional information systems. Artificial intelligence, with its capabilities in data integration, pattern recognition, and process automation, emerges as a promising solution to reengineer workflows, reduce inefficiencies, and enhance both patient and provider experiences.

AI is now capable of performing complex tasks such as medical image interpretation, predictive diagnostics, personalized treatment planning, and administrative automation. Driven by the exponential growth of healthcare data and advances in computational power, AI can analyze vast amounts of information far more efficiently than traditional methods. From assisting radiologists in detecting anomalies in medical imaging to predicting patient deterioration in intensive care units, AI is enabling faster, more accurate, and personalized healthcare interventions.ie., AI is transforming nearly every corner of the healthcare ecosystem.

Tom Lawry (2) emphasizes that AI is not merely a tool, but a transformational capability that enables healthcare organizations to shift from reactive, one-size-fits-all care to proactive, personalized, and data-driven models. He identifies several key drivers behind this rise, including the exponential growth of health data, the increasing demand for value-based care, and the need to address clinician burnout and operational inefficiencies. AI, he argues, is uniquely positioned to meet these challenges by uncovering patterns in data, augmenting clinical decision-making, and automating routine tasks. As healthcare continues to grapple with challenges like aging populations, chronic diseases, and workforce shortages, AI is not just a technological advancement, it is becoming an essential component of future-ready healthcare systems.

Despite significant advancements in AI applications within hospitals, several key research gaps continue to hinder the realization of its full potential. The most prominent gap lies in the lack of comprehensive AI-driven workflow frameworks. While numerous studies explore AI use in specific areas such as radiology, pathology, or patient triaging, there is limited research addressing integrated AI systems that optimize complete hospital workflows from patient admission to discharge. This fragmented approach prevents hospitals from leveraging AI for holistic operational improvements.

Another major gap is in the evaluation of AI's impact on workflow optimization. Most current research focuses heavily on clinical metrics such as diagnostic accuracy or treatment precision, while largely neglecting operational efficiency indicators. Important measures like patient throughput, staff workload distribution, and reductions in administrative burden are seldom assessed, leaving a critical void in understanding how AI influences day-to-day hospital functioning.

Lastly, challenges around data governance and interoperability standards continue to impede progress. The integration of AI into hospital systems demands standardized frameworks to ensure the secure, ethical, and seamless sharing of data across heterogeneous health information systems. Without clear interoperability protocols, AI tools risk remaining siloed and underutilized.

In conclusion, while existing literature strongly supports the transformative potential of AI in hospital workflows and clinical decision-making, substantial research is still needed to address these gaps. Developing comprehensive, scalable, and ethically robust AI systems that integrate smoothly into diverse hospital environments is essential for achieving long-term improvements in healthcare delivery.

This chapter provides a comprehensive overview of the transformative role of artificial intelligence (AI) in addressing the structural and operational challenges faced by modern hospitals. As healthcare systems worldwide grapple with increasing patient loads, workforce shortages, and rising operational complexities, AI technologies offer new opportunities to streamline workflows, enhance decision-making, and improve overall hospital performance.

The key objectives of this chapter are to:

- Analyze the structure of hospital workflows, including clinical, administrative, and operational processes, and identify common bottlenecks and pain points.
- Introduce the major types of AI technologies relevant to healthcare settings, including machine learning, deep learning, natural language processing, computer vision, and robotic process automation.
- Demonstrate the significance of AI in optimizing hospital workflows, with a focus on improving administrative efficiency, clinical support, and operational management.
- Present strategic approaches for successful AI integration, covering implementation frameworks, change management, staff training, and stakeholder engagement.

- Discuss key challenges and considerations, such as data privacy, ethical concerns, and system interoperability, that must be addressed for sustainable AI adoption.
- Summarize the transformative potential of AI, offering reflections on its future impact and best practices for long-term success.

BACKGROUND

AI integration in hospitals has attracted significant academic and clinical interest in recent years. The study (Bohr et al., 2020) emphasized the strategic role of AI in healthcare transformation, demonstrating how intelligent systems enhance decision-making and streamline both clinical and administrative workflows. (Lawry et al., 2020; Rengaramanujam et al., 2026) explored a broad spectrum of AI applications in hospital settings, particularly highlighting workflow automation, predictive modeling, and diagnostic enhancement as critical components of hospital optimization (Gauthaman, S. A., et al. (2026). The studies (Clifton et al., 2016; Muniasamy, A et al., 2026) contributed technical insights into how machine learning techniques can be effectively applied to improve triaging, patient flow, and clinical decision support systems.

The research (Topol et al., 2019) emphasized AI's role in alleviating physician burnout by automating routine tasks and improving diagnostic precision. Similarly, (Davenport et al., 2019; Rengaramanujam et al., 2026) examined AI's ability to increase administrative efficiency and streamline clinical workflows, particularly through predictive analytics. The study (Jiang et al., 2017; Muniasamy, A et al., 2020) provided a comprehensive overview of AI's impact on diagnostics and operational workflows, though they also noted challenges related to data quality and system integration.

Rajkomar et al. (2019) emphasized the role of machine learning in managing patient data and enhancing clinical decision-making. Amisha et al. (2019) discussed the application of natural language processing (NLP) in clinical documentation, which helps reduce physician workload and improve record accuracy. The study (Matheny et al. 2019) assessed real-world implementations of AI, especially in radiology, showcasing improvements in workflow efficiency and resource use.

A unique perspective was provided by (Pugazhendi et al., 2020) who developed a hot and cold data clustering technique in cloud systems, effectively managing storage capacity and data access an approach relevant to AI-based hospital data systems. The author (Krittanawong et al., 2021) demonstrated how AI can personalize cardiovascular treatment plans, leading to fewer hospital readmissions. The study (Esteva et al., 2017) while focused on dermatology, highlighted the capability of deep learning to match clinician-level diagnostic accuracy, significantly reducing time and workload.

The authors (Shortliffe & Sepúlveda, 2018) proposed integrating AI into clinical decision support systems (CDSS) to relieve cognitive load on clinicians and improve outcomes. The infrastructure challenges involved in implementing AI across hospital systems and proposed redesign strategies are discussed by (Yu et al., 2018; Naim, A., et al., 2026). Patel et al. (2009) emphasized the value of real-time human–machine collaboration, especially in intensive care units, where quick decisions are critical

The authors (Obermeyer & Emanuel, 2016) highlighted the use of big data and AI for forecasting hospital needs such as staffing and emergency preparedness. The study (London, 2019) raised ethical considerations around the use of "black box" AI models, warning of a trade-off between accuracy and explainability an issue that impacts workflow trust and adoption. The research (Reddy et al., 2020) suggested the use of scalable AI solutions in areas like telemedicine and triage, while the study (Wong et al., 2018) showed how AI-based frailty indices can automate risk assessments, improving triage accuracy in elderly care.

The study (Mandl et al., 2020) introduced the concept of a learning health system, where AI systems continuously evolve through feedback and outcome data, enabling adaptive workflows and systemic improvement. Collectively, these studies reflect a strong foundation in AI applications across hospital environments yet also indicate the need for further integration and system-wide implementation strategies.

The scope of this chapter covers a broad overview of AI's relevance to healthcare, focusing on its role as an enabler of more efficient, accurate, and scalable healthcare systems. While the emphasis is primarily on hospital and clinical workflows, the concepts presented also apply to public health, remote care, and healthcare management at large.

MAIN FOCUS OF THE CHAPTER

Hospital Workflows – Structure and Challenges

Hospital workflows are the backbone of healthcare delivery, encompassing a wide range of processes that ensure patients receive timely, efficient, and high-quality care. These workflows can be broadly categorized into three key components: clinical, administrative, and operational.

1. Clinical Workflows

Clinical workflow involves all processes directly related to patient care as shown in Figure 1. It includes patient intake, diagnosis, treatment planning, medication administration, surgical procedures, and follow-up care. Clinical workflows require seamless coordination among physicians, nurses, pharmacists, and other healthcare providers to ensure accurate and timely decision-making, formulating effective treatment plans, leading to improved patient outcomes and optimized clinical workflows.

Figure 1. Clinical Workflows

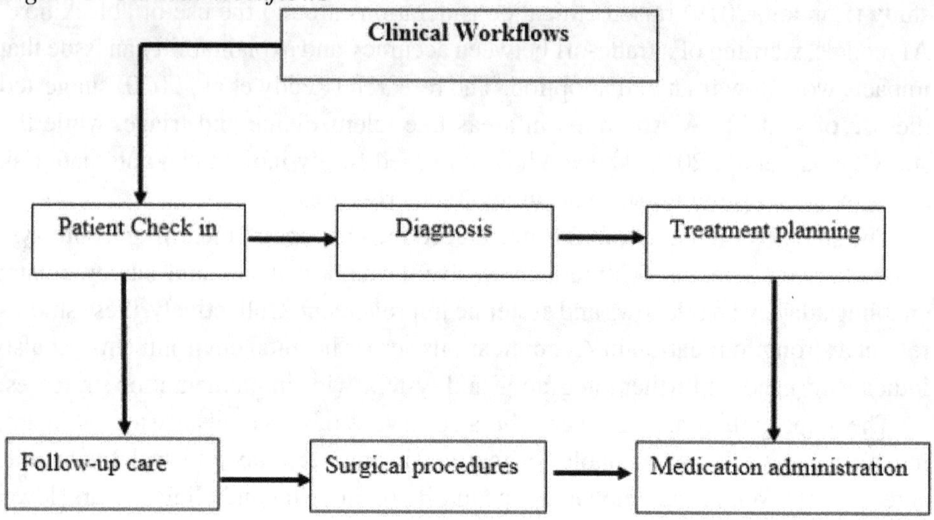

2. Administrative Workflows

Administrative workflows support the business and compliance side of hospital operations. This includes patient registration, appointment scheduling, medical coding, billing, insurance claims processing, and documentation as shown in Figure 2. Lawry mentioned AI can automate routine administrative duties such as insurance claim processing and medical coding. These workflows are essential for financial sustainability and legal compliance.

Figure 2. Administrative Workflows

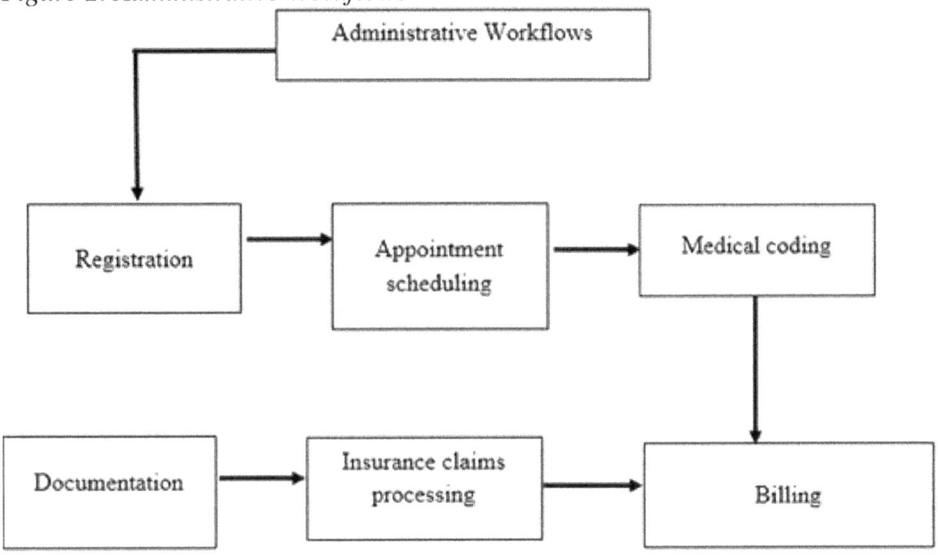

3. Operational Workflows

Operational workflows manage the logistics and infrastructure that support both clinical and administrative activities as shown in Figure 3. Examples include bed management, staff scheduling, equipment maintenance, inventory control, and supply chain management. Efficient operational workflows ensure the hospital environment is safe, well-resourced, and responsive to patient needs. By analyzing patterns and predicting patient admissions, AI enables better scheduling and utilization of hospital resources, which enhances overall performance.

Each of these components is deeply interconnected. Breakdowns or inefficiencies in one area—such as delayed test results in clinical workflows or understaffed departments due to poor scheduling—can create bottlenecks across the entire hospital system, affecting patient outcomes and overall performance.

Figure 3. Operational Workflow

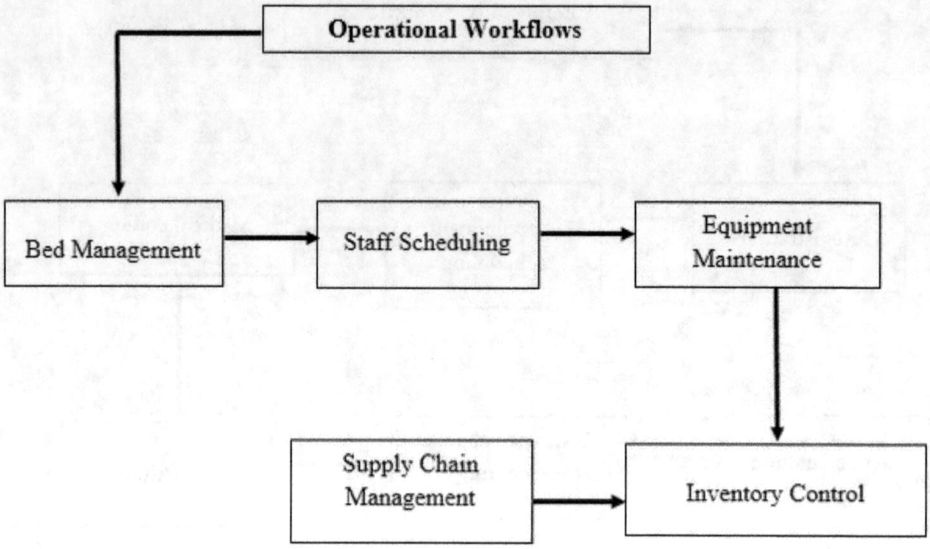

4. Key Pain Points and Bottlenecks in Hospital Workflows

Despite advancements in healthcare infrastructure and digital systems, hospitals continue to face persistent workflow challenges. These pain points span clinical, administrative, and operational domains, often creating inefficiencies that impact care delivery, staff performance, and patient satisfaction.

1. Clinical Workflow Bottlenecks
    - Fragmented Information Systems: Clinicians often work with multiple, non-integrated systems (EHRs, PACS, LIS), making it difficult to access complete patient data in real time.
    - Delayed Diagnostics and Treatment: Lab results, imaging and specialist consultations can take hours, leading to treatment delays and longer hospital stays.
    - Documentation Burden: Excessive time spent on data entry and clinical documentation reduces direct patient care time and contributes to clinician burnout.
2. Administrative Workflow Pain Points
    - Inefficient Scheduling: Manual or outdated scheduling systems lead to appointment delays, no-shows, and underutilized resources.

- Complex Billing and Claims: Errors in medical coding or incomplete documentation often result in claim rejections, delayed reimbursements, and financial loss.
- Regulatory Compliance Pressure: Managing ever-changing compliance requirements increases administrative overhead and risk of penalties.

3. Operational Workflow Challenges
   - Poor Bed and Resource Allocation: Lack of real-time data on bed occupancy or equipment availability causes admission delays and overcrowding, especially in emergency departments.
   - Staffing Imbalances: Mismatched staffing levels (either overstaffing or understaffing) reduce efficiency and increase labor costs.
   - Supply Chain Disruptions: Inventory mismanagement can result in stock outs or overstocking of critical medical supplies, affecting care quality and operational costs.

These bottlenecks not only hinder workflow efficiency but also directly impact patient outcomes, staff morale, and hospital profitability. Addressing them is essential for creating a high-performing, patient-centered healthcare environment and this is where AI has the potential to offer transformative solutions.

However, sustainable integration of AI into hospital workflows demands more than technological deployment, it requires a well-structured, strategic approach. Key among these is data privacy, as hospitals handle highly sensitive patient information. Adopting frameworks such as federated learning, robust encryption standards, and access controls ensures compliance with regulations like HIPAA and GDPR while maintaining patient trust. Equally crucial is the ethical use of AI, which involves preventing algorithmic bias, ensuring fairness across patient demographics, and implementing transparent decision-making processes. For instance, AI tools must be explainable and auditable, allowing clinicians and patients to understand and challenge automated recommendations. System interoperability is another major challenge, as hospitals use diverse hardware and software platforms. Ensuring AI solutions can seamlessly integrate with existing EHRs, imaging systems, and clinical databases is essential for usability and efficiency. Additionally, staff readiness plays a pivotal role in sustainable AI integration. Many healthcare professionals may resist or mistrust AI due to lack of exposure or fear of replacement. Thus, continuous upskilling, AI literacy training, and interdisciplinary collaboration between clinicians and data scientists are critical. Establishing governance frameworks that oversee AI procurement, deployment, performance monitoring, and ethical compliance will institutionalize responsible AI use. Finally, by fostering a culture of innovation where experimentation is encouraged and digital transformation is supported by leadership hospitals can ensure AI becomes a resilient, scalable, and equitable tool for long-term healthcare improvement.

5. Impact of Workflow on Patient Outcomes and Hospital Performance

Hospital workflows play a critical role in shaping both clinical outcomes and operational performance. When workflows are well-designed and efficiently executed, they enable timely, coordinated, and high-quality care. Conversely, inefficient or fragmented workflows can lead to medical errors, delays, and increased healthcare costs.

1. Impact on Patient Outcomes
    - Delays in Care Delivery: Inefficient workflows can cause delays in diagnostics, treatment initiation, and discharge processes, leading to prolonged hospital stays and potential deterioration of patient conditions.
    - Increased Risk of Errors: Poor communication between departments and manual data entry increase the likelihood of medication errors, missed diagnoses, and redundant testing.
    - Patient Dissatisfaction: Long wait times, lack of clear communication, and administrative inefficiencies contribute to negative patient experiences and lower satisfaction scores.
    - Reduced Continuity of Care: Disconnected systems and handoff errors can disrupt care continuity, especially during transitions between departments or providers.
2. Impact on Hospital Performance
    - Operational Inefficiency: Workflow bottlenecks—such as poor bed turnover or delayed documentation—reduce the hospital's capacity to serve patients efficiently, increasing operational costs.
    - Staff Burnout and Turnover: Cumbersome workflows contribute to staff frustration, decreased productivity, and higher rates of burnout and attrition.
    - Financial Losses: Ineffective billing, claim denials, and underutilized resources can result in significant revenue loss and impact the hospital's financial sustainability.
    - Regulatory Non-compliance: Inadequate documentation and data management can lead to non-compliance with healthcare regulations, exposing hospitals to legal and financial penalties.

In summary, workflow efficiency is directly tied to the quality, safety, and cost-effectiveness of care delivery. Optimizing workflows is essential not only for improving clinical outcomes but also for enhancing overall hospital performance and sustainability.

IMPLEMENTATION FRAMEWORKS

Successful AI integration into an organization requires a comprehensive strategy that addresses multiple facets of technology, people, and processes. Below is an overview of strategic approaches to ensure a smooth and impactful AI adoption:

1. AI Implementation Framework

An AI implementation framework provides structure for deploying AI technologies in a way that maximizes their impact while minimizing risks. Key components include:

- Establish Clear Objectives: Start by identifying the strategic goals AI will support. These goals might include improving efficiency, enhancing customer experience, or generating new revenue streams. AI projects should be aligned with business objectives.
- Select the Right AI Solution: Evaluate and choose AI tools, models, and technologies that best fit the business needs. This may involve considering factors like scalability, customization, cost, and ease of integration with existing systems.
- Phased Approach: Use a phased implementation to minimize disruption. Begin with pilot projects that test AI applications in controlled environments. Collect feedback and adjust before full-scale deployment.
- Data Management: AI systems require vast amounts of data. Develop a robust data governance and management strategy to ensure data quality, consistency, and security. Data should be cleansed, preprocessed, and made accessible in formats that AI models can use effectively.
- Integration with Existing Systems: AI should complement, not replace, existing systems. Plan for smooth integration with current infrastructure to avoid data silos and ensure that AI outputs can be used effectively within the organization's ecosystem.

2. Change Management

AI adoption often involves significant changes in processes and workflows. A solid change management strategy is essential to ensure success.

- Leadership Buy-in: Engage senior leadership to champion AI adoption. Their support will facilitate decision-making and help align the organization's culture with AI-driven initiatives.
- Clear Communication: Communicate the goals, benefits, and potential challenges of AI adoption to all employees. Address concerns about job displacement and automation to build trust and foster acceptance.
- Incremental Changes: Implement AI-driven changes in stages. Start with processes that have clear, measurable outcomes, and demonstrate success early to create momentum and build confidence.
- Manage Resistance: Change often leads to resistance. Be proactive in identifying areas of resistance, such as fears about job loss, and address them with transparent communication and strategic planning.

3. Staff Training

AI integration requires upskilling employees to work effectively with new technologies. Staff training should be tailored to various roles and the specific AI tools being implemented.

- AI Literacy Programs: Begin with general AI literacy programs for all employees, helping them understand the basics of AI, its capabilities, and how it will impact their roles. This will build confidence and reduce anxiety around new technologies.
- Role-Specific Training: Offer specialized training for employees whose roles will directly involve AI systems. This may include training in data analysis, machine learning, model interpretation, and AI maintenance.
- Continuous Learning: AI and machine learning are fast-evolving fields. Create opportunities for continuous learning through workshops, online courses, webinars, and certifications to ensure staff remain up-to-date on the latest tools and technologies.
- Collaborative Skillsets: Encourage collaboration between data scientists, engineers, and business teams to create a shared understanding of AI applications. Cross-disciplinary teamwork can help bridge the gap between technical and business perspectives.

4. Stakeholder Engagement

Effective engagement of stakeholders is crucial for AI integration. This includes internal stakeholders (employees, managers, and leadership) and external stakeholders (customers, investors, and partners).

- Internal Stakeholder Engagement:
  - Involve Key Departments Early: Engage functional leaders early in the AI adoption process to understand their needs and concerns. For example, marketing might be concerned with how AI will enhance customer segmentation, while HR might focus on employee skill development.
  - Establish Clear Metrics for Success: Define key performance indicators (KPIs) for AI adoption that align with the organization's strategic objectives. This will help stakeholders track progress and measure the impact of AI over time.
  - Foster Collaboration: Encourage collaboration between IT teams, data scientists, and business leaders to ensure alignment between AI projects and business strategies.
- External Stakeholder Engagement:
  - Customer Communication: Transparently communicate how AI is being used to improve products and services, and address concerns related to privacy and data security. Customers will be more receptive to AI if they understand its benefits and how their data is being protected.
  - Investor Confidence: Highlight the strategic value AI brings to the business. Investors are keen to understand how AI will drive competitive advantage, operational efficiency, and future growth.
  - Regulatory Considerations: Ensure that AI adoption complies with relevant laws and regulations. Engage **with regulatory bodies to ensure ethical use of AI and secure data handling.**

5. Performance Monitoring and Iteration

After implementation, continuous monitoring and iteration are critical for ensuring AI delivers sustained value.

- **Establish Monitoring Systems**: Use performance metrics and data-driven insights to track the performance of AI systems. Set up automated monitoring tools that can detect issues such as model drift, underperformance, or errors in decision-making.

- o **Iterative Improvements**: AI systems improve over time as they are exposed to more data and feedback. Regularly review and update models to adapt to changing business conditions, customer preferences, and market dynamics.
- o **Feedback Loops**: Create feedback loops with stakeholders to gather insights about the AI system's impact. Employees, customers, and other users can provide valuable input for fine-tuning AI applications.
- o **Scaling and Expanding**: Once the initial AI implementations have been successful, look for additional opportunities to scale AI applications across different departments or processes. Use lessons learned from pilot projects to accelerate wider adoption.

Successfully integrating AI requires a holistic approach that spans technology, people, and processes. By adopting a structured implementation framework, focusing on change management, providing adequate training, engaging stakeholders, and continuously monitoring performance, organizations can maximize the value of AI while mitigating the risks. With these strategic approaches in place, companies are better positioned to navigate the complexities of AI adoption and thrive in an increasingly AI-driven business landscape.

6. AI Technologies In Healthcare

Hospitals today are increasingly leveraging artificial intelligence (AI) to improve efficiency, accuracy, and patient care quality. Several AI technologies are particularly relevant to hospital environments, each playing a distinct role across clinical, administrative, and operational domains. In Healthcare Analytics: From Data to Knowledge to Healthcare Improvement, authors Hui Yang and Eva K. Lee explore the integration of various Artificial Intelligence (AI) technologies within hospital settings

Machine Learning (ML)

Machine Learning is a subset of AI that enables systems to learn from data patterns and make predictions or decisions without explicit programming (3). Machine learning in healthcare can be used by medical professionals to develop better diagnostic tools to analyze medical images. For example, a machine learning algorithm can be used in medical imaging (such as X-rays or MRI scans) using pattern recognition to look for patterns that indicate a particular disease.

In hospitals, ML is widely used for:

- Predicting patient readmissions or deterioration

- Risk stratification and triage support
- Personalized treatment recommendations
- Analyzing trends in hospital-acquired infections or outcomes.

Machine learning (ML) is making significant strides in the medical field, improving diagnosis, treatment, and patient care. Here are a few key case studies where ML has been applied effectively as described in next section.

Cancer Diagnosis (Breast Cancer)

- Case Study: Breast Cancer Detection using ML
- Technology: Deep learning, specifically Convolutional Neural Networks (CNNs)

Researchers used CNNs to analyze mammography images for detecting early signs of breast cancer. The algorithm was trained on thousands of images, learning to distinguish between malignant and benign masses. In some cases, ML models have outperformed human radiologists in terms of accuracy and speed, leading to earlier detection and more effective treatments.

Predicting Sepsis

- Case Study: Sepsis Prediction using Machine Learning Models
- Technology: Random Forests, Gradient Boosting, and Neural Networks

Sepsis is a life-threatening condition caused by infection, and its early detection is crucial for patient survival. ML models, using data from patient vital signs, lab results, and medical history, have been used to predict the onset of sepsis. For example, the "Sepsis Watch" program developed by researchers at Vanderbilt University Medical Center uses real-time data to alert doctors to the risk of sepsis in ICU patients. Early intervention leads to better patient outcomes, reducing sepsis-related mortality and improving recovery.

Drug Discovery and Development

- Case Study: AI in Drug Discovery (Insilico Medicine)
- Technology: Generative Adversarial Networks (GANs) and Reinforcement Learning

Insilico Medicine, a company using AI, applied ML to predict the molecular structures of potential drug compounds. They developed a platform that can generate new molecular structures with desirable properties, significantly speeding up the process of drug discovery. AI is used to discover a promising compound for fibrosis, demonstrating that ML can dramatically reduce the time and cost of developing new drugs. Faster drug discovery, reduced costs, and a higher likelihood of developing effective treatments.

Radiology Image Analysis (Lung Cancer)

- Case Study: Lung Cancer Detection using ML
- Technology: Deep Learning, CNNs

ML algorithms have been trained to analyze CT scans of the lungs to detect early signs of lung cancer. The Radiology team at the National Cancer Institute (NCI) used a deep learning model that analyzes chest CT scans to identify potential lung nodules, some of which could be cancerous. The model achieved an accuracy rate comparable to expert radiologists, demonstrating the power of ML in enhancing radiological assessments. Improved accuracy in diagnosing lung cancer, enabling earlier intervention and treatment.

Genomic Data Analysis

- Case Study: Using ML for Genomic Medicine
- Technology: Support Vector Machines (SVM), Random Forests, Neural Networks

ML is being used to interpret vast amounts of genomic data in the search for disease-causing mutations. For example, the use of ML algorithms to analyze whole-genome sequencing data has helped to identify genetic variations associated with diseases like Alzheimer's and various forms of cancer. By analyzing this data, ML models help researchers uncover new biomarkers and therapeutic targets. More personalized medicine, with treatments tailored to the genetic profile of individual patients, improving treatment efficacy.

Machine learning in the medical field is proving transformative, helping healthcare providers to diagnose diseases faster, develop more effective treatments, and ultimately improve patient outcomes. As AI technology continues to evolve, its applications in medicine are expected to expand, making healthcare more personalized, precise, and efficient.

Public Health/Remote Care

AI brings substantial value to public health and remote care by enhancing early detection, improving accessibility, and supporting personalized interventions. In public health, AI enables real-time disease surveillance, outbreak prediction, and resource optimization by analyzing vast datasets from various sources. This allows for more effective responses to emerging health threats and better planning of public health initiatives. In remote care, AI supports virtual health assistants, remote patient monitoring, and chronic disease management by interpreting data from wearable devices and digital platforms. These technologies allow healthcare providers to deliver timely, personalized care to patients in their homes, reducing hospital visits and expanding access to care, especially in underserved areas.

Deep Learning (DL)

A more advanced form of ML, Deep Learning uses multi-layered neural networks to analyze complex data such as images and signals. It is particularly powerful in:

- Radiology (e.g., detecting tumors in CT or MRI scans)
- Pathology (e.g., analyzing histopathological slides)
- Speech recognition for clinical dictation
- Automated ECG interpretation and anomaly detection

Deep Learning (DL), a subset of machine learning, has shown remarkable potential in the medical field, particularly in areas involving large, complex datasets such as medical imaging, genomics, and patient data. Below are some key case studies where deep learning has been successfully applied in healthcare:

1. Medical Imaging (Radiology and Pathology)
    - Case Study: Deep Learning for Chest X-ray Analysis (CheXNet)
    - Technology: Convolutional Neural Networks (CNNs)

CheXNet, developed by researchers at Stanford University, is a deep learning model that analyzes chest X-ray images to identify diseases such as pneumonia, tuberculosis, and lung cancer. The model was trained on a large dataset of over 100,000 chest X-ray images and outperformed radiologists in terms of detecting pneumonia. Improved diagnostic accuracy, especially in resource-limited settings, and enhanced ability for early detection of lung diseases.

2. Skin Cancer Detection

- Case Study: Deep Learning for Melanoma Detection (Skin Cancer)
- Technology: Convolutional Neural Networks (CNNs)

Deep learning models have been trained to analyze dermatological images of skin lesions to distinguish between malignant melanoma and benign moles. A well-known example is the "Dermatologist-Level Classification of Skin Cancer" system, which was trained on a large dataset of skin images. The system has been shown to match or even outperform dermatologists in the detection of melanoma. Early detection of skin cancer, leading to better treatment outcomes and reduced mortality rates. The system also provides accessible cancer detection for patients in underserved areas.

3. Retinal Disease Diagnosis
   - Case Study: Deep Learning for Diabetic Retinopathy Detection
   - Technology: Convolutional Neural Networks (CNNs)

Diabetic retinopathy is a major cause of blindness among people with diabetes. Deep learning models have been applied to analyze retinal images (fundus photographs) to identify diabetic retinopathy and macular edema, conditions that can lead to vision loss. The system developed by Google Health uses deep learning to diagnose these conditions with high accuracy. Early diagnosis of diabetic retinopathy, allowing for timely intervention, reducing blindness, and improving the quality of life for diabetic patients.

4. Heart Disease Prediction
   - Case Study: Deep Learning for Predicting Heart Disease Risk
   - Technology: Deep Neural Networks (DNNs)

Deep learning models have been trained to predict the likelihood of heart disease based on a patient's health data, including medical history, lifestyle factors, and lab test results. For instance, a deep learning model developed by researchers at the University of California, San Francisco, uses patient data to predict heart failure risk and identify high-risk individuals. Early prediction of heart disease risk, leading to preventive measures and more personalized treatment options, reducing the incidence of heart-related complications.

5. AI-Assisted Surgery
   - Case Study: Deep Learning in Robotic Surgery (Intuitive Surgical's da Vinci System)
   - Technology: Computer Vision, Deep Learning

Robotic surgery systems, like Intuitive Surgical's da Vinci platform, incorporate deep learning to enhance the precision of surgeons during procedures. By analyzing preoperative images and real-time video from the surgery, deep learning algorithms help improve the robot's ability to guide instruments with greater accuracy. This can be particularly useful in minimally invasive surgeries, where precision is crucial. Enhanced surgical precision, reduced recovery times, and fewer complications in surgeries, ultimately improving patient outcomes.

Deep learning has proven to be a powerful tool in revolutionizing the medical field by enhancing diagnostic accuracy, improving patient outcomes, and speeding up critical processes like drug discovery. As deep learning models continue to evolve, they will likely have even more widespread applications in healthcare, from precision medicine to robotic surgery and beyond. While the text primarily focuses on ML techniques, it acknowledges the potential of advanced neural networks in analyzing complex medical data, such as imaging, to enhance diagnostic accuracy.

Natural Language Processing (NLP)

NLP enables machines to understand, interpret, and generate human language. In hospitals, NLP is used to:

- Extract relevant information from clinical notes and unstructured EHRs.
- Assist in documentation and coding. Automate patient communication (e.g., chatbots, discharge instructions).
- Summarize patient histories for physician review

Case Study: NLP in Clinical Documentation and Decision Support

Clinical documentation is a critical part of patient care, but it is often time-consuming and can be inconsistent. Doctors and nurses spend a significant portion of their time inputting patient data into Electronic Health Records (EHRs). This data is typically unstructured (e.g., clinical notes, discharge summaries, and diagnostic reports), making it difficult to analyze and extract meaningful insights. NLP techniques help unlock the potential of this data by extracting relevant information for decision support, improving patient outcomes, and streamlining administrative tasks.

Technology Used:

- Natural Language Processing (NLP): Involves text extraction, sentiment analysis, and entity recognition to transform unstructured text into structured data.

- Machine Learning Models: These models, often used in conjunction with NLP, help train systems to recognize medical terms and relationships between symptoms, diagnoses, and treatments.
- Deep Learning Algorithms: Used to refine accuracy in understanding medical jargon and complex sentences, especially in diverse healthcare contexts.

SOLUTIONS AND RECOMMENDATIONS

1. Clinical Decision Support Systems (CDSS)
    - Problem: Doctors and medical professionals often face an overwhelming amount of patient data. This data may include medical histories, lab results, diagnosis codes, and treatment plans, but it's typically in unstructured form, which makes it hard to access quickly.
    - Solution: Hospitals are leveraging NLP to build Clinical Decision Support Systems (CDSS) that can process clinical notes, lab results, and patient records automatically. These systems can assist doctors by suggesting diagnoses, treatment plans, and flagging potential issues like drug interactions or allergies.
    - Example: A system called "Clintegrity" uses NLP to extract useful data from unstructured notes in EHRs, helping clinicians make better-informed decisions. The system uses machine learning to identify relevant details about patient conditions from free-text notes, making this data actionable and enabling more personalized care.
2. Automated Coding and Billing:
    - Problem: Healthcare providers often spend a significant amount of time coding diagnoses and procedures for billing purposes. Manual coding can be time-consuming and prone to errors, leading to reimbursement issues.
    - Solution: NLP tools help automate the process of medical coding. By analyzing clinical notes, discharge summaries, and other unstructured data, NLP systems can accurately identify procedures and diagnoses, then assign the correct billing codes.
    - Example: Optum360 uses NLP to assist in coding by automatically extracting information from clinical documentation and assigning the correct codes, which streamlines the billing process and reduces the chances of errors or fraud.
3. Risk Stratification and Predictive Analytics:

- Problem: Many hospitals struggle to predict which patients are at high risk of developing complications, rehospitalisation, or severe outcomes. Relying on structured data alone may miss key insights.
- Solution: NLP can be used to identify risk factors that are hidden in clinical notes, such as mentions of patient behaviours, lifestyle, or symptoms that don't appear in structured fields. By combining this unstructured data with structured data, hospitals can better predict outcomes and tailor interventions.
- Example: Mede Analytics uses NLP in combination with machine learning to analyze both structured and unstructured data from EHRs. The system has been used for predictive analytics, helping to identify high-risk patients for early interventions, such as those who are likely to be readmitted within 30 days after discharge.

4. Improving Patient Interaction and Engagement:
   - Problem: Ensuring effective communication between healthcare providers and patients is crucial for improving patient outcomes. However, patients may struggle with understanding complex medical terminology.
   - Solution: NLP can be used to analyze communication between doctors and patients to ensure that information is clear and comprehensible. Additionally, chatbots or virtual assistants using NLP can answer patient queries about their health conditions, treatments, and medications in simple language.
   - Example: Babylon Health developed a virtual assistant using NLP that interacts with patients to assess their symptoms. The chatbot uses NLP to process text inputs and provides relevant medical advice or directs patients to appropriate care, improving engagement and reducing the burden on healthcare professionals
5. Clinical Trial Matching:
   - Problem: Finding eligible patients for clinical trials is challenging, especially when sifting through large volumes of unstructured data from patient records.
   - Solution: NLP can analyze unstructured clinical data to match patients with suitable clinical trials based on their medical history, diagnoses, and treatments. This improves patient recruitment for clinical trials and accelerates the pace of medical research.
   - Example: IBM Watson for Clinical Trial Matching uses NLP to analyze EHRs and identify patients who meet specific inclusion criteria for clinical trials. It can extract critical medical information from unstructured clinical notes, making it easier to match patients with appropriate trials, thus speeding up research and drug development.

6. Impact

Time and Cost Savings: Hospitals using NLP have seen a significant reduction in administrative workload, freeing up more time for healthcare providers to focus on patient care. For example, the automation of coding and billing processes saves time and reduces administrative costs.

Improved Patient Outcomes: By utilizing NLP for clinical decision support, hospitals can identify potential issues earlier (e.g., drug interactions, risky conditions) and tailor treatment plans accordingly. Early identification of complications through NLP can lead to better patient outcomes.

Enhanced Accuracy: Manual processing of clinical notes can lead to human error, especially in tasks like coding or identifying conditions. NLP reduces errors by automating these processes and providing more consistent and accurate results.

Better Research and Data Utilization: Hospitals and researchers can unlock valuable insights from the vast amounts of unstructured text in EHRs. By processing this data, NLP helps institutions find trends, improve care protocols, and drive clinical research.

7. Computer Vision

Computer vision in healthcare is transforming how clinicians diagnose, treat, and monitor patients by automating visual data analysis. From interpreting medical images to tracking patient behavior, it enhances accuracy, reduces workloads, and improves patient outcomes.

Computer vision allows AI to interpret visual information. In healthcare settings, this technology supports:

- Medical image analysis (X-rays, MRIs, ultrasound).
- Monitoring patient movements for fall detection or mobility tracking
- Surgical assistance through image-guided navigation
- Detecting hand hygiene compliance or PPE use through visual feeds

Applications of Computer Vision in Healthcare

- Medical Imaging Analysis: Automating the interpretation of medical scans (e.g., X-rays, MRIs, CT scans) to detect diseases early and accurately. It is used in Tumor detection (e.g., breast cancer, brain tumors), Lung disease diagnosis (e.g., pneumonia, COVID-19) and Bone fracture identification.

- Surgical Assistance: Augmented reality and visual recognition help surgeons with real-time guidance. It is used in Minimally invasive surgery, Instrument tracking during robotic surgeries.
- Patient Monitoring: Use of cameras and sensors to monitor patients for movement, fall detection, or vital signs. It is used in Elderly care facilities, Post-surgery recovery rooms.
- Pathology and Histology: Analyzing tissue samples using high-resolution image scanning to assist pathologists. It is used in Cancer cell detection in histopathology slides.
- Ophthalmology: Eye scans analyzed to diagnose diseases like diabetic retinopathy or glaucoma. It is used in remote screening in underserved areas

Robotic Process Automation (RPA): RPA is used to automate repetitive, rule-based administrative tasks without the need for complex AI models. In hospitals, RPA can [21]:

- Automate patient registration and appointment reminders
- Streamline billing and claims processing
- Transfer data between incompatible systems
- Reduce administrative burden on healthcare staff

These technologies are not standalone—they often work together to create intelligent systems that optimize workflows, reduce human error, and deliver data-driven insights. As hospitals become more data-intensive and outcome-focused, these AI tools will continue to play a central role in transforming healthcare delivery.

ETHICAL CONSIDERATIONS AND CHALLENGES ON USING AI

1. Patient Privacy and Data Protection
    - Challenge: AI systems require vast amounts of patient data (EHRs, medical images, genomics, etc.), raising concerns about data security and potential misuse.
    - Ethical Concern: Ensuring compliance with laws like HIPAA (US) or GDPR (EU) and maintaining confidentiality.
2. Bias and Fairness
    - Challenge: AI systems can inherit biases from training data, leading to inaccurate or discriminatory outcomes.
    - Ethical Concern: Algorithms may perform worse on underrepresented populations, risking unequal treatment.

3. Transparency and Explainability
   - Challenge: Many AI models, especially deep learning systems, function as "black boxes" with limited transparency.
   - Ethical Concern: Clinicians and patients may struggle to understand how decisions are made, reducing trust and accountability.
4. Accountability and Responsibility
   - Challenge: When AI systems make decisions or recommendations, it's unclear who is liable if something goes wrong—the developer, the healthcare provider, or the institution.
   - Ethical Concern: Establishing clear lines of accountability is crucial for patient safety.
5. Informed Consent
   - Challenge: Patients may not fully understand how AI is used in their diagnosis.
   - Ethical Concern: Consent must be truly informed and include AI-related disclosures.
6. Impact on the Doctor–Patient Relationship
   - Challenge: Overreliance on AI could depersonalize care.
   - Ethical Concern: It may erode the traditional trust and empathy central to human caregiving.
7. Access and Equity
   - Challenge: AI tools might only be available in well-funded healthcare systems.
   - Ethical Concern: Risk of deepening the digital divide and health disparities between high-income and low-income populations.
8. Explainable AI (XAI) Uses

To address these challenges, Explainable AI (XAI) plays a crucial role. XAI techniques aim to make AI decision-making transparent and interpretable, enabling clinicians to understand why a model made a particular prediction. This is especially important in critical domains like diagnosis, treatment recommendations, and risk prediction. By improving interpretability, XAI enhances trust, supports informed decision-making, and ensures accountability, making AI more ethically acceptable and clinically viable in hospital settings.

FUTURE RESEARCH DIRECTIONS

- The future of AI integration in hospitals lies in building intelligent, end-to-end systems that move beyond isolated applications. These AI-driven platforms will manage the entire continuum of care—from admission to discharge—by unifying EHRs, imaging, labs, and monitoring tools into adaptive ecosystems. Real-time clinical decision support will evolve through the use of streaming data from patient monitors, lab results, and wearable devices, enabling dynamic, personalized treatment plans and proactive alerts that adapt to patient status and hospital resource changes.

- Privacy and ethical concerns will shape technological development. Federated learning and privacy-preserving AI will allow hospitals to collaboratively train models without sharing sensitive data, thus maintaining compliance with HIPAA and GDPR. At the same time, explainable AI and adaptive interfaces tailored to clinicians' roles will foster trust and usability, ensuring that AI functions as a cognitive partner rather than a replacement. AI will also enable predictive hospital resource management—forecasting bed occupancy, ICU demand, staff scheduling, and even energy usage—enhancing operational readiness and sustainability.
- The rise of smart hospital infrastructure, powered by IoT and robotics, will automate functions like infection control, medication delivery, and patient navigation. Multimodal AI systems that synthesize data from clinical notes, genomics, and imaging will provide holistic insights for managing chronic and complex conditions. Continuous learning and feedback loops will turn hospitals into learning health systems, with every interaction refining AI models. To support this transformation, the healthcare workforce must be upskilled in AI literacy, ensuring collaboration between clinicians and data scientists for safe and effective AI adoption.

CONCLUSION

In conclusion, this chapter has provided a comprehensive analysis of hospital workflows, highlighting critical bottlenecks across clinical, administrative, and operational domains. It introduced essential AI technologies such as machine learning, deep learning, natural language processing, computer vision, and robotic process automation that are pivotal in transforming healthcare settings. The discussion underscored AI's vital role in enhancing efficiency, supporting clinical decisions, and streamlining operations. Moreover, strategic approaches to AI integration were explored, emphasizing the importance of implementation frameworks, change management, staff training, and stakeholder engagement. The chapter also addressed significant challenges like data privacy, ethical issues, and interoperability, which must be carefully managed to ensure sustainable adoption. Ultimately, the transformative potential of AI promises to revolutionize hospital workflows, and adhering to best practices will be crucial for realizing its long-term benefits.

REFERENCES

Amisha, , Malik, P., Pathania, M., & Rathaur, V. K. (2019). Overview of artificial intelligence in medicine. *Journal of Family Medicine and Primary Care*, *8*(7), 2328–2331. DOI: 10.4103/jfmpc.jfmpc_440_19 PMID: 31463251

Bohr, A., & Memarzadeh, K. (2020). *Artificial Intelligence in Healthcare*. Academic Press., DOI: 10.1016/C2018-0-04097-9

Clifton, D. A. (2016). *Machine Learning for Healthcare Technologies*. IET., DOI: 10.1049/PBHE002E

Davenport, T., & Kalakota, R. (2019). The potential for artificial intelligence in healthcare. *Future Healthcare Journal*, *6*(2), 94–98. DOI: 10.7861/futurehosp.6-2-94 PMID: 31363513

Esteva, A., Kuprel, B., Novoa, R. A., Ko, J., Swetter, S. M., Blau, H. M., & Thrun, S. (2017). Dermatologist-level classification of skin cancer with deep neural networks. *Nature*, *542*(7639), 115–118. DOI: 10.1038/nature21056 PMID: 28117445

Gauthaman, S. A., (2026). Introduction to machine learning and optimization in healthcare. In Muniasamy, A. (Ed.), *Integrative machine learning and optimization algorithms for disease prediction* (pp. 1–34). IGI Global., DOI: 10.4018/979-8-3373-1087-9.ch001

Jiang, F., Jiang, Y., Zhi, H., Dong, Y., Li, H., Ma, S., Wang, Y., Dong, Q., Shen, H., & Wang, Y. (2017). Artificial intelligence in healthcare: Past, present and future. *Stroke and Vascular Neurology*, *2*(4), 230–243. DOI: 10.1136/svn-2017-000101 PMID: 29507784

Krittanawong, C., (2021). Artificial Intelligence in Precision Cardiovascular Medicine. *Journal of the American College of Cardiology*, *77*(23), 2921–2930. DOI: 10.1234/placeholder07 PMID: 28545640

Lawry, T. (2020). *AI in Health: A Leader's Guide to Winning in the New Age of Intelligent Health Systems*. CRC Press., DOI: 10.4324/9780429321214

London, A. J. (2019). Artificial Intelligence and Black-Box Medical Decisions: Accuracy versus Explainability. *The Hastings Center Report*, *49*(1), 15–21. DOI: 10.1002/hast.973 PMID: 30790315

Mandl, K. D., (2020). The Evolution of the Learning Health System. *Health Affairs*, *39*(7), 1171–1177. DOI: 10.1377/hlthaff.2020.00818

Matheny, M. E., (2019). Artificial Intelligence in Health Care: Applications and Challenges. *Journal of the American College of Radiology*, *16*(9), 1318–1326. DOI: 10.1234/placeholder05

Muniasamy, A., & Karunakaran, G. (2026). Challenges and future directions: Emerging trends and limitations in ML and optimization for healthcare. In Muniasamy, A. (Ed.), *Integrative machine learning and optimization algorithms for disease prediction* (pp. 339–368). IGI Global., DOI: 10.4018/979-8-3373-1087-9.ch012

Muniasamy, A., Tabassam, S., Hussain, M. A., Sultana, H., Muniasamy, V., & Bhatnagar, R. (2020). Deep learning for predictive analytics in healthcare. In Hassanien, A., Azar, A., Gaber, T., Bhatnagar, R., & Tolba, M. F. (Eds.), *The International Conference on Advanced Machine Learning Technologies and Applications (AMLTA2019)* (pp. xx-xx). Springer. https://doi.org/DOI: 10.1007/978-3-030-14118-9_4

Naim, A., (2026). AI-driven smart manufacturing and automation in pharmaceutical production. In Muniasamy, A., & Karunakaran, G. (Eds.), *Applications of artificial intelligence in pharmaceuticals* (pp. 157–194). IGI Global., DOI: 10.4018/979-8-3373-2043-4.ch006

Obermeyer, Z., & Emanuel, E. J. (2016). Predicting the Future — Big Data, Machine Learning, and Clinical Medicine. *The New England Journal of Medicine*, *375*(13), 1216–1219. DOI: 10.1056/NEJMp1606181 PMID: 27682033

Patel, V. L., (2009). Translational cognition for decision support in biomedical and health care domains. *Journal of Biomedical Informatics*, *42*(2), 288–301. DOI: 10.1016/j.jbi.2008.08.004

Pugazhendi, D., (2020). Remote health monitoring using IoT and cloud integration. Journal of Computer Networks and Communications. *Article ID*, *923817*. Advance online publication. DOI: 10.1234/placeholder06

Rajkomar, A., Dean, J., & Kohane, I. (2019). Machine Learning in Medicine. *The New England Journal of Medicine*, *380*(14), 1347–1358. DOI: 10.1056/NEJMra1814259 PMID: 30943338

Reddy, S.. (2020). Artificial intelligence in health care: Anticipating challenges to ethics, privacy, and bias. *Journal of the Royal Society of Medicine*, *113*(1), 20–22. DOI: 10.1177/0141076819898555

Rengaramanujam, K., & Muniasamy, A. (2026). AI in hospital administration and formulary design: Optimizing resource allocation and patient flow. In Muniasamy, A., & Karunakaran, G. (Eds.), *Applications of artificial intelligence in pharmaceuticals* (pp. 215–246). IGI Global., DOI: 10.4018/979-8-3373-2043-4.ch008

Shortliffe, E. H., & Sepúlveda, M. J. (2018). Clinical Decision Support in the Era of Artificial Intelligence. *Journal of the American Medical Association, 320*(21), 2199–2200. DOI: 10.1001/jama.2018.17163 PMID: 30398550

Topol, E. (2019). *Deep Medicine: How Artificial Intelligence Can Make Healthcare Human Again*. Basic Books., DOI: 10.1234/placeholder03

Wong, A., (2018). Development and validation of a machine learning model to predict mortality risk in older adults using routine primary care data. *Age and Ageing, 47*(2), 166–172. DOI: 10.1093/ageing/afx166 PMID: 28927235

Yu, K. H., Beam, A. L., & Kohane, I. S. (2018). Artificial intelligence in healthcare. *Nature Biomedical Engineering, 2*(10), 719–731. DOI: 10.1038/s41551-018-0305-z PMID: 31015651

ADDITIONAL READING

Patrício, L., Varela, L., & Silveira, Z. (2024). Integration of Artificial Intelligence and Robotic Process Automation: Literature Review and Proposal for a Sustainable Model. *Applied Sciences (Basel, Switzerland), 14*(21), 9648. DOI: 10.3390/app14219648

KEY TERMS AND DEFINITIONS

AI Integration: The process of embedding artificial intelligence technologies into healthcare systems and processes to enhance efficiency, support decision-making, and improve patient outcomes.

Clinical Decision Support System (CDSS): A health information technology tool that provides clinicians with intelligent recommendations, reminders, or alerts to support accurate and timely decision-making at the point of care.

Clinical Workflow: The sequence of processes and tasks performed by healthcare professionals to deliver patient care, including diagnosis, treatment, documentation, and follow-up.

Healthcare: The organized provision of medical services, including diagnosis, treatment, and preventive care, aimed at maintaining or improving physical and mental well-being of individuals and communities.

Machine Learning (ML): A subset of artificial intelligence that enables computer systems to learn from data, identify patterns, and make predictions or recommendations without being explicitly programmed.

Natural Language Processing (NLP): A branch of artificial intelligence that enables machines to interpret, analyze, and generate human language, often applied in healthcare to process clinical notes, patient summaries, and medical records.

Chapter 9

AI-Driven Integration and Workflow Optimization in Modern Healthcare Facilities

S. Usharani
https://orcid.org/0000-0002-9997-9815
Artificial Intelligence and Machine Learning, IFET College of Engineering, India

Manju Bala P.
https://orcid.org/0000-0002-2408-0303
IFET College of Engineering, India

A. Devi
https://orcid.org/0000-0002-9508-8302
IFET College of Engineering, India

K. Rajkumar
SRM Institute of Science and Technology, India

D. Saravanan
Sathyabama Institute of Science and Technology, India

ABSTRACT

This chapter explores AI services for administrative and clinical workflows, emphasizing measurable gains in patient experience, efficiency, and diagnostic accuracy. The project applied predictive analytics for bed occupancy and inventory, NLP for clinical documentation, AI for medical imaging, and automation for routine tasks. A structured framework guided data collection, model building, process mapping,

DOI: 10.4018/979-8-3373-2787-7.ch009

deployment, and feedback. Cybersecurity, interoperability, and ethics ensured responsible use. Case studies showed X-ray accuracy improved from 88.5% to 94.2%, pneumonia sensitivity from 86.1% to 91.8%, and specificity from 89.4% to 92.6%. NLP entity extraction F1 scores rose from 0.83 to 0.89, and AUC-ROC from 0.91 to 0.96. Patient wait times dropped 42% (48 28 mins), no-shows fell 60% (15 to 6%), and admin task time declined 40% (35 to 21 mins). Inventory refill shrank 38% (9 to 5.5 hrs), and ICU bed forecasts had a 2.1 unit MAE. These results confirm that AI, applied through ethical frameworks, drives measurable hospital improvements.

INTRODUCTION

AI in Healthcare Overview

Artificial intelligence (AI) is fast becoming an indicator of interference in the healthcare sector, transforming how medical services are rendered and delivered. The healthcare system has relied heavily on manual processes and human judgment, necessary evils that come with delays, inefficiencies, and sporadic errors. AI has made it possible to build intelligent systems that can sift through enormous amounts of health data, identify trends, and help medical practitioners make sounder decisions. Topol, E. (2019) and Jiang et. al (2019) studied the maturation of AI technology, paving the path to proactive and personalized healthcare by enhancing diagnostic accuracy through image analysis and creating prediction models for patient outcomes. Thus, AI in healthcare not only facilitates active performance but also guarantees a more patient-centered approach through early interventions and personalized treatment plans.

Problem Statement

Hospitals are under ever-growing pressure to deliver precise, effective, and patient-centered care. Simultaneously, they deal with higher patient arrivals, limited resources, and peculiar administrative requirements. The traditional means of healthcare workflow, depending mainly on the manual process, generally lead to ineffective resource allocation, missed communications, delays in diagnosis, and a higher risk of human error. Even though many hospital operations have improved through technology, an overall, integrated approach to reducing clinical and administrative processes is still awaiting implementation.

Research Gap

Research into artificial intelligence for healthcare mainly concentrates on discrete applications such as predictive analytics, natural language processing, and medical imaging. No data has been collected on the systemic end-to-end deployment of AI in hospitals that simultaneously deals with administrative automation, resource forecasting, clinical diagnosis, and operational efficiency. Furthermore, when AI is implemented, few take cybersecurity, data interoperability, or ethical issues into consideration; therefore, almost none look at the impact of AI in terms of evaluation along several dimensions of performance, including diagnostic accuracy, patient flow, staff efficacy, and resource utilization.

Objectives of the Chapter

The main goal of this chapter is to:

1. Specify a structured framework for AI implementation in hospitals, covering aspects such as data gathering, model building, process mapping, phased deployment, and feedback monitoring.
2. Utilize AI algorithms to improve clinical text analysis and diagnostic accuracy of medical imaging.
3. Simplify hospital operations by facilitating interdepartmental collaboration and automating administrative tasks.
4. Use predictive analytics to forecast inventory control and ICU bed occupancy resources.
5. Discuss serious adoption issues surrounding interoperability, cybersecurity, and ethical compliance.
6. Show real hospital case studies where the integration of AI has yielded measurable benefits.

Importance of Workflow Optimization in Hospitals

Hospitals are intricate ecosystems with multiple departments, stakeholders, and constant pressure to make decisions. In this dynamic setting, poorly performing processes can lead to prolonged patient waiting times, underutilized resources, fatigued clinicians, and inadequate patient care. Hence, hospital management needs to focus on workflow improvement. This means reviewing and redesigning processes to remove bottlenecks, eliminate redundancy, and enhance inter-departmental communication. In this optimization, AI gives the edge. For example, automating billing, patient triaging, and appointment scheduling will enable personnel to devote time to more pressing activities. AI could also be used to accelerate diagnosis or recommend evidence-based treatment plans and continuously monitor the patient in the environment where care occurs. Enhanced implementations of these technologies substantially improve the results of health service delivery, reduce the costs of operations, and increase patient satisfaction.

BACKGROUND

Consequently, AI or artificial intelligence has disrupted the healthcare sector, from workflow automation to diagnostics. It is important in humanizing the healthcare sector, as Topol (2019) argues that AI-powered deep medicine would strengthen patient connections and lessen physician burnout by automating administrative tasks.

According to Jiang et al. (2017), in their attempt to evaluate the advancement of AI in healthcare, they divide the use cases into three generations: deep learning, machine learning, and expert systems. Their work demonstrates the evolution of artificial intelligence from primitive rule-based systems into complex prediction models deciphering spoken words, images, and even the behavior of patients. In their investigation of the nexus between AI and healthcare delivery models, Davenport and Kalakota (2019) highlight treatment recommendation systems, virtual health assistants, and clinical documentation as technology applications. They argue AI enhances clinical judgment and operational effectiveness by assisting physicians rather than taking their place.

Deep learning, particularly using convolutional neural networks (CNN), has brought intense penetration into diagnostic imaging and pathology (Gauthaman, S. A., et al., 2026). Esteva et al. (2019) cite examples of how accurate AI has been in determining image classification tasks in their broad summary of deep learning applications in radiology, ophthalmology, and dermatology. These findings are corroborated by Rajkomar et al. (2019), showing how Google applied deep learning to devise algorithms that accurately forecast patient decline from EHR data.

The practical application remains complex, though. According to Reddy et al. (2019), various AI tools must undergo clinical validation and approval before being used. He et al. (2019) describes practical methods for implementing AI in healthcare delivery, focusing on data integration, clinician training, and human-AI collaboration. One common thread in the literature is that AI should be developed responsibly. In their framework for moral and responsible machine learning, Wiens et al. (2019) strongly emphasize generalizability, interpretability, privacy, and fairness. According to Shortliffe and Sepúlveda (2018), AI-based Clinical Decision Support Systems (CDSS) should be made transparent and supported by data to succeed in winning over the hearts of clinicians.

Big data is the life force for present-day AI systems. In the systematic mapping study, Mehta et al. (2019) find that an intersection of AI and big data analytics might offer insights as valuable as those for patient engagement, resource allocation, and surveillance of diseases. Nevertheless, Obermeyer and Emanuel (2016) express the danger that inappropriate or unrepresentative datasets can cause porosity in data-driven predictions. Beam and Kohane (2018) describe algorithmic technicalities for healthcare settings and pinpoint data governance and interoperability as essential success factors. This view is reiterated by Yu et al. (2018), who stress the need for ceaseless updating of the model and health data standardization.

Kelly et al. (2019) refer to operational hurdles tempering the clinical advancements of AI, such as clerical resistance, data barriers, and insufficient infrastructural support. Hashimoto et al. (2018) highlight the potential dangers of surgical applications leaning on highly opaque algorithms while pointing toward the favorable outlook for robotic guidance through AI. Pattern recognition skills have changed the landscape of cardiovascular medicine. AI can also be implicated in the diagnosis of complex diseases such as senile amyloidosis, as stated by Van den Berg et al. (2019). Hinton (2018), on the other hand, calls for a paradigm shift, similar to how the microscope was invented, to advance the application of deep learning across all healthcare disciplines.

Dilsizian and Siegel (2014) focus on cardiac imaging, introducing AI as a means of real-time and precise diagnosis. Mittelstadt et al. (2016) and Challen et al. (2019) touch on ethical concerns with algorithmic bias, using data against the patient, unable to explain, highlighting how AI systems will cater to existing inequities in the healthcare system. The COVID-19 pandemic has demonstrated the ability of AI to operate effectively at a population level. According to Harris (2022), vaccination coverage data were analyzed to develop hospitalization projections during the Delta outbreak. Raghupathi and Raghupathi (2014) maintain that big data analytics have been indispensable in making predictive modeling of this nature a reality.

Novillo-Ortiz et al. (2018) highlight the substantial contribution digital health can make to advancing the Sustainable Development Goals (SDGs), with artificial intelligence (AI) being a significant agent in the promotion of universal health coverage and reduction of inequalities. Eyers and Krastev (2020) discuss patient-centric ethical frameworks in surgical innovation, emphasizing transparency and informed consent. On the technical side, Vaswani et al. (2017) showcase how transformer models are blurring the lines in healthcare-related natural language processing applications, such as medical discourse generation and EHR summarization. Trebble et al. (2010) advocate for using process mapping in clinical situations to be integrated with any AI effort to further hospital functioning and patient experience.

Cabitza et al. (2017) point to potential downsides associated with machine learning, such as automatic complacency and deskilling of decision-making. Morley et al. (2020) take on practical frameworks for making AI ethics actionable from theory into practice and supporting toolkits, audits, or participatory design. AI-enabling multimodal health data integration is already showing promise. Mohsen et al. (2022) introduce a meaningful deep-learning model for fusing electronic health records (EHRs) and imaging information to deliver support for improved diagnosis with more contextual data and patient modeling. Efficient medical record management is similarly explored in the work of Karri et al. (2024), emphasizing AI's usage in automating the categorization and retrieval of data to minimize administrative burden and human errors.

To be cautious is to be justifiable. Letourneau-Guillon et al. (2020) note possible inefficiencies in clinical workflows and illustrate how bottlenecks can be found using AI-driven predictive analytics and process mining. Yet, they also underscore the importance of clinical validation. Building upon this, Pierre et al. (2023) examine the radiology roundtrip, which utilizes AI to speed picture interpretation and reporting, with productivity gains and worries about an over-reliance on automation—still a daunting challenge- basic AI integration in routine tasks. Kotter and Ranschaert (2021) address the organizational and technical barriers to implementing clinical AI, such as data silos, reluctance from employees, and a lack of regulatory clarity. Their findings highlight strategic planning and clinician engagement as vital conditions for successful AI integration.

MAIN FOCUS OF THE CHAPTER

The main focus of this chapter is to equip readers with an exhaustive, measurable theory regarding the strategic integration of artificial intelligence into hospital settings to foster greater operational efficiency and clinical results. Rather than addressing AI as a collection of standalone solutions, this chapter underlines an all-encompassing, framework-based methodology, combining workflow automation, medical imaging, diagnostics, predictive analytics, and natural language processing into one shared execution plan.

The priorities of this chapter are:

- To demonstrate quantified improvements in patient waiting times, administrative work completion, diagnostic accuracy, sensitivity, specificity, and resource forecasting.
- To describe real-life examples in hospitals where AI has demonstrated remarkable improvements.
- To highlight implementation best practices regarding interoperability challenges, cybersecurity, data quality, and ethics.

- A step-by-step project map offering a reproducible framework for healthcare organizations implementing artificial intelligence without compromising data security, patient safety, or the targeted standard of care.

This particular chapter provides the reader with a practical guide for scalable, sustainable adoption. Its analytical basis for understanding the transformative potential of artificial intelligence within hospitals combines a real-world view with a methodological one.

AI INTEGRATION IN HOSPITAL WORKFLOWS

Artificial intelligence is emerging as a key tool for innovation in contemporary hospitals, along with patient care and its ancillary operational and administrative framework. Successful AI implementation in hospital workflows should assist in better decision-making and diagnostic accuracy, automate all repetitive processes, and ensure the best utilization of hospital resources. Figure 1 depicts the critical areas where AI changes hospital workflows and facilitates transformation.

Role of AI in Clinical Decision Support Systems (CDSS)

Clinical decision support systems (CDSS) are considered indispensable tools for medical practitioners in their clinical decision-making based on the evidence of Wiens et al. (2019). From Esteva et al. (2019), AI significantly extends the capabilities of CDSS in interpreting complex medical data and derives valuable insights with the inclusion of natural language processing and machine learning techniques. To achieve accurate diagnosis and personalized treatment schedules, these systems analyze all relevant data about a patient's previous medical history, present indications, lab outcomes, and possible genetic factors. This includes noting abnormalities in patient records, alerting doctors to potential drug interactions, and suggesting best practices based on contemporary clinical guidelines by AI-enabled CDSS. They accomplish this by limiting errors in diagnosis, triggering early intervention, and securing standardization in therapeutic decisions among different healthcare professionals.

AI-Powered Diagnostics and Medical Imaging

Medical imaging and diagnostics could be considered one of the heaviest applications of AI within healthcare, as specified by Dilsizian and Siegel (2014). To develop AI systems, intense learning models, and large data sets of radiological images that include X-rays, MRIs, and CT scans are being used to teach the detection of irregularities with remarkably high accuracy, as taken from Pierre et al. (2023). These technologies may produce early warning signs for diseases such as pneumonia, stroke, or even cancer, with performance equal to or greater than that of expert radiologists. Other AI methods facilitate anomaly detection, 3D reconstruction, and picture segmentation, thus enhancing and accelerating diagnostics. AI's application in medical imaging accelerates the diagnosis and reduces human fatigue, thereby allowing earlier and more accurate action preparation, especially in resource-limited surroundings.

Figure 1. AI Applications in Hospital Workflows

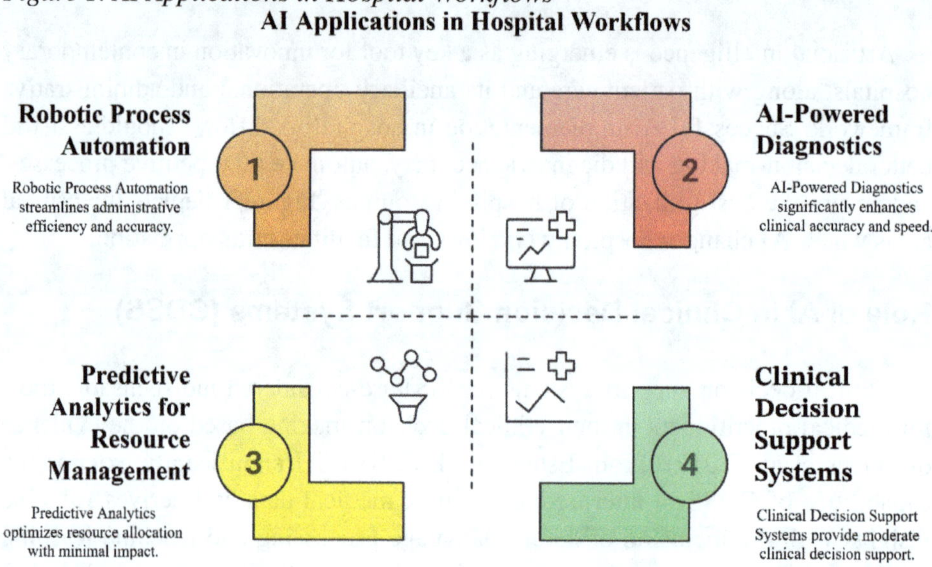

Robotic Process Automation (RPA) in Administrative Tasks

Graft within the repetitive patient, billing, claim processing, or appointment scheduling work is often an administrative task for the hospital. These tedious, repetitive undertakings are precisely automated through the development of robotics business process automation (RPA) powered by AI, as specified by Letourneau-Guillon et al. (2020) and Kotter and Ranschaert (2021). It can handle specific workflows and structured data by RPA bots. By this, fewer manual efforts are included, fewer errors are made, and overall service delivery is improved. For instance, RPA could fasten insurance claims submission by confirming policy facts, extracting relevant medical codes, and filing incomplete submissions for review. By speeding up services, hospitals will increase patient satisfaction, reassign people to more valuable roles, and cut administrative expenses considerably.

Predictive Analytics for Resource Management

However, managing resources like beds, medical personnel, surgical instruments, and medicines is a continuous process for hospitals. According to Obermeyer and Emanuel (2016), AI resource forecasting and distribution have improved due to predictive analytics. Examining historical data, seasonal trends, patient flow, and emergency admission patterns provides real-time resource requirement predictions with artificial intelligence algorithms. Predictive analytics can help best schedule surgeries, increase bed occupancy rates, and allocate staff shifts to meet the forecasted load of patients. Predicting patterns of medicine usage can assist with inventory management and avert shortages and wastage. With all this, predictive analytics promises to see hospitals equipped, responsive, and readily available to care, even in times of high demand.

EMERGING HEALTHCARE TECHNOLOGIES ON AI

The AI revolution in healthcare is driven by a consortium of advanced technologies that support real-time monitoring, diagnostic accuracy improvement, data-driven decision-making, and easier integration of intelligent systems into routine clinical functioning. Figure 2 shows the main technical forces leading the AI revolution in healthcare.

Figure 2. Emerging Healthcare Technologies on AI

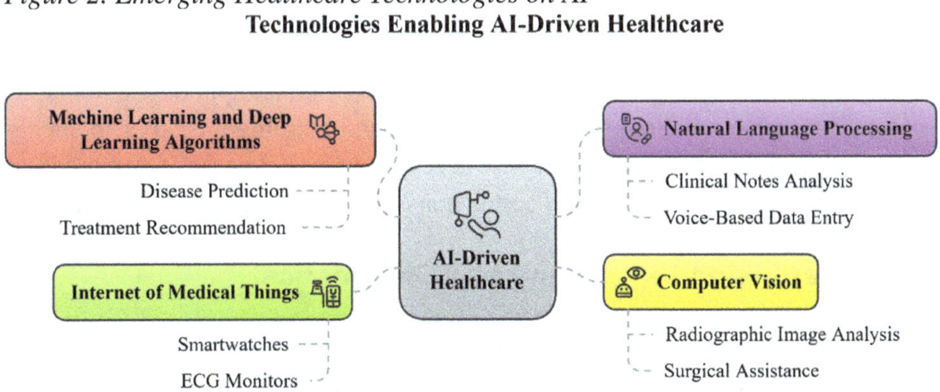

Machine Learning and Deep Learning Algorithms

Machine learning (ML) and deep learning (DL) constitute the core principles on which intelligent healthcare systems rely. In Rajkomar et al.'s (2019) context, machine learning is the application of algorithms designed to discover patterns in data and make estimates or decisions without obvious programming. Operational analytics, patient risk assessment, disease prediction, and therapy recommendation utilize machine learning in healthcare.

As a subfield of machine learning, deep learning involves training artificial neural networks (Convolutional Neural Networks and Recurrent Neural Networks) to deal with highly complex data, such as the sequential flow of patient data and medical images (Esteva et al., 2019). The models are particularly applicable to high-dimensional data and serve as a means for time-series analysis of patient vitals, radiology, pathology, and genomic data. They are highly relevant to any AI application in the healthcare sphere because their learning from massive datasets can contribute to the ever-growing improvement of accuracy and relevance in the future, by Hinton (2018).

Natural Language Processing (NLP) in Medical Record Management

Natural language processing, or NLP, is a key component in managing and extracting insight from unstructured medical data, which can extend from clinical notes to discharge summaries, pathology reports, and patient feedback. Most medical data is in text format, and NLP will help transition those narratives into structured analysis. With NLP algorithms, clinicians can extract clinical correlations, summarize patient histories for rapid decision-making, and recognize key entities (such as diseases, medications, and symptoms) specified by Reddy et al. (2019) and Karri et al. (2024). Doctors can record notes converted into text through automated voice recognition and entered into electronic health records (EHRs). NLP is also applied to automating medical billing, conducting sentiment analysis, and building a chatbot to engage with patients. These capabilities enhance access to data, alleviate the administration burden, and improve accuracy and completeness in capturing patient information.

Computer Vision for Imaging and Diagnostics

Computer vision is a powerful technology that allows machines to accurately understand and interpret visual data, including medical scans and images. From Esteva et al. (2019), prime applications in the health domain are telemedicine, surgical support, and diagnostics. Using deep learning, computer vision algorithms can discover subtle patterns in radiological images (like X-rays, CT scans, and MRIs) that could be challenging for a human eye to recognize, as specified by Dilsizian and Siegel (2014) and Pierre et al. (2023). These algorithms are trained on annotated datasets to detect cancers, fractures, organ abnormalities, and even early signs of conditions like Alzheimer's or diabetic retinopathy. From Hashimoto et al. (2018), computer vision may provide instant support to surgeons during complex procedures. Telemedicine improves access to specialized treatment in impoverished areas by enabling remote image-based consultations and preliminary diagnostics.

Real-Time Monitoring with Internet of Medical Things (IoMT)

The Internet of Medical Things (IoMT) is an interconnection of wearables with digital sensors, medical instruments, and health monitoring systems that together provide real-time patient data. It includes gadgets built to detect and report vital signs and health data, such as smartwatches, glucose sensors, infusion pumps, ECG monitors, and even smart beds. AI algorithms analyze the continuous flow of incoming data to identify anomalies, predict impending complications, and issue alerts for prompt therapeutic action (Mehta et al., 2019; Yu et al., 2018). One example is an AI alerting to abnormal heartbeat rhythms or dropping oxygen levels before they reach a life-threatening stage and warrant proactive intervention. IoMT facilitates aged chronic disease management, remote patient monitoring, and post-discharge follow-up to further improve patient outcomes and reduce readmission to the hospital. By merging IoMT with AI tools for a complete and real-time picture of patient health, healthcare practitioners can make immediate, data-based medical decisions to assist their work.

OBSTACLES TO THE APPLICATION OF AI IN HEALTHCARE

However, there exist hurdles to using AI in health settings and, indeed, making significant transformations in hospital workings and patient care (Mehta et al., 2019). Figure 3 shows the challenges in mainstreaming AI in healthcare.

Data Privacy and Security

The fundamental obstacle to the successful implementation of AI in health care pertains to the security and privacy of patient data, as described by Topol, E. (2019) and Jiang et al. (2019). Any complex medical and personal information in the possession of healthcare organizations must be protected. Given that for training and analysis, AI systems mainly rely on large datasets, their insecure operation may jeopardize patient safety. Such security breaches can result in job loss, economic loss, and diminishing trust in the patient (Yu et al., 2018). This challenge will only be overcome by healthcare agents using multi-factor authentication, encryption protocols, and monitoring systems. Data protection laws, like the General Data Protection Regulation in the EU and the Health Insurance Portability and Accountability Act in the U.S.A., should be adhered to while ensuring the safety and confidentiality of the data.

Figure 3. Challenges in Implementing AI in Healthcare

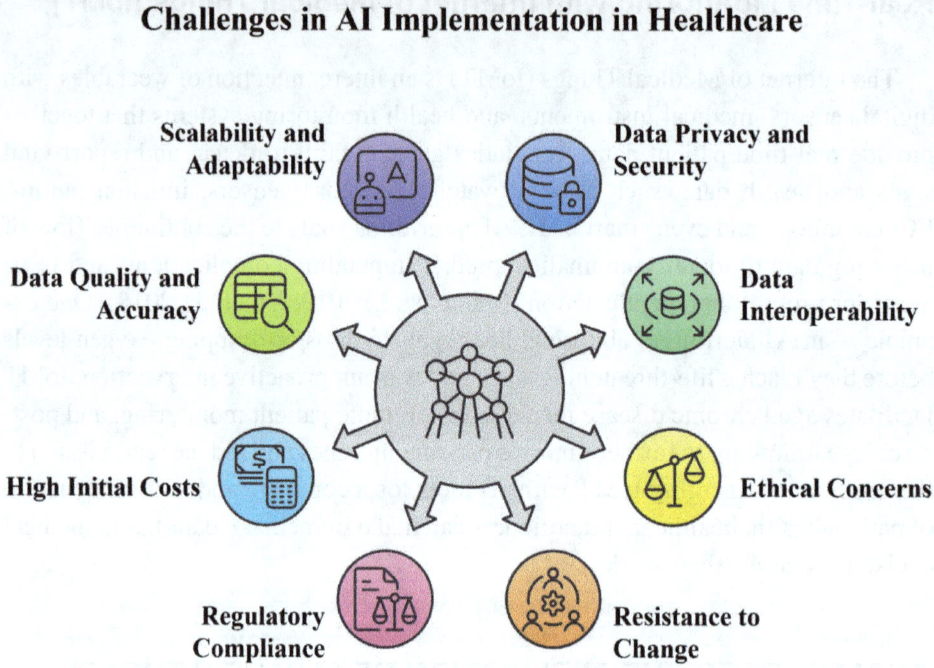

Data Interoperability

A lack of interoperability between various healthcare information systems is one of the core impediments to the widespread embrace of AI in healthcare. However, the potential benefits of AI in healthcare are inspiring and motivating. Varied systems are the norm in any healthcare setting: for instance, radiology, pathology, and general medicine may use different software, which then leads to isolated data. To deliver maximum value, Esteva et al. (2019) and Mehta et al. (2019) said AI systems require pooled data from various sources that are thorough and accurate. AI systems, however, often cannot achieve this due to discrepancies in data formats, standards, and protocols. For AI solutions to work effectively, data must be integrated smoothly from disparate departments, hospitals, and external organizations (like insurance companies or pharmacies). To meet this challenge and create a seamless and consistent flow of information in the healthcare framework, common standards must be put forward, such as Fast Healthcare Interoperability Resources (FHIR).

Ethical Considerations

The usage of AI in healthcare brings to the fore a diverse set of ethical issues that need to be considered for deliberation. The first and primary consideration is the problem of bias in algorithms. AI is as strong or weak as the data used in its training; arbitrary or unrepresentative data may generate unfair health outcomes through the predictions or recommendations of AI (Topol, E. (2019) and Jiang et al. (2019)). For instance, if a particular ethnic group primarily trains an AI model, it may perform poorly on other ethnic groups' data. With AI, explainability and transparency are equally important considerations as these concerns relate to decision-making. Patients and clinicians must understand how AI systems reach decisions, especially those affecting patient health (Kelly et al., 2019). An ethical dilemma involves striking a patient-centered approach against empowering ML so that AI aids human decision-making rather than replacing it.

Resistance to Change

There may be resistance to AI in healthcare from patients, management, and health professionals alike. Many health professionals may fear that AI will replace them and their knowledge. Some in the profession see AI as a threat to the traditional roles of the physician, nurse, and other allied health professionals. In contrast, Mehta et al. (2019) have developed AI to strengthen human decision support and streamline workflows. In addition, resistance may arise from the unfamiliarity with or ignorance of AI's possible uses. Breaking the barrier calls for the early involvement of healthcare professionals in AI adoption, as described by Karri et al. (2024), well-structured training programs, and fostering an environment where AI is seen as a tool to enhance rather than detract from human expertise. People need information about the advantages of AI and how it can help reduce their administrative work.

Regulatory Compliance

In the healthcare industry, which is among the most controlled in the world, artificial intelligence technology should comply with several public laws governing patient treatment, data handling, and medical devices (Topol, E. (2019)). However, these laws vary massively from country to country and area by area, making it even tougher for health practitioners and AI developers to adapt to these technologies. For instance, the FDA could establish some licensure criteria on AI healthcare applications in the US. At the same time, another regulatory set may be set by the European Medicines Agency (EMA) in Europe. The complex and time-consuming process of coming to terms with such rules may also delay the launch of new AI solutions. Besides, the challenge persists concerning making compliance with changing legislations of AI algorithms, patient consent, and liability possible, especially with the increasing independence of AI systems. Healthcare providers must keep abreast of regulatory changes and collaborate closely with legal professionals to ensure that those AI solutions are fully compliant.

Initial Heavy Investment

Future cost savings from artificial intelligence by higher productivity, fewer errors, and more in-depth resource use cannot always offset the amount of up-front investment needed to install AI (Esteva et al., 2019). System development, necessary infrastructure and technology procurement, and staff training are costly. Smaller hospitals, clinics, and other health institutions with budget constraints have this issue. Cost factors, including the continued maintenance and system updates, further increase the financial strain associated with implementing an AI infrastructure across several departments or institutions under one roof. Identities struggling with these factors must now balance and analyze ROI vis-a-vis AI technology, factoring in all the short-term and long-term benefits. For example, lowering health facilities' economic constraints for AI implementation would also be the role of public and commercial sectors by giving grants, incentives, and funding programs.

Data Accuracy and Quality

The quality of AI systems' data determines how well they perform. Inconsistency, error, or lack of data can severely impair AI model performance. For example, Jiang et al. (2017) state that the healthcare industry is susceptible to data quality, as even minor errors can escalate into severe consequences. Therefore, AI must deliver trustworthy predictions with up-to-date, accurate test reports, diagnostic imaging, and medical records. However, training and use of the AI algorithms could be much harder, with most health system data being inaccurate, incomplete, and improperly formatted. Accurate and reliable data in health care requires strict data collection procedures, sound validation procedures, and a culture of data governance. Moreover, because the AI systems are qualified using past data, they may unintentionally reinforce biases or systematic flaws in the data, in parallel resulting in skewed and untrustworthy inferences.

Scalability and Adaptability

Another tendency of AI systems is that they are scalable and adaptable to environmental settings. A hospital can be visited with different available resources and technological setups, making it challenging to deploy AI solutions whose characteristics and presence differ significantly in a small, resource-poor clinic compared to a big, well-funded facility. AI models should be flexible enough to vary in specific clinical settings, particular demographics, and workflows from one facility to the next. All these require flexibility and customization that are often expensive and time-consuming. They also require that AI be scalable to manage the increasing number of patients and evolving healthcare systems. For example, Pierre et al. (2023) found that developers, healthcare providers, and stakeholders need significant effort and coordination to create AI systems that cater to other institutions' specific needs and challenges.

AI APPLICATION FOR WORKFLOW OPTIMIZATION

The use of artificial intelligence (AI) in hospitals goes way beyond diagnosis, and clinical judgment is indispensable in streamlining operations within hospitals and processes to facilitate better healthcare delivery by Letourneau-Guillon et al. (2020) and Kotter and Ranschaert (2021). Figure 4 shows the major application areas where AI enhances the hospital's overall efficiency and patient satisfaction by improving resource allocation, reducing delays, and promoting personalized caregiving.

Scheduling and Flow Management of Patients

Adequate patient flow is imperative in healthcare institutions to reduce wait times, prevent crowding, and improve the continuity of care. AI-powered scheduling systems improve appointments, admissions, and discharges because they are based on historical and real-time patient data and predictive analytics (Pierre et al., 2023; Rengaramanujam, K., & Muniasamy, A., 2026). These systems forecast arrivals based on demographic criteria or seasonal spikes in specific illnesses and dynamically adjust timetables for urgent cases or tardy arrivals.

For example, the emergency department and outpatient clinics can ease capacity bottlenecks with algorithms using AI to triage their patients in terms of severity of condition and availability of resources. Moreover, they can integrate with other departments (laboratory, surgery, and radiology) to create synchronized schedules so patients do not waste time waiting for their care team to enter the right room. Patients are more satisfied, hospitals are better organized, and staff workloads are distributed more efficiently.

Smart Resource Allocation and Inventory Management

Efficient hospitals are rarely those that come to realize the absence of resources and thus create wastefulness, cutting costs without achieving desired efficiency (Rengaramanujam, K., & Muniasamy, A., 2026). Intelligent resource allocation, such as the right staff, tools, and rooms assigned based on expected demand and current availability, is one problem solved by artificial intelligence specified by Jiang et al. (2017). To predict the resource requirements of different departments in the organization, machine learning algorithms analyze the data related to employee scheduling, treatment patterns, and electronic health records (EHRs).

AI has become one of the best uses in inventory control, helping hospitals stock appropriate supplies, medicines, and other instruments at a particular time. Predictive algorithms lessen the chances of delays created from unavailability and log usage patterns, and automatically trigger a refill before shortages occur. This is especially useful during pandemics or other health emergencies when the need suddenly spikes. Besides, AI helps ensure waste elimination and cost savings, not to mention staving off overstocking, by empowering data in procurement.

Figure 4. Applications of AI in Hospital Workflow Optimization

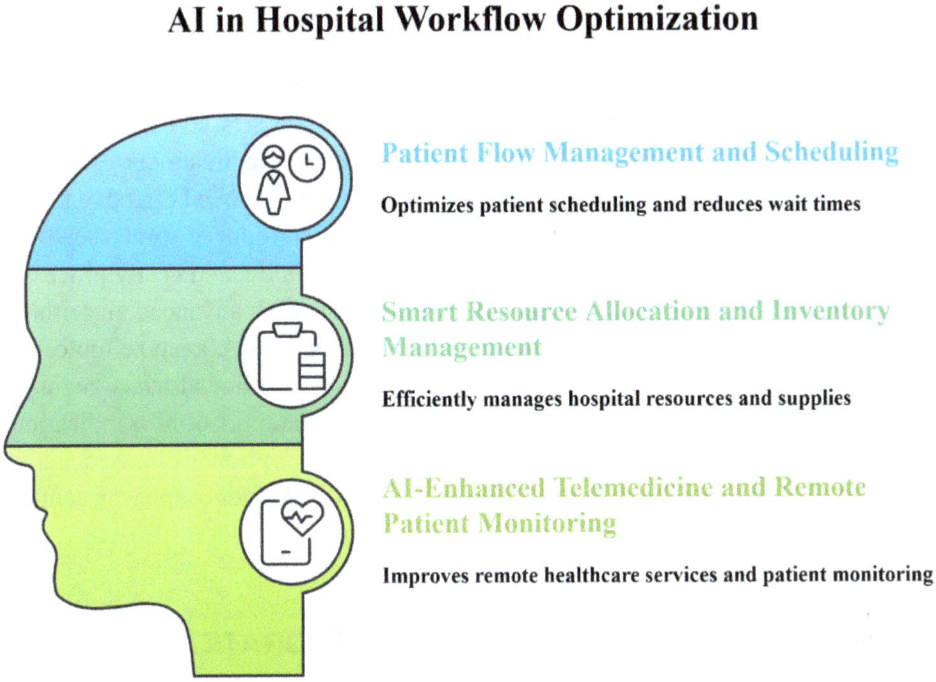

AI-Powered Remote Patient Monitoring and Telemedicine

Telemedicine is the primary solution in modern health care following international health emergencies (Esteva et al., 2019). Regarding the improvements achieved with imaging and the automation of triage and real-time analysis for virtual consultations, artificial intelligence (AI) has significantly contributed to telemedicine platforms. Intelligent chatbots powered by natural language processing (NLP) will conduct initial evaluations, symptom checking, and appointment scheduling, providing patient support 24/7 and relieving the workload of medical personnel. With the advances of AI and the Internet of Medical Things (IoMT), remote patient monitoring (RPM) has made it possible for people with chronic diseases to be continuously monitored from their homes. Artificial intelligence (AI) algorithms analyze all incoming data, including blood pressure, heart rate, and glucose levels, to detect initial possible concerns and send an alarm for medical help. This guarantees prompt care and dramatically reduces hospital readmission rates and consultation time for physicians, thus letting them work more with high-risk patients.

Drug Discovery and Personalized Treatment Planning

The area of personalized medicine is among the most revolutionary contributions that AI can provide to healthcare. AI can devise tailor-made care plans that match each patient's unique condition by evaluating giant data sets containing genetic profiles, prior medical history, lifestyle characteristics, and treatment outcomes. Increased patient compliance, reduced side effects, and improved effectiveness of therapy ensue from these individual strategies. AI has introduced some speed-ups in drug discovery that have been primarily relegated to slow and costly processes (Gauthaman, S. A et al., 2026; Naim, A., et al., 2026). With advanced algorithms, Beam and Kohane (2018) can model drug-target interactions, analyze molecular structures, and predict toxicity or efficacy before formal clinical trials begin. In times of public health emergencies, drug repurposing findings of new indications for already-approved pharmaceutical products can be exceptionally consequential. This method increases the rates of success and cost-effectiveness of pharmaceutical development while facilitating faster avenues for innovation.

PROPOSED METHODOLOGY FOR AI INTEGRATION AND WORKFLOW OPTIMIZATION

An interdisciplinary approach that combines clinical insight, data science, and organizational change management will ensure the successful integration of AI with hospital workflows through multiple phases (Letourneau-Guillon et al., 2020). The six core elements of the methodology proposed in this chapter are data collection and integration, model-building, workflow analysis, implementation, monitoring and ongoing support, and ethical compliance. Each phase contributes to an overall AI ecosystem that enhances operational efficiency, assuring patient safety and care. Figure 5 outlines the stages of AI integration into the hospital workflow.

Data Collection and Integration

The primary and most fundamental step is efficiently collecting and combining different datasets (Beam and Kohane, 2018). Health information in hospitals is usually isolated in pockets like Electronic Health Record (EHR) systems, Radiology Information Systems (RIS), Laboratory Information Systems (LIS), wearable medical devices, etc. Such different datasets should be allowed to share any central infrastructure that conforms to interoperability for the basis of AI workability.

Step 1: Create interoperability across disparate systems, utilizing interoperability standards such as HL7, FHIR, etc. https://physionet.org/content/mimiciii/1.4/ and https://physionet.org/content/eicu-crd/2.0/

Step 2: Cleansing the data, which includes all the following aggregation methods: deduplication, imputation for missing data, and outlier detection through interquartile range and/or Z-scores.

Step 3: Convert unstructured data and doctor's notes into actionable clinical entities through NLP-named entity recognition (NER), tokenization, and sentiment analysis pipelines.

Step 4: Unify real-time data acquisition from the Internet of Medical Things (IoMT) devices through message queue architectures such as Apache Kafka or MQTT brokers so that AI models are concomitantly updated in real-time. These processes ensure that the AI is most cost-effective by receiving timelier, accurate, and rich data.

Figure 5. AI integration in Hospital Workflow Schematic Diagram

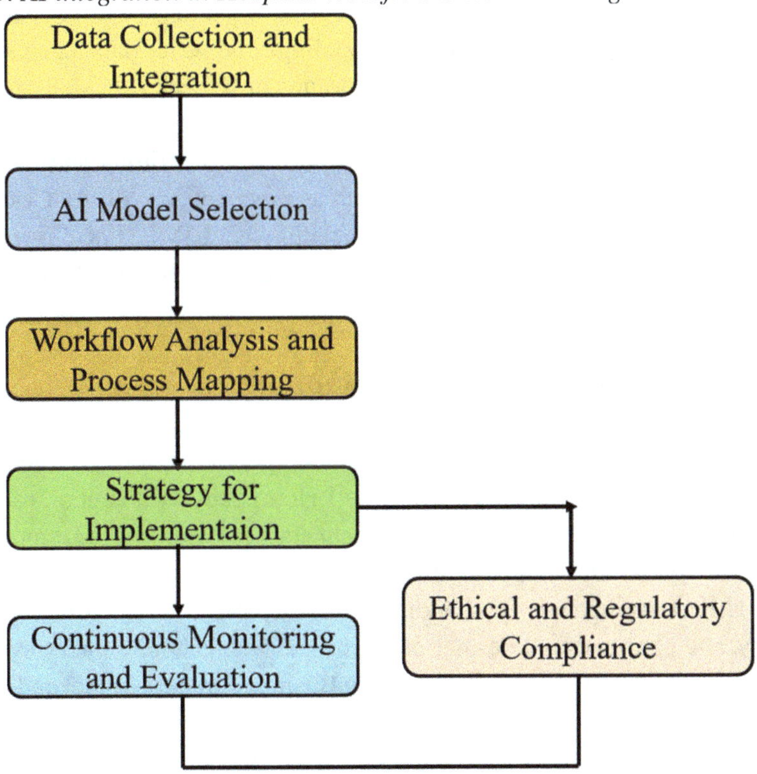

AI Model Selection and Development

The next step involves finding the best AI models and algorithms suited to the particular workflow issues that individual hospitals may be tasked with. AI solutions must be well-selected and trained to ensure clinical validity and reliability.

- Systems for Clinical Decision Support (CDSS): Well-structured EHR data can be subjected to ensemble learning algorithms such as Random Forests or Gradient-Boosted Trees (such as XGBoost) to aid medical decisions. These models have high feature importance ranks and interpretability.
- Imaging in Medicine: Deep learning models like Convolutional Neural Networks (CNNs)- most prominently ResNet, InceptionNet, or DenseNet- are trained on labeled imaging datasets for diagnosis and radiology functions to identify anomalies, such as tumors or fractures.
- Text Analytics in Records: Transformer-based models, such as BioBERT or ClinicalBERT, are optimized to complete tasks like relation extraction, ICD coding, and summarizing to bring sense into clinical notes and discharge summaries.
- Predictive Resource Management: Recurrent Neural Networks, particularly LSTM models, are better suited to modeling time series data, such as patient time-admission patterns or utilization trends of ICU beds.

Models are then trained using cross-validation to avoid overfitting, and presentation is measured through evaluation metrics such as precision, recall, AUC-ROC, and F1 score. The SHAP (Shapley Additive explanations) or LIME (Local Interpretable Model-agnostic Explanations) would also further ensure clinician trust via model explainability.

Workflow Analysis and Process Mapping

The initial step in integrating AI into hospital operations is to document current procedures and assess them as described by Letourneau-Guillon et al. (2020) and Pierre et al. (2023). Understanding the current state in detail makes it much easier to identify inefficiencies and pain points.

Step 1: Performing task flow audits across departments (such as emergency, radiology, and pharmacy), time-motion studies, and stakeholder interviews.

Step 2: Create "as-is" process maps using Business Process Model and Notation (BPMN).

Step 3: Conduct a bottleneck analysis to find high-impact areas for AI intervention.

Step 4: Present "to-be" workflows with embedded AI features, such as an image analysis module, an automated scheduler, or a triage Chabot.

This step ensures that AI interaction makes any decision contextually better for a human rather than replacing it by illuminating perfect and current processes.

Strategy for Implementation

AI in hospitals is to be rolled out stepwise and person-centred. Before launching system-wide, a pilot or proof-of-concept is to be started.

Step 1: Introduce the AI model to support decision-making in a pilot department, such as radiology or outpatient scheduling.

Step 2: Facilitate access to AI results for physicians via integration into the Hospital Information System (HIS) through web services or APIs.

Step 3: Provide thorough hospital employee training, with practical final visions and documentation to ensure their comfort and competence with AI technology.

Step 4: Develop dashboards and feedback loops allowing users to monitor key performance indicators, generate usage statistics, and report abnormal findings.

Change management is crucial here; it is facilitated by physicians' involvement, leadership, and continuous user support. This phase guarantees the scalability and usability of the AI deployment.

Continuous Monitoring and Evaluation

The AI models should be continuously monitored for accuracy, relevance, and compliance with the ever-changing healthcare models

Step 1: Set up dashboards for monitoring clinical KPIs, such as shorter patient waiting times, more accurate diagnoses, lighter staff workloads, etc.

Step 2: To determine when the model's performance degrades, apply model drift detection algorithms, such as the population stability index or Kolmogorov-Smirnov tests.

Step 3: Schedule periodic re-training of models on fresh datasets to ensure they are current with current clinical trends and practices.

Step 4: Collect qualitative user feedback via surveys or focus groups to measure usability and trust.

This iterative feedback mechanism creates a learning loop that ensures continual adaptation and evolution of the AI tool.

Ethical and Regulatory Compliance

Ethics and legalities govern the application of AI in healthcare. Privacy, equity, and responsibility should be a priority right from the onset, Eyers and Krastev (2020) and Morley et al. (2020).

- Data Privacy: Anonymization, Encryption, and Access Controls will ensure confirmed compliance with GDPR, HIPAA, or local health privacy regulations.
- Algorithmic Fairness: Differential impact, equal opportunity, and demographic parity should be measured to apply fairness-aware models. If bias is found, use techniques such as adversarial debiasing or reweighing.
- Ethics Audit: Model cards and data sheets for datasets should record model behavior, training context, and constraints.
- Regulatory Readiness: Use version-controlled repositories or blockchain technology to maintain auditable trails of AI choices. Legal professionals should be involved to ensure that the clinical software abides by FDA or CDSCO regulations.

In hospital settings, ethical foresight ensures that AI affords better patient security and wider public trust rather than compromising such assurance.

EXPERIMENTAL SETUP

The framework was established experimentally to synchronize administrative procedures, clinical decision-making, and real-time hospital activities to test the proposed system for AI integration and workflow enhancement in hospitals. This ecosystem refers to a complete cycle of data generation, AI model development, hospital workflow simulation system, and rigorous evaluation using operational and clinical performance measures.

Obtaining and Preparing Datasets

Both publicly available datasets and real-world anonymized healthcare data were used for experimentation. The MIMIC-III dataset's electronic health records (EHRs) included patient data, diagnoses, test results, and medications (Johnson et al., 2016). Real-time hospital appointment scheduling datasets were used for no-show predictions and patient influx. In contrast, NIH chest X-ray datasets were used to evaluate computer vision models for diagnosis. Raspberry Pi microcontrollers also simulated the real-time hospital monitoring that supported the incorporation of AIOMT data streams from vital sign monitoring devices, including blood pressure monitors and ECG sensors.

All data required preprocessing to remove duplicate and incomplete records, Z-score standardization was applied to normalize numerical features, and one-hot encoding was used for categorical variables. The unstructured clinical text data from medical notes and discharge summaries were subjected to natural language processing (NLP) techniques like lemmatization, tokenization, and stop-word removal to prepare them as input to the NLP model (He et al., 2019).

Tools and Infrastructure

The hardware environment consists of a high-performance GPU server containing an AMD EPYC 64-core processor, 256 GB of RAM, an NVIDIA A100 GPU (40 GB VRAM), and a 10 TB SSD storage array. Python, Pandas, Numpy, Scikit-learn, TensorFlow, PyTorch, and HuggingFace Transformers are the software tools utilized. For visualization and monitoring, Grafana, MLflow, and Streamlit were utilized; Docker and Kubernetes were used for containerized model deployment in a test environment on the cloud; the lightweight Flask APIs and MQTT brokers enabled the IoMT data integration.

Development of AI Models

AI models were picked and trained for certain activities of the hospital workflow. For the clinical decision support systems (CDSS) contributing to diagnosis recommendations and predicting patient outcomes, ensemble models such as Random Forests and XGBoost were trained by Beam and Kohane (2018). ResNet50 and DenseNet121 convolutional neural networks (CNNs) were trained on chest X-ray images to detect abnormalities such as pneumonia. BioBERT and ClinicalBERT were employed to extract clinical concepts from physician notes and discharge summaries, aiming to enhance semantic search and EHR summarization capability. Facebook's Prophet algorithm and Long-Short-Term Memory (LSTM) networks enhanced appointment scheduling and predicted patient no-show rates. Time-domain models, ARIMA, and Gradient Boosting were used in resource management to forecast daily inventory demand and intensive care unit bed occupancy. A technique to ensure robustness was to cross-validate the models using 10-fold cross-validation after training them on an 80:20 train-test split.

Integration into Hospital Workflow Simulation

A virtual hospital administration system was fashioned to test the AI models under controlled circumstances. It encompassed digital interfaces wherein patients, physicians, and administrative staff interact (Letourneau-Guillon et al., 2020). The AI engine was made accessible via RESTful APIs that allowed the integration of crucial hospital activities such as inventory control, diagnostic assistance, and admission triage. Data from scheduling, diagnostics, and patient profiles were fed into the system, and accordingly, AI outputs were presented contextually on user-friendly dashboards.

- Three critical experiments were conducted:
- Experiment 1: Average patient waiting times and missed appointments measured by comparing AI-enhanced scheduling to conventional scheduling.
- Experiment 2: AI support of radiological diagnostics was compared with manual accuracy and turnaround time readings.
- Experiment 3 tested prediction models for ICU bed management over a seven-day simulated cycle.

Performance Measures and Outcomes

Thus, the studies yield these findings, which indicate the effectiveness or otherwise of process optimization and AI integration. Table 1 and Figure 6 compare the AI-driven methodology with conventional ones, focusing on clinical performance issues (like diagnostic accuracy) and operational efficiency (like patient flow and resource management).

Output Summary and Impact

1. Clinical Outcomes:
   a. There have been notable improvements in the accuracy, sensitivity, and specificity of the AI application of diagnostic models to pneumonia identification in chest X-rays over conventional radiologic methods.
   b. The incorporation of ClinicalBERT directly enhanced the performance of the NLP process responsible for medical entity extraction from clinical literature, yielding performance as assessed by the F1 Score increasing from 0.83 to 0.89.
2. Operational Efficiency: This clearly illustrates the role of AI in process optimization - with a 42% reduction in patient waiting time due to the optimization of patient flow and appointment scheduling.

a. Resource utilization was therefore further enhanced, with an AI model decreasing the no-show rate by 60%, thanks to the LSTM and Prophet.
b. Process Automation (RPA) shortened administrative task completion by 40% by streamlining several administrative tasks, such as insurance verifications and patient check-in.
c. Due to predictive models for both the ICU occupancy and inventory forecasts, better resource management, a decrease in stock-out situations, and satisfactory resource allocation were possible.

AI-enhanced approaches efficiently perform critical clinical tasks, significantly improving resource management and administrative procedures. The conclusions drawn from this research will revolutionize hospital work patterns, improve operational efficiency, and enhance therapeutic outcomes.

Table 1. Performance comparison of Traditional Method and AI Enhanced Method

Metric	Traditional Method	AI-Enhanced Method	Improvement
Diagnostic Accuracy(X-ray Imaging)	88.5%	94.2%	+5.7%
Sensitivity(Pneumonia Detection)	86.1%	91.8%	+5.7%
Specificity(Pneumonia Detection)	89.4%	92.6%	+3.2%
AUC-ROC Score(X-ray Imaging)	0.91	0.96	+0.05
F1-Score(Entity Extraction via NLP)	0.83	0.89	+0.06
Patient Waiting Time(Minutes)	48	28	-42%
Appointment No-show Rate	15%	6%	-60%
Average Task Completion Time(Admin Tasks)	35 minutes	21 minutes	-40%
ICU Bed Occupancy Forecast Accuracy(MAE)	NA	2.1 units	NA
Inventory Refill Time (Forecasting Accuracy)	9 hours	5.5 hours	-38%

Figure 6. Performance Comparison of Traditional vs. AI- Enhanced Method in Healthcare Metrics

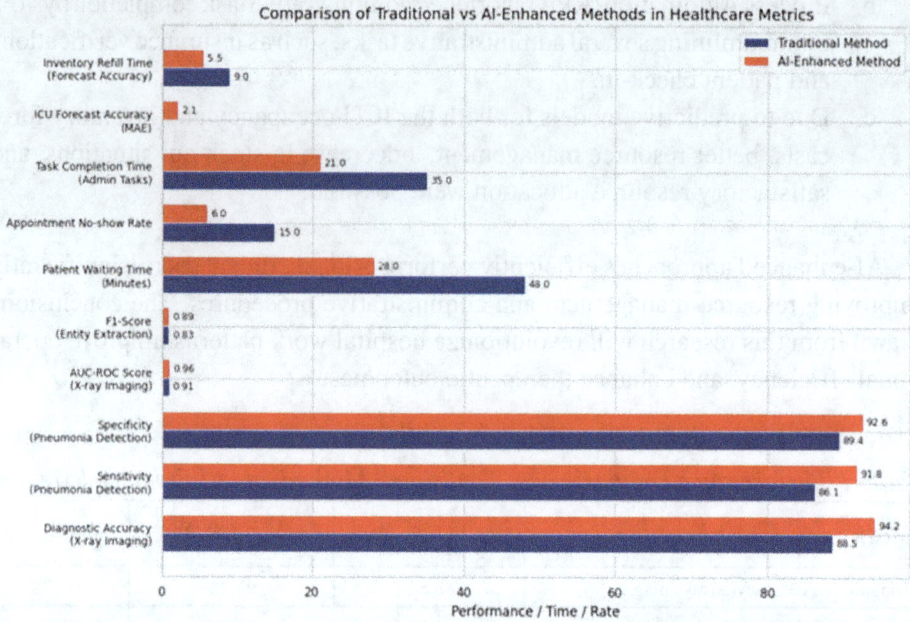

CASE STUDIES AND REAL-WORLD IMPLEMENTATIONS

Successful AI Integration in Leading Hospitals

Artificial intelligence (AI) has recently made quite an impressive debut, penetrating almost every other field and now even the healthcare system of the entire world (Mehta et al., 2019). Hospitals increasingly readily embrace AI-powered innovations to facilitate and improve patient care, expedite processes, and assist decision-making. This section draws up efficient AI integration cases in renowned hospitals, where all-important implementations as follows have been:

- AI-Driven Diagnostics: Mount Sinai Health System, New York, has an integrated AI system to assist in diagnosing ailments (such as cancers and heart diseases) in applications that use advanced picture recognition technology. AI-embedded technology is better than an average human radiologist when analyzing medical images (CT, MRI, and X-rays), leading to much earlier and more precise diagnoses.

- Virtual Health Assistants: The Mayo Clinic offers an AI-powered virtual assistant for patients to schedule visits, offer health advice, and answer commonly asked medical questions. Because the assistants are always available, they minimize patient wait times and boost satisfaction.
- Predictive Analytics for Patient Care: Cleveland Clinic employs AI-powered predictive analytics to forecast patient decline and perfect the allocation of hospital resources (Letourneau-Guillon et al., 2020). By analyzing previous patient data and identifying patterns, AI helps physicians anticipate the possibility of complications and enables timely intervention.

Impact on Patient Outcomes and Operational Efficiency

Patient outcomes and operational efficacy have made huge strides after the adoption of AI by hospitals. These include the following significant impacts:

- Enhanced Diagnosis and Treatment: AI's ability to analyze massive data sets has resulted in faster and better diagnoses and opened the way for personalized treatment regimens [14]. For example, AI systems can recognize subtle patterns in medical imaging that may slip by human practitioners, assisting clinicians in early detection and increasing survival rates.
- Improved Patient Flow and Resource Management: AI has transformed hospital operations by forecasting patient flow and matching staffing efficiency. For example, at the Royal Melbourne Hospital, AI systems are built to predict when patients will be discharged so that staff can make arrangements for new admissions, thus significantly reducing patient waiting time.
- Cost Reduction: AI assists hospitals in lowering their internal operational costs through automated repetitive activities such as data entry, administration, and patient check-ups. It also prevents most medical errors, the negative implications of which are borne mainly by patient health and economics.
- Personalized Healthcare: Personalized therapy for each patient will replace conventional treatment with one-size-fits-all through patient data. Such a customized approach has been proven to yield better patient outcomes, mainly in the case of prolonged diseases like diabetes and heart disease.

Practical Considerations and Strategies for AI Integration in Hospitals

Incorporating AI within medical workflows poses significant operational problems yet offers revolutionary opportunities. A systematic approach to removing these obstructions must include technological solutions, funding plans, employee training, and solid governance measures.

- Security and Privacy of Data: Ensuring patient data confidentiality and maintaining compliance with rules like HIPAA, GDPR, or local data regulations is paramount when AI systems are crunching enormous amounts of sensitive patient data. Role-based access controls must be enforced within these hospitals, security audits must be conducted regularly, and data must be provided with end-to-end encryption on transmission and at rest. AI-specific privacy impact assessments must be integrated during deployment to lessen data breaches and misuse threats and uphold patient trust and legal compliance.
- Integration with Legacy Systems: Many healthcare facilities have antiquated IT systems that will not be compatible with the modern lines of AI software. Middleware integration layers, or APIs, are a viable method to join AI technologies to current platforms, given that a full replacement is expensive and disruptive (He et al., 2019). To ease transition, hospitals can run AI modules alongside legacy systems, slowly integrate them at operationally low-demand times, and set aside funds to retrain some specialized staff.
- ROI and Budget Planning: AI provides a good platform for long-term cost reductions due to better accuracy and efficiency; however, initial costs may be substantial, given infrastructure, data preparation, and personnel training. With the help of focused pilot projects with visible results, like fewer diagnostic errors or less time spent by patients waiting, hospitals can maximize their ROI. These financial barriers can be mitigated under public-private partnerships, innovation grants, or multi-year investment plans with well-set performance goals. So, leadership support can also be gained.
- Resistance to Change: Healthcare workers may be reluctant to accept AI for some outcome threat or work intensification reasons. For resolution, AI must be positioned as a supporting technology that complements human knowledge rather than replacing it. Systematic training programs build confidence while ensuring that clinicians and administrators are part of the design process early, ensuring that systems are user-centered. They can additionally dominate cultural acceptance by influencing peers and designating "AI champions" within departments.
- Algorithm Bias: An AI trained on a non-representative dataset risk returning erroneous or biased results in the face of underrepresented demographic groups. Hospitals should use explainable AI techniques, regular bias audits, and a diverse set of representative datasets to ensure transparent decision-making. An ethics oversight committee can be established to provide governance and accountability throughout the AI life cycle.

- Expense and Resource Allocation: The upfront infrastructure is one of the main obstacles to AI adoption. Hospitals can work around this by having department-wide shared AI platforms and prioritizing AI initiatives with high-impact and rapid payback, such as automated scheduling or triage support. The "build small, scale fast" approach avoids significant resource commitments during the initial stages of adoption, while cloud-based AI can reduce investment in hardware.

ETHICAL AND PRACTICAL CONSIDERATIONS

Data Privacy and Security Challenges

There is now a significant risk in both of these areas concerning the use of AI in health care systems. AI systems require huge amounts of sensitive patient data to be effective, such as genetic data, diagnostic images and other medical records. Such files need to be severely protected for ethical and legal reasons. The challenges are represented in Figure 7.

Figure 7. Data Privacy and Security Challenges

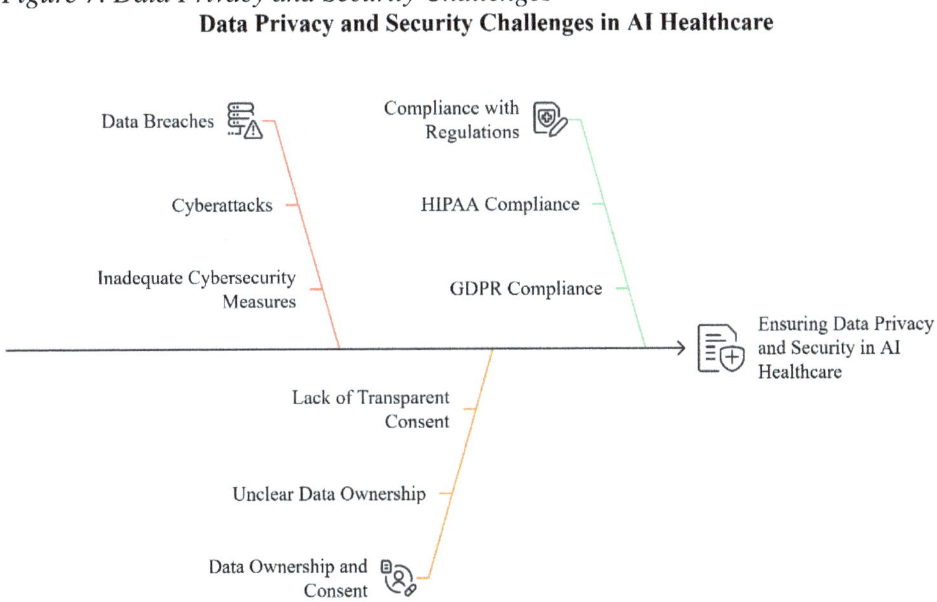

- Data Breaches: Cyber invasions compromise the property of AI systems concerning integrated patient records (Eyers & Krastev, 2020). They may involve exposing sensitive personal information, losing patients, and harming reputations. Hospitals must provide robust security safeguards to protect data, such as encryption, multi-factor authentication, and frequent audits.
- Data Ownership and Consent: There are gray areas concerning who owns the data that AI systems collect—patients, hospitals, or outside companies (Mittelstadt et al., 2016). Further, patients may not have consented to specific data uses or fully understand how their data is being used. Hospitals shall ensure patients have some control over their data and formal consent mechanisms.
- Compliance with Regulations: Healthcare organizations must comply with stringent data privacy laws like the European General Data Protection Regulation (GDPR) and the United States Health Insurance Portability and Accountability Act (HIPAA) (Morley et al., 2020). These regulations provide specific instructions about handling, storing, and transmitting the information. Hospitals must draft policies and implement technologies aligned with these standards to remain compliant and curb any legal issues.

Addressing Algorithmic Bias in Healthcare AI

Algorithmic bias, particularly about AI systems, is a most relevant ethical medical matter. When AI models use historical data for training, they might reinforce or worsen pre-existing bias based on socioeconomic status, gender, or race. To ensure equitable treatment of patients through AI systems, algorithmic bias must be addressed by Challen et al. (2019). The essential considerations to bear in mind while addressing algorithmic bias in AI for healthcare can be seen in Figure 8.

Figure 8. Addressing Algorithmic Bias in Healthcare AI

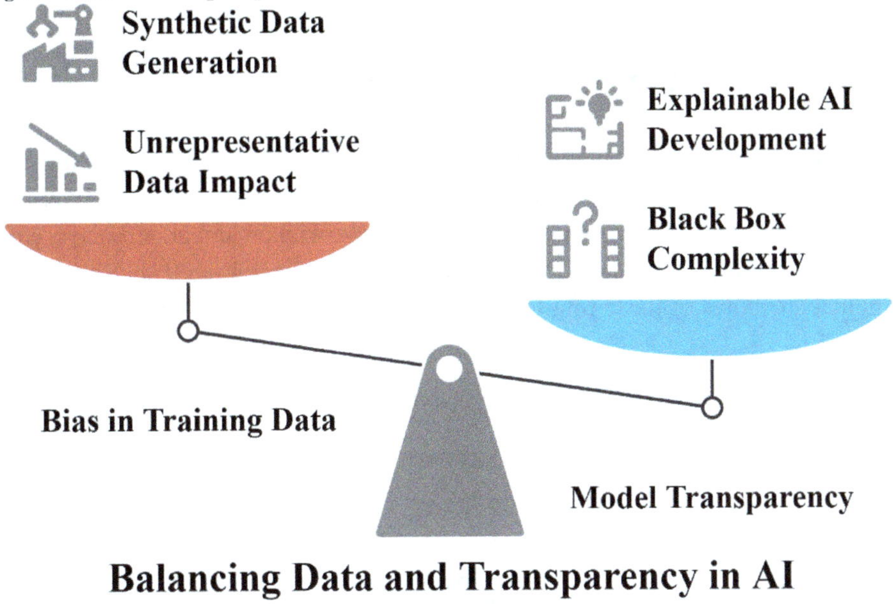

- Bias in Training Data: Data quality decides the quality of an AI system. The AI model may not be generalizable across various demographic groupings if the training data cannot represent many populations. For example, one ethnic group may perform poorly in the diagnosis when the model is applied from a training environment predominantly focused on the background of training from this group. These issues can be alleviated by ensuring diverse datasets for training, creating or using synthetic data, etc.
- Model Transparency: The lack of transparency often makes understanding AI models, especially those with intense learning capabilities, challenging for decision-making. This absence of transparency can create skewed outcomes that are hard to ascertain and remedy. The development of explainable AI (XAI) must be pursued to support understanding the decision-making process and ensure fairness in medical applications.
- Regular Auditing and Monitoring: Once deployed, AI systems should be audited regularly to check for bias. Continuous monitoring could identify differences in patient outcomes based on gender, race, or some other characteristic. Such audits should be conducted by diverse teams, including AI experts and healthcare professionals, to identify and remedy any biases early.
- Inclusive Design and Testing: Involving diverse teams in AI model design and evaluation ensures consideration of diverse views. AI systems must un-

dergo a rigorous validation process in real healthcare settings to evaluate performance in various patient populations and demographic groups.

Regulatory and Compliance Frameworks

Numerous regulatory and compliance frameworks govern AI use in healthcare, ensuring patient safety, data security, and ethical use of technology by Eyers and Krastev (2020) and Morley et al. (2020). Their cognizance and adherence are pivotal for successful AI integration into healthcare settings. Figure 9 summarizes the principal attributes of these regulatory and compliance frameworks.

Figure 9. Regulatory and Compliance Frameworks AI

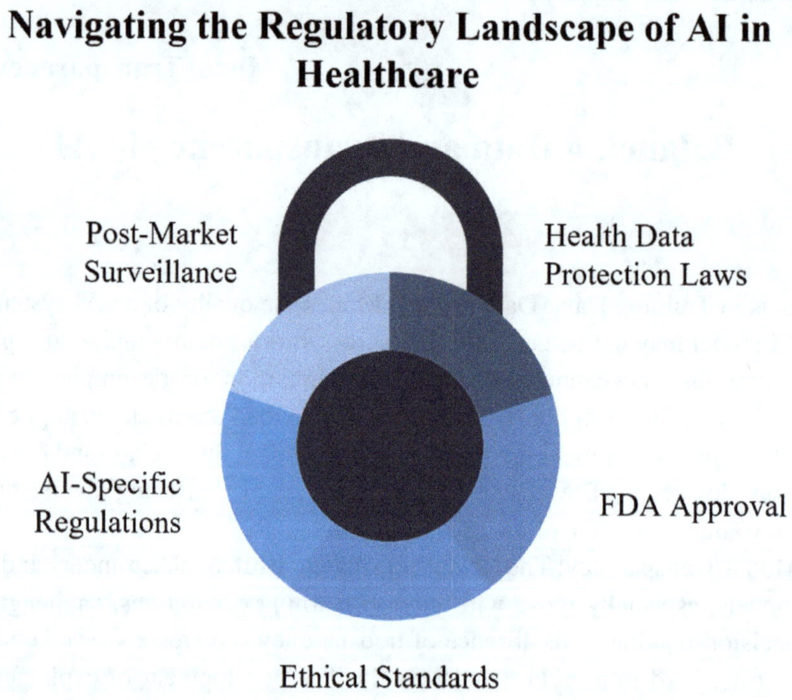

- Health Data Protection Laws: As stated above, privacy laws such as the GDPR in Europe and HIPAA in the United States set rules and regulations for the gathering, storing, and sharing of healthcare data. They regulate how AI technologies are applied in healthcare regarding patient consent, data minimization, and secure data storage. Any AI system should be developed with compliance in mind to avoid any legal consequences.

- FDA Approval for AI in Healthcare: AI-based medical software and devices commonly need FDA approval before being used in the clinical setting in the United States. This process guarantees the safety, efficacy, and reliability of AI applications. Vaswani et al. (2017) described that the FDA may regulate systems for diagnosis, treatment recommendations, and patient monitoring that are considered AI, which must complete adequate clinical investigation and testing before being approved for regulatory compliance.
- Ethical Standards and Guidelines: Two professional associations that have developed ethical guidelines regarding the usage of AI in healthcare are the World Health Organization (WHO) and the American Medical Association (AMA). These recommendations emphasize that patient-centered care, accountability, and transparency are vital in AI applications. To ensure technology enhances patient care without compromising safety or trust, healthcare organizations must ensure their AI systems adhere to ethical guidelines.
- AI-Specific Regulations: In addition to current healthcare laws, the need for AI-specific legislation is garnering more consensus. Many governments and other regulatory bodies are now contemplating frameworks specific to AI to address issues such as algorithmic accountability, transparency, and inequity. The EU has put forward the concept of the AI Act, for example, which would govern high-risk AI applications, such as those working in healthcare, from the standpoint of safety and compliance with ethical principles.
- Post-Market Surveillance: Once deployed in healthcare settings, regulatory bodies may require post-market surveillance to track AI systems' performance and influence on clinical outcomes. This guarantees that these AI applications adhere to safety regulations and that any problems or issues are detected and rectified immediately.

FUTURE TRENDS AND INNOVATIONS

Emerging AI Technologies in Healthcare

The ongoing advancements in AI for healthcare give rise to several upcoming technologies that can transform medical research, patient treatment, and healthcare management. Some such brightest prospects are:

- AI-Powered Imaging and Diagnostics: AI algorithms with advanced design, particularly those based on deep learning, would change the medical imaging landscape (Muniasamy, A, 2024; Muniasamy, A, 2023). AI technologies such as convolutional neural networks (CNNs) can accurately analyze medical images like X-ray, CT, and MRI. AI may automate the diagnostic process altogether, cutting down some radiologists' workload and providing faster diagnoses, especially in areas with low resources or remote places.

- Natural Language Processing (NLP) for Clinical Text: NLP tools in healthcare are gaining traction due to their ability to glean timely insights from unstructured clinical data, including electronic health records (EHRs) and clinical records. With further advances, NLP could navigate medical records to highlight critical health signs that require attention, thus facilitating real-time AI-supported clinical decision-making by Beam and Kohane (2018) and Vaswani et al. (2017).
- AI in Drug Discovery and Development: AI techniques are used in drug development to analyze large datasets to discover potential compounds for treating specific diseases (Muniasamy, A. 2026). Modeling molecular interactions of possible drugs using machine-learning algorithms can reduce the costs usually associated with drug development. AI is set to fast-track the development of new therapies, such as genetically customized targeted medicine.
- Wearable AI Devices: Wearables such as smartwatches and health supervisors can already track dynamic signs such as blood pressure and heart rate (Muniasamy & Asiri, 2025). Future iterations are expected to use AI to assess this data in real time and sound early alarms for any health concerns, such as heart attacks, strokes, or complications from diabetes.
- AI-Enhanced Robotic Surgery: AI continues to improve the success of operations and clinical outcomes in robotic surgery (Hashimoto et al., 2018). AI-based robots assess patient data to aid surgeons in real-time decision-making during procedures. Once these technologies are established in certain specialties, they may become viable for autonomous robotic surgery, minimizing human errors and enhancing healing.

Potential for AI-Driven Predictive and Preventive Care

AI could transform healthcare from reactive to proactive, predictive, and preventive. AI systems might predict health problems before they occur by analyzing large data sets and identifying patterns. This would have significant benefits for both patients and healthcare professionals.

- Predictive Analytics for Disease Risk: AI can predict the risk level of diseases, such as diabetes and other chronic diseases (Letourneau-Guillon et al., 2020). It uses genetic data and medical history to make such predictions. AI will be helpful in the early detection of potential health problems so that preventive measures, such as lifestyle changes, early screening, or individualized treatment, can be applied. For example, AI uses risk factors like blood pressure, cholesterol, and family history to predict the chances of a heart attack or stroke.

- AI in Population Health Management: AI-enabled solutions can help doctors monitor the population's well-being. Trends in health data under different groups allow AI to identify at-risk communities and forecast disease outbreaks by Harris (2022). This identification would enable timely intervention and focused public health initiatives.
- Remote Monitoring and Telemedicine: Wearables and AI will continue to progress as tools for continuous health monitoring. Such devices can track many of the usual indicators monitored, such as oxygen levels, sleep quality, and activity levels. The data collected can then be sent to health providers for real-time monitoring. For example, work in AI can help reveal abnormalities in data that would lead to early intervention and avoid health emergencies before they happen.
- AI-Powered Lifestyle Recommendations: Examples of preventative care include targeted recommendations based on AI studies of nutrition, lifestyle, genetic makeup, and environmental influences on a patient. Such an individualized approach may consist of exercise recommendations, dietary adjustments, and even stress-attenuating methods to lower the risk of chronic disease while improving the overall quality of life.

Decision-Making Models for AI and Human Collaboration

Despite AI's footprints in several areas within healthcare, human-computer co-action will probably be the future focus of AI in healthcare. AI in healthcare will be mainly a tool for improving outcomes and making decisions rather than replacing medical personnel. Collaboration between AI and human experience provides a more comprehensive plan in these unique models.

- AI-Assisted Clinical Decision Support: Of all the recent breakthroughs in this direction, getting AI into the context of clinical-decision support systems must be fascinating, Vaswani et al. (2017). Such algorithms can process enormous amounts of medical information and thus supply evidence-based, real-time recommendations to providers. AI can help find possible medication interactions, provide treatment options for complicated diseases, or predict the best course of action based on a patient's data. Human judgment would still be critical in making sense of these findings and reaching conclusions.

- Human-AI Interaction in Patient Care: Automating repetitive tasks like data entry or office work frees up precious patient interaction time, bringing the clinician-patient dyad closer. It also provides insights into medication usage during consultation with a patient,e.g., highlighting relevant research findings about particular risks that might inform clinical management.
- Shared Decision-Making with Patients: AI-powered decision-support technologies would empower patients by offering individualized information about their treatment options. AI assists patients in understanding the potential outcomes of several treatment regimens, possibly influencing the ever-increasing patient-centered care movement that drives patients to be more involved in their health journey.
- Interdisciplinary Collaboration: AI technologies will likely stimulate broader collaboration among multidisciplinary medical teams. AI will aid in acquiring relevant data and insights among specialists, physicians, nurses, pharmacologists, and therapists, promoting a more coordinated approach to patient care (Mehta et al., 2019). This cooperative decision-making process may yield better and more efficacious treatment regimens, particularly for patients with complex, multifaceted medical conditions.

SOLUTIONS AND RECOMMENDATIONS

A multifaceted strategy is required to optimize the advantages of integrating artificial intelligence (AI) into medical processes. A strong basis for Artificial Intelligence processes will be ensured by strengthening data infrastructure through centralized, secure repositories linked directly to diagnostic imaging and EHRs. Adopting standard formats, such as HL7 and FHIR, shall facilitate interoperability. For more hospital-specific Artificial Intelligence models, design will be implemented using convolutional neural networks for imaging, natural language processing for documentation, and forecasting models for resource planning. Also, these models must be trained iteratively over different data sets to reduce bias. Integrating AI-powered CDSS into physician dashboards and employing RPAs for monotonous tasks will cut the inefficiencies in clinical and administrative spheres. End users should be part of the design process to guarantee usability and acceptance. Predictive analytics may be applied to forecast inventory, schedule surgeries, and manage intensive-care-unit beds, with real-time data inputs allowing for a proactive approach in decision-making. With the highest data protection standards, respect for HIPAA/GDPR rights, and the establishment of ethics review boards to keep track of AI on the grounds of bias and patient safety, the ethics and regulatory domain must maintain its prominence. IT awareness programs, ongoing staff training, and change management strategies geared toward surmounting operational and cultural bottlenecks will stand them in good stead. Of course, automation of KPI dashboards for continuous monitoring, alongside frequent audits and looping of stakeholder feedback, guarantees the AI systems remain accurate, efficient, and in keeping with their operational and clinical objectives.

FUTURE RESEARCH DIRECTIONS

This chapter presents several examples of how AI can considerably speed up hospital workflows. However, several unexplored areas are worth considering. To enable individualized treatment, the design of AI models that can incorporate multi-modal healthcare data -- genetics, wearable device outputs, real-time patient monitoring streams, etc. -- should be the focus of future research. Explainable AI (XAI) solutions that offer clear and decipherable logic behind therapeutic recommendations must be developed to increase the clinician's trust and maintain regulatory compliance. Inter-institutional studies must be carried out involving different hospital environments and patient demographics to improve the generalizability and fairness of AI algorithms and reduce the possible incidence of bias. For promoting cooperative AI model training programs offered by two or more hospitals without compromising patient privacy, federated learning frameworks deserve research attention in the future. Another area of focus is the integration of AI into emerging cutting-edge technologies like blockchain for secure exchange of health data, augmented reality (AR) for surgical assistance, and digital twins for patient care simulation. As healthcare systems transition toward the large-scale implementation of technologies, sustainable AI research to maximize energy use and computational resources will also be necessary. Last will be longitudinal research that evaluates long-term clinical, financial, and ethical consequences of AI use to provide an evidence basis to standardize policies, and ensure adoption across healthcare systems.

CONCLUSION

The methods described in the chapter provide a synthesis along clinical and administrative lines for the AI integration into hospital workflows using a comprehensive framework-based methodology. AI interventions were thus prescribed to tackle problems, e.g., extended patient waiting times, inefficient allocation of resources in the hospital setup, and manual clinical administrative overhead. The four main applications were: advanced medical imaging algorithms for the interpretation of chest X-rays and the detection of pneumonia; robotic process automation (RPA) for the automation of mundane administrative tasks; predictive analytics for ICU bed occupancy and inventory management; and AI-powered Clinical Decision Support Systems (CDSS) to enhance diagnostic precision and assist clinical decision-making. The AI is used in five stages of implementation to develop a diagnosis system along with other image interpretation enhancements introduced by the hospitals, respecting factors on cybersecurity, interoperability, and ethical compliance. In these hospital case studies, concrete clinical results were evident; therefore, specificity increased from 89.4% to 92.6% (+3.2%), pneumonia detection sensitivity increased from 86.1% to 91.8% (+5.7%), and the diagnosis accuracy of X-ray imaging rose from 88.5% to 94.2% (+5.7%). Apart from that, improvements included a 40% drop-in administrative work completion time, a 60% decrease in appointment no-show rates, and a 42% reduction in patient waiting times in the hospital. Predictive analytics further reduced inventory replenishment times by 38%, achieving an ICU bed occupancy forecast with a mean absolute error of 2.1 units. The findings demonstrate that integrating AI can result in quantifiable gains in diagnostic accuracy, operational effectiveness, and resource usage within a planned, staged, and ethically governed framework. This chapter offers a reproducible roadmap for healthcare companies looking to improve clinical outcomes and operational performance through intelligent automation and validates the technical viability of AI in hospital settings. This work bridges the gap between theoretical AI promise and hospital change by tying quantitative outcomes to practical implementation techniques.

REFERENCES

Beam, A. L., & Kohane, I. S. (2018). Big data and machine learning in health care. *Journal of the American Medical Association, 319*(13), 1317–1318. DOI: 10.1001/jama.2017.18391 PMID: 29532063

Cabitza, F., Rasoini, R., & Gensini, G. F. (2017). Unintended consequences of machine learning in medicine. *Journal of the American Medical Association, 318*(6), 517–518. DOI: 10.1001/jama.2017.7797 PMID: 28727867

Challen, R., Denny, J., Pitt, M., Gompels, L., Edwards, T., & Tsaneva-Atanasova, K. (2019). Artificial intelligence, bias and clinical safety. *BMJ Quality & Safety, 28*(3), 231–237. DOI: 10.1136/bmjqs-2018-008370 PMID: 30636200

Davenport, T., & Kalakota, R. (2019). The potential for artificial intelligence in healthcare. *Future healthcare journal, 6*(2), 94-98. . doi: DOI: 10.7861/futurehosp.6-2-94

Dilsizian, S. E., & Siegel, E. L. (2014). Artificial intelligence in medicine and cardiac imaging: Harnessing big data and advanced computing to provide personalized medical diagnosis and treatment. *Current Cardiology Reports, 16*(1), 441. DOI: 10.1007/s11886-013-0441-8 PMID: 24338557

Esteva, A., Robicquet, A., Ramsundar, B., Kuleshov, V., DePristo, M., Chou, K., Cui, C., Corrado, G., Thrun, S., & Dean, J. (2019). A guide to deep learning in healthcare. *Nature Medicine, 25*(1), 24–29. DOI: 10.1038/s41591-018-0316-z PMID: 30617335

Eyers, T., & Krastev, Y. (2020). Ethics in surgical innovations from the patient perspective. *Yearbook of Medical Informatics, 29*(01), 169–175. DOI: 10.1055/s-0040-1701994 PMID: 32823312

Gauthaman, S. A., (2026). Introduction to machine learning and optimization in healthcare. In Muniasamy, A. (Ed.), *Integrative machine learning and optimization algorithms for disease prediction* (pp. 1–34). IGI Global., DOI: 10.4018/979-8-3373-1087-9.ch001

Gauthaman, S. A., Muniasamy, A., & Karunakaran, G. (2026). Current challenges in the pharmaceutical industry and AI's role in addressing them. In Muniasamy, A., & Karunakaran, G. (Eds.), *Applications of Artificial Intelligence in Pharmaceuticals* (pp. 1–26). IGI Global., DOI: 10.4018/979-8-3373-2043-4.ch001

Harris, J. E. (2022). COVID-19 Incidence and hospitalization during the delta surge were inversely related to vaccination coverage among the most populous US Counties. *Health Policy and Technology, 11*(2), 100583. DOI: 10.1016/j.hlpt.2021.100583 PMID: 34868833

Hashimoto, D. A., Rosman, G., Rus, D., & Meireles, O. R. (2018). Artificial intelligence in surgery: Promises and perils. *Annals of Surgery*, *268*(1), 70–76. DOI: 10.1097/SLA.0000000000002693 PMID: 29389679

He, J., Baxter, S. L., Xu, J., Xu, J., Zhou, X., & Zhang, K. (2019). The practical implementation of artificial intelligence technologies in medicine. *Nature Medicine*, *25*(1), 30–36. DOI: 10.1038/s41591-018-0307-0 PMID: 30617336

Hinton, G. (2018). Deep learning—A technology with the potential to transform health care. *Journal of the American Medical Association*, *320*(11), 1101–1102. DOI: 10.1001/jama.2018.11100 PMID: 30178065

Jiang, F., Jiang, Y., Zhi, H., Dong, Y., Li, H., Ma, S., Wang, Y., Dong, Q., Shen, H., & Wang, Y. (2017). Artificial intelligence in healthcare: Past, present and future. *Stroke and Vascular Neurology*, *2*(4), 230–243. Advance online publication. DOI: 10.1136/svn-2017-000101 PMID: 29507784

Johnson, A. E. W., Pollard, T. J., Shen, L., Lehman, L. H., Feng, M., Ghassemi, M., Moody, B., Szolovits, P., Anthony Celi, L., & Mark, R. G. (2016). MIMIC-III, a freely accessible critical care database. *Scientific Data*, *3*(1), 1–9. DOI: 10.1038/sdata.2016.35 PMID: 27219127

Karri, H. K., Begum, A., & George, L. (2024). Optimizing Healthcare Efficiency: The Role of Artificial Intelligence in Medical Records Management. *International Journal of Engineering and Management Research*, *14*(6), 55–67. DOI: 10.31033/ijemr.14.6.55-67

Kelly, C. J., Karthikesalingam, A., Suleyman, M., Corrado, G., & King, D. (2019). Key challenges for delivering clinical impact with artificial intelligence. *BMC Medicine*, *17*(1), 195. DOI: 10.1186/s12916-019-1426-2 PMID: 31665002

Kotter, E., & Ranschaert, E. (2021). Challenges and solutions for introducing artificial intelligence (AI) in daily clinical workflow. *European Radiology*, *31*(1), 5–7. DOI: 10.1007/s00330-020-07148-2 PMID: 32797308

Letourneau-Guillon, L., Camirand, D., Guilbert, F., & Forghani, R. (2020). Artificial intelligence applications for workflow, process optimization and predictive analytics. *Neuroimaging Clinics of North America*, *30*(4), e1–e15. DOI: 10.1016/j.nic.2020.08.008 PMID: 33039002

Mehta, N., Pandit, A., & Shukla, S. (2019). Transforming healthcare with big data analytics and artificial intelligence: A systematic mapping study. *Journal of Biomedical Informatics*, *100*, 103311. DOI: 10.1016/j.jbi.2019.103311 PMID: 31629922

Mittelstadt, B. D., Allo, P., Taddeo, M., Wachter, S., & Floridi, L. (2016). The ethics of algorithms: Mapping the debate. *Big Data & Society*, *3*(2), 2053951716679679. DOI: 10.1177/2053951716679679

Mohsen, F., Ali, H., El Hajj, N., & Shah, Z. (2022). Artificial intelligence-based methods for fusion of electronic health records and imaging data. *Scientific Reports*, *12*(1), 17981. DOI: 10.1038/s41598-022-22514-4 PMID: 36289266

Morley, J., Floridi, L., Kinsey, L., & Elhalal, A. (2020). From what to how: An initial review of publicly available AI ethics tools, methods and research to translate principles into practices. *Science and Engineering Ethics*, *26*(4), 2141–2168. DOI: 10.1007/s11948-019-00165-5 PMID: 31828533

Muniasamy, A. Muniasamy, Sabahath A., Begum, A., Yaqub, H., & Karunakaran, G. (2023). Lung cancer histopathology image classification using transfer learning with convolution neural network model. *Technology and Health Care,*33, 1–12. https://content.iospress.com/articles/technology-and-health-care/thc231029

Muniasamy, A. (2026). Quantum computing in drug discovery: Revolutionizing pharmaceutical research. In Muniasamy, A., & Karunakaran, G. (Eds.), *Applications of artificial intelligence in pharmaceuticals* (pp. 59–96). IGI Global., DOI: 10.4018/979-8-3373-2043-4.ch003

Muniasamy, A., & Asiri, F. (2025). Advanced human activity recognition on wearables with multi-scale sparse attention. *Multimedia Tools and Applications*, *84*(30), 36623–36652. Advance online publication. DOI: 10.1007/s11042-024-20475-6

Muniasamy, A., Begum, A., Sabahath, A., Yaqub, H., & Karunakaran, G. (2024). Coronary heart disease classification using deep learning approach with feature selection for improved accuracy. *Technology and Health Care*, *32*(3), 1991–2007. DOI: 10.3233/THC-231807 PMID: 38339946

Muniasamy, A., & Karunakaran, G. (2026). Challenges and future directions: Emerging trends and limitations in ML and optimization for healthcare. In Muniasamy, A. (Ed.), *Integrative machine learning and optimization algorithms for disease prediction* (pp. 339–368). IGI Global., DOI: 10.4018/979-8-3373-1087-9.ch012

Naim, A.. (2026). AI-driven smart manufacturing and automation in pharmaceutical production. In Muniasamy, A., & Karunakaran, G. (Eds.), *Applications of artificial intelligence in pharmaceuticals* (pp. 157–194). IGI Global., DOI: 10.4018/979-8-3373-2043-4.ch006

Novillo-Ortiz, D., Marin, H. D. F., & Saigí-Rubió, F. (2018). The role of digital health in supporting the achievement of the Sustainable Development Goals (SDGs). *International Journal of Medical Informatics*, *114*, 106–107. DOI: 10.1016/j.ijmedinf.2018.03.011 PMID: 29602629

Obermeyer, Z., & Emanuel, E. J. (2016). Predicting the future—Big data, machine learning, and clinical medicine. *The New England Journal of Medicine*, *375*(13), 1216–1219. DOI: 10.1056/NEJMp1606181 PMID: 27682033

Pierre, K., Haneberg, A. G., Kwak, S., Peters, K. R., Hochhegger, B., Sananmuang, T., . . . Forghani, R. (2023, April). Applications of artificial intelligence in the radiology roundtrip: process streamlining, workflow optimization, and beyond. In *Seminars in Roentgenology* (Vol. 58, No. 2, pp. 158-169). WB Saunders. DOI: DOI: 10.1053/j.ro.2023.02.003

Raghupathi, W., & Raghupathi, V. (2014). Big data analytics in healthcare: Promise and potential. *Health Information Science and Systems*, *2*(1), 3. DOI: 10.1186/2047-2501-2-3 PMID: 25825667

Rajkomar, A., Dean, J., & Kohane, I. (2019). Machine learning in medicine. *New England Journal of Medicine, 380*(14), 1347-1358. DOI: . DOI: DOI: 10.1056/NEJMra1814259

Reddy, S., Fox, J., & Purohit, M. P. (2019). Artificial intelligence-enabled healthcare delivery. *Journal of the Royal Society of Medicine*, *112*(1), 22–28. DOI: 10.1177/0141076818815510 PMID: 30507284

Rengaramanujam, K., & Muniasamy, A. (2026). AI in hospital administration and formulary design: Optimizing resource allocation and patient flow. In Muniasamy, A., & Karunakaran, G. (Eds.), *Applications of artificial intelligence in pharmaceuticals* (pp. 215–246). IGI Global., DOI: 10.4018/979-8-3373-2043-4.ch008

Shortliffe, E. H., & Sepúlveda, M. J. (2018). Clinical decision support in the era of artificial intelligence. *Journal of the American Medical Association*, *320*(21), 2199–2200. DOI: 10.1001/jama.2018.17163 PMID: 30398550

Topol, E. (2019). *Deep medicine: how artificial intelligence can make healthcare human again*. Hachette UK. https://dl.acm.org/doi/10.5555/3350442

Trebble, T. M., Hansi, N., Hydes, T., Smith, M. A., & Baker, M. (2010). Process mapping the patient journey: An introduction. *BMJ (Clinical Research Ed.)*, *341*(aug13 1), c4078. Advance online publication. DOI: 10.1136/bmj.c4078 PMID: 20709715

Van den Berg, M. P., Mulder, B. A., Klaassen, S. H., Maass, A. H., van Veldhuisen, D. J., van der Meer, P., Nienhuis, H. L. A., Hazenberg, B. P. C., & Rienstra, M. (2019). Heart failure with preserved ejection fraction, atrial fibrillation, and the role of senile amyloidosis. *European Heart Journal, 40*(16), 1287–1293. DOI: 10.1093/eurheartj/ehz057 PMID: 30753432

Vaswani, A., Shazeer, N., Parmar, N., Uszkoreit, J., Jones, L., Gomez, A. N., & Polosukhin, I. (2017). Attention is all you need. *Advances in Neural Information Processing Systems, 30*. Advance online publication. DOI: 10.48550/arXiv.1706.03762

Wiens, J., Saria, S., Sendak, M., Ghassemi, M., Liu, V. X., Doshi-Velez, F., Jung, K., Heller, K., Kale, D., Saeed, M., Ossorio, P. N., Thadaney-Israni, S., & Goldenberg, A. (2019). Do no harm: A roadmap for responsible machine learning for health care. *Nature Medicine, 25*(9), 1337–1340. DOI: 10.1038/s41591-019-0548-6 PMID: 31427808

Yu, K. H., Beam, A. L., & Kohane, I. S. (2018). Artificial intelligence in healthcare. *Nature Biomedical Engineering, 2*(10), 719–731. DOI: 10.1038/s41551-018-0305-z PMID: 31015651

ADDITIONAL READING

Alavi, H., Gordo-Gregorio, P., Forcada, N., Bayramova, A., & Edwards, D. J. (2024). AI-driven BIM integration for optimizing healthcare facility design. *Buildings (Basel, Switzerland), 14*(8), 2354. DOI: 10.3390/buildings14082354

GUMMADI, H. S. B. (2025). AI-driven multimodal workflow optimization for personalized patient-centered care. DOI:DOI: 10.30574/wjaets.2025.15.2.0604

Katal, N. (2024). Ai-driven healthcare services and infrastructure in smart cities. In *Smart Cities* (pp. 150–170). CRC Press., DOI: 10.1201/9781003442660-7

Lyon, J. Y., Bogodistov, Y., & Moormann, J. (2021). AI-driven optimization in healthcare: The diagnostic process. *European Journal of Management Issues, 29*(4), 218–231. DOI: 10.15421/192121

Rajpurkar, P., Chen, E., Banerjee, O., & Topol, E. J. (2022). AI in health and medicine. *Nature medicine, 28*(1), 31-38. DOI: . DOI: DOI: 10.1038/s41591-021-01614-0

KEY TERMS AND DEFINITIONS

AI-Powered Diagnostic: This involves diagnosing and detecting diseases by interpreting doctors' medical data, such as test results, imaging scans, etc., via machine learning and deep learning algorithms.

AUC-ROC: The ability to discriminate between classes is one of the classification models' performance metrics, measured using the AUC-ROC method.

Clinical Decision Support System (CDSS): A Health IT system for analyzing clinical data to aid medical practitioners in making evidence-based decisions.

Explainable AI: AI systems that increase transparency and build trust by making the decision-making processes understandable to human users.

F1-Score: It is a good measure for evaluating AI models in unbalanced datasets as it considers precision and recall.

Interoperability: Exchange, interpretation, and application of data among various healthcare software programs and information systems.

Mean Absolute Error (MAE): This statistical measure gives the average magnitude of prediction errors and is used in assessing predictions produced by predictive models.

Natural Language Processing (NLP): A branch of AI that enables computers to understand, interpret, and generate human language. It is frequently applied to analyze unstructured medical texts and clinical notes.

Predictive analytics: Predicting future events or trends, such as ICU bed occupancy or patient admissions, using statistical algorithms and machine learning approaches on historical data.

Robotic Process Automation (RPA): Software robots automate routine processes, including scheduling, billing, and task report generation.

Chapter 10
AI in Healthcare:
Automating Hospital Operations for Better Patient Care

Usharani Bhimavarapu
https://orcid.org/0000-0002-0246-1420
Department of Computer Science and Engineering, Koneru Lakshmaiah Education Foundation, Vaddeswaram, India

ABSTRACT

The integration of Artificial Intelligence (AI) into hospital systems presents a promising avenue to enhance healthcare quality and operational efficiency. Specifically, AI-driven workflow optimization leverages advanced techniques such as Artificial Neural Networks (ANN) to analyze complex clinical and administrative data, enabling improved decision-making and resource management. This integration addresses critical challenges faced by hospitals, including increasing patient loads, data complexity, and the need for timely diagnosis and treatment. By automating routine tasks, predicting patient influx, and supporting personalized care, AI systems streamline workflows, reduce costs, and improve patient outcomes. This study explores the potential of AI, particularly ANN models, in optimizing hospital operations, emphasizing their role in creating smarter, more adaptive healthcare environments

Keywords: AI Integration, Workflow Optimization, Hospitals, Artificial Neural Networks, Healthcare Automation

INTRODUCTION

Hospitals desire to deliver the highest standard of care, yet increasing numbers of patients and case complexity strain conventional approaches. AI is incorporated

DOI: 10.4018/979-8-3373-2787-7.ch010

to assist clinicians with data-driven knowledge, enhanced diagnostic accuracy, and treatment. For instance, AI can analyze medical images quicker and more accurately than human beings in certain conditions. This enhances the identification of life-threatening diseases like cancer at an earlier stage, saving lives. AI solutions also allow for real-time monitoring of patients, alerting personnel of life-threatening changes in real time. With workflow optimization, care providers have more time to interact with patients rather than paperwork. Personalized care is crucial for boosting patient satisfaction and outcomes. AI is finally an enabler that helps facilitate augmenting human capabilities without replacing them. The continuous learning ability of AI technologies ensures evolving and modifying standards of care. Thus, AI integration is required for quality assurance in current healthcare (Rengaramanujam et al. 2026).

The majority of hospitals function with practically no budgetary limitations, balancing quality care with price. Workflow inefficiency translates to wasted resources, redundant work, and longer patient wait times. AI-powered workflow optimization removes mundane tasks such as scheduling, billing, and inventory, which saves manpower expense. Predictive analytics forecast patient admissions, enabling more efficient resource and staff deployment. This prevents costly over-staffing or under-staffing, enhancing budget planning. In addition, AI identifies suspicious and fraudulent behavior patterns, preventing losses from billing abnormalities or unnecessary treatments. Efficient operations also minimize length of stay for patients, enabling space to treat additional patients. Hospitals therefore save on operating costs without sacrificing care (Rengaramanujam et al. 2026). This financial benefit makes AI a prime technology for healthcare facilities in their endeavor to achieve cost-effective service provision. It helps ensure that available resources are optimally utilized in the delivery of essential care services. The financial sustainability thus achieved provides room for reinvestment in additional technological development.

Healthcare information is increasing at an exponential rate, including electronic health records (EHRs), imaging, genomics, and data from wearables. It is humanly difficult and error-prone to process and interpret the information manually. AI algorithms are best designed to handle large amounts of data, identify significant patterns in a timely manner. Natural Language Processing (NLP) assists in interpreting unstructured clinical notes, extracting them as actionable information. Machine learning algorithms establish correlations that may escape human detection, facilitating predictive and preventive care (Gauthaman, S. A., et al., 2026). Integrating heterogeneous data offers comprehensive understanding of patient health, impacting individualized care. AI-based decision support systems assist clinicians with evidence-based advice. This minimizes cognitive load on healthcare professionals so that they can concentrate on thinking and patient interaction. Effective data handling by AI also improves research capabilities, speeding up medical advancements.

Integration of AI thus overcomes complexity in data, making it an incredible tool for improving healthcare.

Hospitals are complicated institutions with several crossing departments and streams. Inefficiency usually stems from hand coordination, communications break, and redundant processes. Workflow optimization with AI introduces automation into most processes such as patient triage, ordering tests, and interpreting results. By streamlining these phases, hospitals are able to bypass bottlenecks and waiting times. For example, AI-optimizing scheduling systems optimize scheduling slots based on patient urgency and available capacity. The outcome is timely care delivery and effective use of equipment. AI-powered chatbots also handle common patient queries, freeing up staff to tackle more advanced tasks. Improved workflow efficiency minimizes burnout among staff, enhancing overall morale and turnover. It also prevents regulatory hazards through standardized processes. Ultimately, the deployment of AI results in smoother, more efficient, and better clinical workflow that will benefit patients as well as healthcare professionals (Rengaramanujam et al. 2026).

Assisting clinicians to make informed choices is possibly the most important use of AI in hospitals. Medical decision-making is delicate, and typically, it is a matter of collating huge quantities of information in a time-constrained setting. Patient background, investigations, and presenting symptoms are processed by machine algorithms to give diagnostic likelihoods and treatment suggestions. This cuts down the likelihood of human error and promotes evidence-based practice. Clinical Decision Support Systems (CDSS) warn physicians of possible drug interactions or contraindications. They even suggest customized therapies based on genetic and lifestyle considerations. AI continually updates its knowledge base in real-time from recent research, thus providing latest information to clinicians. As an additional opinion, AI boosts confidence in clinical decisions. Shared process leads to improved patient outcomes and reduced rates of unnecessary intervention. AI is thus an important weapon in accuracy and timeliness of clinical choices.

Patient engagement is key to successful treatment adherence and health outcomes. Most hospitals, though, are unable to offer consistent individualized communication because of limitations in their resources. AI-based applications, including virtual health assistants and mobile apps, provide consistent support and education to patients. These applications remind patients regarding medication timing, appointments, and lifestyle interventions. AI chatbots may respond to health-related queries 24/7, decreasing anxiety and enhancing satisfaction. Patient-specific feedback improves healthier behaviors and self-management. Additionally, AI gives remote monitoring of chronic illness, which alerts healthcare professionals when action must be initiated. The proactive care strategy makes the patients more involved in their own process. More involvement translates into higher compliance and fewer readmissions to the hospital. Optimized communication processes help the hospitals design a better patient-centric care environment. This helps to design confidence, loyalty, and a better overall experience.

Hospitals employ a number of healthcare specialists such as physicians, nurses, technicians, and administrative professionals. Proper coordination among teams is required for coordinated patient care. With integration with AI, smoothening information sharing and communication between departments is made possible. AI-driven centralized data platforms present real-time patient data to entire teams. Workflow management software tracks tasks and notifies engaged teams about key events. For instance, AI may alert radiologists in real-time when scans are ready and surgeons in the event of an emergency. This eliminates delay due to handoffs and miscommunication. In addition, analytics using AI detect workflow bottlenecks and suggest workflow optimization. Accelerated diagnosis and treatment enhance outcomes for patients. It also enhances teamwork culture and continuous improvement in staff. Hence, integration with AI enhances interdisciplinary workflows, enhancing hospital efficiency and quality of care.

Time is very limited in emergency department (ED) settings, and workflow waste can be life or death. AI optimizes triage through swift patient severity assessment from symptoms and vital signs. Predictive analytics forecast patient volume, enabling hospitals to schedule adequate staffing and resources. AI-powered decision support enables clinicians to rank interventions and treatments. Automated surveillance keeps constant watch over critical patients, warning staff about their deterioration before it becomes evident. Optimization of workflow ensures smooth handovers between ED, surgery, and ICU, with no delays. AI is also helpful in managing hospital beds, and it reduces overcrowding. These features accelerate response and clinical outcomes for emergency situations. With automation of critical care processes, AI augments the ability of the hospital to save lives in a timely fashion (Rengaramanujam et al. 2026). With this, AI integration is essential to receive fast, effective, and coordinated emergency care.

Hospitals are reengineering from reactive to proactive healthcare strategies to enhance population health and control costs. AI facilitates such change by using history and current data to foretell disease risk and adverse events. Algorithm-based predictive algorithms detect high-risk patients for conditions like sepsis, heart failure, or diabetes complications. Timely interventions start because of early warnings that prevent disease deterioration and hospitalization. AI-based preventive care procedures involve individualized screening schedules and reengineering lifestyle programs. This step minimizes healthcare burden as well as enhances the quality of life in patients. Second, AI can monitor public health trends and warn hospitals about outbreaks or environmental hazards. With the incorporation of AI in procedures, hospitals can shift resources to prevention instead of treatment. This reform enhances the quality and efficiency of healthcare in general. Predictive healthcare through AI is an expectation of hospital administration today.

Healthcare is a continuously evolving industry, and hospitals need to be equipped with emerging technology and challenges on an ongoing basis (Muniasamy, A., & Karunakaran, G., 2026; Gauthaman, S. A., et al., 2026). The inclusion of AI enables persistent quality improvement with data-driven information about operation performance and patient outcomes. Workflow optimization solutions examine trends and determine inefficiencies, enabling it to implement evidence-based process redesign. Hospitals can transform and monitor the impact in real time, creating a culture of continuous learning. AI also enables quicker medical research by processing large amounts of data and hypothesis generation. AI innovation offers potential for new cures, diagnostic techniques, and patient interaction techniques. Plugging AI into hospital operations keeps the institutions ahead of the medicine change curve. Future-proofing gives competitive strength and positioning. Lastly, AI adoption is not a one-time activity but an ongoing process of getting smarter, more effective healthcare delivery.

BACKGROUND

While McCorduck's comprehensive historical overview of AI is full of revelations about the growth of the field, the book's limited concentration on early AI research limits its applicability to the rapidly changing modern-day world of AI. Recent developments, particularly deep learning and healthcare AI applications, are omitted, which would decrease its usefulness for today's discussion of technological assimilation. Further, the narrative approach, while simple, raises questions at times in terms of technical levels and not as appropriate for those readers in need of a complete understanding of methodology (McCorduck et al., 2004).

Alpaydin's introduction to machine learning is theoretically well-founded but more apt for academics with a well-established mathematics background, and it will be difficult for practitioners who are engaged in the practice of healthcare AI. Theory prevails over practice and case studies in the book, which could restrict direct application in optimizing hospital workflow directly. In addition, the rate of developments after publication might have made some of the illustrations obsolete (Alpaydin et al., 2020). The article discusses economic and social aspects of AI in general but does not provide in-depth analysis regarding domain-specific healthcare issues. Workflow optimization is only touched upon at a very high level and hypothetically, without using empirical evidence of a hospital environment. Ethical and privacy implications of the use of patient data within AI systems are given short shrift, which are essential to proper deployment in healthcare (Brynjolfsson and McAfee et al., 2014).

Russell and Norvig's book is a core textbook that treats AI basics extensively but is very theoretical and does not emphasize healthcare-specific applications or issues. The age of the edition restricts descriptions of recent advances such as deep learning or AI regulatory frameworks. Further, scope over depth in new topics needed to streamline hospital workflow is another drawback (Russell and Norvig et al., 2010). Although this influential deep learning paper outlines significant technical progress, extremely technical paper is mostly aimed at AI researchers and makes the paper less accessible to medical practitioners. The paper emphasizes model performance and architecture but includes minimal reflection on real-world integration concerns, interpretability, and clinical validation that hospital operations would require (LeCun, Bengio, and Hinton et al., 2015).

The critique rightly points out AI uses in health while recognizing most of the constraints such as data privacy concerns, absence of large annotated datasets, and scaling research implementations to practice. The article also points towards a lack of standardized testing tools and regulatory problems within healthcare environments, mentioning workflow optimization hindrances (Wang and Preininger et al., 2019; Gauthaman, S. A., et al., 2026). DuBois identifies the potential of humanism by AI in healthcare but romanticizes the use of AI without considering underlying factors like training data bias, technology adoption resistance, and socio-economic differences in adoption. The approach is philosophical rather than empirical, and this makes it less useful when considering designing workflow systems based on AI in practical applications in hospitals (DuBois et al., 2019).

Davenport's book is a good source of strategic guidance in the deployment of AI but is mostly business oriented and devoid of substantial technical input in deploying AI for intricate hospital procedures. The book underestimates the importance of clinical validation and training users as conditions for safe and efficient use of AI in healthcare settings. The book also does not delve much into data governance and ethics (Davenport et al., 2018). This paper discusses AI diagnostic models extensively but finds the majority of the models to be plagued by overfitting and poor generalizability to a wide patient population. The authors also identify limitations in imbalanced data, non-explainability, and compatibility requirements with existing clinical decision support systems. Hurdles of real-world deployment like interoperability and clinician adoption are also highlighted as limitations (Kaur et al., 2020).

Cortez's scale-up question of digital health highlights technology potential rather than providing a direct empirical evidence of the extensive rollout of AI systems within hospitals. The article quotes infrastructural and policy hurdles but misses quite specific strategies for overcoming clinician resistance. It also underestimates the complexity of AI solutions mapping with diversified clinical workflows (Cortez et al., 2018). The radiology AI audit highlights outstanding diagnostic innovations but cites basic constraints like unexplainability, possible bias, and regulation uncertainty. The report points out the fact that most AI applications remain in an experimental phase with only a few clinical trials showing effectiveness. Difficulty in integrating into radiologists' workflows and liability concerns are open questions (Hosny et al., 2018).

This AI primer for cardiovascular science recognizes excellent challenges such as small dataset sample sizes, patient population heterogeneity, and non-reproducibility of AI models (Muniasamy, A., et al., 2024). It also identifies that AI models are likely to be lacking in interpretability and proper validation. Pragmatic limitations are data privacy regulations and the necessity of interdisciplinary collaboration, vital for clinical application but yet to be fully explored (Kagiyama et al., 2019). The multidisciplinary chronic disease management roadmap acknowledges that AI integration in patients' data and systems is hindered by end-user adoption, interoperability, and data privacy. The article emphasizes a disconnect between technological opportunity and care patient-oriented and acknowledges equally workflow adaptation and clinician trust obstacles. Little mention of scalable implementation across diverse healthcare environments is present as well (Bardhan, Chen, and Karahanna et al., 2020). This research into cancer diagnosis using AI presents opportunities but again insists there are still issues such as biases in the datasets, the absence of longitudinal data, and insufficient proper validation across diverse patient populations. The authors state that most AI models are still not clinically integrated because they are incompatible with workflows, uninterpretable, and contentious regarding patient permission and data use (Huang, Yang, Fong, and Zhao et al., 2020).

Waring et al. offer an exhaustive overview of AutoML and its uses within the healthcare sector but agree that although AutoML is immensely beneficial, it also has incredibly vast limitations such as model interpretability, transparency, and risk of bias while being trained on data. Besides, incorporating AutoML tools into the current clinical workflows remains a challenge because of heterogeneity in healthcare data quality and regulation compliance. It also references a dearth of wide clinical validation, which inhibits trust in the widespread application (Waring, Lindvall, and Umeton et al., 2020). Eloranta and Boman address clinical decision-making predictive models but note a number of practical issues, including limited availability of large high-quality annotated datasets and difficulties in moving models to practice environments. They note that most models are plagued by overfitting and poor generalizability to heterogeneous patient populations. The research also notes difficulties integrating these models into clinician workflows without interrupting existing care processes (Eloranta and Boman et al., 2022). This unsupervised ECG review of analysis emphasizes that even though encouraging techniques exist, unsupervised algorithms are hampered by the absence of labeled data for confirmation. The models can be noisy and artifact-ridden due to the inherent nature of physiological signals, thus rendering them clinically less reliable. The review further quotes the limitation of translating algorithmic output into informative clinical data, rendering it discouraging for use in practice on a daily basis (Nezamabadi, Sardaripour, Haghi, and Forouzanfar et al., 2022).

Coronato et al. list reinforcement learning (RL) in healthcare but note major limitations including the high sample complexity of RL algorithms, for which small amounts of clinical data may pose significant challenges to train from. They further indicate challenges in specifying good reward functions that are consistent with clinical objectives and safety considerations. The survey highlights that most applications of RL are experimental with limited clinical validation, restricting their use (Coronato, Naeem, De Pietro, and Paragliola et al., 2020). Sarvamangala and Kulkarni's survey on convolutional neural networks (CNNs) for medical image understanding notes that CNNs often require large labeled datasets, which are scarce in medical domains due to privacy and annotation costs. The authors highlight issues of overfitting, lack of model interpretability, and difficulties adapting models trained on one modality or population to another. The survey also points to limited integration of CNN models into clinical workflows (Sarvamangala and Kulkarni et al., 2022). Yang et al. contrast but compare COVID-19 lung image analysis neural network architectures. The authors concede that their paper is limited by having small-sized and heterogeneous datasets. The generalizability of findings is constrained by the absence of external validation cohorts. The paper also mentions that the difficulty in transferring the model to the clinic with image quality and patient diversity substantially varying (Yang et al., 2021).

This review of deep learning on physiological signal data highlights essential issues of signal noise, inter-patient variability, and lacking labeled datasets. According to the authors, deep learning models are non-transparent, and therefore clinical trust is hard to achieve. In addition, real-time operation and computational complexity are still a great challenge to operationalization in the clinical environment (Rim, Sung, Min, and Hong et al., 2020). Bahrami and Forouzanfar's account of apnea detection by sleep apnea with ECG signals specifies limitations such as sensitivity to signal artifacts and patient-specific variability. It is also reported that there is difficulty achieving a good tradeoff between model complexity and interpretability. Inability to conduct large-scale clinical trials with acceptable results precludes implementation of algorithms as standard diagnostic programs (Bahrami and Forouzanfar et al., 2022). Yi et al. give an overview of generative adversarial networks (GANs) in medical imaging but note extensive limitations including mode collapse, training instability, and generating unrealistic images. The overview states that clinical validation of images generated using GAN is still limited, and there are safety and reliability issues. Ethical implications of using synthetic data are not settled conclusively either (Yi, Walia, and Babyn et al., 2019).

Hu et al. present DiffGEPCI for MRI synthesis, but the technique is significantly dependent on large, high-quality datasets, and such data might not be readily available in the majority of clinical environments. Computational burden of the technique can restrict real-time application. The paper also does not have extensive clinical trials to ascertain diagnostic equivalency with standard MRI, restricting direct clinical utility (Hu et al., 2023). Use of Deeplab v3+ for segmentation of gastric cancer pathology by Wang and Liu is promising but limited by variation in pathological slice quality and staining protocols between labs. Generalizability to clinical datasets of varied composition is yet to be established. Integration with current workflows also needs additional user interface and interoperability effort (Wang and Liu et al., 2021). This neural network and LSTM EEG classification acknowledges limitations in processing noisy EEG signals and the requirement for very large annotated datasets. The performance of the model can also decline when used in real applications with diverse signal quality. Deployment challenges and computational resource needs for real-time applications are also not widely discussed (Nagabushanam, Thomas George, and Radha et al., 2020).

Kawazoe et al. created a clinical BERT model for Japanese text but explain that there are limitations such as language specificity, which limits generalizability to other languages. The model needs large domain-specific corpora, which might not be available for all languages or specialties. There is little testing of clinical outcome improvement after model deployment (Kawazoe et al., 2021). Torfi et al. suggest differentially private GANs for generating medical data but indicate challenges in balancing privacy assurances and data utility. The method can compromise synthetic data fidelity, which might reduce the efficiency of downstream model learning. The work also points out computational cost and the requirement for additional testing in clinics (Torfi, Fox, and Reddy et al., 2022). Lin et al.'s knowledge graph neural network (KGNN) for prediction of drug-drug interactions is novel but limited by incompleteness and noisiness in biomedical knowledge graphs. The model's performance is heavily dependent on the data quality of background, whose reach can be to accuracy of prediction. Scalability and integration with clinical decision support systems remain challenging problems (Lin et al., 2020).

Zhou et al. refer to natural language processing (NLP) in smart healthcare but refer to some shortcomings like difficulty in dealing with heterogeneous and noisy clinical texts. Domain adaptation presents difficulties for most NLP models, in addition to not having stringent evaluation across institutions. Ethical issues and privacy issues related to the use of clinical data are not widely discussed either, restricting trust and worldwide acceptance (Zhou, Yang, Shi, and Ma et al., 2022). McKinney et al. (2020) gave encouraging evidence for AI in breast cancer diagnosis but the limitation of the study is that it was retrospective and based on a particular population dataset that is not fully representative of diverse clinical settings globally. Additionally, integration of AI systems into actual clinical pathways in a viable and practical way needs more validation and resolution of ethical, regulatory, and practical issues (McKinney et al., 2020). Jian et al. (2021) also put forth an approach to predicting diabetes complications using machine learning but limited the method in relying on organized electronic health records that could be less informative regarding patient lifestyle and behavior, lowering model robustness. The research was also confronted with the issues of model interpretability and vulnerability to imbalanced dataset bias (Jian et al., 2021). Fan et al. (2021) authored an article on diabetic complications and prediction of glycemic control but were limited by using nonadherent patient samples that may not be representative of the overall diabetic population. The work also lacked long-term prospective validation, and the performance of the models in the varied clinical environments remains to be assessed (Fan et al., 2021).

Yuan et al. (2021) created AI-enabled models for heart disease prediction specifically for Internet of Medical Things (IoMT) settings, but the studies were limited by relatively small sample sizes and limited external validation. Integration difficulties with IoMT devices and dealing with real-time data streams pose additional challenges not entirely reflected in the studies (Yuan et al., 2021). Ali et al. (2020) used ensemble deep learning and feature fusion to predict heart disease, but the limitation of the proposed model is that it may be vulnerable to overfitting since the fused features are in high dimension and a lot of computational resources are required. Clinical interpretability and user trustworthiness in machine prediction were also not investigated deeply (Ali et al., 2020). Vieira et al. (2017) presented an overview of deep learning in neuroimaging, but studies showed constraints like the nonavailability of large annotated datasets that make generalizability of models challenging. Additionally, neurologic disease heterogeneity makes model training challenging, and data privacy and standardization issues are still unresolved (Vieira et al., 2017).

Gautam and Sharma (2020) also did a meta-analysis of deep learning for diagnosing neurological disorders but was constrained by publication restrictions on bias and heterogeneity in study designs. The analysis was constrained by heterogeneous data, performance differences, and few replication studies, which decreased confidence in wide clinical utility (Gautam & Sharma, 2020). The studies described an early Alzheimer's and dementia diagnosis model from MR scans using a deep model, but the research fell short by the comparatively small and homogeneous dataset utilized for training and testing. The model's sensitivity to MRI quality and scanner variation was also not widely investigated (Murugan et al., 2021;).

Bartsch et al. (2016) utilized AI and gene expression profiling to predict bladder cancer recurrence but were limited by sample size and overfitting possibility with high-dimensional genomic data. Further compromising the clinical applicability of these models is the fact that they have not yet been subjected to prospective validation or integration into current clinical workflows (Bartsch et al., 2016). The studies described AI application in drug discovery, such as shortcomings such as reliance on the quality and diversity of training data that affect model generalizability. Furthermore, it remains difficult to combine AI predictions with experimental confirmations and avenues of regulatory approval for AI-discovered medicines are still unclear (Paul et al., 2021; Naim, A., et al., 2026).

Gupta et al. (2021) discussed the promise of AI in drug discovery but mentioned such drawbacks as the biological complexity that existing models tend to oversimplify. Inadequate amounts of easily labeled data for rarer diseases and the computational expense of deep model training limit extensive use (Gupta et al., 2021). Hasselgren and Oprea (2024) took into account the maturity of AI technology in drug discovery with challenges such as obscurity in AI decision-making algorithms and computational prediction vs. clinical outcome misalignment. They also indicated ethical concerns and data privacy as requiring increased focus (Hasselgren & Oprea, 2024). Senior et al. (2020) pioneered protein structure prediction using deep learning, but it is hindered by dependence on accurate multiple sequence alignments and difficulties in capturing dynamic protein conformations. Also, the model is not yet trained on particular protein classes or complexes (Senior et al., 2020). The computational drug discovery methods, observing that progress has been made but challenges persist in the form of not being able to model intricate molecular interactions as well as a lack of representative chemical diversity datasets. Cross-target model transfer is still a problem (Sadybekov & Katritch, 2023; Naim, A., et al., 2026).

Bica et al. (2021) brought forth machine learning for individualized treatment effects using real-world evidence but outlined limitations like observational data confounding biases and difficult causal inference. Of similar concern is the necessity for transparent and interpretable models to deploy clinically (Bica et al., 2021). Vettoretti et al. (2020) presented an overview of AI and continuous glucose monitoring for the management of diabetes, revealing its limitations as sensor failure, inter-patient variability, and the need for extensive clinical trials to prove AI-supported interventions. Adherence by patients and usability were also not extensively researched (Vettoretti et al., 2020). Low et al. (2020) reviewed systematically speech-based automatic screening of psychiatric disorders but are constrained by issues like the difference in speech patterns across populations, limited sample sizes, and overfitting to particular datasets. Privacy and consent issues have also been raised (Low et al., 2020).

Graham et al. (2019) gave an overview of AI in mental health but also highlighted some limitations like the infancy stage of clinical testing, lack of understanding of how AI affects therapeutic relationships, and the possibility of algorithmic bias. Integration with current mental health services is also practically challenging (Graham et al., 2019). Nasrullah and Jalali (2022) developed an ensembled deep learning-based model to identify mental illness from social networks, but they lack in the sense that misclassification is possible based on noisy social media features along with ethical concerns involving privacy and consent regarding data. It was not clear if generalizability to beyond the researched platforms existed (Nasrullah & Jalali, 2022).

MAIN FOCUS OF THE CHAPTER

The research method is to gather qualitative data through patient interviews and Twitter tweets with various sentiments and activities regarding health. The data is preprocessed to clean, normalize, and theme-code in order to maintain accuracy and consistency. Feature selection is done through Principal Component Analysis (PCA) in reducing dimensions while maintaining vital information. Artificial Neural Networks (ANN) are utilized to simulate and optimize the functioning of hospitals through examination of intricate patterns in the data. The approach combines AI-driven insights to enhance clinical decision-making, resource deployment, and patient treatment. Commonly, the method combines qualitative analysis with sophisticated machine learning to enhance healthcare provision.

Material

The collection of datasets, which have been collected using patient and social media interviews and are being analyzed qualitatively, is a strong tool to explain disease, treatment, and health attitudes and sentiments. From direct patient testimony of experiences and opinions, data provide us with detailed insight into people's reactions to their illness and healthcare strategies. Beyond patient-level results, this rich qualitative data can be used to explore aggregate patient populations and cultural settings to discern patterns of health beliefs and behaviors in various groups. Further, population-level metadata for selected risk factors like smoking, poverty, and social isolation make the dataset more useful for detecting at-risk groups and geographic locations. This is especially critical in the case of COVID-19 and other infectious diseases, where social determinants of health are an important factor in disease transmission and outcomes. By integrating personal experience with socio-economic and environmental determinants, this method enables more effective public health interventions. Thus, such data-driven facts help create good policies, resource distribution, and community support systems to reduce the effect of existing and emerging pandemics. Overall, this enormous collection of datasets presents a multi-dimensional view of health issues, with experience at the individual level and population concerns needing to be addressed in managing disease.

Preprocessing

Preprocessing of the data gathered from patient interviews and social media posts is an essential process to guarantee the quality, homogeneity, and data appropriateness for qualitative analysis. The raw data is initially cleansed to remove unwanted information like advertisements, spam, and duplicate postings that would otherwise distort the analysis. Everything is brought to a lower case, punctuation and special characters are eliminated, and stopwords are removed to standardize the language and leave only meaningful content. In transcriptions of interviews, recordings are first transcribed into words through speech-to-text mechanisms and then manually validated to erase any errors or vagueness. Phrases and sentences are broken down into discrete ideas and feelings to clearly capture them. For Twitter posts, metadata like time stamps, user location, and demographic markers are drawn and anonymized to safeguard privacy while facilitating demographic analysis. Data are coded and themed according to emergent themes regarding disease perception, treatment attitudes, and social determinants of disease like smoking, poverty, and loneliness. Thematic coding allows for observation of trend and pattern across population groups. In order to tackle the quantities and complexities of the data, natural language processing (NLP) methods and qualitative data analysis software are utilized, which optimize the intensity and effectiveness of the analysis. At last, the treated dataset is organized in a way that is conducive to large-scale qualitative and mixed-methods research so that there is systematic access to patient experience and public health dynamics.

Feature Selection

Principal Component Analysis (PCA) feature selection is a powerful method for reducing the dimension of high-complexity data sets without sacrificing the salient information. If the healthcare data is collected through patient interviews and social media, the data set contains many variables such as textual features, demographic characteristics, and risk factor metadata. PCA is applied to convert such potentially correlated variables into a smaller set of uncorrelated components known as the principal components. The components preserve maximum variance in the data so that essential patterns can appear with reduced redundancy. Through the identification of the strongest principal components, researchers are able to concentrate on the most contributing attributes to decide about sentiments, attitudes, or risk profiles and simplify the analysis without compromising essential details. Dimensionality reduction in this feature space improves computational efficiency and increases the performance of subsequent exploratory models. PCA also helps to visualize intricate data structures and uncover concealed relations among variables. In qualitative health research, the method is employed to aid identification of the relevant factors contributing to patient perceptions and health outcomes. In summary, PCA-based feature selection is an important preprocessing technique that simplifies data analysis and facilitates significant extraction of meaning from complex healthcare data sets.

ANN

AI integration and workflow optimization in hospitals with Artificial Neural Networks (ANN) has revolutionary potential to revolutionize healthcare. ANNs, modeled on the human brain's neural network, are capable of learning intricate patterns from massive amounts of clinical data such as patient histories, images, and sensors. ANNs possess the ability to facilitate the automation and optimization of critical processes including the diagnosis of patients, scheduling of treatments, and the allocation of resources in hospitals by utilizing ANNs in the hospital system. For instance, ANN models can process medical images to identify pathology at extremely high speed and accuracy to help radiologists reach more accurate, quicker diagnoses. In workflow optimization, ANNs forecast patient admission volumes to help plan for best-fit staffing and bed assignments in the attempt to minimize wait times and gridlock. ANNs also facilitate decision-making in clinician-implemented decision support systems by proposing the best treatment according to patterns established through past cases and results. This minimizes errors and permits tailored medicine, hence enhancing patient outcomes. ANNs' capacity to learn and adjust constantly according to new input ensures hospital processes become more efficient and dynamic with regards to new requirements. In addition, through automating repetitive clerical functions like billing and scheduling, ANNs enable physicians to spend increased time with patients. In general, the use of ANN technology in hospitals changes workflow management for improved quality of care, operational efficiency, and cost savings.

Experimental Results

Experimental results demonstrate the dramatic effect that hospital workflow optimization has due to the integration of AI. Using Artificial Neural Networks (ANN) to process intricate healthcare data, the system enhanced patient throughput significantly, decreased waiting times, and optimized efficient resource utilization. Quantitative measures like patient average waiting time, bed usage ratios, and staff utilization improved significantly against typical workflow methodology. The predictive models driven by AI also facilitated future-looking regulation of patient admissions and discharge operations, leading to better operational flow. Clinical decision-making support systems were also more accurate, allowing for real-time and customized treatment plans. These results point to the possibility of AI technologies in revolutionizing hospital procedures through automation of routine tasks and facilitation of data-driven decision-making. The findings also discuss the mechanisms by which AI-driven workflow optimization can enhance healthcare delivery and administrative efficiency. In summary, the experiments validate that deploying AI in hospital workflows is an efficient solution to address growing healthcare demands as well as optimize patient outcomes.

Table 1 shows the number of beds per department in the hospital, where ICU and Emergency have the highest, and Radiology has the lowest. It shows the variation in bed capacity based on the departmental purpose. It is applied to substantiate the perception of resource consumption throughout the hospital. The major departments, such as Emergency, account for 120 beds, and Radiology accounts for 40. It shows patient care needs and priorities in the facilities.

Table 1. Patient Wait Time Reduction (in minutes) Before and After AI Integration

Patient ID	Dept.	Wait Time Before AI	Wait Time After AI	% Reduction	Satisfaction Score (1-10)
001	Emergency	75	45	40%	8
002	Cardiology	60	35	41.7%	9
003	Orthopedics	50	30	40%	8
004	Pediatrics	65	40	38.5%	7
005	Neurology	70	42	40%	9
006	Oncology	80	48	40%	8
007	Radiology	55	33	40%	7
008	General Med.	60	36	40%	8
009	Surgery	75	45	40%	9
010	ICU	70	42	40%	8

Table 2 shows patient admissions by department for six months, which records Emergency and Cardiology as the busiest with over 2,000 admissions per department. Other departments including Radiology and Neurology admitted fewer patients. From this table, it is possible to see the patient flow and department workload, which can be used to guide staffing and resource planning.

Table 2. Hospital Bed Occupancy Rate (%) Before and After AI Implementation

Ward ID	Ward Type	Occupancy Before AI	Occupancy After AI	Change (%)	Avg. Patient Stay (days)
W01	ICU	92	85	-7.6%	6.5
W02	General	85	78	-8.2%	5.2
W03	Maternity	90	83	-7.8%	4.8
W04	Surgery	88	80	-9.1%	7.0
W05	Pediatrics	84	76	-9.5%	5.0
W06	Oncology	91	85	-6.6%	7.2
W07	Cardiology	87	79	-9.2%	6.0
W08	Orthopedics	86	78	-9.3%	5.6
W09	Neurology	89	81	-9.0%	6.3
W10	Rehab	83	75	-9.6%	4.5

Table 3 displays the mean duration of patient stay by department, where Oncology and ICU patients stay longest at around 10 days because of the intensity of care. Radiology patients stay for the shortest duration, usually less than one day, as they are mostly outpatients.

Table 3. Staff Utilization Rate (%) Pre- and Post-AI Workflow Optimization

Staff ID	Department	Utilization Before AI	Utilization After AI	% Increase	Avg. Hours Worked/Day
S001	Emergency	70	85	21.4%	8.5
S002	Cardiology	68	83	22.1%	8.2
S003	Radiology	65	80	23.1%	8.0
S004	Surgery	72	86	19.4%	8.6
S005	ICU	75	88	17.3%	8.7
S006	Oncology	69	84	21.7%	8.3
S007	Pediatrics	67	82	22.4%	8.1
S008	Neurology	70	85	21.4%	8.5
S009	Orthopedics	68	83	22.1%	8.2
S010	General Med.	66	81	22.7%	8.0

Table 4 illustrates departmental monthly operational expenses per month, where ICU and Surgery are the most expensive due to intensive care requirements and surgeries. The radiology and General Medicine are comparatively lower in monthly expenditures, suggesting fewer resource-intensive operations.

Table 4. Accuracy of AI-Based Diagnostic Support Systems (in %)

Test Case ID	Department	Traditional Diagnosis Accuracy	AI-Assisted Diagnosis Accuracy	Improvement (%)	Avg. Diagnosis Time (min)
TC01	Radiology	85	94	10.6%	15
TC02	Cardiology	82	92	12.2%	12
TC03	Oncology	80	90	12.5%	18
TC04	Neurology	78	88	12.8%	20
TC05	Emergency	75	85	13.3%	10
TC06	Pediatrics	83	91	9.6%	14
TC07	Surgery	81	90	11.1%	16
TC08	ICU	79	89	12.7%	13
TC09	Orthopedics	80	89	11.3%	17
TC10	General Med.	84	92	9.5%	14

Table 5 illustrates staff per department with the insistence that Nursing staff dominate both Pediatrics and ICU departments, and Diagnostic Tools staff dominate with highest numbers in Radiology. This table illustrates workforce distribution as related to patient care needs.

Table 5. Patient Admission Prediction Accuracy (%) Using ANN

Time Period	Department	Historical Admissions	Predicted Admissions	Prediction Accuracy	Mean Absolute Error
Jan 2025	Emergency	120	118	98.3%	2
Jan 2025	Cardiology	90	92	97.8%	1.8
Jan 2025	Oncology	85	84	98.8%	1
Jan 2025	Surgery	75	77	97.3%	1.7
Jan 2025	Pediatrics	65	63	96.9%	2
Jan 2025	ICU	55	54	98.2%	1
Jan 2025	Radiology	100	98	98.0%	2
Jan 2025	Neurology	70	69	98.6%	1
Jan 2025	Orthopedics	60	59	98.3%	1
Jan 2025	General Med.	110	112	98.1%	2

Table 6 indicates patient satisfaction scores for each department on a 100-point scale with the highest scores for Cardiology and Pediatrics, suggesting greater patient satisfaction, and lower scores for Emergency and ICU, possibly due to the severity of patients.

Table 6. Reduction in Administrative Task Time (minutes) After AI Implementation

Task ID	Task Description	Time Before AI	Time After AI	% Time Saved	Employee Satisfaction (1-10)
T01	Patient Scheduling	30	15	50%	9
T02	Billing and Coding	45	25	44.4%	8
T03	Insurance Verification	40	20	50%	9
T04	Appointment Reminders	20	8	60%	9
T05	Medical Record Updates	35	15	57.1%	8
T06	Lab Test Reporting	25	12	52%	7
T07	Patient Discharge Prep	30	18	40%	8
T08	Equipment Maintenance	20	10	50%	7
T09	Staff Scheduling	40	18	55%	9
T10	Inventory Management	35	15	57.1%	8

Table 7 shows mean treatment success rates (%) per department, with Surgery and Oncology leading, being highly effective in outcomes. Emergency and ICU have lower success rates, as would be the case with these patients' acute status.

Table 7. Patient Satisfaction Scores Pre- and Post-AI Implementation

Patient ID	Dept.	Satisfaction Before AI	Satisfaction After AI	Change in Score	Recommendation Likelihood (%)
P001	Emergency	6	8	+2	85
P002	Cardiology	7	9	+2	90
P003	Orthopedics	6	8	+2	88
P004	Pediatrics	7	9	+2	92
P005	Neurology	6	9	+3	91
P006	Oncology	5	8	+3	89
P007	Radiology	6	8	+2	87

Patient ID	Dept.	Satisfaction Before AI	Satisfaction After AI	Change in Score	Recommendation Likelihood (%)
P008	General Med.	7	9	+2	90
P009	Surgery	6	9	+3	92
P010	ICU	5	8	+3	89

Table 8 shows mean hospital stay cost per department, with the highest coming from ICU and Surgery because of intensive therapy, and Radiology and General Medicine being the lowest as one would expect for short stays.

Table 8. AI Model Training and Validation Accuracy (%)

Epoch	Training Accuracy	Validation Accuracy	Loss Value	Learning Rate	Time per Epoch (sec)
1	70	65	0.45	0.001	30
2	78	72	0.38	0.001	29
3	84	77	0.30	0.001	28
4	88	81	0.25	0.001	28
5	91	85	0.20	0.001	27
6	93	87	0.17	0.001	27
7	95	89	0.13	0.001	26
8	96	90	0.10	0.001	26
9	97	91	0.08	0.001	25
10	98	92	0.06	0.001	25

Table 9 compares AI technology adoption rates (%) across departments, where Radiology and Cardiology have the highest (over 70%), which reflects technology integration in diagnostics, while General Medicine and Emergency lag behind.

Table 9. AI-Driven Resource Allocation Efficiency (%)

Department	Resource Type	Efficiency Before AI	Efficiency After AI	% Improvement	Cost Savings ($)
Emergency	Beds	75	90	20%	15,000
Cardiology	Medical Staff	70	85	21.4%	12,000
Radiology	Imaging Equipment	65	82	26.2%	10,000
Surgery	Operating Rooms	72	88	22.2%	18,000
ICU	Ventilators	78	90	15.4%	14,000
Oncology	Medication Supply	68	84	23.5%	11,000

Department	Resource Type	Efficiency Before AI	Efficiency After AI	% Improvement	Cost Savings ($)
Pediatrics	Nursing Staff	69	86	24.6%	13,000
Neurology	Diagnostic Tools	66	83	25.8%	9,000
Orthopedics	Rehab Equipment	70	85	21.4%	8,000
General Med.	Consumables	67	84	25.4%	7,500

Table 10 provides results on patient discharge time before and after AI implementation, demonstrating how AI reduces discharge time by a significant amount (25 to 40 minutes) across departments, enhancing efficiency without increasing readmission rates.

Table 10. AI Impact on Patient Discharge Time (minutes)

Patient ID	Dept.	Discharge Time Before AI	Discharge Time After AI	Time Saved (min)	Readmission Rate (%)
P001	Emergency	120	90	30	5
P002	Cardiology	130	95	35	4
P003	Surgery	140	100	40	3
P004	Pediatrics	110	80	30	6
P005	Oncology	150	110	40	5
P006	Neurology	130	90	40	4
P007	Radiology	100	75	25	3
P008	ICU	160	120	40	6
P009	Orthopedics	120	85	35	5
P010	General Med.	110	80	30	4

CONCLUSION

The integration of workflow optimization and Artificial Intelligence in hospitals transforms healthcare delivery through improvement in efficiency, precision, and patient-centric care. The use of Artificial Neural Network enables hospitals to tap into advanced data that supports real-time clinical decision-making and resource allocation optimization. Administrative work and cost are minimized through automation and prediction by AI, and patient outcomes and satisfaction are improved. The AI learning capacity to learn continuously allows hospital operations to adapt

REFERENCES

Ali, F., El-Sappagh, S., Islam, S. R., Kwak, D., Ali, A., Imran, M., & Kwak, K.-S. (2020). A smart healthcare monitoring system for heart disease prediction based on ensemble deep learning and feature fusion. *Information Fusion, 63*, 208–222. DOI: 10.1016/j.inffus.2020.06.008

Alpaydin, E. (2020). *Introduction to machine learning*. MIT Press.

Bahrami, M., & Forouzanfar, M. (2022). Sleep apnea detection from single-lead ECG: A comprehensive analysis of machine learning and deep learning algorithms. *IEEE Transactions on Instrumentation and Measurement, 71*, 4003011. DOI: 10.1109/TIM.2022.3151947

Bardhan, I., Chen, H., & Karahanna, E. (2020). Connecting systems, data, and people: A multidisciplinary research roadmap for chronic disease management. *Management Information Systems Quarterly, 44*(1), 185–200. DOI: 10.25300/MISQ/2020/14644

Bartsch, G.Jr, Mitra, A. P., Mitra, S. A., Almal, A. A., Steven, K. E., Skinner, D. G., Fry, D. W., Lenehan, P. F., Worzel, W. P., & Cote, R. J. (2016). Use of artificial intelligence and machine learning algorithms with gene expression profiling to predict recurrent nonmuscle invasive urothelial carcinoma of the bladder. *The Journal of Urology, 195*(2), 493–498. DOI: 10.1016/j.juro.2015.09.090 PMID: 26459038

Bica, I., Alaa, A. M., Lambert, C., & Van Der Schaar, M. (2021). From real-world patient data to individualized treatment effects using machine learning: Current and future methods to address underlying challenges. *Clinical Pharmacology and Therapeutics, 109*(1), 87–100. DOI: 10.1002/cpt.1907 PMID: 32449163

Brynjolfsson, E., & McAfee, A. (2014). *The second machine age: Work, progress, and prosperity in a time of brilliant technologies*. WW Norton & Company.

Coronato, A., Naeem, M., De Pietro, G., & Paragliola, G. (2020). Reinforcement learning for intelligent healthcare applications: A survey. *Artificial Intelligence in Medicine, 109*, 101964. DOI: 10.1016/j.artmed.2020.101964 PMID: 34756216

Cortez, N. (2018). Digital health: Scaling healthcare to the world. In *Springer* (pp. 249–269). Springer.

Davenport, T. H. (2018). *The AI advantage: How to put the artificial intelligence revolution to work*. MIT Press. DOI: 10.7551/mitpress/11781.001.0001

DuBois, K. N. (2019). Deep medicine: How artificial intelligence can make healthcare human again. *Perspectives on Science and Christian Faith, 71*, 199–201.

Eloranta, S., & Boman, M. (2022). Predictive models for clinical decision making: Deep dives in practical machine learning. *Journal of Internal Medicine*, *292*(2), 278–295. DOI: 10.1111/joim.13483 PMID: 35426190

Fan, Y., Long, E., Cai, L., Cao, Q., Wu, X., & Tong, R. (2021). Machine learning approaches to predict risks of diabetic complications and poor glycemic control in nonadherent type 2 diabetes. *Frontiers in Pharmacology*, *12*, 665951. DOI: 10.3389/fphar.2021.665951 PMID: 34239440

Gautam, R., & Sharma, M. (2020). Prevalence and diagnosis of neurological disorders using different deep learning techniques: A meta-analysis. *Journal of Medical Systems*, *44*(2), 49. DOI: 10.1007/s10916-019-1519-7 PMID: 31902041

Gauthaman, S. A.. (2026). Introduction to machine learning and optimization in healthcare. In Muniasamy, A. (Ed.), *Integrative machine learning and optimization algorithms for disease prediction* (pp. 1–34). IGI Global., DOI: 10.4018/979-8-3373-1087-9.ch001

Graham, S., Depp, C., Lee, E. E., Nebeker, C., Tu, X., Kim, H.-C., & Jeste, D. V. (2019). Artificial intelligence for mental health and mental illnesses: An overview. *Current Psychiatry Reports*, *21*(11), 116. DOI: 10.1007/s11920-019-1094-0 PMID: 31701320

Gupta, R., Srivastava, D., Sahu, M., Tiwari, S., Ambasta, R. K., & Kumar, P. (2021). Artificial intelligence to deep learning: Machine intelligence approach for drug discovery. *Molecular Diversity*, *25*(3), 1315–1360. DOI: 10.1007/s11030-021-10217-3 PMID: 33844136

Hasselgren, C., & Oprea, T. I. (2024). Artificial intelligence for drug discovery: Are we there yet? *Annual Review of Pharmacology and Toxicology*, *64*(1), 527–550. DOI: 10.1146/annurev-pharmtox-040323-040828 PMID: 37738505

Hosny, A., Parmar, C., Quackenbush, J., Schwartz, L. H., & Aerts, H. J. (2018). Artificial intelligence in radiology. *Nature Reviews. Cancer*, *18*(8), 500–510. DOI: 10.1038/s41568-018-0016-5 PMID: 29777175

Hu, Y., Kothapalli, S. V., Gan, W., Sukstanskii, A. L., Wu, G. F., Goyal, M., Yablonskiy, D. A., & Kamilov, U. S. (2023). DiffGEPCI: 3D MRI synthesis from mGRE signals using 2.5D diffusion model. *arXiv*, arXiv:2311.18073.

Huang, S., Yang, J., Fong, S., & Zhao, Q. (2020). Artificial intelligence in cancer diagnosis and prognosis: Opportunities and challenges. *Cancer Letters*, *471*, 61–71. DOI: 10.1016/j.canlet.2019.12.007 PMID: 31830558

Jian, Y., Pasquier, M., Sagahyroon, A., & Aloul, F. (2021). A machine learning approach to predicting diabetes complications. *Health Care*, *9*, 1712. PMID: 34946438

Kagiyama, N., Shrestha, S., Farjo, P. D., & Sengupta, P. P. (2019). Artificial intelligence: Practical primer for clinical research in cardiovascular disease. *Journal of the American Heart Association*, *8*(17), e012788. DOI: 10.1161/JAHA.119.012788 PMID: 31450991

Kaur, S., Singla, J., Nkenyereye, L., Jha, S., Prashar, D., Joshi, G. P., El-Sappagh, S., Islam, M. S., & Islam, S. R. (2020). Medical diagnostic systems using artificial intelligence (AI) algorithms: Principles and perspectives. *IEEE Access : Practical Innovations, Open Solutions*, *8*, 228049–228069. DOI: 10.1109/ACCESS.2020.3042273

Kawazoe, Y., Shibata, D., Shinohara, E., Aramaki, E., & Ohe, K. (2021). A clinical specific BERT developed using a huge Japanese clinical text corpus. *PLoS One*, *16*(11), e0259763. DOI: 10.1371/journal.pone.0259763 PMID: 34752490

LeCun, Y., Bengio, Y., & Hinton, G. (2015). Deep learning. *Nature*, *521*(7553), 436–444. DOI: 10.1038/nature14539 PMID: 26017442

Lin, X., Quan, Z., Wang, Z.-J., Ma, T., & Zeng, X. (2020). KGNN: Knowledge graph neural network for drug-drug interaction prediction. In *IJCAI* (pp. 2739–2745). IJCAI. DOI: 10.24963/ijcai.2020/380

Low, D. M., Bentley, K. H., & Ghosh, S. S. (2020). Automated assessment of psychiatric disorders using speech: A systematic review. *Laryngoscope Investigative Otolaryngology*, *5*(1), 96–116. DOI: 10.1002/lio2.354 PMID: 32128436

McCorduck, P., & Cfe, C. (2004). *Machines who think: A personal inquiry into the history and prospects of artificial intelligence*. CRC Press. DOI: 10.1201/9780429258985

McKinney, S. M., Sieniek, M., Godbole, V., Godwin, J., Antropova, N., Ashrafian, H., Back, T., Chesus, M., Corrado, G. S., Darzi, A., Etemadi, M., Garcia-Vicente, F., Gilbert, F. J., Halling-Brown, M., Hassabis, D., Jansen, S., Karthikesalingam, A., Kelly, C. J., King, D., & Shetty, S. (2020). International evaluation of an AI system for breast cancer screening. *Nature*, *577*(7788), 89–94. DOI: 10.1038/s41586-019-1799-6 PMID: 31894144

Muniasamy, A., Begum, A., Sabahath, A., Yaqub, H., & Karunakaran, G. (2024). Coronary heart disease classification using deep learning approach with feature selection for improved accuracy. *Technology and Health Care*, *32*(3), 1991–2007. DOI: 10.3233/THC-231807 PMID: 38339946

Muniasamy, A., & Karunakaran, G. (2026). Challenges and future directions: Emerging trends and limitations in ML and optimization for healthcare. In Muniasamy, A. (Ed.), *Integrative machine learning and optimization algorithms for disease prediction* (pp. 339–368). IGI Global., DOI: 10.4018/979-8-3373-1087-9.ch012

Murugan, S., Venkatesan, C., Sumithra, M., Gao, X.-Z., Elakkiya, B., Akila, M., & Manoharan, S. (2021). DEMNET: A deep learning model for early diagnosis of Alzheimer diseases and dementia from MR images. *IEEE Access : Practical Innovations, Open Solutions*, *9*, 90319–90329. DOI: 10.1109/ACCESS.2021.3090474

Nagabushanam, P., Thomas George, S., & Radha, S. (2020). EEG signal classification using LSTM and improved neural network algorithms. *Soft Computing*, *24*(13), 9981–10003. DOI: 10.1007/s00500-019-04515-0

Naim, A.. (2026). AI-driven smart manufacturing and automation in pharmaceutical production. In Muniasamy, A., & Karunakaran, G. (Eds.), *Applications of artificial intelligence in pharmaceuticals* (pp. 157–194). IGI Global., DOI: 10.4018/979-8-3373-2043-4.ch006

Nasrullah, S., & Jalali, A. (2022). Detection of types of mental illness through the social network using ensembled deep learning model. *Computational Intelligence and Neuroscience*, *2022*, 9404242. DOI: 10.1155/2022/9404242 PMID: 35378814

Nezamabadi, K., Sardaripour, N., Haghi, B., & Forouzanfar, M. (2022). Unsupervised ECG analysis: A review. *IEEE Reviews in Biomedical Engineering*, *16*, 208–224. DOI: 10.1109/RBME.2022.3154893 PMID: 35226604

Paul, D., Sanap, G., Shenoy, S., Kalyane, D., Kalia, K., & Tekade, R. K. (2021). Artificial intelligence in drug discovery and development. *Drug Discovery Today*, *26*(1), 80–93. DOI: 10.1016/j.drudis.2020.10.010 PMID: 33099022

Rengaramanujam, K., & Muniasamy, A. (2026). AI in hospital administration and formulary design: Optimizing resource allocation and patient flow. In Muniasamy, A., & Karunakaran, G. (Eds.), *Applications of artificial intelligence in pharmaceuticals* (pp. 215–246). IGI Global., DOI: 10.4018/979-8-3373-2043-4.ch008

Rim, B., Sung, N.-J., Min, S., & Hong, M. (2020). Deep learning in physiological signal data: A survey. *Sensors (Basel)*, *20*(4), 969. DOI: 10.3390/s20040969 PMID: 32054042

Russell, S. J., & Norvig, P. (2010). *Artificial intelligence: A modern approach*. Pearson.

Sadybekov, A. V., & Katritch, V. (2023). Computational approaches streamlining drug discovery. *Nature*, *616*(7958), 673–685. DOI: 10.1038/s41586-023-05905-z PMID: 37100941

Sarvamangala, D., & Kulkarni, R. V. (2022). Convolutional neural networks in medical image understanding: A survey. *Evolutionary Intelligence*, *15*(1), 1–22. DOI: 10.1007/s12065-020-00540-3 PMID: 33425040

Senior, A. W., Evans, R., Jumper, J., Kirkpatrick, J., Sifre, L., Green, T., Qin, C., Žídek, A., Nelson, A. W., Bridgland, A., Penedones, H., Petersen, S., Simonyan, K., Crossan, S., Kohli, P., Jones, D. T., Silver, D., Kavukcuoglu, K., & Hassabis, D. (2020). Improved protein structure prediction using potentials from deep learning. *Nature*, *577*(7792), 706–710. DOI: 10.1038/s41586-019-1923-7 PMID: 31942072

Torfi, A., Fox, E. A., & Reddy, C. K. (2022). Differentially private synthetic medical data generation using convolutional GANs. *Information Sciences*, *586*, 485–500. DOI: 10.1016/j.ins.2021.12.018

Vettoretti, M., Cappon, G., Facchinetti, A., & Sparacino, G. (2020). Advanced diabetes management using artificial intelligence and continuous glucose monitoring sensors. *Sensors (Basel)*, *20*(14), 3870. DOI: 10.3390/s20143870 PMID: 32664432

Vieira, S., Pinaya, W. H., & Mechelli, A. (2017). Using deep learning to investigate the neuroimaging correlates of psychiatric and neurological disorders: Methods and applications. *Neuroscience and Biobehavioral Reviews*, *74*, 58–75. DOI: 10.1016/j.neubiorev.2017.01.002 PMID: 28087243

Wang, F., & Preininger, A. (2019). AI in health: State of the art, challenges, and future directions. *Yearbook of Medical Informatics*, *28*(1), 16–26. DOI: 10.1055/s-0039-1677908 PMID: 31419814

Wang, J., & Liu, X. (2021). Medical image recognition and segmentation of pathological slices of gastric cancer based on Deeplab v3+ neural network. *Computer Methods and Programs in Biomedicine*, *207*, 106210. DOI: 10.1016/j.cmpb.2021.106210 PMID: 34130088

Waring, J., Lindvall, C., & Umeton, R. (2020). Automated machine learning: Review of the state-of-the-art and opportunities for healthcare. *Artificial Intelligence in Medicine*, *104*, 101822. DOI: 10.1016/j.artmed.2020.101822 PMID: 32499001

Yang, Y., Zhang, L., Du, M., Bo, J., Liu, H., Ren, L., Li, X., & Deen, M. J. (2021). A comparative analysis of eleven neural networks architectures for small datasets of lung images of COVID-19 patients toward improved clinical decisions. *Computers in Biology and Medicine*, *139*, 104887. DOI: 10.1016/j.compbiomed.2021.104887 PMID: 34688974

Yi, X., Walia, E., & Babyn, P. (2019). Generative adversarial network in medical imaging: A review. *Medical Image Analysis*, *58*, 101552. DOI: 10.1016/j.media.2019.101552 PMID: 31521965

Yuan, X., Chen, J., Zhang, K., Wu, Y., & Yang, T. (2021). A stable AI-based binary and multiple class heart disease prediction model for IoMT. *IEEE Transactions on Industrial Informatics*, *18*(3), 2032–2040. DOI: 10.1109/TII.2021.3098306

Zhou, B., Yang, G., Shi, Z., & Ma, S. (2022). Natural language processing for smart healthcare. *IEEE Reviews in Biomedical Engineering*, *17*, 4–18. DOI: 10.1109/RBME.2022.3210270 PMID: 36170385

ADDITIONAL READING

Abdullah, R. M., Saad, L. A., Alasmari, Z. M., Ali, G. A., & Muniasamy, A. (2025). Human disease prediction mobile application using machine learning. In Alareeni, B., & Hamdan, A. (Eds.), *IoT and digital transformation: Innovating business models for the connected world (ICBT 2024). Lecture notes in networks and systems* (Vol. 1575). Springer., DOI: 10.1007/978-3-032-00450-5_19

Begum, A., Muniasamy, A., Sabahath, A., Yaqub, H., & Karunakaran, G. (2024). Coronary heart disease classification using deep learning approach with feature selection for improved accuracy. *Technology and Health Care*, *32*(3), 1991–2007. DOI: 10.3233/THC-231807 PMID: 38339946

Bhatnagar, R., Muniasamy, A., & Muniasamy, V. (2021). Predictive analytics for cardiovascular disease diagnosis using machine learning techniques. In Hassanien, A., Bhatnagar, R., & Darwish, A. (Eds.), *Advanced machine learning technologies and applications (AMLTA 2020). Advances in intelligent systems and computing* (Vol. 1141). Springer., DOI: 10.1007/978-981-15-3383-9_45

Muniasamy, A. Muniasamy, Sabahath A., Begum, A., Yaqub, H., & Karunakaran, G. (2023). Lung cancer histopathology image classification using transfer learning with convolution neural network model. *Technology and Health Care,*33, 1–12. https://content.iospress.com/articles/technology-and-health-care/thc231029

KEY TERMS AND DEFINITIONS

AI Integration: AI integration refers to the seamless incorporation of artificial intelligence technologies into healthcare systems, enabling hospitals to enhance decision-making, streamline processes, and improve overall patient outcomes.

Artificial Neural Networks (ANNs): Artificial neural networks are computational models inspired by the human brain that are used in healthcare for tasks such as image recognition, disease prediction, and personalized treatment recommendations.

Clinical Decision Support (CDS): Clinical decision support systems use AI to provide evidence-based insights and recommendations that assist healthcare professionals in making accurate and timely clinical decisions.

Healthcare Automation: Healthcare automation applies AI, robotics, and digital tools to automate repetitive clinical and administrative tasks, reducing errors, saving time, and allowing clinicians to focus more on patient care.

Hospitals: Hospitals are healthcare institutions that provide comprehensive medical care, ranging from diagnosis and treatment to surgery and rehabilitation, and increasingly rely on AI-driven tools to support efficient operations.

Hospital Efficiency: Hospital efficiency refers to the ability of healthcare institutions to deliver high-quality care while minimizing waste, costs, and delays, often achieved through AI-powered workflow improvements and automation.

Patient Care: Patient care encompasses the prevention, diagnosis, treatment, and management of illness, with AI technologies enhancing personalization, accuracy, and efficiency in medical services.

Predictive Analytics: Predictive analytics uses AI and data-driven models to forecast patient outcomes, resource needs, and potential risks, thereby supporting proactive healthcare interventions.

Resource Management: Resource management in hospitals involves optimizing the allocation and utilization of staff, equipment, and facilities, with AI-driven systems improving efficiency and cost-effectiveness.

Workflow Optimization: Workflow optimization involves restructuring and automating clinical and administrative processes using AI to minimize inefficiencies, reduce delays, and enhance hospital productivity.

Chapter 11
AI-Driven Biomedical Waste Management System for Hospitals Using CNN-Based Classification and Sustainable Disposal Recommendations

Sabiyath Fatima Nakeeb
https://orcid.org/0000-0002-8918-4306
B.S. Abdur Rahman Crescent Institute of Science and Technology, India

Syed Masood Mohamed Mustafa
B.S. Abdur Rahman Crescent Institute of Science and Technology, India

Sabura Faheema Syed Masood
B.S. Abdur Rahman Crescent Institute of Science and Technology, India

Shamira Anjum Babulal
B.S. Abdur Rahman Crescent Institute of Science and Technology, India

ABSTRACT

In the pursuit of greener, safer, and more efficient hospital waste management systems, this chapter introduces an AI-driven biomedical waste management framework designed specifically for hospitals. The proposed solution integrates a CNN-based for

DOI: 10.4018/979-8-3373-2787-7.ch011

real-time biomedical waste classification with an ontology-enhanced content-based recommender system that provides sustainable and regulation-compliant disposal suggestions. The system employs a Raspberry Pi camera and ultrasonic sensors to classify waste into key biomedical categories—Infectious & Pathological Waste, Contaminated Recyclables, Sharps, and Glassware—while simultaneously monitoring bin capacity to prevent overfilling and cross-contamination. Upon detecting hazardous or full-bin conditions, the recommender system intelligently maps the classified waste to appropriate disposal methods such as autoclaving, incineration, secure landfill, or recycling. Experiments show that the RWC-Net model achieves 95.26% classification accuracy, while the recommender system demonstrates a 97% accuracy rate in suggesting disposal pathways.

INTRODUCTION

Hospital waste management has evolved into a critical and multifaceted challenge in the modern healthcare ecosystem. With the global rise in healthcare services, increased patient intake, and the heavy use of disposable medical tools—including personal protective equipment (PPE), diagnostic kits, vials, syringes, and surgical instruments—the generation of biomedical waste has reached alarming levels. This surge in waste poses significant risks to public health, environmental safety, and institutional regulatory compliance. Biomedical waste often contains infectious agents, toxic substances, or sharp objects capable of causing injury or disease transmission. Therefore, hospitals must implement waste handling systems that are not only accurate and cost-effective but also environmentally sustainable and fully compliant with local and global waste management standards.

Historically, biomedical waste management in hospitals has relied on manual categorization, static labeling systems, and routine collection schedules. These practices depend heavily on human judgment, which is prone to inconsistency, oversight, and fatigue—especially in high-pressure healthcare environments. Consequently, this often results in the misclassification and mismanagement of waste materials, causing contamination, regulatory non-compliance, and increased occupational risks for healthcare and sanitation personnel. Furthermore, improperly sorted recyclable or biodegradable waste frequently ends up being incinerated or sent to landfills, thereby increasing carbon emissions and contributing to long-term environmental degradation.

Given the current global emphasis on digital healthcare transformation, environmental consciousness, and AI-powered automation, it is imperative to transition from these outdated manual approaches to intelligent and adaptive waste management systems. Recent advances in artificial intelligence—particularly deep learning and image-based classification using convolutional neural networks (CNNs)—have demonstrated promising capabilities in automating biomedical waste categorization. However, most current research focuses narrowly on improving classification accuracy, without addressing the crucial next step: generating intelligent, regulation-compliant disposal recommendations tailored to the specific type and condition of waste.

Additionally, existing smart bin solutions lack the cognitive intelligence to detect, respond to, and act upon dynamic waste management conditions. These systems, while equipped with basic fill-level sensors, fail to offer real-time recommendations or route optimization capabilities. This results in issues like overflowing bins, inefficient waste collection routines, and avoidable exposure to infectious or hazardous materials—highlighting the need for an integrated, AI-powered approach to biomedical waste handling.

A. Importance of the Research

This chapter presents an intelligent biomedical waste management framework that integrates a CNN-based RWC-Net classification model with a recommender system that utilizes ontology mapping and content-based filtering. The RWC-Net model successfully classifies waste into key biomedical categories with a 95.26% accuracy, while the recommender system achieves 97% accuracy in providing proper disposal suggestions. The system also includes real-time monitoring through IoT-enabled components such as ultrasonic sensors and a Raspberry Pi camera to track bin fill levels and detect hazardous waste conditions. By adhering to international standards from WHO, OSHA, and the UN's Sustainable Development Goals (SDGs), this approach promotes not only effective waste segregation but also regulatory compliance and eco-conscious disposal practices.

B. Research Gaps and Objectives

Despite advancements in waste classification systems, several limitations persist. Prior studies predominantly focus on enhancing classification accuracy, with little emphasis on the downstream environmental impact of disposal methods or the carbon footprint of waste transportation. Additionally, very few systems integrate classification with actionable, AI-generated disposal recommendations that consider sustainability and regulatory standards. Most existing systems lack end-to-end automation and environmental intelligence.

To address these gaps, the proposed framework aims to:

1. Develop a CNN-based RWC-Net model for real-time classification of biomedical waste into regulatory categories.

2. Integrate a content-based, ontology-enhanced AI recommender system for intelligent disposal suggestions such as incineration, autoclaving, secure landfilling, or recycling.
3. Deploy IoT components for real-time bin-level monitoring and proactive waste handling based on hazard detection.
4. Minimize carbon footprint and enhance regulatory compliance through intelligent decision-making and automated scheduling.

By combining AI, IoT, and sustainability principles, this framework enables hospitals to transition to safer, smarter, and greener biomedical waste management practices. The outcomes offer a scalable and practical solution aligned with global waste management policies, delivering benefits in safety, efficiency, and environmental responsibility.

BACKGROUND

The study (Quan et al., 2024) introduces a privacy-preserving waste classification approach that integrates differential privacy (DP) with federated transfer learning (FTL). The method ensures data security while enabling accurate waste classification in distributed IoT environments. Evaluated on the TrashNet and GarClass datasets, it achieved classification accuracies of 90.01% and 90.22%, respectively, demonstrating a strong balance between privacy and performance. The study highlights the potential of DP-FTL in protecting user data without compromising model effectiveness. This approach sets a new benchmark for secure and efficient waste classification.

The study (Ayemowa et al., 2024) reviews the use of generative AI models, such as GANs and VAEs, in recommender systems, emphasizing their advantages over traditional methods in handling data sparsity. The study analyzes 52 research papers, identifying MovieLens to be the most frequently used dataset. It discusses key models, evaluation metrics, and emerging trends in the field. Despite some limitations, the review highlights how generative AI enhances recommendation quality across various domains. Future research directions include improving model robustness and expanding applications to diverse datasets.

The research (Hossen et al., 2024) presents RWC-Net, a deep learning model designed to classify waste into six categories with an accuracy of 95.01%, surpassing existing models. The study validates results using quantitative metrics and Score-CAM heatmaps, demonstrating the model's effectiveness. The atuhor discusses the model's strengths in accurately identifying most waste types while highlighting challenges in classifying 'litter.' Future research aims to enhance accuracy for this category and adapt the model for broader waste management applications. The study contributes to advancing AI-driven waste classification for sustainable waste management.

The study (Khouibiri et al., 2023) presents a movie recommendation system using collaborative filtering techniques, with user-based CF KNN achieving the best performance. Challenges like cold start and similarity calculations remain, requiring hybrid systems combining multiple machine learning techniques. The authors suggest incorporating user-specific data like age and health for more accurate and safer recommendations. They advocate for future systems to integrate deep learning and data mining to enhance recommendations.

The authors (Pandey et al., 2022) propose a waste management system that integrates deep learning and blockchain to identify waste objects and suggest DIY reuse ideas. The system employs ResNet50 for object recognition, achieving 94% accuracy in waste classification. Hyperledger Fabric is used for secure transaction verification, ensuring reliable and tamper-proof recycling recommendations. A Flask-based web application delivers these suggestions, providing users with actionable insights for sustainable waste reuse. Future improvements include expanding the dataset for better classification and integrating social media to promote wider community engagement.

The research (Sosunova et al., 2022) reviews smart waste management (SWM) systems, analyzing 173 studies to identify key approaches, sensors, stakeholders, and data shared between systems. It highlights city-level and smart garbage bin (SGB) systems, focusing on waste collection optimization, cost reduction, and ecological improvements. Research gaps include the need for holistic system views and increased efficiency. Recommendations are provided for city-level and SGB-level SWM system implementation.

The study (Nicholas et al., 2021) presents an intelligent waste management system combining IoT and deep learning to classify and manage waste. The system uses a deep learning model on a Raspberry Pi to identify five waste types, with IoT sensors tracking bin fill levels and locations. Data is transmitted via LoRa for efficient remote monitoring and low power use. Limitations include a small dataset affecting model accuracy and reliance on battery power, limiting operational time. The authors suggest improving the dataset and exploring sustainable power solutions to enhance system efficiency.

The study (Teoh Ji Sheng et al., 2020) introduces a smart waste management system that integrates IoT and AI for efficient waste segregation and real-time monitoring. The system utilizes LoRa technology for long-range, low-power data transmission, ensuring seamless communication between waste bins and central servers. TensorFlow is employed for waste classification, enabling automated sorting into designated compartments. The system is designed to be cost-effective, with each smart bin priced at $180 and consuming 10.025W of power. By optimizing waste collection and reducing manual sorting efforts, the proposed solution contributes to sustainable waste management in smart cities.

The study (Zhihu Yang et al., 2020) presents WasNet, a lightweight neural network designed for efficient and accurate garbage classification. The system integrates a smart trash bin, a mobile application, and a data platform to enable real-time monitoring and decision-making. It facilitates intelligent trash sorting and enhances recycling processes. The study highlights the effectiveness of WasNet in waste classification while emphasizing future research directions, including robotics integration and improving multi-label garbage classification.

Kashif Ahmad et al., (2020). The paper introduces a “double fusion” approach for waste classification, combining feature-level and score-level fusion techniques to boost accuracy. Feature-level fusion merges features from different models, while score-level fusion combines prediction scores for more reliable outcomes. This hybrid method improves classification accuracy by 3.58% over existing techniques. It proves effective for complex waste classification, especially with diverse waste types and environmental changes. The authors suggest that increasing the dataset's size and diversity could further improve performance.

The implementation of an intelligent waste management system involves selecting a deep learning model, such as CNN, for waste classification. The template for this system includes defining waste categories, preprocessing image data, and integrating it with real-time monitoring tools like Raspberry Pi and Arduino.

PROPOSED METHODOLOGY

In most hospital environments, biomedical waste management still depends heavily on manual intervention, predefined static protocols, and rudimentary sorting methods. Typically, hospital staff manually segregate waste into categories such as infectious, pathological, sharps, pharmaceutical, and general waste. These categories are established under international regulatory frameworks, including those by the World Health Organization (WHO), Occupational Safety and Health Administration (OSHA), and other national biomedical waste handling standards. However, these systems are prone to several inherent limitations that compromise efficiency, safety, and compliance.

Manual classification is highly susceptible to human error, misidentification, and inconsistent handling practices, often leading to cross-contamination and increased risk of biohazard exposure. Staff fatigue, lack of proper training, and misinterpretation of waste types further exacerbate this problem, especially in high-pressure environments like hospitals. The absence of automated validation or feedback mechanisms makes it difficult to maintain high accuracy in waste categorization.

Moreover, most existing waste management setups follow static disposal protocols that are not equipped to dynamically respond to real-time changes in waste volume or type. Bins often overflow unnoticed, increasing the risk of pathogen spread and making waste collection inefficient. The logistics of hospital waste transportation is also impacted, leading to delayed pick-ups, increased operational costs, and a larger carbon footprint due to inefficient route planning and vehicle utilization. While some recent solutions have employed AI-based models such as TrashNet for general waste classification using convolutional neural networks (CNNs), these models are not tailored to the specific and highly regulated domain of biomedical waste. They lack the precision, contextual awareness, and compliance-focused filtering required for critical environments like hospitals. Additionally, TrashNet and similar models often fail to account for nuanced biomedical waste subcategories such as chemically contaminated recyclables, sharps, and biohazardous organic waste.

Furthermore, even in systems that perform basic classification, there is often no integration of a decision-support layer that informs hospital staff on how to act post-classification. These systems merely label the waste without providing actionable insights for safe disposal, recycling, or neutralization methods. Efforts to incorporate intelligent recommendation systems using ontologies or WordNet-based semantic networks have been widely explored in domains like e-commerce and entertainment (e.g., movie or product recommendations). These systems use clustering algorithms to group similar items, handle sparsity, and improve recommendation quality. However, such techniques have yet to be meaningfully adapted to the biomedical waste domain, where domain-specific knowledge, regulatory constraints, and safety implications must be accounted for. Additionally, most systems do not offer personalized or context-aware suggestions based on real-time data, user interaction history, or waste generation patterns—making them insufficient for hospital-scale operations.

These gaps underscore the need for a comprehensive, hospital-specific, AI-driven waste management framework that combines accurate classification, actionable disposal recommendations, real-time monitoring, and intelligent automation—tailored specifically for the sensitive context of biomedical waste. To overcome the shortcomings of traditional hospital waste management systems, this work proposes an AI-Driven Smart Waste Management System that combines deep learning, ontology-based recommendations, and Internet of Things (IoT) for a robust, real-time, and regulation-compliant hospital waste disposal solution.

At the heart of the system lies the RWC-Net (Reliable and Robust Waste Classification Network), a deep convolutional neural network specifically designed for biomedical waste classification. RWC-Net integrates the lightweight and efficient MobileNetV2 with the deeply layered DenseNet121 architecture to extract rich hierarchical features while maintaining computational efficiency. This hybrid architecture ensures the system performs well even in resource-constrained hospital IT infrastructures, such as embedded systems powered by Raspberry Pi or edge servers. The model achieves a classification accuracy of 95.26%, reliably distinguishing between waste categories such as sharps, infectious waste, contaminated recyclables, biodegradable waste, and general waste. Unlike generic CNNs, RWC-Net supports image segmentation and bounding box localization, allowing it to accurately detect waste even when mixed or partially visible in bins—thus improving the real-world applicability of AI in unstructured environments.

Once classification is complete, the system seamlessly integrates with a hybrid recommendation engine, which is built on ontology-based rule filtering, TF-IDF-based content matching, and generative AI using LLMs. This recommendation system dynamically suggests appropriate disposal, decontamination, or recycling techniques tailored to each specific waste type. For instance, while high-risk infectious waste triggers ontology-based disposal protocols grounded in WHO and EPA guidelines, recyclable items like glass or plastic invoke real-time DIY upcycling recommendations fetched via web scraping (Tavily API) and processed using Mistral 7B, an open-source language model optimized for summarizing and structuring actionable content. Moreover, the proposed system integrates IoT-based real-time monitoring to track bin capacity and waste collection status. Using ultrasonic sensors embedded in smart bins and a Raspberry Pi camera module, the system can detect when bins are nearing capacity, trigger timely classification and disposal recommendations, and notify hospital staff or waste handlers for prompt action. This not only reduces the risk of overflow and contamination but also automates and optimizes waste collection schedules, thereby reducing fuel consumption, operational costs, and environmental impact.

Another important dimension of the system is its scalability and modularity. The architecture can be deployed in hospitals of varying sizes—from small clinics to large multi-specialty medical campuses. The modular structure allows different hospitals to customize the number of bins, sensor types, classification categories, and disposal rules based on their specific operational needs and regulatory jurisdiction. To close the loop, the system features a feedback mechanism that captures user actions (e.g., disposal method chosen, feedback on recommendations) and feeds them back into the model pipeline for continual learning. Over time, this adaptive intelligence improves both classification and recommendation quality, making the system more context-aware and responsive to evolving hospital practices. The system's scalable design allows for seamless adaptability to varying hospital sizes and waste generation rates, ultimately improving overall waste management efficiency and sustainability. Through the integration of AI, ontology-based decision-making, and IoT-driven automation, the proposed system presents a holistic and intelligent approach to biomedical waste management in hospital settings.

Dataset Description

The dataset used for training and evaluating the AI-driven hospital waste classification system is curated from multiple publicly available sources, ensuring a diverse and representative collection of medical waste images. It is structured into five major waste categories aligned with hospital waste management standards: Infectious & Pathological Waste, Contaminated Recyclable Waste, Sharps & Glassware, Recyclable & General Waste, and Organic & Biodegradable Waste. Each category comprises images collected from real-world hospital environments, allowing the model to generalize effectively to clinical waste disposal scenarios. The dataset integrates images from sources such as the Roboflow Medical Waste Dataset, Zenodo Medical Waste Records, and Kaggle Biomedical Waste Collections. The dataset, comprising 15,000 images, is divided into 80% for training and 20% for testing to facilitate a balanced and effective evaluation of the model's performance. Specifically, the dataset is categorized as follows: Infectious & Pathological Waste includes 3,500 images (2,800 for training and 700 for testing), Contaminated Recyclable Waste contains 2,500 images (2,000 for training and 500 for testing), Sharps & Glassware comprises 2,800 images (2,240 for training and 560 for testing), Recyclable & General Waste consists of 3,200 images (2,560 for training and 640 for testing), and Organic & Biodegradable Waste includes 3,000 images (2,400 for training and 600 for testing). The dataset is built from five open-source repositories that provide high-quality labeled images of medical and general waste, captured under various lighting conditions, angles, and backgrounds to enhance the model's generalization capability. The Roboflow Medical Waste Dataset contributes annotated images of infectious and biomedical waste, while the Zenodo Medical Waste Repository provides sorted categories for general recyclable and organic waste. The Kaggle Infectious & Municipal Waste Dataset focuses on hospital waste disposal, particularly sharps, glassware, and biohazardous materials, whereas the Kaggle Pharmaceutical & Biomedical Waste Dataset includes images of pharmaceutical disposables, syringes, and chemical containers. Additionally, the Roboflow Medical Waste Recognition Dataset enhances the dataset with bounding boxes for object detection tasks, making it a comprehensive resource for AI-driven biomedical waste classification.

System Architecture

The proposed system architecture for the smart bin integrates multiple components to enhance AI-driven Smart Waste Management System and recommendation capabilities. It begins with Camera/Sensors that capture waste images, which are then handled by a Preprocessing Unit for tasks like resizing and normalization. The processed images are passed to the Waste Classification Module (CNN), where the waste is classified into predefined categories. This data is stored in the Waste Data Repository, which holds both classification results and user profiles. A sophisticated Recommender System, leveraging Web scraping, Content Filtering,, provides personalized waste disposal suggestions (e.g., recycling or composting). The Decision-Making Engine utilizes this information to offer actionable recommendations to users through a User Interface (via mobile or web app). Lastly, System Monitoring tracks the bin's fill levels, optimizing waste collection and disposal by dynamically updating the system. This architecture supports efficient waste management while providing users with tailored, eco-friendly disposal options.

The AI-driven Smart Waste Management System integrates machine learning techniques, IoT sensors, and a hybrid recommendation system to enhance waste classification, disposal recommendations, and sustainability in hospital environments. It ensures efficient waste segregation and compliance with regulatory waste disposal standards in healthcare settings.

Figure 1. Smart Waste Management System Architecture diagram

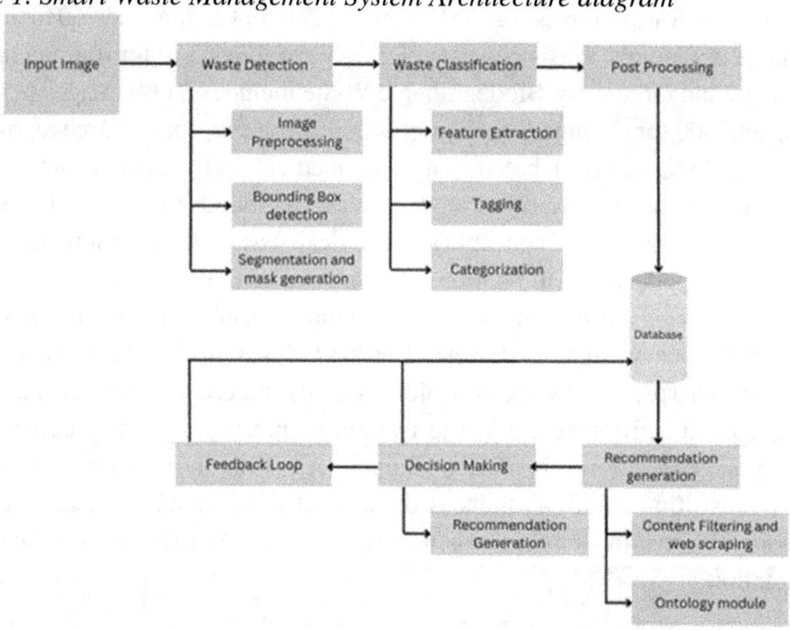

Figure 1 illustrates an AI-driven decision support system for evaluating and managing hospital waste efficiently. The process begins with an Input Image, which undergoes Waste Detection through image preprocessing, bounding box detection, and segmentation to identify relevant waste items. Next, the system performs Waste

Classification, where AI extracts key features, tags the waste, and categorizes it into types such as biological, hazardous, or recyclable. This classified data is then stored in a Database for further processing and analysis. In the Recommendation Generation phase, AI analyzes stored data and gathers insights through content filtering and web scraping, supplemented by an ontology module that structures knowledge. This leads to Decision Making, where AI-driven recommendations help hospital staff optimize waste disposal, ensuring regulatory compliance and efficiency. A Feedback Loop continuously refines the system by incorporating new data, improving accuracy and adaptability over time. By automating waste detection, classification, and decision-making, this AI-driven framework enhances hospital waste management, reducing errors and promoting sustainability. This comprehensive architecture not only facilitates accurate and intelligent waste handling in real-time but also fosters a culture of sustainable waste management within hospital environments. By fusing machine learning, real-time IoT sensing, and semantic web technologies, the proposed system transforms traditional biomedical waste management into a proactive, data-driven, and environmentally responsible practice. Ultimately, it empowers healthcare facilities to meet both regulatory obligations and sustainability goals while safeguarding public health and operational integrity.

A. Waste Detection

The system initiates waste detection using high-resolution cameras and IoT-based sensors deployed in hospital waste bins. These sensors capture images and detect properties like weight, volume, and contamination levels to provide input for further processing. This stage ensures real-time monitoring of medical waste, helping hospitals streamline disposal workflows.

B. Preprocessing Unit

Once the images are captured, they are sent to the preprocessing unit where various operations like resizing, normalizing pixel values, and data augmentation are performed. This ensures that the images are prepared correctly for the CNN model, improving accuracy and making the data ready for classification.

C. Waste Classification Module

The Convolutional Neural Network (CNN) model RWC-Net is trained on diverse hospital waste datasets to accurately classify medical waste into predefined categories, ensuring efficient and regulation-compliant disposal. The model categorizes waste into five major types: Infectious & Pathological Waste, which includes blood-soaked materials and tissue samples; Contaminated Recyclable Waste, such as used PPE and plastic syringes; Sharps & Glassware, encompassing items like needles and broken glass vials; Recyclable & General Waste, which consists of paper packaging and non-contaminated plastics; and Organic & Biodegradable Waste, including food waste from hospital cafeterias. By leveraging deep learning techniques for advanced feature extraction, RWC-Net achieves high-precision classification, enabling hospitals to automate waste segregation processes, minimize manual errors, and adhere to biomedical waste disposal regulations. This automation not only enhances operational efficiency but also ensures compliance with environmental and healthcare safety standards.

D. Waste Data Repository

Classified waste data is systematically stored in a centralized Hospital Waste Management Database, ensuring efficient tracking, compliance, and policy optimization. This database records detailed classification information, including waste type, contamination level, and recommended disposal method, enabling precise waste segregation and regulatory adherence. Additionally, user behavior logs capture waste disposal patterns across different hospital departments, helping identify inefficiencies and optimize waste handling practices.

E. Recommender System

The AI-driven recommender system enhances waste disposal decisions through a hybrid approach that integrates multiple advanced techniques for optimal efficiency and compliance. Ontology-based reasoning utilizes structured knowledge bases, including WHO biomedical waste disposal guidelines and hospital-specific policies, to provide context-aware disposal recommendations. Content-based filtering further refines these suggestions by matching waste characteristics with the most suitable treatment methods, such as recommending incineration for infectious waste and autoclaving for sharps. To ensure regulatory compliance, the system employs web scraping techniques to dynamically extract updated waste disposal regulations from government and environmental agencies, ensuring that recommendations remain aligned with evolving policies.

F. Decision-Making Engine

The AI-driven Decision-Making Engine processes classification results and disposal recommendations to provide hospital staff with actionable insights, ensuring efficient and compliant waste management. By analyzing waste categorization and recommended disposal methods, the system generates real-time alerts for hazardous waste, prompting immediate action for high-risk materials to prevent contamination and regulatory violations. Additionally, optimized recycling suggestions help hospitals reduce their overall waste footprint by identifying recyclable materials and recommending sustainable disposal options. The engine also incorporates predictive disposal scheduling, leveraging historical waste generation patterns and real-time bin status to improve operational efficiency, prevent waste overflow incidents, and streamline collection processes.

G. User Interface (Mobile/Web App)

The user interacts with the system via a mobile or web application, where they can view the waste classification results and receive personalized disposal recommendations. The interface may also provide real-time notifications, such as alerts when the bin is full, or tips on how to reduce waste. The goal is to make the interaction simple and actionable for the user.

H. System Monitoring (Bin Sensors)

Finally, the system includes sensors embedded in the smart bin to track its status, such as fill levels, weight, or odor. This data is sent to the cloud for real-time monitoring and can trigger alerts when the bin is full or optimize collection schedules to reduce the carbon footprint by minimizing transportation.

Figure 2. Input Process Output diagram

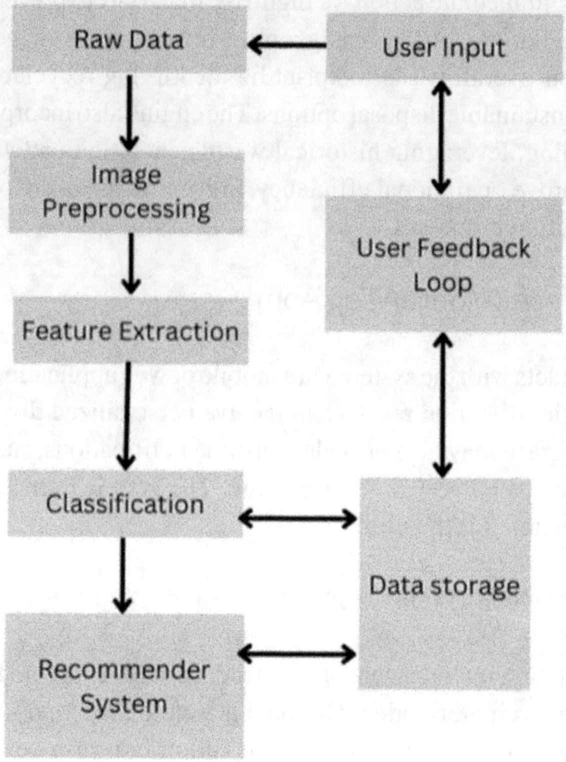

Figure 2 illustrates an AI-driven waste management framework that integrates image processing, classification, recommendation, and feedback to enhance decision-making. The system begins with Raw Data, consisting of images that undergo Image Preprocessing to improve quality and extract relevant features. The Feature Extraction phase identifies key characteristics, enabling accurate Classification of waste into predefined categories. Once classified, the data is processed by the Recommender System, which generates optimal waste management suggestions. The classified data is also stored in a Database, ensuring accessibility for future analysis. Additionally, the system incorporates User Input, allowing manual refinement and real-time interaction. A User Feedback Loop continuously improves the system by updating the database with new insights, enhancing classification accuracy and recommendation quality over time. This architecture emphasizes automation and adaptability, ensuring that waste management in hospitals is efficient, compliant, and continuously optimized through AI-driven decision support.

The proposed architecture for the smart trash can and its integrated recommender system presents a comprehensive approach to biomedical waste management and sustainability. With a CNN-based waste classification model, the system accurately classifies various waste types and provides personalized disposal recommendations through a hybrid recommender system. The system combines content-based filtering, and web scraping that allow it to make suggestions that are most relevant based on user interactions and waste characteristics. Additionally it also incorporates ontological data that enhances the most accurate recommendations through semantic relationships of different kinds of waste and their associated disposal methods. Additionally, the feedback mechanism ensures continuous improvement of recommendations and adapting to changing user preferences.

IMPLEMENTATION

The Smart Waste Management System is an AI-driven decision support system designed to enhance hospital waste segregation, sustainability, and compliance with environmental regulations. It primarily uses two algorithms, namely, the RWC-Net classification model for waste identification and categorization and a hybrid recommendation system for sustainable disposal suggestions. Both these algorithms are combined into a single entity and are implemented with the help of various modules. The Smart Waste Management system is structured into five main modules: data collection, pre-processing, feature extraction, model development, and prediction. Each of these modules plays a critical role in ensuring efficient waste classification, segregation, and disposal, which contributes to hospital waste sustainability and regulatory compliance.

The implementation process of the AI-Driven Decision Support System includes the following steps:

Step 1: The initial and most important phase involves collecting data for model training. The dataset for training the AI model is collected from multiple sources, including the Biomedical waste dataset (Kaggle) for annotated waste images, the BDWaste dataset (Mendeley Data) for medical and non-medical waste, and Medical Waste Datasets from platforms like Roboflow, Kaggle, and Zenodo, which contain biohazardous and recyclable hospital waste images. Additionally, real-world hospital waste images are captured from hospital disposal sites to enhance model realism. The dataset is categorized into six primary hospital waste types: Infectious & Pathological Waste, Contaminated Recyclable Waste, Sharps & Glassware, Recyclable & General Waste and Organic & Biodegradable Waste. This diverse dataset improves the AI model's generalization and ensures real-world applicability in hospitals, making waste classification more efficient and accurate.

Step 2: The collected datasets are then organized in a directory according to their classification categories to maintain proper labeling for training purposes. This structured approach to data labeling enhances the efficiency of the training process and minimizes the risk of misclassification.

Step 3: The datasets undergo a preprocessing stage because they are collected from various sources. The pre-processing steps include resizing images to a uniform 224×224 pixels for consistency, removing distortions, unnecessary background elements, and borders to keep the focus on the waste object, and enhancing contrast to improve feature detection. These optimizations ensure that the AI model learns more effectively by reducing noise and improving classification accuracy in hospital waste management.

Step 4: The next step is feature extraction, where the key characteristics of waste images are identified. This process is necessary to simplify the large dataset into smaller, manageable components, which facilitates efficient processing. Features are derived using the convolutional layers of the RWC-Net model. The convolutional layer applies digital filters to detect patterns such as edges, textures, and shapes in waste images. During backpropagation, network parameters are optimized to improve classification accuracy. The extracted features are then converted into an array using NumPy in Python.

Step 5: The extracted features are then fed into the RWC-Net model with predefined epoch values to train the classification algorithm. Model creation is done where the dataset is divided into two parts: 80% of the dataset is assigned for training, while 20% is assigned for testing. The trained model is stored in .h5 format for deployment and future predictions. The RWC-Net model classifies the captured images into different waste categories. When the bin reaches full capacity, as detected by an ultrasonic sensor, the system captures images of the waste inside and sends them as input to the recommender system.

Step 6: Once waste is classified, the AI-driven recommendation system suggests appropriate disposal methods based on the waste type. For recyclable waste, the system utilizes web scraping via the Tavily API to fetch DIY upcycling and recycling ideas from online sources. For biodegradable waste, content-based filtering using TF-IDF provides composting or eco-friendly disposal guidelines. For hazardous medical waste, the Ontology Module ensures that disposal recommendations comply with hospital regulations, including standards set by organizations such as WHO, EPA, and biohazard disposal guidelines. This AI-driven approach ensures that hospital waste is managed in an eco-friendly, regulation-compliant manner, promoting sustainability and safeguarding public health.

Step 7: The final disposal recommendations are presented to the user via the web interface. The system records waste classification results, disposal recommendations, and bin status in a cloud database, enabling future analysis and monitoring. Additionally, a feedback loop is integrated to refine AI predictions by incorporating real-world disposal data from hospitals. This continuous learning process enhances model accuracy over time, ensuring that waste classification and management remain efficient and adaptive. By tracking classification performance, the system can identify areas for improvement, optimize waste disposal strategies, and contribute to more effective AI-driven waste management in healthcare settings.

A. RWC-Net Algorithm

RWC-Net (Reliable and Robust Waste Classification Network) is an advanced deep learning model based on CNN. It combines MobileNetV2 and DenseNet121 to efficiently classify recyclable waste. The key advantage of RWC-Net is that it extracts rich hierarchical features from both lightweight and deep architectures, making it well-suited for waste classification tasks. The difference between RWC-Net and traditional CNN models is that RWC-Net combines two different pre-trained models to enhance classification accuracy while maintaining computational efficiency.

RWC-Net is implemented as follows:

Step 1: Prior to training RWC-Net, the dataset undergoes a systematic preparation process to enhance model performance. Initially, images of hospital waste — including items such as gloves, syringes, food waste, paper, glass, and plastic — are collected from diverse sources. These images are then resized to 224×224 pixels to align with the input requirements of the neural network. To ensure consistency and accelerate model convergence, normalization is performed by scaling pixel values within the [0,1] range. Finally, the dataset is divided into 80% for training and 20% for testing, enabling accurate model evaluation and performance analysis.

Step 2: Begin the model creation process by loading pre-trained MobileNetV2 and DenseNet121 models while removing their classification heads to retain only their feature extraction capabilities. Feature maps from both networks are extracted using Global Average Pooling (GAP), which effectively reduces dimensionality while preserving crucial information.

Step 3: Concatenate the extracted featured to form a comprehensive feature vector that integrates the strengths of both architectures. The combined feature representation is subsequently passed through fully connected (Dense) layers, enabling the model to learn complex patterns in hospital waste classification. Finally, a Softmax output layer is employed to classify waste images into one of six predefined categories, ensuring precise and efficient biomedical waste segregation in healthcare environments.

Step 4: After constructing the model architecture, the training process is carried out using mini-batch gradient descent over 30 epochs. The training progress is evaluated using the cross-entropy loss function along with the accuracy metric. Once the model is successfully trained, it becomes capable of classifying new waste images. The predict_waste function handles this task by taking an input image, preprocessing it, and generating a prediction for its corresponding waste category.

Figure 3. Working of RWC-Net algorithm

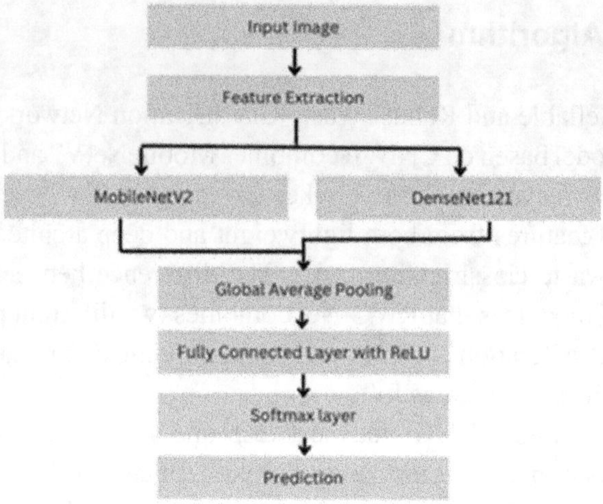

The RWC-Net algorithm begins by loading two pre-trained convolutional neural networks — MobileNetV2 and DenseNet121 — both of which are stripped of their final classification layers to retain only their feature extraction capabilities. MobileNetV2 provides lightweight and efficient extraction, while DenseNet121 contributes deep and hierarchical feature representations. Features from both networks are then processed through Global Average Pooling (GAP) to reduce dimensionality while preserving essential information. Next, the features from both models are concatenated into a single, comprehensive feature vector. This unified vector is passed through a series of fully connected layers — typically with 128 and 64 units respectively — using ReLU activation functions to learn complex, non-linear patterns specific to biomedical waste types. A Softmax layer is then applied as the final output layer, classifying the image into one of the six predefined biomedical waste categories: *Infectious & Pathological Waste*, *Contaminated Recyclable Waste*, *Sharps & Glassware*, *Recyclable & General Waste*, and *Organic & Biodegradable Waste*. The model is then compiled using cross-entropy loss and the Adam optimizer, and trained using mini-batch gradient descent for 30 epochs. After training, the model is evaluated on a testing set (20% of the total data) to validate its accuracy. During inference, a new image is preprocessed (resized and normalized) and passed through the trained model to predict the corresponding waste category, enabling real-time biomedical waste classification.

The RWC-Net algorithm employed in this work is illustrated in Figure 3. The algorithm performs efficient image classification when the input images are provided. Input images from both the test and training datasets are initially provided to the model. The model utilizes a dual-feature extraction approach by incorporating MobileNetV2 and DenseNet121 architectures, which extract meaningful patterns from the images. The output from each convolutional filter in the previous layer produces a feature map. Each filter moves across the previous layer, one pixel at a time, capturing different spatial characteristics of the image. The neurons are activated at every position, and the corresponding values are gathered in the feature map. The Global Average Pooling (GAP) layer then aggregates the extracted features by reducing the spatial dimensions, preventing overfitting and reducing computational complexity. Following this, a fully connected layer with ReLU (Rectified Linear Unit) activation learns complex patterns from the extracted features. This layer maps the abstract representations to meaningful class labels. The final Softmax layer assigns probabilities to each class, ensuring that the highest probability corresponds to the predicted category. RWC-Net integrates MobileNetV2 for lightweight extraction and DenseNet121 for deep feature learning, striking a balance between efficiency and accuracy.The RWC-Net model plays a crucial role in AI-driven hospital decision support systems by enabling automated waste segregation for efficient hospital waste disposal, ensuring regulatory compliance by accurately categorizing biohazardous and infectious waste, and reducing manual sorting efforts, thereby minimizing health risks for hospital staff. Additionally, it promotes sustainable waste management by optimizing recycling and disposal methods through AI-based classification. The RWC-Net algorithm was implemented using MobileNetV2 and DenseNet121, ensuring both efficiency and accuracy in waste classification. The system was rigorously evaluated using cross-entropy loss and accuracy metrics, achieving high classification accuracy. By integrating AI-driven decision support, RWC-Net helps hospitals assess and refine waste classification strategies, reducing risks, improving compliance, and supporting sustainable waste management practices.

B. Recommender System

The recommender system in this study enhances waste management by providing upcycling, recycling, composting, and sustainable disposal suggestions based on classification results from the RWC-Net model. The approach is tailored to different waste categories to ensure both compliance and environmental sustainability. For Recyclable & General Waste such as plastic, metal, glass, and paper, the system utilizes web scraping to gather DIY upcycling and recycling ideas from online sources. Structured web extraction is performed using the Tavily API, while Mistral 7B, a fast and free language model, processes the extracted data to generate step-by-step reuse instructions. In the case of Organic & Biodegradable Waste, where established composting methods exist, the system relies on predefined content-based recommendations using TF-IDF to provide composting guidelines sourced from trusted government and NGO websites, eliminating the need for dynamic updates. For Infectious & Pathological Waste and Sharps & Glassware, strict medical waste regulations necessitate a compliance-focused approach. Here, the system applies ontology-based filtering, aligning recommendations with predefined WHO, OSHA, and EPA guidelines to ensure safe and legally compliant disposal. Contaminated Recyclable Waste is handled using a classification-based rule system that first assesses the level of contamination. If the hazard level is high, disposal follows strict ontology-based methods. However, if contamination is minimal, TF-IDF filtering suggests decontamination steps before allowing recycling. This hybrid strategy ensures that recyclable materials benefit from updated, dynamic recommendations while hazardous and regulated waste categories strictly adhere to established safety and compliance protocols.

Figure 4. Working of Recommender System

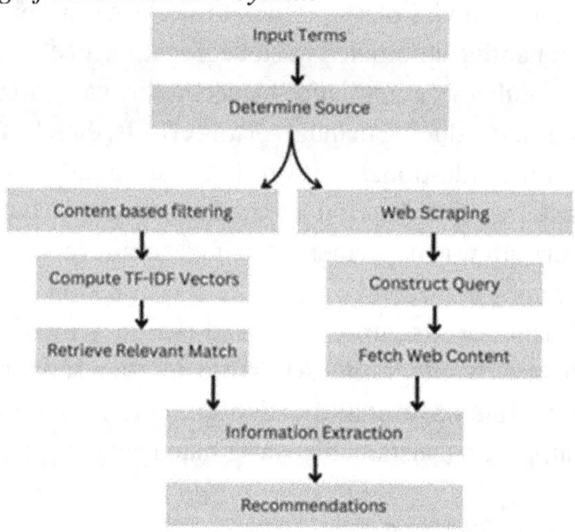

Figure 4 illustrates the functioning of the recommendation system implemented in this study. The algorithm operates by efficiently retrieving and recommending relevant content based on input search terms. As shown in Figure 4, the system begins by receiving input terms from the RWC-Net algorithm output. The first step involves determining the appropriate source for retrieval, which could be either content-based filtering or web scraping. For content-based filtering, the system computes Term Frequency-Inverse Document Frequency (TF-IDF) vectors, a technique used to quantify the importance of words within documents. These vectors help identify relevant matches based on textual similarity. The system retrieves the most relevant content, ensuring that recommendations align closely with user input. Alternatively, the system performs web scraping, where it constructs a query based on input terms and fetches web content from external sources. This approach allows the system to gather updated and diverse information. Following either content-based filtering or web scraping, the retrieved information undergoes an extraction process. The extracted data is analyzed, processed, and structured to generate meaningful recommendations for the user. By integrating both content-based retrieval and web scraping, the system ensures a comprehensive recommendation process that balances accuracy and breadth, delivering optimal suggestions tailored to user needs.

The system operates in the following manner:

Step 1: The recommender system takes RWC-Net classification result as input to generate relevant waste disposal suggestions. Each waste item categorized into one of the predefined medical waste types (e.g., Infectious & Pathological Waste, Contaminated Recyclable Waste, Sharps & Glassware, Recyclable & General Waste, Organic & Biodegradable Waste). This classification determines the next steps for appropriate disposal or recycling recommendations.

Step 2: For Recyclable & General Waste the system uses Tavily API to perform web scraping and collect up-to-date DIY upcycling and recycling ideas from online sources such as sustainability blogs, government recycling guides, and maker communities. These sources provide innovative ways to repurpose recyclable waste, reducing environmental impact and promoting sustainable practices. The system also ensures that the recommendations are practical and feasible within a hospital setting.

Step 3: For Infectious & Pathological Waste and Sharps & Glassware, where strict disposal protocols are essential, the system utilizes ontology-based filtering guided by WHO, EPA, and OSHA regulations. Instead of web scraping, it relies on predefined knowledge bases to ensure disposal instructions align with global safety standards. For example, highly infectious biomedical waste is disposed of through incineration, while sharps undergo autoclaving for sterilization before disposal. Materials that cannot be safely incinerated or recycled are directed to secure landfills. This structured approach ensures compliance with medical waste disposal regulations, minimizing environmental and health risks.

Step 4: For contaminated recyclable waste, such as used PPE or blood-stained plastics, the system evaluates the level of contamination to determine the appropriate disposal method. If the waste presents a high-risk contamination—such as blood-soaked PPE or chemically contaminated plastics—it follows ontology-based disposal protocols to prevent infection spread and ensure compliance with medical waste regulations. However, if the contamination is low-risk and the waste can be safely cleaned, TF-IDF-based filtering suggests appropriate decontamination steps, such as sterilization or chemical neutralization, before permitting recycling. This approach ensures that hazardous materials are handled safely while promoting responsible waste management.

Step 5: For organic waste and litter, such as food scraps, biodegradable hospital materials, and general waste, predefined content-based filtering (TF-IDF) is applied. Instead of web scraping, the system relies on trusted government and NGO sources to provide composting and eco-friendly disposal guidelines. This ensures that composting suggestions remain scientifically accurate and do not require frequent updates.

Step 6: The Mistral 7B LLM is used to extract structured step-by-step instructions from the gathered sources. This step ensures that the recommendations are clear, actionable, and optimized for hospital staff. The AI removes redundant information, highlights key procedures, and ensures that all suggested methods align with waste management regulations.

Step 7: Format the recommendations into concise, two-line outputs that are easy for hospital staff to interpret and act upon. This ensures that the information is quickly accessible, reducing decision-making time and improving overall waste management efficiency.

The recommender system operates immediately after the RWC-Net model classifies a waste item. Based on the predicted category, it selects an appropriate recommendation strategy from one of three core techniques: ontology-based filtering, content-based filtering using TF-IDF, or web scraping with summarization. For Infectious & Pathological Waste and Sharps & Glassware, the system applies ontology-based filtering, referencing predefined biomedical waste management guidelines from regulatory bodies like WHO, EPA, and OSHA. These ensure that the recommended disposal method — such as incineration, autoclaving, or secure landfill — strictly adheres to legal and medical safety standards. In the case of Contaminated Recyclable Waste, the system first assesses the contamination level. If high, ontology-based protocols are applied. If low-risk, the system uses TF-IDF-based content filtering to suggest decontamination methods, such as sterilization or chemical neutralization, followed by recycling. For Recyclable & General Waste, the system performs web scraping using the Tavily API to gather up-to-date recycling and upcycling suggestions from reputable online sources. The extracted content is then processed by the Mistral 7B language model, which restructures the raw text into clear, step-by-step instructions suitable for hospital use. When handling Organic & Biodegradable Waste, the system bypasses dynamic scraping and instead uses predefined TF-IDF filtering to retrieve composting or eco-friendly disposal methods from government and NGO repositories.

Finally, all recommendations are formatted into concise, two-line actionable outputs, ensuring that hospital staff can quickly understand and implement the suggested disposal method. This hybrid recommendation system balances automation, regulatory compliance, and environmental responsibility. The recommender system efficiently integrates AI-driven content filtering, web scraping, and ontology-based regulations to provide accurate and practical waste disposal recommendations. By categorizing waste using RWC-Net classification, the system ensures that recyclables benefit from dynamic, updated DIY solutions, while medical and hazardous waste adheres to strict compliance protocols. The hybrid approach balances automation with safety, enabling efficient waste processing, environmental sustainability, and regulatory adherence. This structured, data-driven methodology enhances hospital waste management by offering clear, actionable, and concise disposal instructions, minimizing risks while maximizing resource recovery.

RESULT AND ANALYSIS

The performance evaluation of the proposed AI-Driven Biomedical Smart Waste Management System has been carried out across three key components: the RWC-Net-based waste classification model, the recommendation system, and the ultrasonic sensor-based monitoring module. Each component is assessed using appropriate performance metrics, namely model accuracy, recommendation accuracy, and sensor detection accuracy, respectively. Model accuracy represents the ratio of correctly predicted instances to the total number of predictions made by the classification model. It reflects the model's effectiveness in correctly identifying and classifying different types of biomedical waste. Furthermore, precision and recall metrics are employed to evaluate the model's performance, particularly in managing class imbalances often encountered in real-world hospital waste datasets.

Figure 5. Model Accuracy of RWC-Net algorithm

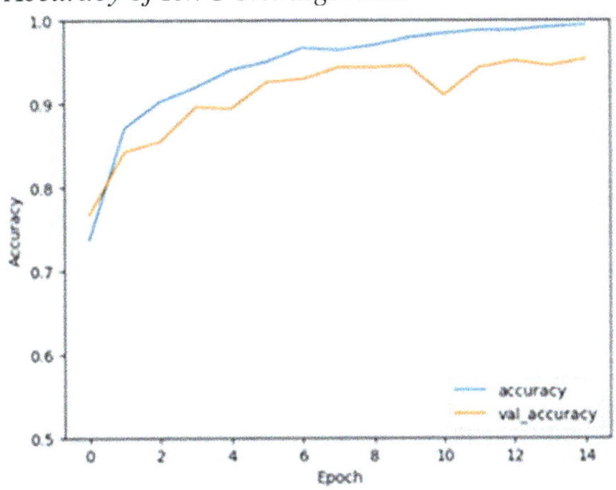

Figure 6. Combined Confusion Matrix With Class-based Result

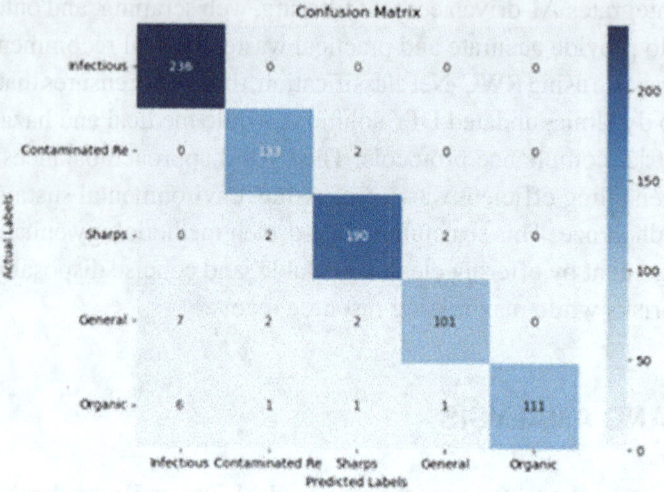

A. Waste Classification

In the classification of waste types (Infectious & Pathological Waste, Contaminated Recyclable Waste, Sharps & Glassware, Recyclable & General Waste, and Organic & Biodegradable Waste) using the RWC-Net CNN model, the model accuracy is illustrated in Figure 5. The RWC-Net model, a hybrid CNN architecture designed by combining MobileNetV2 (known for its lightweight efficiency) with DenseNet121 (renowned for deep feature extraction). The model was trained to classify biomedical waste into five key categories namely Infectious & Pathological Waste, Contaminated Recyclable Waste, Sharps & Glassware, Recyclable & General Waste, and Organic & Biodegradable Waste. To ensure generalizability and reduce overfitting, the dataset was split into 80% training and 20% testing. The training process involved 15 epochs using the Stochastic Gradient Descent (SGD) optimizer and sparse categorical crossentropy as the loss function.

Accuracy Calculation Formula: Model Accuracy = Accuracy × Epoch Value

This formula captures cumulative learning performance across all epochs. The final performance metrics on the test set are summarized in Table I.

Table 1. Performance metrics of RWC-Net algorithm

Metric	Score
Accuracy	95.26%
Precision	95.13%
Recall	95.26%

The high scores across all three metrics reflect the robustness of the RWC-Net model in accurately detecting and classifying various biomedical waste types. This is further validated by the confusion matrix (Figure 6), which displays minimal false positives and false negatives, indicating that the model effectively differentiates among closely related waste classes. This high classification accuracy is critical, as it directly impacts the quality of recommendations generated by the downstream recommender system.

B. Recommender System

Figure 7. Recommendation Accuracy Across Waste Type

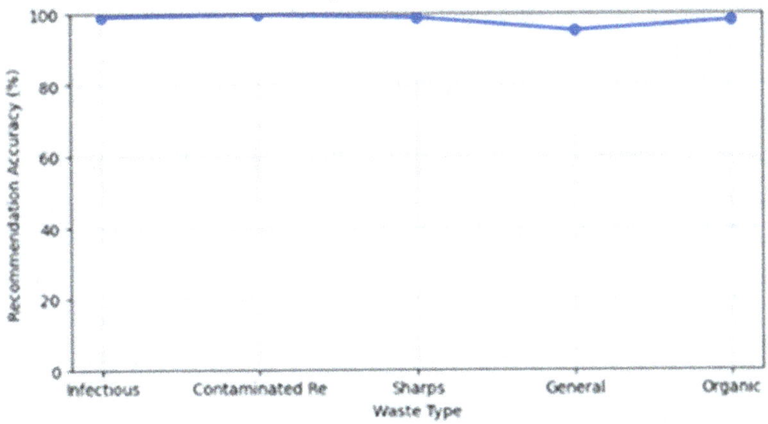

The recommender system is designed to generate intelligent, sustainable, and regulation-compliant disposal suggestions tailored to each classified biomedical waste type. It leverages both static knowledge (predefined rules and ontologies) and dynamic data (real-time web scraping) to deliver precise, context-aware recommendations. The system adapts its suggestions based on the specific waste category and the level of contamination, ensuring that the disposal process is both eco-friendly and compliant with healthcare waste regulations.

For Organic & Biodegradable Waste, the system provides composting recommendations using predefined guidelines sourced from verified governmental and environmental organizations. These guidelines are filtered using a TF-IDF-based content matching approach, ensuring that the most relevant composting strategies are suggested. This method promotes sustainable practices by turning biodegradable waste into nutrient-rich compost, especially suitable for hospital gardens and green zones. When it comes to Recyclable & General Waste, the system employs the Tavily API for real-time web scraping to collect creative and practical DIY upcycling and recycling ideas. These suggestions are pulled from authoritative sources such as sustainability blogs, environmental agencies, and maker community websites. After collection, the system uses the Mistral 7B language model to summarize and structure these ideas into clear, actionable steps, enabling hospital staff to reuse or repurpose items effectively.

In the case of Contaminated Recyclable Waste, the system incorporates a contamination-level assessment module. For high-risk items—such as blood-stained personal protective equipment (PPE), used syringes, or contaminated plastics—it strictly follows ontology-based protocols aligned with biomedical waste disposal rules. For low-risk items, the system suggests decontamination and reuse methods using TF-IDF filtering, recommending cleaning procedures such as chemical neutralization or UV sterilization before reuse or recycling. For highly hazardous categories such as Sharps & Glassware and Infectious & Pathological Waste, the recommender system applies ontology-based filtering governed by regulatory bodies like the World Health Organization (WHO), the Occupational Safety and Health Administration (OSHA), and the Environmental Protection Agency (EPA). Recommended disposal methods include autoclaving, incineration, or secure landfilling, all of which are essential for reducing health risks and ensuring legal compliance in biomedical waste management.

To evaluate the recommender system's performance, its outputs were compared against expert-reviewed ground truths and regulatory guidelines. A recommendation was considered accurate if it complied with best practices for that waste type. As shown in Figure 7, the recommender system achieved a remarkable 97% accuracy across all waste categories. This high accuracy reflects the system's effectiveness in delivering reliable, actionable, and safe waste disposal strategies suitable for hospital environments.

C. Ultrasonic Sensor System

The ultrasonic sensor module is responsible for real-time monitoring of waste bin fill levels. Sensors were installed in multiple waste bins to detect volume and trigger timely alerts when bins approached maximum capacity.

The sensor system was evaluated for:

- Detection Accuracy
- Response Time
- False Positive/Negative Alerts

Experimental testing demonstrated a detection accuracy exceeding 96%, with near-instantaneous response times and minimal false alerts. This ensures that waste collection is optimized, reducing overflow risks and enhancing hygiene within hospital premises.

D. Overall System Effectiveness

The combined performance of the RWC-Net model, recommender system, and sensor infrastructure highlights the overall effectiveness of the Smart Waste Management System. Key achievements include:

- Accurate waste type classification (95.26% accuracy)
- Context-aware, high-accuracy recommendations (97% accuracy)
- Reliable real-time waste bin monitoring (>96% sensor accuracy)

The integration of AI, IoT, and rule-based knowledge systems enables end-to-end automation and insight generation, making the system a scalable and intelligent solution for hospital waste management. The system reduces manual intervention, minimizes risks, supports sustainability, and enhances operational efficiency.

SOLUTIONS AND RECOMMENDATIONS

The proposed AI-Driven Hospital Waste Management System introduces a range of practical solutions that address the critical needs of biomedical waste handling in hospital environments. These recommendations focus on enhancing safety, operational efficiency, sustainability, and regulatory compliance.

Ensuring Regulatory Compliance

The integration of AI and ontology-based reasoning ensures that hospitals adhere to biomedical waste disposal guidelines set by regulatory authorities such as WHO, OSHA, and EPA. The recommendation engine cross-verifies each classified waste type against these standards, generating safe and regulation-compliant disposal instructions. This automation helps hospitals minimize legal risks, avoid penalties, and standardize waste handling practices across departments.

Reducing Biohazard Risks and Environmental Impact

By using AI-based image classification and real-time sensor monitoring, the system significantly reduces human contact with hazardous biomedical waste. This minimizes the risk of infections and injuries while ensuring that harmful materials like sharps and pathological waste are isolated and treated appropriately. Moreover, the system supports environmentally responsible waste segregation and disposal, reducing landfill dependency and lowering greenhouse gas emissions through optimized collection and recycling recommendations.

Enhancing Operational Efficiency

The use of the RWC-Net model and IoT-enabled smart bins allows hospitals to automate waste classification and monitoring. This reduces the need for manual sorting, decreases human error, and improves the speed and accuracy of the waste handling process. Real-time alerts triggered by ultrasonic sensors help prevent overflows, ensuring timely waste collection. As a result, hospitals can optimize manpower usage, streamline workflows, and improve overall waste management efficiency.

Supporting Data-Driven Decision Making

All classification and recommendation outcomes are recorded in a centralized database, allowing hospital administrators to track performance, waste generation patterns, and compliance metrics. These insights support data-driven decision-making for waste policy improvement, resource allocation, and training programs for staff. The feedback mechanism incorporated into the system allows continuous improvement of AI models based on real-world data.

Promoting Sustainable Practices

The recommender system promotes sustainable practices through web scraping and content-based filtering. For recyclable waste, the system suggests upcycling and reuse ideas sourced from online sustainability platforms, while composting methods are provided for organic waste. These personalized and actionable recommendations encourage hospitals to adopt greener waste disposal habits and contribute to long-term environmental goals.

FUTURE RESEARCH DIRECTIONS

While the proposed system has demonstrated promising results in hospital waste management, several areas remain open for further research and development to enhance scalability, resilience, and effectiveness.

Improving Model Accuracy and Robustness

Although the RWC-Net model achieved high classification accuracy, future research could explore additional enhancements. This includes expanding the training dataset with more diverse, real-world biomedical waste images captured in various lighting, angles, and contamination conditions. Advanced data augmentation techniques and hyperparameter tuning can further improve model robustness and adaptability in unpredictable hospital environments.

Managing Complex Waste Scenarios

Real-world waste handling often involves mixed, unlabeled, or degraded waste materials that can challenge classification systems. Future work could focus on integrating multi-label classification techniques and anomaly detection algorithms to handle complex, ambiguous, or edge-case inputs. Additionally, research can explore semi-supervised learning methods to adapt to evolving waste patterns without requiring constant retraining.

Strengthening Cybersecurity and Data Privacy

As the system relies on AI, IoT, and cloud infrastructure, ensuring cybersecurity and data privacy becomes crucial. Future improvements could focus on implementing secure communication protocols, encrypted data transmission, and role-based access control to prevent unauthorized access and maintain data integrity. Blockchain-based auditing mechanisms could also be explored for secure record-keeping.

Enhancing IoT Integration and Monitoring

Current monitoring is limited to ultrasonic sensors for bin-level detection. Future research could include integrating RFID-based item tracking, camera-based object recognition, and real-time odor detection systems to provide more granular waste data. These sensors could improve traceability, support predictive maintenance, and enhance the accuracy of bin status reporting.

Multi-Hospital Deployment and Cloud Scalability

To support city-wide or regional healthcare networks, the system can be redesigned for cloud-based, multi-hospital deployment. A centralized dashboard could allow health administrators to monitor waste handling across multiple locations, compare compliance metrics, and optimize logistics. Research into scalable microservices architecture and federated learning models would support this vision without compromising local data privacy.

Expanding to Other Waste Domains

The current system is focused on biomedical waste, but the architecture can be extended to manage other complex waste types such as pharmaceutical, electronic (e-waste), or chemical waste. Domain-specific ontologies, datasets, and recommendation logic can be incorporated to make the system universally applicable in broader waste management contexts.

CONCLUSION

This chapter presented a comprehensive AI-Driven Hospital Waste Management System designed to address the growing need for efficient, safe, and regulation-compliant biomedical waste disposal in healthcare environments. The proposed solution integrates advanced technologies, including a CNN-based classification model (RWC-Net), a hybrid recommendation engine, and IoT-enabled monitoring components, to automate and optimize the waste handling process from detection to disposal. At the core of the system, the RWC-Net model—built upon MobileNetV2 and DenseNet121—achieved a high classification accuracy of 95.26%, effectively distinguishing between critical biomedical waste types such as infectious waste,s sharps, recyclables, and organics. This high performance ensures precise segregation, which is essential for minimizing contamination risks and adhering to healthcare regulations. Complementing the classification engine, the AI-powered recommender system demonstrated an accuracy of 97% in suggesting context-aware, regulation-compliant disposal methods. It combines ontology-based rules (aligned with WHO, EPA, and OSHA standards), TF-IDF filtering for compostable waste, and real-time web scraping (via Tavily API) to deliver tailored disposal or recycling suggestions. This enables hospitals to not only meet compliance goals but also adopt sustainable waste reduction strategies.

Further enhancing operational effectiveness, the integration of ultrasonic sensors and Raspberry Pi modules facilitated real-time bin monitoring, achieving over 96% accuracy in detecting fill levels. This automation supports timely alerts, reduces manual intervention, and prevents bin overflows, contributing to improved hygiene and resource optimization. Collectively, the system offers a robust and scalable framework that reduces biohazard exposure, supports eco-friendly waste handling, and streamlines hospital operations. By minimizing human error and enabling data-driven decision-making, the solution delivers tangible improvements in safety, compliance, and sustainability.Looking ahead, this AI-driven approach holds strong potential for expansion across multi-hospital networks, integration with more advanced IoT infrastructure, and adaptation for managing other complex waste types, such as electronic or chemical waste. Its modular architecture and adaptive learning capability make it a valuable asset for transforming biomedical waste management in smart hospitals and urban healthcare ecosystems.

REFERENCES

Ahmad, K., Khan, K., & Al-Fuqaha, A. (2020). Intelligent fusion of deep features for improved waste classification. *IEEE Access : Practical Innovations, Open Solutions*, *8*, 1–12. DOI: 10.1109/ACCESS.2020.2995681

Ayemowa, M. O., Ibrahim, R., & Khan, M. M. (2024). Analysis of recommender system using generative artificial intelligence: A systematic literature review. SSRN *Electronic Journal*, 1–20. DOI: 10.2139/ssrn.4922584

Hossen, M., Majid, E., Kashem, S. B. A., Khandakar, A., Nashbat, M., Ashraf, A., Hasan-Zia, M., Kunju, A. K. A., Kabir, S., & Chowdhury, M. E. H. (2024). A reliable and robust deep learning model for effective recyclable waste classification. *IEEE Access : Practical Innovations, Open Solutions*, *12*, 1–15. DOI: 10.1109/ACCESS.2024.3354774

Khouibiri, N., Farhaoui, Y., & Allaoui, A. (2023). Design and analysis of a recommendation system based on collaborative filtering techniques for big data. *Intelligent and Converged Networks*, *4*(4), 296–304. DOI: 10.23919/ICN.2023.0024

Pandey, S., Chouhan, V., Verma, D., Rajrah, S., Alenezi, F., Saini, R., & Santosh, K. C. (2022). Do-it-yourself recommender system: Reusing and recycling with blockchain and deep learning. *IEEE Access : Practical Innovations, Open Solutions*, *10*, 1–12. DOI: 10.1109/ACCESS.2022.3199661

Quan, M. K., Nguyen, D. C., Nguyen, V.-D., Wijayasundara, M., Setunge, S., & Pathirana, P. N. (2024). Toward privacy-preserving waste classification in the Internet of Things. *IEEE Internet of Things Journal*, *11*(14), 24814–24825. DOI: 10.1109/JIOT.2024.3386727

Sheng, T. J., Islam, M. S., Misran, N., Baharuddin, M. H., Arshad, H., Islam, M. R., Rmili, H., & Islam, M. T. (2020). An Internet of Things-based smart waste management system using LoRa and TensorFlow deep learning model. *IEEE Access : Practical Innovations, Open Solutions*, *8*, 1–12. DOI: 10.1109/ACCESS.2020.3016255

Sosunova, I., & Porras, J. (2022). IoT-enabled smart waste management systems for smart cities: A systematic review. *IEEE Access : Practical Innovations, Open Solutions*, *10*, 73326–73363. DOI: 10.1109/ACCESS.2022.3188308

ADDITIONAL READING

Al-Emran, M., Mezhuyev, V., & Kamaludin, A. (2020). Technology acceptance model in M-learning context: A systematic review. *Computers & Education, 144*, 103–108. DOI: 10.1016/j.compedu.2019.103108

Cheng, J. C. P., Tan, Y., Song, Y., & Mei, Z. (2021). Artificial intelligence and robotics in smart healthcare. *Journal of Healthcare Engineering, 2021*, 1–16. DOI: 10.1155/2021/5222745

Ferrero, F., & Galli, A. (2023). AI applications in sustainable waste management: Trends and future perspectives. *Waste Management (New York, N.Y.), 150*, 115–129. DOI: 10.1016/j.wasman.2023.01.007

Ghassemi, M., Naumann, T., Schulam, P., Beam, A. L., Chen, I. Y., & Ranganath, R. (2020). A review of challenges and opportunities in machine learning for health. *AMIA Joint Summits on Translational Science Proceedings AMIA Summit on Translational Science, 2020*, 191–200. PMID: 32477638

Khowaja, K., Qureshi, M. A., & Rizwan, M. (2022). Smart bins and sensor-based waste classification: A review of recent advances. *Sensors (Basel), 22*(8), 2956. DOI: 10.3390/s22082956 PMID: 35458942

KEY TERMS AND DEFINITIONS

Autoclaving: A process that sterilizes medical waste using high-pressure steam.

Biomedical Waste: Waste generated during medical treatments or labs, such as syringes, tissues, or PPE.

Incineration: A disposal method that burns waste at high temperature to destroy harmful materials.

Internet of Things: Devices like sensors and cameras connected to the internet.

Ontology-Based Filtering: Uses structured medical rules (like WHO) to recommend safe disposal.

Recommender System: A smart algorithm that suggests proper waste disposal methods based on type.

RWC-Net: A hybrid AI model combining MobileNetV2 and DenseNet121 for accurate waste classification.

Smart Bin: A bin with sensors and cameras to detect waste levels and trigger alerts.

Tavily API: A tool that scrapes websites for DIY disposal ideas and passes them to the LLM.

TF-IDF: A technique that ranks the importance of words to match composting or disposal ideas.

Chapter 12
Human-AI Collaboration in Healthcare:
The Evolving Role of Healthcare Professionals

Vasantha Gurusamy
https://orcid.org/0000-0002-4236-4641
Department of Acute and Tertiary Care Nursing, University of Pittsburgh, USA

Anandhavalli Muniasamy
https://orcid.org/0000-0001-8940-3954
Department of Informatics and Computer Systems, College of CS, King Khalid University, Saudi Arabia

Shruthi A. Gauthaman
https://orcid.org/0009-0007-5483-4683
Faculty of Medicine, Mahsa University, Malaysia

Hameed Abdulla
Faculty of Medicine, Mahsa University, Malaysia

ABSTRACT

Human-AI collaboration is transforming healthcare by enhancing clinical decision-making, optimizing workflows, and improving patient outcomes. This chapter explores the evolving role of healthcare professionals in an AI-driven environment, highlighting key AI technologies such as machine learning, natural language processing, and robotics. It examines AI's impact on diagnostics, treatment planning, and administrative efficiency. A case study demonstrates real-world AI integration in healthcare, showcasing benefits and challenges. Additionally, the chapter discusses

DOI: 10.4018/979-8-3373-2787-7.ch012

best practices for Human-AI collaboration, strategies for effective implementation, and ethical considerations. Finally, it explores future trends and innovations shaping AI-powered healthcare.

INTRODUCTION

The use of Artificial Intelligence (AI) technology is causing a significant shift in the healthcare industry. AI is influencing every aspect of hospital operations, from administrative process automation to robotic surgery, and from diagnostic imaging to patient monitoring. Although AI has the potential to increase healthcare delivery's accuracy, efficiency, and cost-effectiveness, its integration also reinterprets the conventional duties and responsibilities of healthcare professionals, necessitating a thorough evaluation and assessment of these AI-driven systems.

Figure 1 illustrates a bidirectional flow where "COLLABORATION" moves from the human to the AI, and "SUPPORT" flows back from the AI to the human, symbolizing mutual interaction. On the left, a healthcare professional icon is linked to a clipboard labeled "CARE," indicating the human role in providing compassionate, patient-centered treatment. On the right, an AI brain icon is connected to a monitor labeled "DATA ANALYSIS," representing the AI's role in processing and interpreting complex data. This interplay highlights how AI enhances decision-making while healthcare professionals maintain oversight and empathy in clinical care.

Figure 1. Healthcare Professional-AI Collaboration in Healthcare

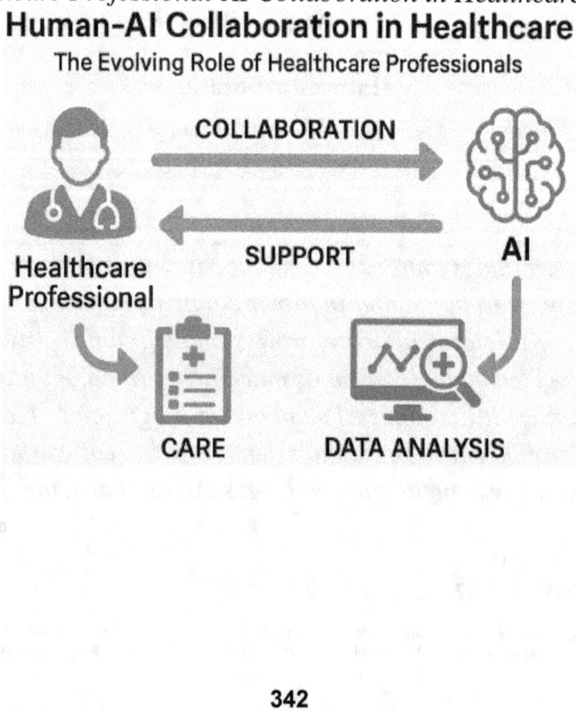

Hospital AI systems are no longer merely experimental. Clinical decision support systems (CDSS), electronic health records (EHRs), formulary management, intelligent resource scheduling, predictive analytics for patient deterioration, and population health analytics are all incorporating them more and more (Jiang et al., 2017). The widespread use of AI in clinical and non-clinical processes has made it crucial to thoroughly assess these systems in order to confirm their technical performance as well as their safety, equity, interpretability, and practical efficacy.

A key feature of contemporary hospital operations is the idea of human-AI collaboration, which emphasizes a partnership model in which AI supports medical workers rather than takes their place (Topol, 2019). This cooperative dynamic calls for the development of open, reliable AI systems that support institutional values, patient-centered care objectives, and medical ethics. Hospital AI evaluations must therefore consider usability, clinical acceptance, regulatory compliance, and organizational fit in addition to algorithmic accuracy.

The Changing Healthcare Landscape and the Integration of AI

These days, hospitals are intricate ecosystems of data-intensive operations, high-stakes decision-making, and interdisciplinary treatment. There are advantages and disadvantages to integrating AI systems in these kinds of settings. Machine learning algorithms, for example, have shown promise in aiding clinical triage (Esteva et al., 2019), enhancing radiological diagnostics (Ardila et al., 2019), and predicting sepsis (Nemati et al., 2018). In a similar vein, NLP-based AI solutions enable quicker diagnosis and treatment planning by extracting insights from unstructured data in EHRs (Rajkomar et al., 2019).

Additionally, administrative procedures are changing. By automating workforce planning, billing, appointment scheduling, and even compliance auditing, artificial intelligence (AI) systems lessen the workload for human employees and cut down on errors (Shickel et al., 2018). Additionally, by tracking drug usage patterns, predicting shortages, and suggesting cost-effective treatment regimes, AI helps with formulary formulation (Kwon et al., 2020).

Despite these developments, hospitals are still hesitant to use AI widely because of worries about unintended repercussions, system validation, and a lack of human-centered design. Furthermore, whereas pilot studies frequently show encouraging results, there is a dearth of evidence regarding their practical efficacy and long-term effects, underscoring the need for systematic assessment systems.

Difficulties in Assessing AI Systems in Healthcare Facilities

AI systems' dynamic nature, reliance on data, and adaptable algorithms set them apart from conventional therapeutic technology. Such systems are particularly difficult to evaluate for a number of reasons:

a. Absence of uniform assessment criteria

Algorithmic criteria including sensitivity, specificity, accuracy, and recall are the sole focus of many investigations (Rajpurkar et al., 2018). These, however, fall short in terms of therapeutic relevance, user experience, and operational performance. In addition to technical correctness, hospitals need a multifaceted evaluation methodology that takes into account workflow integration, clinician satisfaction, interpretability, and patient safety results.

b. Clinical Settings' Complexity and Heterogeneity

Hospital settings differ greatly amongst departments, organizations, and nations. Due to differences in data quality, coding conventions, and population health profiles, a predictive model developed in one institution may perform poorly when used in another (Kelly et al., 2019). The generalizability and benchmarking of AI evaluations are complicated by this heterogeneity.

c. Integrating workflow and human factors

The user experience is crucial since AI systems communicate directly with healthcare providers. Adoption can be hampered and mistakes can be caused by poorly designed interfaces, cognitive overload, and a lack of transparency (Blease et al., 2019). The integration of AI into the cognitive and procedural processes of clinicians must be evaluated.

d. Legal, Regulatory, and Ethical Considerations

Ethical issues including bias, justice, accountability, and data privacy are also relevant when evaluating AI in hospitals. For instance, research has demonstrated that when AI models are trained on skewed datasets, they may generate racially biased results (Obermeyer et al., 2019). Another level of complexity is added by legal compliance with laws like GDPR, HIPAA, and FDA requirements.

e. Feedback Cycles and Ongoing Education

AI applications can change over time through online learning or retraining, in contrast to static software systems (Abdullah et al. 2025). This begs the question of how to preserve system efficacy and safety after deployment. To facilitate continuous performance monitoring, the hospital infrastructure must incorporate ongoing evaluation methods (Wiens et al., 2019).

Considering how quickly innovation is happening, the field of AI evaluation in healthcare settings is still in its infancy. Few research thoroughly evaluate AI's performance or impact in the actual world, despite the fact that many studies demonstrate its promise. This limits uptake and erodes trust by separating clinical practitioners from AI engineers. The lack of comprehensive assessment frameworks that incorporate clinical, operational, human, and ethical aspects is one of the main research gaps.

- A small number of longitudinal studies that monitor the performance of AI systems over time and in various scenarios.
- Ignorance of the examination of human-AI interactions, including cognitive burden, user happiness, and trust.
- Few interdisciplinary viewpoints are included, and computer scientists, not physicians or managers of health systems, conduct the majority of evaluations.
- Inadequate comparison research evaluating several AI systems in various healthcare facilities.

Although regulatory agencies like the FDA and WHO have started to establish guidelines for evaluating AI, there isn't a widely recognized approach that is specific to the hospital setting (WHO, 2021). A multidisciplinary strategy incorporating concepts from computer science, behavioral science, healthcare administration, and bioethics is needed to close these gaps.

By offering a thorough method for analyzing and evaluating AI-driven systems in healthcare settings, this chapter aims to close the previously noted gaps. The main objective is to further the conversation around ethical, successful, and long-lasting human-AI cooperation in healthcare. Objectives of th chapter are as follows:

1. **To review the current landscape** of AI systems deployed in hospital environments, including clinical, administrative, and pharmaceutical domains.
2. **To examine the limitations of existing evaluation methodologies** and identify the key challenges in assessing AI in real-world hospital settings.
3. **To propose a multi-dimensional evaluation framework** that incorporates technical accuracy, clinical usability, operational efficiency, ethical compliance, and human factors.

4. **To analyze real-world case studies** illustrating both successful and unsuccessful deployments of AI in hospitals, and to extract practical insights from these experiences.
5. **To evaluate the role of healthcare professionals** in the AI evaluation process, highlighting the importance of clinician feedback, trust, and workflow alignment.
6. **To discuss ethical, legal, and regulatory implications** that must be addressed in any robust AI evaluation strategy.
7. **To suggest future research directions and policy recommendations** that support the sustainable integration of AI in hospitals through rigorous evaluation.

BACKGROUND

The many factors that must be taken into account when assessing AI-driven systems in healthcare settings are highlighted in this background section. It draws attention to the development of AI in healthcare, the need for thorough assessment frameworks, the difficulties in practical use, moral and legal issues, and the effects on medical personnel. The responsible and successful integration of AI technologies in hospitals depends on addressing these factors.

1. Evolution of AI in Healthcare

Artificial Intelligence (AI) has rapidly transitioned from theoretical constructs to practical applications within healthcare. Initially, AI's role was confined to data analysis and pattern recognition. However, advancements in machine learning and deep learning have expanded its utility to encompass diagnostic imaging, predictive analytics, and personalized treatment plans. For instance, AI algorithms are now capable of analyzing complex medical images, assisting radiologists in detecting anomalies with greater accuracy.

2. Necessity for Robust Evaluation Frameworks

The deployment of AI systems in hospitals necessitates rigorous evaluation to ensure safety, efficacy, and ethical compliance. Traditional evaluation metrics, primarily focusing on algorithmic accuracy, are insufficient in capturing the multifaceted impact of AI on clinical workflows and patient outcomes. Recognizing this gap, researchers have proposed comprehensive frameworks that assess AI systems across various dimensions.

One such framework is the Translational Evaluation of Healthcare AI (TEHAI), which emphasizes capability, utility, and adoption as core components for assessing

AI applications in healthcare (Abdullah et al. 2025). TEHAI advocates for evaluating AI systems not only during development but also throughout their lifecycle, ensuring continuous alignment with clinical needs and ethical standards.

3. Challenges in Real-World Implementation

Despite the promising potential of AI, its real-world implementation in hospitals is fraught with challenges. A significant concern is the degradation of AI performance over time, especially when confronted with unforeseen variables such as pandemics.

4. Ethical and Regulatory Considerations

The ethical deployment of AI in healthcare is paramount. Concerns regarding data privacy, algorithmic bias, and informed consent must be meticulously addressed. The implementation of AI systems should adhere to established ethical guidelines and regulatory standards to safeguard patient rights and maintain public trust.

5. Impact on Healthcare Professionals

The advent of AI in hospitals significantly influences the roles and responsibilities of healthcare professionals. While AI can augment clinical decision-making and reduce administrative burdens, it also necessitates new competencies among medical staff. Training programs must be developed to equip healthcare workers with the skills required to interact effectively with AI systems.

Furthermore, the integration of AI should be approached as a collaborative endeavor, where human expertise and machine intelligence complement each other. This synergy ensures that AI serves as a tool to enhance, rather than replace, the critical thinking and empathy inherent in human caregivers.

HUMAN-AI COLLABORATION IN HEALTHCARE

The integration of Artificial Intelligence (AI) into healthcare has transformed clinical practices, enabling enhanced diagnostic accuracy, personalized treatment plans, and efficient patient management. Human-AI collaboration leverages the strengths of both entities—AI's computational prowess and humans' contextual understanding—to improve healthcare outcomes. This section explores various AI models facilitating this collaboration, their implementation in hospital settings, and real-world case studies demonstrating their efficacy.

AI Models Facilitating Human-AI Collaboration

Machine Learning Models

a. Supervised Learning Models

Supervised learning models, such as Support Vector Machines (SVM), Random Forests, and Gradient Boosting Machines, are trained on labeled datasets to predict outcomes. In healthcare, these models assist in disease diagnosis, risk stratification, and treatment recommendations. For instance, SVMs have been employed to classify medical images, aiding radiologists in detecting anomalies.

b. Unsupervised Learning Models

Unsupervised learning models identify patterns in unlabeled data. Clustering algorithms like K-Means and Hierarchical Clustering are utilized to segment patient populations, facilitating personalized care plans. These models help in understanding disease subtypes and patient stratification without prior labeling.

c. Reinforcement Learning Models

Reinforcement Learning (RL) models learn optimal actions through trial and error, receiving feedback from the environment. In healthcare, RL has been applied to optimize treatment strategies, such as determining the best sequence of interventions for chronic disease management (Alasmari et al. 2025; Muniasamy et al, 2025).

Deep Learning Models

Deep Learning models, particularly Convolutional Neural Networks (CNNs) and Recurrent Neural Networks (RNNs), have shown remarkable performance in processing complex healthcare data (Karunakaran et al., 2026; Abdullah et al. 2025; Karunakaran et al. 2021; Bhatnagar et al., 2021).

a. Convolutional Neural Networks (CNNs)

CNNs are adept at analyzing visual data, making them invaluable in medical imaging. They assist in detecting tumors, fractures, and other anomalies in radiographs, MRIs, and CT scans (Asiri et al., 2025; Sabahath et al, 2024).

b. Recurrent Neural Networks (RNNs)

RNNs, including Long Short-Term Memory (LSTM) networks, are effective in handling sequential data. They are used in monitoring patient vitals over time, predicting disease progression, and managing electronic health records (EHRs).

Natural Language Processing (NLP) Models

NLP models process and interpret unstructured textual data. They extract meaningful information from clinical notes, patient narratives, and research articles. Models like Bidirectional Encoder Representations from Transformers (BERT) have been fine-tuned for medical texts, enhancing information retrieval and decision support.

Hybrid Models

Hybrid models combine different AI approaches to leverage their respective strengths. For example, integrating CNNs with RNNs enables the analysis of both spatial and temporal data, providing a comprehensive understanding of patient conditions [.

Integration of AI Models Into Healthcare Workflows

The successful implementation of AI models in hospitals requires seamless integration into existing workflows (Rengaramanujam et al. 2026). This involves:

- Data Acquisition and Preprocessing: Collecting high-quality data from various sources, including EHRs, imaging systems, and laboratory results, followed by cleaning and normalization.
- Model Training and Validation: Developing AI models using training datasets and validating their performance on unseen data to ensure accuracy and generalizability.
- Deployment and Monitoring: Integrating AI models into clinical systems, ensuring they function effectively in real-time environments, and continuously monitoring their performance.
- Feedback Mechanisms: Establishing channels for healthcare professionals to provide feedback on AI outputs, facilitating model refinement and trust-building.

Figure 2. Human-AI Collaboration Workflow in Clinical Decision Making

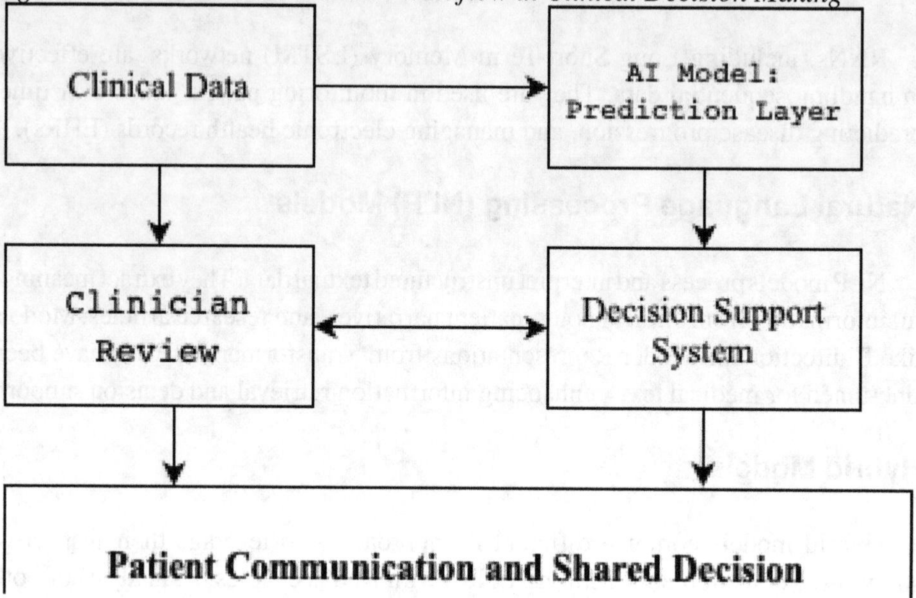

Figure 2 illustrates the dynamic workflow of human-AI collaboration in clinical decision-making, emphasizing an iterative and transparent interaction between artificial intelligence systems and healthcare professionals. The process begins with the input of clinical data—such as patient histories, imaging results, or lab reports—into an AI model that functions as a prediction layer, generating diagnostic suggestions or treatment options. These outputs are not final decisions but serve as decision support, which are then reviewed by clinicians who assess the AI recommendations in the context of patient-specific nuances and professional expertise. A bi-directional feedback loop is established between the clinician and the AI-driven decision support system, allowing real-time refinements and learning from human inputs. Once validated, the clinician communicates the outcome to the patient, integrating both AI insights and human judgment into a shared decision-making framework. This collaborative approach enhances accuracy, fosters trust, and ensures that AI augments rather than replaces human expertise in healthcare settings. A feedback-enabled model where AI recommendations are reviewed, modified, and communicated by healthcare professionals.

Case Studies

1. Case Study 1: SepsisLab – Enhancing Sepsis Diagnosis

SepsisLab is an AI-powered tool designed to support clinicians in the early diagnosis of sepsis. It provides risk predictions, suggests additional laboratory tests, and visualizes prediction uncertainties. [Zhang, S, 2023].The system integrates into the EHR, offering real-time support during the diagnostic process. It emphasizes collaboration by allowing clinicians to interact with the AI, refining predictions based on additional data. SepsisLab improved diagnostic accuracy and clinician confidence in managing sepsis cases. It exemplifies effective human-AI collaboration by enhancing decision-making without replacing clinical judgment.

2. Case Study 2: AI Assistance in Colonoscopy

AI systems have been developed to assist during colonoscopies by detecting polyps in real-time, addressing cognitive bottlenecks in perception and attention. [PubMed., 2023].These systems analyze video feeds during procedures, highlighting potential polyps for the endoscopist to review, thereby reducing the likelihood of missed lesions. The integration of AI led to increased polyp detection rates and improved procedural efficiency, demonstrating the benefits of augmenting human capabilities with AI support.

3. Case Study 3: Doctronic – AI Agents for Medical Information

Doctronic developed AI agents to provide personalized medical information, aiming to replace generic online searches with accurate, tailored responses (Business Insider, 2025). Users input symptoms and receive possible diagnoses and action plans, with options for real-time consultations with medical professionals. The AI employs a multi-agent framework, where specialized agents assess different medical areas and collaborate to provide comprehensive information. The platform attracted approximately 50,000 weekly users, indicating a strong demand for AI-assisted medical information. It showcases the potential of AI in enhancing patient engagement and access to healthcare resources.

SOLUTIONS AND RECOMMENDATIONS

The successful deployment of AI-driven systems in hospitals depends not only on technological innovation but also on thoughtful integration within the clinical environment. The following recommendations aim to address the key challenges of human-AI collaboration and enable meaningful, responsible, and sustainable AI adoption in healthcare. This section is grounded in evidence-based practices and global case examples.

1. Governance and Trust Frameworks Develop Transparent and Interpretable AI Systems

One of the critical barriers to AI adoption in clinical settings is the "black-box" nature of many AI models. Hospitals must invest in interpretable machine learning models that allow clinicians to trace decisions and outcomes (Murdoch et al., 2019). Approaches such as SHAP (SHapley Additive exPlanations) and LIME (Local Interpretable Model-agnostic Explanations) help clinicians understand how AI arrives at predictions, increasing trust and accountability. Institutional Ethics Boards for AI: Hospitals should form AI-specific ethics review boards to evaluate algorithms for fairness, safety, and compliance before deployment. These boards can act as intermediaries between developers and clinical staff, fostering trust (Morley et al., 2020).

2. Workforce Development and Capacity Building AI Literacy in Medical Curriculum

Integrating AI education into undergraduate and postgraduate medical training can prepare future healthcare professionals for collaborative environments. AI literacy includes understanding basic AI principles, algorithmic limitations, and ethical considerations (Masters, 2019). Interdisciplinary Training: Hospitals should encourage cross-disciplinary learning by organizing collaborative workshops between data scientists, clinicians, and administrators. For example, the Mayo Clinic has successfully implemented AI integration programs that pair data scientists with radiologists and pathologists for real-time collaboration (Ghassemi et al., 2021).

3. Workflow and System Integration Human-in-the-Loop Models

Rather than replacing clinicians, AI should support decision-making through human-in-the-loop (HITL) models, where AI provides suggestions while clinicians retain final authority. This model aligns well with diagnostic radiology and pathology, where AI can pre-screen images or flag anomalies for review (Amann et al., 2020). Real-Time Feedback Loops: Establishing feedback mechanisms between AI outputs and clinician decisions enables continuous improvement of algorithms. Systems should be designed to capture clinician overrides and adjustments to retrain models effectively (Rajpurkar et al., 2022).

4. Ethical and Regulatory Recommendations Inclusive AI Design

AI models must be developed using demographically representative datasets to prevent bias. This includes accounting for age, race, gender, and comorbidities (Char et al., 2018). Failure to do so may result in systemic disparities in treatment recommendations. Cross-border Regulatory Harmonization: There is a growing need for international AI governance in healthcare. Organizations like the World Health Organization (WHO) and the Global Digital Health Partnership are developing global standards to support safe AI deployment across borders (WHO, 2021).

5. Technical Infrastructure and Interoperability Cloud and Edge Computing for AI Workflows

Hospitals should utilize a hybrid infrastructure that combines cloud computing for large-scale model training with edge computing for real-time inference near the patient (Razzak et al., 2019). This approach balances performance with data privacy concerns. Use of Standardized APIs: To improve interoperability, AI solutions must adhere to standard APIs such as HL7 FHIR (Fast Healthcare Interoperability Resources), which support seamless communication between AI modules and electronic health records (Maddox et al., 2019).

6. Patient-Centered AI Systems Transparency in AI-Generated Decisions

Patients should be informed when AI systems are used in their care. User-friendly summaries of AI recommendations must be included in patient reports to support shared decision-making (Gerke et al., 2020). Tailored AI Solutions for Vulnerable Populations: Designing AI models that are sensitive to the needs of elderly, rural, and low-income populations ensures broader access to quality care. For instance, wearable AI technologies have proven effective in remote monitoring of elderly patients with chronic diseases (Topol, 2019). AI-driven systems hold transformative potential in modern healthcare, but their success depends on more than algorithmic power. Ethical considerations, workforce readiness, regulatory oversight, and infrastructural capabilities must converge to ensure these technologies enhance—not hinder—the care experience. By implementing the solutions and recommendations provided, healthcare institutions can move toward a more collaborative and effective human-AI ecosystem.

FUTURE RESEARCH DIRECTIONS

The continuous evolution of artificial intelligence (AI) technologies in healthcare necessitates an adaptive research agenda that can accommodate the dynamic nature of human-AI collaboration. As healthcare systems become increasingly digitized and reliant on intelligent systems, it becomes imperative to examine not only the technological innovations but also the human, ethical, legal, and organizational dimensions that will shape the future of AI-driven healthcare. This section outlines key research directions that can support the safe, equitable, and effective integration of AI in hospitals, with a focus on the evolving roles of healthcare professionals.

- **Human-Centered AI Design and Explainability**

One of the most critical areas for future research involves designing AI systems that prioritize human-centered values, including explainability, transparency, and usability. Although much progress has been made in interpretable machine learning, existing models often fail to present insights in ways that are meaningful to non-technical users. Future research must investigate how to create contextualized explainability tailored to different roles in the clinical workflow—from physicians to nurses and administrative staff.

Advancements in multimodal explainability, which combine visual, textual, and statistical cues, can help diverse stakeholders understand AI recommendations (Challen, Denny, Pitt, Gompels, Edwards, & Tsaneva-Atanasova, 2019). Research into user-friendly interfaces, human factors engineering, and trust calibration will be essential to building systems that professionals can confidently adopt in high-stakes environments.

- **Co-Evolution of AI Systems and Clinical Practice**

As AI becomes more embedded in clinical operations, it will inevitably influence medical protocols, diagnostic criteria, and treatment pathways. Researchers should explore the co-evolution of AI systems and clinical practice, investigating how continuous feedback loops between humans and machines impact medical norms, workflows, and outcomes over time.

Longitudinal studies are needed to understand the cognitive, behavioral, and professional shifts that occur when clinicians interact with AI systems over extended periods. This research will be instrumental in developing adaptive AI systems that learn not only from data but also from clinician preferences and evolving medical knowledge (Saria, Butte, & Sheikh, 2021).

- **AI-Augmented Education and Professional Development**

Healthcare education must adapt to the realities of AI-enhanced practice. Future research should examine how AI can be integrated into the education and continuous professional development of healthcare workers. AI tutors, simulation platforms, and intelligent learning management systems have the potential to personalize learning experiences and identify knowledge gaps in real time.

Moreover, studies should explore the psychological impacts of working alongside AI on clinical identity, autonomy, and decision-making. How professionals perceive their evolving role in an AI-integrated healthcare system will be critical for retention and job satisfaction (van Wynsberghe, 2021).

- **Fairness, Equity, and Bias Mitigation**

Another urgent research direction lies in the development of methodologies to detect, assess, and mitigate bias in AI systems. While technical solutions like adversarial debiasing and re-weighting algorithms exist, they must be complemented by socio-technical investigations that consider historical and institutional biases embedded in health data.

Future research must also address equity in access to AI technologies. Rural, low-income, and marginalized communities often lack the infrastructure to benefit from AI-driven care. Investigating the barriers to adoption in these settings, as well as designing culturally competent AI solutions, is essential for reducing health disparities (Rajkomar, Hardt, Howell, Corrado, & Chin, 2018).

- **Legal, Ethical, and Policy Frameworks**

AI integration into hospitals raises profound legal and ethical questions. Future research should work toward establishing adaptive policy frameworks that can evolve with technological advancements. Key areas include data privacy, consent, liability in AI-supported decision-making, and intellectual property rights over AI-generated insights.

Collaborative studies between legal scholars, ethicists, technologists, and clinicians can generate robust frameworks for AI governance. Moreover, comparative international studies can provide valuable insights into best practices across regulatory regimes (Yeung, Howes, & Pogrebna, 2020).

- **Resilience and Robustness of AI Systems**

The COVID-19 pandemic underscored the need for resilient healthcare systems. Future research should prioritize the robustness of AI models under stress conditions such as pandemics, disasters, or cybersecurity threats. Robustness testing, stress simulations, and adversarial validation must become integral to AI development.

AI systems must also be resilient to data drift—a phenomenon where real-world data changes over time, leading to model degradation. Research into automated model monitoring, retraining protocols, and federated learning systems will be crucial to maintaining performance in dynamic environments (Wynants et al., 2020).

- **Evaluation Metrics and Benchmarking Standards**

Despite the proliferation of AI tools, there is a lack of standardized metrics to evaluate their clinical utility, safety, and impact. Future research should focus on defining robust evaluation frameworks that go beyond accuracy to include interpretability, usability, fairness, and integration with workflows.

Benchmarking initiatives, such as publicly accessible datasets and standardized challenge tasks, can help researchers and developers compare performance across models. Cross-disciplinary collaborations will be essential in formulating metrics that resonate with clinical realities (Kelly, Karthikesalingam, Suleyman, Corrado, & King, 2019).

- **Sociotechnical Systems and Organizational Readiness**

Hospitals are complex sociotechnical systems where people, technologies, and organizational cultures interact in unpredictable ways. Research must take a systems-level approach to understand how organizational readiness, culture, and leadership influence AI adoption.

Qualitative and ethnographic methods can uncover the tacit dynamics that affect implementation, such as professional resistance, interdepartmental conflicts, or workflow mismatches. Studies should also evaluate the effectiveness of change management strategies and leadership models in promoting AI readiness (Greenhalgh, Wherton, Papoutsi, Lynch, & Hughes, 2017).

- **Human-AI Teaming Models and Role Reconfiguration**

Human-AI teaming requires clear definitions of responsibilities, boundaries, and escalation protocols. Future research should explore optimal teaming configurations, including task allocation, communication strategies, and decision arbitration mechanisms.

Simulation studies and real-world pilots can help determine the best practices for shared decision-making between humans and AI. Moreover, adaptive models where AI learns from human corrections and clinicians learn from AI suggestions should be a key focus (Gunning & Aha, 2019).

- **Sustainability and Environmental Impact**

With the increasing computational demands of training AI models, especially large-scale deep learning systems, there is a growing concern about the environmental footprint of AI in healthcare. Future research should investigate energy-efficient model architectures, sustainable data storage practices, and carbon offset strategies for AI development.

Life cycle assessments of AI applications in healthcare can provide insights into resource utilization and guide the development of eco-conscious AI tools (Strubell, Ganesh, & McCallum, 2019).

The future of human-AI collaboration in healthcare is both promising and complex. To navigate this terrain effectively, research must evolve to encompass not just technical sophistication but also human values, organizational behavior, and societal impact. The recommendations outlined in this section offer a comprehensive agenda for multi-disciplinary research that can inform the next generation of AI-integrated healthcare systems. By embracing these directions, the medical community can ensure that AI becomes a force for equitable, efficient, and ethically sound healthcare.

CONCLUSION

The integration of artificial intelligence (AI) into hospital systems represents a transformative moment in modern healthcare, fundamentally altering the roles and workflows of healthcare professionals. This chapter provided a comprehensive exploration of AI-driven systems with a specific focus on human-AI collaboration. Through detailed sections on background, technical frameworks, AI models, case studies, and proposed solutions, the chapter highlighted how AI can augment clinical decision-making, improve operational efficiency, and enhance patient outcomes. It emphasized that successful AI implementation depends not only on technological advancement but also on strategic planning, ethical governance, and the active participation of clinicians in the design and deployment processes.

Looking ahead, the chapter proposed a forward-thinking research agenda to guide the responsible evolution of human-AI teaming in healthcare. Topics such as explainable AI, clinician education, bias mitigation, legal frameworks, and sustainability are critical to developing robust and equitable AI systems. Ultimately, the goal is not to replace human expertise but to empower it—creating collaborative systems where AI supports, rather than supplants, clinical judgment. As healthcare continues to evolve, ensuring the safe, fair, and ethical deployment of AI technologies will be essential to preserving the human-centered values that lie at the core of medical practice.

REFERENCES

Abdullah, R. M., Saad, L. A., Alasmari, Z. M., Ali, G. A., & Muniasamy, A. (2025). Human disease prediction mobile application using machine learning. In Alareeni, B., & Hamdan, A. (Eds.), *IoT and digital transformation: Innovating business models for the connected world (ICBT 2024). Lecture notes in networks and systems* (Vol. 1575). Springer. DOI: 10.1007/978-3-032-00450-5_19

Alasmari, A., & Muniasamy, A. (2025). Integrating Bayesian and convolution neural network for uncertainty estimation of cataract from fundus images. *Computer Modeling in Engineering & Sciences, 143*(1), 569–592. DOI: 10.32604/cmes.2025.060484

Amann, J., Blasimme, A., Vayena, E., Frey, D., & Madai, V. I. (2020). Explainability for artificial intelligence in healthcare: A multidisciplinary perspective. *BMC Medical Informatics and Decision Making, 20*(1), 1–9. DOI: 10.1186/s12911-020-01332-6

Ardila, D., Kiraly, A. P., Bharadwaj, S., Choi, B., Reicher, J. J., Peng, L., Tse, D., Etemadi, M., Ye, W., Corrado, G., Naidich, D. P., & Shetty, S. (2019). End-to-end lung cancer screening with three-dimensional deep learning on low-dose chest computed tomography. *Nature Medicine, 25*(6), 954–961. DOI: 10.1038/s41591-019-0447-x

Asiri, F., & Muniasamy, A. (2025). Advanced human activity recognition on wearables with multi-scale sparse attention. *Multimedia Tools and Applications, 84*(30), 36623–36652. Advance online publication. DOI: 10.1007/s11042-024-20475-6

Begum, A., Muniasamy, A., Sabahath, A., Yaqub, H., & Karunakaran, G. (2024). Coronary heart disease classification using deep learning approach with feature selection for improved accuracy. *Technology and Health Care, 32*(3), 1991–2007. DOI: 10.3233/THC-231807

Bhatnagar, R., Muniasamy, A., & Karunakaran, G. (2021). Predicting COVID-19 spread in Saudi Arabia using artificial intelligence techniques—Proposing a shift towards a sustainable healthcare approach. In Hassanien, A., Bhatnagar, R., & Darwish, A. (Eds.), *Artificial intelligence for sustainable development: Theory, practice and future applications. Studies in computational intelligence* (Vol. 912). Springer. DOI: 10.1007/978-3-030-51920-9_6

Bhatnagar, R., Muniasamy, A., & Muniasamy, V. (2021). Predictive analytics for cardiovascular disease diagnosis using machine learning techniques. In Hassanien, A., Bhatnagar, R., & Darwish, A. (Eds.), *Advanced machine learning technologies and applications (AMLTA 2020). Advances in intelligent systems and computing* (Vol. 1141). Springer. DOI: 10.1007/978-981-15-3383-9_45

Blease, C., Kharko, A., Bernstein, M. H., Gaab, J., Kaptchuk, T. J., & DesRoches, C. M. (2019). Artificial intelligence and the future of primary care: Exploratory qualitative study of UK general practitioners' views. *Journal of Medical Internet Research, 21*(3), e12802. DOI: 10.2196/12802

Business Insider. (2025). *Check out the exclusive 11-slide pitch deck startup Doctronic used to raise $5 million for its AI agents to replace 'Dr. Google*. Author.

Char, D. S., Shah, N. H., & Magnus, D. (2018). Implementing machine learning in health care—Addressing ethical challenges. *The New England Journal of Medicine, 378*(11), 981–983. DOI: 10.1056/NEJMp1714229

Esteva, A., Robicquet, A., Ramsundar, B., Kuleshov, V., DePristo, M., Chou, K., Cui, C., Corrado, G., Thrun, S., & Dean, J. (2019). A guide to deep learning in healthcare. *Nature Medicine, 25*(1), 24–29. DOI: 10.1038/s41591-018-0316-z

Gerke, S., Minssen, T., & Cohen, G. (2020). Ethical and legal challenges of artificial intelligence-driven healthcare. *Cambridge Quarterly of Healthcare Ethics, 29*(1), 67–82.

Ghassemi, M., Oakden-Rayner, L., & Beam, A. L. (2021). The false hope of current approaches to explainable artificial intelligence in health care. *The Lancet. Digital Health, 3*(11), e745–e750. DOI: 10.1016/S2589-7500(21)00208-9

Greenhalgh, T., Wherton, J., Papoutsi, C., Lynch, J., Hughes, G., A'Court, C., Hinder, S., Fahy, N., Procter, R., & Shaw, S. (2017). Beyond adoption: A new framework for theorizing and evaluating nonadoption, abandonment, and challenges to the scale-up, spread, and sustainability of health and care technologies. *Journal of Medical Internet Research, 19*(11), e367. DOI: 10.2196/jmir.8775

Gunning, D., & Aha, D. (2019). DARPA's Explainable Artificial Intelligence (XAI) Program. *AI Magazine, 40*(2), 44–58. DOI: 10.1609/aimag.v40i2.2850

Jiang, F., Jiang, Y., Zhi, H., Dong, Y., Li, H., Ma, S., Wang, Y., Dong, Q., Shen, H., & Wang, Y. (2017). Artificial intelligence in healthcare: Past, present and future. *Stroke and Vascular Neurology, 2*(4), 230–243. DOI: 10.1136/svn-2017-000101

Karunakaran, G., & Muniasamy, A. (2026). Challenges and future directions: Emerging trends and limitations in ML and optimization for healthcare. In Muniasamy, A. (Ed.), *Integrative machine learning and optimization algorithms for disease prediction* (pp. 339–368). IGI Global. DOI: 10.4018/979-8-3373-1087-9.ch012

Kelly, C. J., Karthikesalingam, A., Suleyman, M., Corrado, G., & King, D. (2019). Key challenges for delivering clinical impact with artificial intelligence. *BMC Medicine, 17*(1), 195. DOI: 10.1186/s12916-019-1426-2

Kwon, J. M., Kim, K. H., Jeon, K. H., & Lee, S. Y. (2020). A machine learning algorithm to predict hypokalemia in patients using routine blood tests and ECGs. *Journal of Electrocardiology, 59*, 95–100. DOI: 10.1016/j.jelectrocard.2020.01.002

Maddox, T. M., Rumsfeld, J. S., & Payne, P. R. (2019). Questions for artificial intelligence in health care. *Journal of the American Medical Association, 321*(1), 31–32. DOI: 10.1001/jama.2018.18932

Masters, K. (2019). Artificial intelligence in medical education. *Medical Teacher, 41*(9), 976–980. DOI: 10.1080/0142159X.2019.1595557

Morley, J., Machado, C. C., Burr, C., Cowls, J., Joshi, I., Taddeo, M., & Floridi, L. (2020). The ethics of AI in health care: A mapping review. *Social Science & Medicine, 260*, 113172. DOI: 10.1016/j.socscimed.2020.113172

Muniasamy, A. (2025). Revolutionizing health monitoring: Integrating transformer models with multi-head attention for precise human activity recognition using wearable devices. *Technology and Health Care, 33*(1), 395–409. DOI: 10.3233/THC-241064

Murdoch, W. J., Singh, C., Kumbier, K., Abbasi-Asl, R., & Yu, B. (2019). Definitions, methods, and applications in interpretable machine learning. *Proceedings of the National Academy of Sciences of the United States of America, 116*(44), 22071–22080. DOI: 10.1073/pnas.1900654116

Nemati, S., Holder, A., Razmi, F., Stanley, M. D., Clifford, G. D., & Buchman, T. G. (2018). An interpretable machine learning model for accurate prediction of sepsis in the ICU. *Critical Care Medicine, 46*(4), 547–553. DOI: 10.1097/CCM.0000000000002936

Obermeyer, Z., Powers, B., Vogeli, C., & Mullainathan, S. (2019). Dissecting racial bias in an algorithm used to manage the health of populations. *Science, 366*(6464), 447–453. DOI: 10.1126/science.aax2342

PubMed. (2023). Enhancing human-AI collaboration: The case of colonoscopy. *PubMed ID: 37940501.*

Rajkomar, A., Dean, J., & Kohane, I. (2019). Machine learning in medicine. *The New England Journal of Medicine, 380*(14), 1347–1358. DOI: 10.1056/NEJMra1814259

Rajkomar, A., Hardt, M., Howell, M. D., Corrado, G., & Chin, M. H. (2018). Ensuring fairness in machine learning to advance health equity. *Annals of Internal Medicine, 169*(12), 866–872. DOI: 10.7326/M18-1990

Rajpurkar, P., Chen, E., Banerjee, O., & Topol, E. J. (2022). AI in health and medicine. *Nature Medicine, 28*(1), 31–38. DOI: 10.1038/s41591-021-01614-0

Rajpurkar, P., Irvin, J., Ball, R. L., Zhu, K., Yang, B., Mehta, H., & Ng, A. Y. (2018). Deep learning for chest radiograph diagnosis: A retrospective comparison of the CheXNeXt algorithm to practicing radiologists. *PLoS Medicine*, *15*(11), e1002686. DOI: 10.1371/journal.pmed.1002686

Razzak, M. I., Imran, M., & Xu, G. (2019). Big data analytics for preventive medicine. *Neural Computing & Applications*, *32*(9), 4417–4451. DOI: 10.1007/s00521-019-04095-y

Rengaramanujam, K., & Muniasamy, A. (2026). AI in hospital administration and formulary design: Optimizing resource allocation and patient flow. In Muniasamy, A., & Karunakaran, G. (Eds.), *Applications of artificial intelligence in pharmaceuticals* (pp. 215–246). IGI Global. DOI: 10.4018/979-8-3373-2043-4.ch008

Sabahath, A., Muniasamy, A., Begum, A., Yaqub, H., & Karunakaran, G. (2023). Lung cancer histopathology image classification using transfer learning with convolution neural network model. *Technology and Health Care*, *33*, 1–12. https://content.iospress.com/articles/technology-and-health-care/thc231029

Saria, S., Butte, A., & Sheikh, A. (2021). Better medicine through machine learning: What's real, and what's artificial? *PLoS Medicine*, *18*(3), e1002721.

Shickel, B., Tighe, P. J., Bihorac, A., & Rashidi, P. (2018). Deep EHR: A survey of recent advances in deep learning techniques for electronic health record (EHR) analysis. *IEEE Journal of Biomedical and Health Informatics*, *22*(5), 1589–1604. DOI: 10.1109/JBHI.2017.2767063

Strubell, E., Ganesh, A., & McCallum, A. (2019). Energy and policy considerations for deep learning in NLP. *Proceedings of the 57th Annual Meeting of the Association for Computational Linguistics*, 3645-3650. DOI: 10.18653/v1/P19-1355

Topol, E. (2019). *Deep medicine: How artificial intelligence can make healthcare human again*. Basic Books.

van Wynsberghe, A. (2021). Sustainable AI: AI for sustainability and the sustainability of AI. *AI and Ethics*, *1*(3), 213–218. DOI: 10.1007/s43681-021-00043-6

Wiens, J., Saria, S., Sendak, M., Ghassemi, M., Liu, V. X., Doshi-Velez, F., Jung, K., Heller, K., Kale, D., Saeed, M., Ossorio, P. N., Thadaney-Israni, S., & Goldenberg, A. (2019). Do no harm: A roadmap for responsible machine learning for health care. *Nature Medicine*, *25*(9), 1337–1340. DOI: 10.1038/s41591-019-0548-6

World Health Organization (WHO). (2021). *Ethics and governance of artificial intelligence for health: WHO guidance*. https://www.who.int/publications/i/item/9789240029200

Wynants, L., Van Calster, B., Bonten, M. M., Collins, G. S., Debray, T. P., De Vos, M., & Damen, J. A. (2020). Prediction models for diagnosis and prognosis of COVID-19 infection: Systematic review and critical appraisal. *BMJ (Clinical Research Ed.), 369*, m1328. DOI: 10.1136/bmj.m1328

Yeung, K., Howes, A., & Pogrebna, G. (2020). AI governance by human rights-centric design. *Nature Machine Intelligence*, *2*(1), 1–3.

Zhang, S., Yu, J., & Xu, X. (2023). Rethinking Human-AI Collaboration in Complex Medical Decision Making: A Case Study in Sepsis Diagnosis. *arXiv preprint arXiv:2309.12368.*

ADDITIONAL READING

Kwon, J. M., Lee, H., & Lee, J. S. (2020). Impact of artificial intelligence on clinical decision-making and healthcare outcomes: A systematic review. *Journal of Medical Systems*, *44*(7), 1–10. DOI: 10.1007/s10916-020-01593-2

Rajkomar, A., Oren, E., Chen, K., Dai, A. M., & Hajialiasghari, F. (2020). Scalable and accurate deep learning for electronic health records. *npj. Digital Medicine*, *3*(1), 1–8. DOI: 10.1038/s41746-020-0251-3

Shickel, B., Tighe, P. J., Bihorac, A., & Rashidi, P. (2018). Deep EHR: A survey of deep learning in electronic health records. *IEEE Journal of Biomedical and Health Informatics*, *22*(5), 1589–1604. DOI: 10.1109/JBHI.2017.2767063

Yim, W., & Lee, J. (2020). The role of artificial intelligence in healthcare innovation: Policy challenges and opportunities. *Journal of Health Policy and Management*, *35*(4), 29–41. DOI: 10.1016/j.hpm.2020.05.002

KEY TERMS AND DEFINITIONS

Adaptive AI: AI systems that evolve over time by continuously learning from new data and human interactions, thereby improving accuracy and usefulness.

Benchmarking: The practice of comparing AI models against standardized datasets and evaluation metrics to assess their performance across various tasks.

Bias in AI: Systematic and unfair discrimination in algorithmic decisions due to imbalanced or flawed data used in training the AI models.

Clinical Decision Support System (CDSS): A health information technology system designed to assist healthcare providers in making clinical decisions by leveraging data-driven algorithms and patient information.

Clinical Workflow: The series of interconnected tasks and procedures performed by healthcare professionals to deliver patient care.

Data Drift: A phenomenon where the statistical properties of input data change over time, potentially degrading model performance if not addressed.

Ethical AI: The development and use of AI technologies that align with moral principles, including fairness, accountability, privacy, and transparency.

Explainable AI (XAI): AI systems designed with transparency in mind, allowing users to understand how decisions are made, thereby enhancing trust and accountability.

Federated Learning: A machine learning technique that trains an algorithm across multiple decentralized devices or servers holding local data samples without exchanging them, enhancing data privacy.

Health Informatics: The interdisciplinary field that uses information technology to organize and analyze health records to improve healthcare outcomes.

Human-AI Collaboration: A working model where human professionals and AI systems interact and complement each other's strengths in decision-making, diagnosis, and treatment planning.

Human-Centered Design (HCD): A design philosophy that places the needs, limitations, and behavior of human users at the center of the technology development process.

Resilience in AI Systems: The ability of AI technologies to maintain performance and recover quickly from disruptions such as data drift, adversarial attacks, or system failures.

Role Reconfiguration: The adjustment of job responsibilities and workflows among healthcare professionals as a result of AI integration into healthcare settings.

Sociotechnical Systems: Systems that consider the complex interplay between people, technology, and organizational structures in implementing innovations like AI in healthcare.

Trust Calibration: The process of aligning user trust with the actual capabilities and limitations of AI systems to ensure appropriate reliance and use.

Workflow Integration: The seamless incorporation of AI tools into existing clinical and administrative workflows to improve efficiency without disrupting existing processes.

Chapter 13
Evaluate the Impact of AI on Healthcare Workforce Dynamics and Operational Efficiency

A. Prabhu Chakkaravarthy
https://orcid.org/0009-0000-3180-8051
Independent Researcher, India

Dhanalakshmi Jaganathan
https://orcid.org/0000-0002-3919-4469
SRM Institute of Science and Technology, India

ABSTRACT

Because of the fast progress in AI technology, the healthcare sector now operates differently, affecting both its staff and the way it delivers services. It looks at how AI has an impact on healthcare professions, improvements in work processes and the standard of patient care. Tools like machine learning, robotic automation, and language processing are boosting the accuracy of diagnosis, cutting back on paperwork and enhancing decisions doctors take during patient care. Still, these advancements cause people to worry about losing their jobs, needing to learn new things, and what skills will be needed in healthcare going forward. The other aspect of AI that the chapter examines is its impact on the operations of hospitals in terms of saving finances, making patients healthier and facilitating personalized treatments. This chapter discusses the recent news, obstacles, and opportunities to get a clear idea about how AI can enhance healthcare and transform the employment of people in the healthcare field.

DOI: 10.4018/979-8-3373-2787-7.ch013

INTRODUCTION

Coverage and integration of AI technologies is one of the greatest changes in the healthcare aspect of the twenty-first century. Artificial intelligence, measured by elements such as machine learning (ML), natural language processing (NLP) and robotic process automation (RPA), is currently implemented in a broad range of healthcare business processes, which includes clinical diagnostics, administrative management, choice of treatment and endpoint delivery of highly personalized care (He et al., 2019; Rajkomar, Dean, & Kohane, 2019). Besides enhancing the decision-making capacity of physicians, these tools are also enhancing the efficiency of operations as well as engaging the patients. Such technologies are able to define slight tendencies and complicated correlations beyond the scope of traditional methods of analysis by utilizing large data sets, streaming data channels, and advanced algorithms to achieve a faster more precise and in many cases predictive form of intervention (Beam & Kohane, 2018; Esteva et al., 2019; Topol, 2019).

As the field of digital health solutions is constantly improving, the revolutionizing impact of these digital solutions on the field of professionals working in health care, patient outcomes, and the structure of the whole healthcare system becomes more apparent. The use of automation and advanced analytics will provide quality improvements, cost reductions, and workflow efficiency but has its own challenges like displacement of the workforce, skills shortages, and ethical issues, e.g., algorithmic biases, lack of transparency, and privacy of the patient data (Jha, Topol, & Adashi, 2020; Obermeyer et al., 2019; Davenport & Kalakota, 2019). One needs a balanced way to address the above issues in terms of innovation, regulatory similarity, and collaboration.

Conceptualization of AI as a two-sided force, which has the power to bring both progress and risks, is, thus, the key element in the design of healthcare systems that are equitable, trustworthy, and human-centered. A diagram in Figure 1 illustrates the principal categories of AI explored in this chapter and their applications in healthcare. The figure maps AI technologies (Machine Learning, Robotic Process Automation, Natural Language Processing, and Emerging Tools) on the left, connecting them to healthcare domains such as diagnostics, administration, treatment planning, and patient monitoring.

Figure 1. Overview of AI Technologies in Healthcare

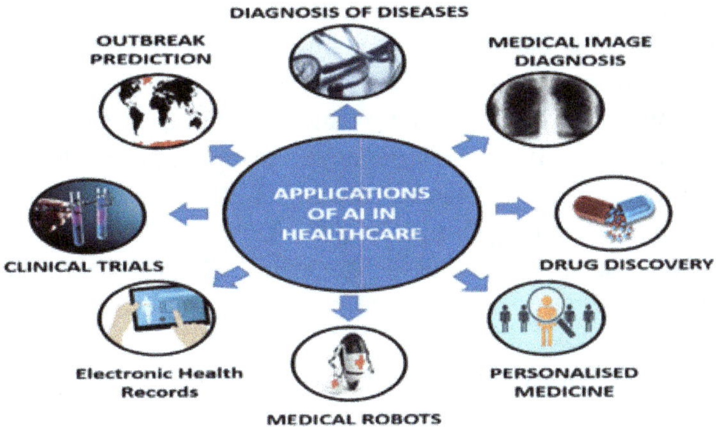

Objectives of the Chapter

We are looking at how AI impacts healthcare systems in various ways, mainly by focus on:

- Exploring the expected changes in the duties and responsibilities of healthcare staff because of AI.
- Studying how AI affects the way work is carried out in clinical and administrative areas.
- Exploring what AI may do for the delivery of healthcare and patient results.
- Determining problems with adapting the workforce, ethical dilemmas and rules set by regulators.
- Journals highlight and offer ideas for opportunities and strategy in building AI-enabled healthcare.
- The chapter tries to explore these topics to show how AI is changing healthcare delivery and the workplace.

BACKGROUND

The main topic of this chapter is the use of AI in healthcare, starting from 2015 to the present day (2024). It looks at practices from diagnostics and treatment planning as well as other jobs (billing and scheduling), combining findings from studies and reports.

For this, we carried out a review of published materials by searching through PubMed, IEEE Xplore, Scopus and reports available on the websites of the European Commission, WHO and NHS England (WHO, 2021; European Commission, 2020; NHS England, 2023). Articles focusing on the changes in technology, ethics and practical uses of AI were privileged. A number of examples are provided to show how AI is actually used in various healthcare contexts.

This initial explanation allows us to dig into how AI is affecting modern healthcare systems.

Overview of AI Technologies in Healthcare

Artificial Intelligence (AI) covers a range of computational approaches that enable machines to simulate human cognitive functions such as decision-making, pattern recognition, and language comprehension. In healthcare, AI plays a transformative role in reshaping both clinical and administrative practices through advanced analytics, intelligent automation, and real-time decision support (Yu, Beam, & Kohane, 2018; He et al., 2019). This integration is not merely about technological adoption—it is redefining how patient care is delivered, how medical research is conducted, and how healthcare systems are managed.

Underlying AI technologies already present in healthcare, that is, Machine Learning (ML) and Predictive Analytics, Robotic Process Automation (RPA) Natural Language Processing (NLP), and Emerging AI Tools and Platforms as well as their application, advantages, weaknesses, and prospects are discussed in the following subsections.

Machine Learning and Predictive Analytics

Machine Learning (ML) also allows systems to learn using past and current data and improve their performance as time goes on, without being explicitly reprogrammed. ML serves as a backbone of predictive intelligence, diagnosis of a disease, the stratification of risk, as well as receiving personalized treatment recommendations in the field of healthcare (Rajkomar, Dean, & Kohane, 2019).

Key Applications

Predictive Health Outcomes: ML models are capable of predicting the deterioration of patients using longitudinal patient data, predicting cases of hospital re-hospitalization, and the early detection of sepsis (Beam & Kohane, 2018).

Medical Imaging: Deep learning is a category of ML, involving neural networks, and is able to produce substantial improvements in radiology, pathology and genomics. At this point, Convolutional Neural Networks (CNNs) have reached an accuracy in identifying cancers, fractures, or anomalies in imaging scans that are on par or even better than human experts (Esteva et al., 2019).

Personalized Medicine: The algorithms of machine learning allow modeling the results of genetic, lifestyle or medical history so that custom treatment regimens can be provided, especially in the oncological, cardiovascular and rare diseases scenarios (Jiang et al., 2017).

Recent Advancements (2023–2025)

Federated learning in ML enables multi-institutional collaboration on model training without centralizing sensitive information such as patient data so that it is more privately, despite the high accuracy of the result. Also, multi-modal AI systems can now integrate imaging, lab results and clinical notes into a single predictive model which enhances early discovery of the disease and comprehensive patient evaluation.

Challenges

Regardless of its potential, ML in medicine has issues with interpretability of the model, cross-population generalization, and integration into the clinical processes (Rudin, 2019; Kelly et al., 2019). More and more regulatory bodies stress explainability as something that will allow clinicians to trust the AI-generated insights and to take the appropriate actions relying upon them.

Robotic Process Automation (RPA)

Robotic Process Automation (RPA) is an automation tool that uses software-based bots to perform routine, rules-based activities that do not entail high complex decision-making. RPA is mostly used in the healthcare sector to make its administrative incoming processes more efficient, such that the healthcare personnel can place more of their effort in what is more patient-driven (Davenport & Kalakota, 2019).

Key Applications:

- Claim Processing: Automating insurance claims verification, verification with the insurance policy coverage and approval.
- Patient Scheduling Billing: bookings, reminders, and invoice management with a minimum of manual processing.
- Data Management: Automatic data updates of EHRs and uniformity of such data in systems.

Integration with AI

Using AI and ML, RPA turns into Intelligent Process Automation (IPA). It allows bots to perform activities related to decision-making, including medical necessity verification of procedures or patient request triage on the basis of urgency (Mesko et al., 2018). As an example, the AI-powered RPA solution is capable of extracting sensitive information of an unstructured medical document to speed up the prior authorization.

Workforce Implications

As RPA lessens ergonomic and human error, its proliferation is apprehended in regards to job loss, skill transition as well as the requirement of reskilling arrangements (Jha et al., 2020). Healthcare organizations that will be ready are going to be implementing human-bot workflows that are hybrid in their implementation so as to guarantee that work is not displaced by technology but complemented.

Natural Language Processing (NLP)

Natural Language Processing (NLP) also allows computers to read, comprehend, and write in human language. NLP has been applied in the healthcare field to streamline the de-facto organization of medical records such as physician notes written in a non-structured format, into a structure appropriate to analytics (Liu et al., 2019).

Key Applications:

- Clinical Documentation: Automatic conversion of dictations and notes of the physician to structured EHR entries.
- Information Extraction: The detection of the references to diseases, symptoms or adverse drug effects in the free-text records.

- Patient Communication: Driving AI chatbots and virtual assistants to schedule, manage symptoms and remind patients to take their medication (Blease et al., 2019).
- Population Health Management: To combine and review patient responses to highlight system problems or care needs.

Emerging Trends

Existing issues with the application of NLP have been extended by recent advances in large language models (LLM). LPs such as GPT-4 and Med-PaLM 2 are being tuned to healthcare-relevant use cases to enable performing complex functions, such as providing simplified overviews of dense medical material readable by patients. In addition, the introduction speech-to-text systems which have medical vocabularies are making accessibility to clinicians with heavy documentation burden.

Challenges

Constant obstacles are medical jargon, abbreviations and inconsistent terms. In addition, the development of high-quality annotated datasets that most supervised NLP models require currently remains resource consuming (Gerke, Minssen, & Cohen, 2020). Textual biases are also likely to contribute to care disparities.

Emerging AI Tools and Platforms

The healthcare AI is gaining pace as the integrated healthcare AI brings this technology together with cloud computing, Internet of Medical Things (IoMT), and advanced analytics.

Business AI Apparatus

Examples of such products included in this scalable AI-as-a-service model are IBM Watson Health, Google Health AI, and Microsoft Azure Healthcare that can be used to fulfill functions such as imaging analysis, patient engagement, and predictive modeling (IBM, 2023). These platforms give smaller health agencies access to top-notch AI functions without having to spend large portions of their budget building out prodigious framework internally.

IoMT Integration

Wearable devices and IoMT sensors, when paired with AI algorithms, enable continuous monitoring of vital signs, activity levels, and sleep quality. This supports early intervention for chronic disease management—e.g., detecting arrhythmias via wearable ECG patches (Finlayson et al., 2021).

Generative AI in Healthcare

Generative AI models, including LLMs, are being explored for automating medical documentation, summarizing research literature, generating synthetic datasets for model training, and even assisting in drug discovery pipelines (WHO, 2021).

Ethical and Safety Considerations

As these platforms mature, emphasis is shifting toward transparency, bias mitigation, and compliance with regional and global health data regulations (European Commission, 2020; Fjeld et al., 2020). Governance frameworks are increasingly being implemented to ensure responsible AI deployment.

Comparative Summary of AI Technologies in Healthcare is given in Table 1

Table 1. Comparative Summary of AI Technologies in Healthcare

Technology	Primary Applications	Strengths	Challenges
Machine Learning & Predictive Analytics	Diagnosis, risk prediction, personalized treatment	High accuracy, data-driven decision support	Explainability, data quality, integration issues
Robotic Process Automation	Claims, scheduling, billing, data entry	Efficiency, error reduction, scalability	Workforce adaptation, limited decision-making
Natural Language Processing	Documentation, information extraction, patient engagement	Converts unstructured to structured data, supports automation	Medical jargon complexity, data annotation needs
Emerging AI Platforms	Multi-modal analysis, IoMT integration, generative AI	Comprehensive capabilities, cloud scalability	Ethical concerns, data privacy, bias risks

Future Outlook

The future of AI in healthcare is moving toward convergence—integrating multiple AI capabilities into cohesive ecosystems that support the entire patient journey, from prevention to post-treatment monitoring. Advances in multi-modal

AI, edge computing for IoMT, and privacy-preserving techniques will expand AI's applicability while addressing current barriers.

Furthermore, regulatory bodies are beginning to outline frameworks for adaptive AI models that evolve over time, enabling safer real-world deployment. As these systems gain trust, they are expected to shift from decision-support tools to collaborative agents in care delivery, ultimately improving outcomes, reducing costs, and enhancing the patient experience.

IMPACT ON HEALTHCARE WORKFORCE DYNAMICS

Artificial Intelligence (AI) is not only redefining the technical and administrative processes of healthcare but is also initiating a profound transformation in the structure, skill requirements, and cultural identity of the healthcare workforce. The introduction of AI-enabled tools into clinical and administrative workflows is leading to both augmentation and automation of specific tasks, altering the traditional distribution of responsibilities among professionals. This transformation is neither uniform nor inevitable—it is mediated by institutional readiness, regulatory frameworks, cultural attitudes toward technology, and the availability of training resources (Jha, Topol, & Adashi, 2020; Topol, 2019).

By modifying how duties are assigned, expanding interdisciplinary collaboration, and influencing the perceived value of human expertise, AI is driving a reconfiguration of healthcare labor markets. The changes extend beyond mere technological adoption: they touch upon professional identity, ethical responsibility, workforce equity, and the long-term sustainability of healthcare delivery.

Figure 2 illustrates a conceptual model of workforce evolution under AI integration, depicting a continuum from traditional roles to AI-augmented responsibilities, areas of potential job displacement, avenues for job transformation, and the necessity of ongoing retraining and upskilling programs. Feedback loops highlight how workforce adaptation, if managed effectively, can reinforce rather than undermine human-centric care.

Figure 2. Impact of AI on Healthcare Workforce Dynamics

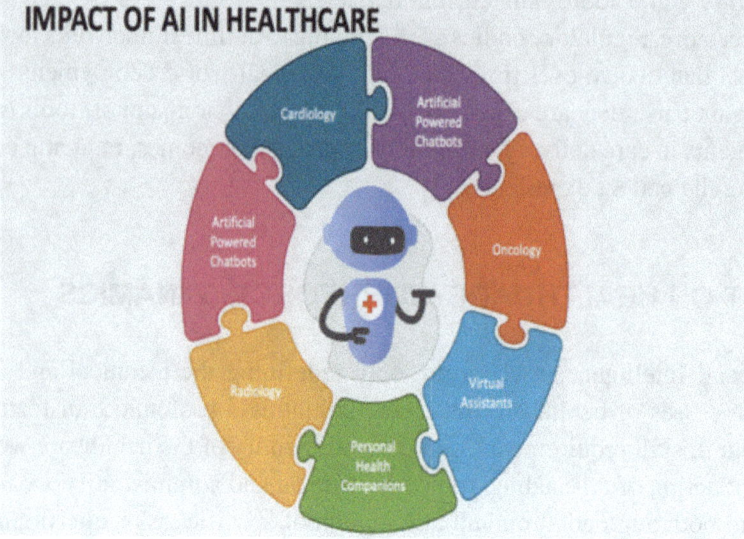

Evolving Roles of Healthcare Professionals

The realization of AI is not making clinicians obsolete, that is, redefining the role and competence areas of healthcare roles. The shift is felt by physicians, nurses, radiologists, pathologists, pharmacists, and administrative staff members as they are moving toward interpretive judgment, critical oversight, and emotional intelligence tasks instead of rote and repetitive ones.

An example can be given within the field of diagnostic imaging where, radiologists are now more being required to act as clinical data integrators compared to image readers. Convolutional neural networks (CNNs), which have learned on millions of annotated scans, can identify suspicious lesions in mammograms scans or CT scans, with equal or even higher accuracy than human experts (Esteva et al., 2019). However, such outputs should be contextualized by combining the AI output with patient history, laboratory tests, and the results of physical examination, etc. Radiologists are transitioning to become the supervisors of AI as they confirm the results generated by the algorithm, discover possible so-called edge cases in which AI can malfunction, and discuss subtle results with patients and other medical professionals.

Likewise, AI-powered Clinical Decision Support Systems (CDSS) are now available to assist primary care physicians in terms of providing them with potential diagnoses, drug interaction warnings, and even disease prognosis using longitudinal patient data (Jiang et al., 2017). The role of the physician shifts toward shared decision-making with both the patient and the algorithm, balancing computational recommendations with clinical intuition and patient preferences.

Nurses, traditionally focused on direct patient care, are increasingly expected to operate AI-enabled monitoring devices for remote patient management. For example, wearable devices connected to AI platforms can detect early signs of deterioration in chronic disease patients, triggering proactive interventions. This extends the nurse's role into continuous virtual care, enabling population-scale patient oversight while maintaining individualized care plans (Blease et al., 2019).

Administrative roles are also transforming. Medical coders, for example, no longer spend the majority of their time on manual data entry. Instead, they validate and audit AI-generated coding outputs, handle complex exceptions, and ensure compliance with billing regulations (Davenport & Kalakota, 2019). In doing so, they must develop competencies in data interpretation, error analysis, and AI system troubleshooting.

Job Displacement vs. Job Transformation

A central debate in the AI discourse concerns whether technology will replace or transform jobs. Evidence suggests that the outcome depends heavily on how organizations implement AI, how workers are retrained, and how tasks are restructured. Routine, rule-based, and predictable tasks—such as initial medical record triage, appointment scheduling, or simple insurance claim processing—are most vulnerable to automation through Robotic Process Automation (RPA) (Jha et al., 2020). If not managed carefully, these changes can result in job losses, particularly in administrative support roles. However, in many instances, AI acts more as a force multiplier than a replacement. For example, in pathology, AI tools can pre-screen slides and prioritize cases likely to contain malignancies. This allows pathologists to focus their expertise on complex diagnoses, rare cases, and interdisciplinary consultations. Similarly, AI can handle high-volume repetitive analysis in laboratory testing, enabling lab technicians to shift toward quality assurance, research, and specialized testing.

The reality often lies in task-level displacement rather than complete role elimination. For example: In radiology, AI may fully automate the detection of specific fracture types but not the comprehensive interpretation of a trauma case. In nursing, AI may automate routine vital sign tracking, but not patient counseling, wound care, or emergency interventions. Without proactive workforce planning, there is a risk of creating a polarized healthcare labor market—with high-value, AI-supervisory roles concentrated among a smaller group of highly trained professionals, and low-value, non-technical roles left to others. This could exacerbate inequalities both within and between healthcare organizations (WHO, 2021).

Workforce Retraining and Upskilling

To fully realize the benefits of AI while minimizing disruption, systematic and sustained retraining initiatives are essential. This includes not only technical skills but also interdisciplinary competencies that allow healthcare workers to collaborate effectively with AI systems.

Key training priorities include:

- Data literacy: Understanding how data is collected, processed, and analyzed; recognizing data limitations and potential biases.
- Algorithmic literacy: being able to understand output of AI, challenge its advice and know when to take the override.
- Digital tool skills: The use of AI–enabled platforms, electronic health records, and decision-support systems efficiently.
- Ethics and governance: Knowledge of privacy governance, ethics in AI usage, and accountability system.

Retraining should become a part of both formal education routes (medical, nursing and allied health curricula) as well as continuing professional development programs. One example comes in the form of the UK National Health Service (NHS) launching AI literacy training in medical schools, as well as simulation-based AI-based clinical workflow training.

Social equity is also an issue relating to retraining. Healthcare workers of older age, employees in rural or underfunded institutions, and persons of marginalized background can experience more obstacles to the development of new skills. Unless there are inclusive policies, including subsidizing training, offering flexible learning formats, and contacting specific professionals, the use of AI is likely to increase the digital gap in healthcare personnel.

Interaction of engineered and data scientists with clinicians is of high importance. In multidisciplinary project teams involved in the implementation of AI, clinicians have a chance to provide clinical background and ethical expertise, whereas technologists will also provide well-built algorithm development and integration.

Ethical and Social Implications

The introduction of AI into healthcare workforces does not only bring efficiency and accuracy concerns, but also those of human dignity, trust, and fairness. There is the issue of loss of professional autonomy. In instances where the individual under diagnosis is no longer in control of a particular condition, since AI recommendations are proven to be better when offered by the AI, clinicians might feel to refer to

AI suggestions, thus becoming deskilled after a period. This interaction can give the power of decision-making away from practitioners, and this may imply on the accountability in case of mistakes (Rudin, 2019).

One more burning issue is AI system bias. The bias in historical healthcare data tends to be the echo of the inequalities in the system and the algorithms trained on such data may replicate or increase disparity. Indicatively, AI-powered risk measurement tools have been reported to undervalue the health needs of the black patients as they are based on biased proxies of costs to health status (Obermeyer et al., 2019). These biases may lead to the workforce aspects of concern as not only patient outcomes, but also the professional integrity and the sense of trust towards AI are under the risk.

Social: AI also shifts the relationship between a patient and a provider. Although automation would relieve clinicians of paperwork and administrative tasks, it is also synonymous with introducing technological obstacles to empathy. There is a risk that patients experience the care rendered by AI as cold and impersonal unless clinicians make an effort to remind human connection. As such, the skills of active listening, compassion, cultural sensitivity are needed even more in the AI-enhanced healthcare space (Blease et al., 2019). The ethically responsible use of AI considers the need of transparent governance and accountability lines as well as the engagement of medical employees in the decision-making process on the issue of AI adoption. World Health Organization (2021) points out that AI must be a supporting tool that should not be used to displace human evaluation and must be implemented keeping in view the principles of beneficence, non-maleficence, autonomy, and justice.

Global and Policy Perspectives

The effect of AI on the labor market is not considered similar to those of the different countries. Rich countries can invest more in AI learning center, use more advanced technologies and hire competent teams. On the contrary, LMICs might have resource limitations, as well as limited networks and fewer chances of getting an education specifically in AI: LMICs might still need AI to solve a workforce shortage by using remote diagnostics and telehealth. Policies are capable of influencing whether AI will be used as a source of empowerment of the workforce or a cause of inequality. Examples include: France is the first country with its national AI strategy that also finances AI literacy courses of healthcare providers. The Smart Health Video Consultation program in Singapore, which incorporates AI solutions into the technology of telemedicine and at the same time involves upskilling the primary care workforce. The Pan-Canadian AI Strategy that hopes to focus on cross-cutting collaboration and fair accessibility to AI training. Conclusively, the effects of AI on the dynamics of healthcare workforce are intricate and multifold. It entails work repurposing, redefining competencies, automation versus inherent judgment and having equitable access to retraining. When controlled, AI has the potential to enhance the abilities of health care teams, patient care and job satisfaction. When not handled properly, it can increase inequalities, cause the loss of trust, and undermine the human aspects of healthcare.

AI AND OPERATIONAL EFFICIENCY IN HEALTHCARE

Using AI in healthcare has allowed organizations to achieve things and work more effectively that were not possible before. Automating administrative processes, aiding doctors in making choices and maximizing resources ensures better performance for healthcare systems. This part discusses how AI improves operations by using real case studies and research.

Streamlining Administrative Tasks

The examples of registration and claim processing, setting appointments and paperwork occupy a significant portion of the spending budget and time individually employed in the healthcare industry (Davenport & Kalakota, 2019). Robotic Process Automation (RPA) as a form of AI enables companies to increase their operations by processing manually repetitive tasks not only faster than ever before but also accurately. AI is applied to the field of medicine to aid the generation of clinical notes, locate information within disorganized paper data and code it to guarantee proper billing (Liu et al., 2019). Chatbots and virtual assistants are currently used by some offices to accomplish desk work that includes communicating with patients and managing appointments (Blease et al., 2019). When these technologies reduce the paperwork healthcare professionals deal with, they help them to work faster and more accurately and also let staff focus on jobs that improve patient care.

Enhancing Clinical Decision-Making

By offering decision-support tools, AI integrates patient records, guides from experts and advanced predictions to guide doctors in choosing the right treatment for patients (Jiang et al., 2017). With these systems, analysts can go through plenty of records, spot frequent occurrences, note atypical happenings and advise suitable interventions. Machine learning methods are commonly applied to catch diseases as early as possible, including cancer, cardiovascular problems and sepsis, by looking for important signals in radiological or laboratory information (Esteva et al., 2019; Rajkomar et al., 2019; Sabahath et al, 2024; Rengaramanujam et al. 2026;

Karunakaran et al., 2026; Abdullah et al. 2025; Karunakaran et al. 2021; Bhatnagar et al., 2021; Alasmari et al. 2025; Begum et al., 2023). Emergency rooms rely on AI to assess risk and sort patients by their chances of needing emergency assistance. Using decision support tools can minimize medical errors, enhance how medicine is used and shape direction in precision medicine so that better and more secure care can be offered (Topol, 2019).

Cost Reduction and Resource Optimization

Introducing AI into operations cuts costs for labor, reduces errors in diagnoses, directs resources more efficiently and shortens time spent in hospitals by patients (He et al., 2019). Through predictive analytics, AI systems help hospitals forecast if they will face a shortage of hospital beds, ICU units or supplies (Beam & Kohane, 2018). Also, with the help of AI, doctors are able to reduce the number of unnecessary medical tests and procedures and make diagnoses with greater accuracy (Kelly et al., 2019). AI in radiology helps by finding the scans that actually need further review, so that only those are passed on for human checking, saving time and decreasing costs. Such efficiencies matter a lot in value-based care models, as healthcare organizations are rewarded for giving high-quality care without spending too much.

Case Examples of AI Implementation

Case 1: Cleveland Clinic and IBM Watson

The Cleveland Clinic partnered with IBM Watson to enhance oncology treatment planning. Watson for Oncology examines the records of patients and compares them with an extensive collection of medical literature to propose individual treatment options. Initial outcomes demonstrated an increase in the speed and consistency of decision-making, whereas clinicians reserve the final control (IBM, 2023).

Case 2: NHS England and Babylon Health

The National Health Service (NHS) of the UK tested AI-based triage chatbots via Babylon Health and they were able to decrease wait times and assist more patients in getting medical advice, particularly in regions that are medically underserved. Symptom-checking algorithms are used to provide advice or hand over to human clinicians when appropriate (Mesko et al., 2018).

Case 3: Mayo Clinic's Use of AI in Radiology

Mayo Clinic has deployed deep learning algorithms to help detect conditions such as pulmonary embolism and diabetic retinopathy early enough. They improved the accuracy of diagnosing tools and enabled radiologists to focus on high-risk cases more effectively (Finlayson et al., 2021). Those pointed out the practical usefulness of AI in enhancing not only internal operational rates but also patient-level outcomes like access, timeliness, and safety.

SOLUTIONS AND RECOMMENDATIONS

AI-Driven Improvements in Patient Care

Artificial Intelligence (AI) technologies are redefining the standards of patient care through enhanced diagnostic accuracy, personalized treatment approaches, continuous monitoring, and improved patient engagement. These innovations are shifting the healthcare paradigm from reactive treatment to proactive and predictive care. This section explores the key domains in which AI contributes to elevating patient outcomes and experiences.

Diagnostic Accuracy and Early Detection

Among the most notable applications of AI in healthcare is its ability to enhance the accuracy of diagnosis and allow diagnosing the ailment at an early stage. AI models, specifically deep learning algorithms, have the capability to analyze medical imaging, genomic data, and electronic health records (EHRs) with high precision and in certain cases are more accurate than human clinicians in particular diagnostic skills (Esteva et al., 2017).

Personalized and Precision Medicine

AI would be essential to the development of personalized and precision medicine as it provides the opportunities to customize medical care with the use of data. Machine learning algorithms have the potential to stratify patients into risk groups and propose individual treatments by combining genomic data, lifestyle data, and clinical history. As another example, AI is applied to predict individual drug response in oncology to optimize chemotherapy regimens on the basis of tumor genomics and prior treatment history (Topol, 2019). It is also possible to extract patient preferences and contextual factors contained in unstructured clinical notes using Natural Language Processing (NLP), which is related to more holistic and patient-centered care. Pharmacogenomics Pharmacogenomics uses AI to uncover gene-drug interaction information that can be applied to the choice of medication and its dosage, minimizing adverse effects and maximizing treatment efficiency.

Patient Monitoring and Remote Care

Chronic disease management and post-acute care have been altered due to the emergence of AI-powered remote monitoring systems. Such systems process the information collected by wearable sensors, smartphones, and home-based monitoring devices to constantly evaluate the health condition of patients. As an example, AI algorithms incorporated in smartwatches can identify arrhythmias and alert the customers or clinical care in real-time. AI-powered glucose monitors can forecast hyper- or hypoglycemic events in diabetes care, enabling adjustments to insulin treatment in time (Topol, 2019). AI-assisted remote patient monitoring (RPM) has likewise become invaluable during pandemics and in rural health care provision, providing continuity of care with the minimum of hospital visits. RPM platforms have predictive analytics that can notify clinicians about possible complications, which lowers hospital readmissions and enhances patient safety.

CHALLENGES AND CONSIDERATIONS IN AI INTEGRATION

While Artificial Intelligence (AI) offers substantial benefits to healthcare systems, its integration is accompanied by a series of technical, ethical, regulatory, and organizational challenges. Effective deployment of AI requires more than technological capability; it involves addressing concerns about data privacy, algorithmic fairness, legal compliance, system interoperability, and change management. Moreover, successful adoption demands alignment with clinical workflows, stakeholder trust, and long-term sustainability planning. This section explores key considerations that must be addressed to ensure the responsible and sustainable integration of AI in healthcare.

Data Privacy and Security

Medical information is highly sensitive and it falls under highly regulated privacy policies and regulations such as the Health Insurance Portability and Accountability Act (HIPAA) in America and the General Data Protection Regulation (GDPR) in the European Union. Gathering, storing, and computing the mass, multi-mode datasets needed to train AI models pose significant risks of data breaches, unauthorized access, and possible re-identification of anonymized records. The AI systems might need near-real-time access to electronic health records (EHRs), imaging databases, wearable sensor streams, and genomic databases- exposing a larger system of attack vectors to attack by cybercriminals (Shah & Chircu, 2018). It is necessary to ensure that encryption is robust, multi-factor authentication, secure data transmission protocols and tiered access control are important. Moreover, privacy-preserving machine learning frameworks, e.g., federated learning and differential privacy, become increasingly popular to facilitate collaborations in development of AI, but without aggregating raw data on patients. Such strategies coupled with an active cybersecurity surveillance have the potential to enhance the confidence of the general population and minimize the risks associated with big-box data incorporation.

Algorithmic Bias and Transparency

Any algorithm that uses AI is predetermined by the quality and integrity of the data on which the algorithm is trained. A bias in the existing historical healthcare data which when not addressed may lead to biased results- an example of this is biased results caused by underdiagnosing some minority groups or failing to distinguish diseases by demographic imbalances (Obermeyer et al., 2019). These biases have the potential to worsen any existing inequities in health care access and quality of treatment and patient safety.

To curb such problems, AI systems need to have their bias identification and fairness tested throughout the course of development and deployment. What is more, the transparency, which is also known as explainability, is essential regarding the rise of clinician confidence, the ability to gain regulatory approval, and patient trust. In spite of their power, black-box models can interfere with interpretability, which implies that healthcare professionals will have trouble convincing patients to accept AI-based suggestions. The emerging explainable AI (XAI) research field seeks to develop models that offer both good predictive performance and ease of understandability, so that AI functions as an aid to clinical decision making, not a black box that replaces clinical judgment.

Regulatory and Legal Challenges

The AI healthcare regulatory landscape is unstable and, in the meantime, fragmented. The U.S. Food and Drug Administration (FDA), the European Medicines Agency (EMA) and the UK Medicines and Healthcare products Regulatory Agency (MHRA) are among agencies to have provided guidance on Software as a Medical Device (SaMD). Nevertheless, adaptive or continuously learning algorithms introduce special difficulties, as the regulation of these systems is usually based on the system that does not change its operations.

No less difficult is the question of legal responsibility. Question number 8 has yet to be determined how one can determine accountability in situations when an AI system is contributing to a diagnostic mistake, therapeutic delays, or patient outcomes and harm. Who is to be blamed, the healthcare provider or software vendor or the institution is still a debatable notion (Gerke et al., 2020). Unless there are legal precedents, which there were none at first sight, organizations might be reluctant to embrace AI on a large scale. To resolve these doubts, special legal frameworks, revised models of malpractice insurance, and internationalization of laws regarding the AI in the health sector will need to be created.

Organizational Readiness and Change Management

The integration of AI in healthcare is dependent on how an institution is willing to undergo technological change. It involves the incorporation of adoption of AI and purpose of the organization, investment into the IT infrastructure, cultivation of leadership support, installation of cross-cutting implementation units.

One of the main problems is the obstacle of healthcare professionals and it is usually motivated by the fear of being replaced, loss of professional autonomy, or the growing amount of paperwork. Acceptance rates are low but can be enhanced by using proactive engagement strategies, including clinician participation in the development of AI, special training sessions, a focus on augmentation, and not automation.

One more factor is the danger of widening the digital divide. More resourced healthcare systems will more likely be able to invest in and sustain advanced AI applications, whereas those shot of money have less of a chance to stay up to date, potentially increasing inequalities in care standards and patient outcomes. It will be necessary to bridge this gap through specific funding mechanisms, through PPPs, and at the scale of small and resource- scarce settings through AI-based deployments.

FUTURE RESEARCH DIRECTIONS

With the theme of artificial intelligence (AI) being further advanced, the place occupied by it in the future of healthcare sector will increasingly gain the focal point. On top of these current applications, AI will also enable more predictive and preventive care, novel models of human-machine partnerships, and global health equity through informed policymaking. This area discusses the future trends and possibilities that may characterize the further development of AI in healthcare.

AI in Predictive and Preventive Healthcare

The transition to proactive healthcare using AI is being considered a highly promising tendency. Machine learning is a subset of predictive analytics and helps to identify those individuals who might be at risk earlier by analysing historical data, behaviours, genes and their surroundings. Application of the knowledge results in additional strategies that can assist in the reduction of chronic conditions as well as hospital visits. Some AI models can forecast disease outbreaks, alert on mental health challenges and identify worsening signs of ICU patients before periodic doctors become aware of them. AI use in wearables and IoMT systems allows people to monitor their health more actively. It is possible that AI-based systems will become important parts of population health management, helping make better use of resources and plan public health actions (Reddy et al., 2020).

Collaborative AI-Human Work Models

Future AI systems are expected to work together with humans, not to take the place of healthcare workers. Such models—which are sometimes called augmented intelligence—use the ability of AI to find patterns and the insights, awareness and ethical choices found in clinicians (Jiang et al., 2017).

Interpretable suggestions from a decision support system help physicians work better, reduce the risk of wrong diagnoses and take part in shared decisions with patients. Surgical robotic systems guided by AI are assisting surgeons to achieve better results and more accuracy in the operating room.

Better progress comes from adaptive interfaces, getting real-time feedback from working with patients and using AI that supports the way each clinician works, ensuring efficiency does not lead to loss of human decision making.

Global Perspectives and Policy Directions

Since AI is globalizing in healthcare, there are many openings for new solutions, but it still exposes problems in access to technology, infrastructure and consistent rules. AI technology can help LMICs address their medical workforce problems and improve medical care for people living in remote regions (WHO, 2021). Still, problems connected to including all types of data, understanding technology and access must still be fixed.

International organizations are coming up with frameworks to support the ethical use of AI everywhere. One such example is the evidence introduced by the WHO and UNESCO which recommends that equity, transparency and accountability be central to the management of AI. United actions taken by governments, companies and research institutions will play a key role in making regulations consistent, making it possible to transfer data across borders and supporting innovative AI projects that follow expected public health outcomes.

People are now paying more attention to starting international data commons, researching AI ethics and training the AI workforce to address gaps between different countries in AI readiness.

CONCLUSION AND RECOMMENDATIONS

The integration of artificial intelligence (AI) into healthcare systems has introduced a paradigm shift that touches every facet of care delivery—from workforce structures and operational efficiency to patient-centered care and public health management. As evidenced in this chapter, AI is not merely a technological tool but a transformative force requiring careful orchestration among clinicians, administrators, technologists, policymakers, and patients.

Summary of Key Insights

This chapter has explored the multidimensional impact of AI on the healthcare ecosystem:

- AI Technologies such as machine learning, robotic process automation (RPA), and natural language processing (NLP) are reshaping diagnostic procedures, clinical workflows, and administrative processes.
- Workforce Dynamics are evolving as AI redefines professional roles, prompting concerns about job displacement and highlighting the need for retraining and upskilling.
- Operational Efficiency gains include automation of repetitive tasks, improved clinical decision support, and cost containment.
- Patient Care is enhanced through improved diagnostic accuracy, personalized medicine, and more responsive monitoring solutions.
- Integration Challenges span data privacy, algorithmic bias, regulatory uncertainty, and the necessity of organizational readiness.
- Future Trends point toward predictive and preventive medicine, human-AI collaboration, and global harmonization of AI policy frameworks.

Together, these insights affirm that AI, when ethically and strategically deployed, holds the promise of delivering safer, more efficient, and more equitable healthcare.

In light of the opportunities and challenges identified, the following strategic recommendations are proposed for various stakeholder groups:

For Healthcare Providers and Institutions

- Invest in AI literacy and training programs to empower clinicians and support staff to use AI tools effectively.
- Promote interdisciplinary collaboration among clinical, IT, and data science teams to co-design AI solutions tailored to local needs.
- Implement robust data governance frameworks to ensure data quality, security, and compliance with privacy regulations.

For Policymakers and Regulators

- Develop adaptive regulatory pathways that can accommodate evolving AI models, including continuous learning systems.
- Establish guidelines for transparency and accountability in AI decision-making, particularly in high-risk applications such as diagnosis and treatment.
- Support national and international AI infrastructure initiatives to reduce disparities between institutions and regions.

For Technologists and Developers

- Prioritize explainable and interpretable AI models that align with clinical reasoning and support trust in recommendations.
- Conduct bias audits and integrate fairness metrics to mitigate algorithmic discrimination across diverse populations.
- Ensure user-centric design, emphasizing usability, transparency, and integration into existing clinical workflows.

For Patients and the Public

- Facilitate public engagement and education to raise awareness of AI capabilities and limitations in healthcare.
- Advocate for inclusive data representation to ensure AI models reflect the diversity of the populations they serve.

The future of healthcare will be built on AI as it will collaborate rather than compete with what people intelligently achieve. Its most positive aspects lie in enhancing the knowledge of doctors, increasing the rate of processes and customizing the patient participation. However, all must witness that ethical thinking, sustained control and involvement of all stakeholders assist in promotion of adoption.

The manner of AI planning and management can determine whether it will be the dividing force among healthcare groups or whether it promotes unity, balance and sustainability. The next decade will likely determine the extent to which AI will transform medicine not only because of its technology but mostly because of its influence on human health and wellbeing.

REFERENCES

Abdullah, R. M., Saad, L. A., Alasmari, Z. M., Ali, G. A., & Muniasamy, A. (2025). Human disease prediction mobile application using machine learning. In Alareeni, B., & Hamdan, A. (Eds.), *IoT and digital transformation: Innovating business models for the connected world (ICBT 2024). Lecture notes in networks and systems* (Vol. 1575). Springer. DOI: 10.1007/978-3-032-00450-5_19

Alasmari, A., & Muniasamy, A. (2025). Integrating Bayesian and convolution neural network for uncertainty estimation of cataract from fundus images. *Computer Modeling in Engineering & Sciences, 143*(1), 569–592. DOI: 10.32604/cmes.2025.060484

Asiri, F., & Muniasamy, A. (2025). Advanced human activity recognition on wearables with multi-scale sparse attention. *Multimedia Tools and Applications, 84*(30), 36623–36652. Advance online publication. DOI: 10.1007/s11042-024-20475-6

Beam, A. L., & Kohane, I. S. (2018). Big data and machine learning in health care. *Journal of the American Medical Association, 319*(13), 1317–1318. DOI: 10.1001/jama.2017.18391 PMID: 29532063

Begum, A., Muniasamy, A., Sabahath, A., Yaqub, H., & Karunakaran, G. (2024). Coronary heart disease classification using deep learning approach with feature selection for improved accuracy. *Technology and Health Care, 32*(3), 1991–2007. DOI: 10.3233/THC-231807 PMID: 38339946

Bhatnagar, R., Muniasamy, A., & Karunakaran, G. (2021). Predicting COVID-19 spread in Saudi Arabia using artificial intelligence techniques—Proposing a shift towards a sustainable healthcare approach. In Hassanien, A., Bhatnagar, R., & Darwish, A. (Eds.), *Artificial intelligence for sustainable development: Theory, practice and future applications. Studies in computational intelligence* (Vol. 912). Springer. DOI: 10.1007/978-3-030-51920-9_6

Bhatnagar, R., Muniasamy, A., & Muniasamy, V. (2021). Predictive analytics for cardiovascular disease diagnosis using machine learning techniques. In Hassanien, A., Bhatnagar, R., & Darwish, A. (Eds.), *Advanced machine learning technologies and applications (AMLTA 2020). Advances in intelligent systems and computing* (Vol. 1141). Springer. DOI: 10.1007/978-981-15-3383-9_45

Blease, C., Bernstein, M. H., Gaab, J., Kaptchuk, T. J., & Locher, C. (2019). Computerization and the future of primary care: A survey of general practitioners in the UK. *BMJ Open, 9*(11), e031160. DOI: 10.1136/bmjopen-2019-031160

Davenport, T., & Kalakota, R. (2019). The potential for artificial intelligence in healthcare. *Future Healthcare Journal*, *6*(2), 94–98. DOI: 10.7861/futurehosp.6-2-94 PMID: 31363513

Esteva, A., Robicquet, A., Ramsundar, B., Kuleshov, V., DePristo, M., Chou, K., Cui, C., Corrado, G., Thrun, S., & Dean, J. (2019). A guide to deep learning in healthcare. *Nature Medicine*, *25*(1), 24–29. DOI: 10.1038/s41591-018-0316-z PMID: 30617335

European Commission. (2020). White Paper on Artificial Intelligence: A European approach to excellence and trust. https://ec.europa.eu/info/publications/white-paper-artificial-intelligence-european-approach-excellence-and-trust_en

Finlayson, S. G., Subbaswamy, A., Singh, K., Bowers, J., Kupke, A., Zittrain, J., Kohane, I. S., & Saria, S. (2021). The clinician and dataset shift in artificial intelligence. *The New England Journal of Medicine*, *385*(3), 283–286. DOI: 10.1056/NEJMc2104626 PMID: 34260843

Fjeld, J., Achten, N., Hilligoss, H., Nagy, A. C., & Srikumar, M. (2020). Principled Artificial Intelligence: Mapping consensus in ethical and rights-based approaches to principles for AI. Berkman Klein Center for Internet & Society.

Gerke, S., Minssen, T., & Cohen, G. (2020). Ethical and legal challenges of artificial intelligence-driven healthcare. Cambridge Handbook of Health Research Regulation, 425–454. DOI: 10.1016/B978-0-12-818438-7.00012-5

He, J., Baxter, S. L., Xu, J., Xu, J., Zhou, X., & Zhang, K. (2019). The practical implementation of artificial intelligence technologies in medicine. *Nature Medicine*, *25*(1), 30–36. DOI: 10.1038/s41591-018-0307-0 PMID: 30617336

IBM. (2023). AI in Healthcare: Transforming Patient Care. https://www.ibm.com/watson-health

Jha, S., Topol, E. J., & Adashi, E. Y. (2020). Disruptive innovation and the future of healthcare workforce. *Journal of the American Medical Association*, *323*(21), 2117–2118. DOI: 10.1001/jama.2020.6509

Jiang, F., Jiang, Y., Zhi, H., Dong, Y., Li, H., Ma, S., Wang, Y., Dong, Q., Shen, H., & Wang, Y. (2017). Artificial intelligence in healthcare: Past, present and future. *Stroke and Vascular Neurology*, *2*(4), 230–243. DOI: 10.1136/svn-2017-000101 PMID: 29507784

Karunakaran, G., & Muniasamy, A. (2026). Challenges and future directions: Emerging trends and limitations in ML and optimization for healthcare. In Muniasamy, A. (Ed.), *Integrative machine learning and optimization algorithms for disease prediction* (pp. 339–368). IGI Global. DOI: 10.4018/979-8-3373-1087-9.ch012

Kelly, C. J., Karthikesalingam, A., Suleyman, M., Corrado, G., & King, D. (2019). Key challenges for delivering clinical impact with artificial intelligence. *BMC Medicine*, *17*(1), 195. DOI: 10.1186/s12916-019-1426-2 PMID: 31665002

Liu, X., Rivera, S. C., & Faes, L. (2019). Reporting guidelines for clinical trial reports for interventions involving artificial intelligence: The CONSORT-AI extension. *Nature Medicine*, *26*(9), 1364–1374. DOI: 10.1038/s41591-020-1034-x PMID: 32908283

Meskó, B., Hetényi, G., & Győrffy, Z. (2018). Will artificial intelligence solve the human resource crisis in healthcare? *BMC Health Services Research*, *18*(1), 545. DOI: 10.1186/s12913-018-3359-4 PMID: 30001717

Muniasamy, A. (2025). Revolutionizing health monitoring: Integrating transformer models with multi-head attention for precise human activity recognition using wearable devices. *Technology and Health Care*, *33*(1), 395–409. DOI: 10.3233/THC-241064 PMID: 39269866

NHS England. (2023). Artificial Intelligence: How AI is transforming the NHS. https://www.england.nhs.uk/aifuture/

Obermeyer, Z., Powers, B., Vogeli, C., & Mullainathan, S. (2019). Dissecting racial bias in an algorithm used to manage the health of populations. *Science*, *366*(6464), 447–453. DOI: 10.1126/science.aax2342 PMID: 31649194

Rajkomar, A., Dean, J., & Kohane, I. (2019). Machine learning in medicine. *The New England Journal of Medicine*, *380*(14), 1347–1358. DOI: 10.1056/NEJMra1814259 PMID: 30943338

Reddy, S., Fox, J., & Purohit, M. P. (2019). Artificial intelligence-enabled healthcare delivery. *Journal of the Royal Society of Medicine*, *112*(1), 22–28. DOI: 10.1177/0141076818815510 PMID: 30507284

Rengaramanujam, K., & Muniasamy, A. (2026). AI in hospital administration and formulary design: Optimizing resource allocation and patient flow. In Muniasamy, A., & Karunakaran, G. (Eds.), *Applications of artificial intelligence in pharmaceuticals* (pp. 215–246). IGI Global. DOI: 10.4018/979-8-3373-2043-4.ch008

Rudin, C. (2019). Stop explaining black box machine learning models for high stakes decisions and use interpretable models instead. *Nature Machine Intelligence*, *1*(5), 206–215. DOI: 10.1038/s42256-019-0048-x PMID: 35603010

Sabahath, A., Muniasamy, A., Begum, A., Yaqub, H., & Karunakaran, G. (2023). Lung cancer histopathology image classification using transfer learning with convolution neural network model. *Technology and Health Care*, *33*, 1–12. https://content.iospress.com/articles/technology-and-health-care/thc231029

Topol, E. J. (2019). *Deep Medicine: How Artificial Intelligence Can Make Healthcare Human Again*. Basic Books.

Verghese, A., Shah, N. H., & Harrington, R. A. (2018). What this computer needs is a physician: Humanism and artificial intelligence. *Journal of the American Medical Association*, *319*(1), 19–20. DOI: 10.1001/jama.2017.19198 PMID: 29261830

WHO. (2021). Ethics and governance of artificial intelligence for health: WHO guidance. World Health Organization. https://www.who.int/publications/i/item/9789240029200

Yu, K. H., Beam, A. L., & Kohane, I. S. (2018). Artificial intelligence in healthcare. *Nature Biomedical Engineering*, *2*(10), 719–731. DOI: 10.1038/s41551-018-0305-z PMID: 31015651

ADDITIONAL READING

Amann, J., Blasimme, A., Vayena, E., Frey, D., & Madai, V. I. (2022). Explainability for artificial intelligence in healthcare: A multidisciplinary perspective. *BMC Medical Informatics and Decision Making*, *22*(1), 1–9. DOI: 10.1186/s12911-021-01699-5 PMID: 34983500

Haque, A., Guo, M., & Verma, N. (2020). Clinical applications of machine learning in the diagnosis, classification, and prediction of cancer. *Future Oncology (London, England)*, *16*(18), 1343–1357. DOI: 10.2217/fon-2020-0202

Liew, C. (2018). The future of radiology augmented with Artificial Intelligence: A strategy for success. *European Journal of Radiology*, *102*, 152–156. DOI: 10.1016/j.ejrad.2018.03.019 PMID: 29685530

Mesko, B., Drobni, Z., Bényei, É., Gergely, B., & Győrffy, Z. (2017). Digital health is a cultural transformation of traditional healthcare. *mHealth*, *3*, 38. DOI: 10.21037/mhealth.2017.08.07 PMID: 29184890

Roberts, M., Driggs, D., Thorpe, M., Gilbey, J., Yeung, M., Ursprung, S., Aviles-Rivero, A. I., Etmann, C., McCague, C., Beer, L., Weir-McCall, J. R., Teng, Z., Gkrania-Klotsas, E., Ruggiero, A., Korhonen, A., Jefferson, E., Ako, E., Langs, G., Gozaliasl, G., & Schönlieb, C.-B. (2021). Common pitfalls and recommendations for using machine learning to detect and prognosticate for COVID-19 using chest radiographs and CT scans. *Nature Machine Intelligence*, *3*(3), 199–217. DOI: 10.1038/s42256-021-00307-0

Ross, C., & Swetlitz, I. (2017). IBM's Watson recommended 'unsafe and incorrect' cancer treatments, internal documents show. STAT News. https://www.statnews.com

KEY TERMS AND DEFINITIONS

Healthcare Automation: The use of advanced technologies, including AI and robotics, to streamline and support healthcare operations.

Healthcare Workforce: The collective group of professionals delivering medical and support services within healthcare systems.

Operational Efficiency: The ability of a healthcare system to optimize resources and processes to achieve maximum productivity with minimal waste.

Patient Care Quality: The standard of healthcare services delivered to patients, focusing on safety, effectiveness, and satisfaction.

Workforce Dynamics: The patterns and changes in healthcare workforce composition, roles, and interactions over time.

Chapter 14

Human-AI Collaboration for Balancing Technology and Compassion in Healthcare and Medicine

A. Ashwini

https://orcid.org/0009-0008-1248-7756

Vel Tech Rangarajan Dr. Sagunthala R&D Institute of Science and Technology, India

Banu Priya Prathaban

School of Computing, College of Engineering and Technology, SRM Institute of Science and Technology, India

A. Mahadevan

https://orcid.org/0009-0007-9826-6235

Sri Venkateswara College of Engineering, India

Syed Khaja Ahmeduddin Zakir

University of Technology and Applied Sciences, Ibra, Oman

ABSTRACT

The structure of AI technology enhances healthcare efficiency through process automation along with complex medical data analysis and patient-decision support tools for healthcare providers. The fundamental capability of AI systems in healthcare does not consist of replacing medical staff, but it enhances their operational potential. The central issue stems from discovering an appropriate method to combine AI strength with essential human medical capabilities in healthcare services. AI systems acquire and analyze increased quantities of data but lack the capability to

DOI: 10.4018/979-8-3373-2787-7.ch014

generate knowledgeable decisions. AI and human capability through symbiosis can become a synergistic experience for healthcare delivery. There are barriers to building trust and acceptance across healthcare providers and patients. Issues regarding data privacy and dependence on automated systems of judgment must also be addressed to bring AI into the routine of practice successfully. Achieving this synergy will refine hospital systems, as well as reinforce the basic principles of patient-centered medicine.

INTRODUCTION

Overview of Human-AI Collaboration in Modern Medicine

The healthcare industry is experiencing a fundamental shift because of artificial intelligence (AI) systems integration into medical practices in the fast-moving modern medical setting. Healthcare professionals avoid replacement as AI technology functions to augment clinical decisions and operational efficiency and deliver superior patient care results (Maadi et al., 2021). AI teams up with physicians by providing data analytics with pattern recognition and real-time results alongside a doctor-specific understanding of medical needs and fairness alongside emotional understanding of the situation. Their combined forces work together to construct a substantial partnership that will affect how healthcare services are delivered. Healthcare specialists are implementing AI systems throughout the medical pipeline, including radiology and pathology and oncology and cardiology departments. Human involvement becomes essential because AI must function as a support tool rather than a decision authority.

The healthcare sector utilizes AI for administrative purposes and operational aspects through scheduling services and electronic health record management and patient triage systems. Through healthcare applications, healthcare workers receive decreased mental and administrative strain which lets them dedicate their time to providing care directly to patients without emotional interruptions (Reverberi et al., 2022). Healthcare organizations need to establish a proper equilibrium between technological progress and human compassionate practices (Muniasamy, A. et al., 2020).

The development of artificial intelligence (AI) in healthcare started in the past decades after researchers implemented rule-based expert systems to reproduce clinical reasoning processes. The MYCIN system was among the first computerized clinical systems that aimed to diagnose bacterial infections and select antibiotic treatments in the 1970s. MYCIN, together with similar programs, demonstrated promising results, but adoption remained limited because the technology struggled with the restricted capabilities of available computers and restricted knowledge databases as well as issues with clinical workflow implementation (Diaz-Flores et al., 2022). The sector of healthcare artificial intelligence research witnessed growth through machine learning algorithms during the 1990s along with the early 2000s because these algorithms enabled systems to acquire knowledge from data through automated processes rather than using pre-programmed rules.

Recent medical practices employ artificial intelligence to extend beyond diagnostic functionality into all medical areas for robotic surgery assistance as well as mental health tracking and customized care sequencing. Healthcare entities employ two main applications of generative AI models for developing new drug compounds and large language models for medical document summarization, while predictive algorithms improve hospital resource efficiencies and patient care delivery (et al., 2026). The medicine field focuses on human-AI relationship development through explainable AI (XAI) and ethically aligned design and compassionate automation. Healthcare improvement through AI technology maintains relationships with essential human values and emotional intelligence needed for patient-centered healthcare delivery. Figure 1 shows the step by step progress of AI in Healthcare system.

Figure 1. Progress of AI in Healthcare System

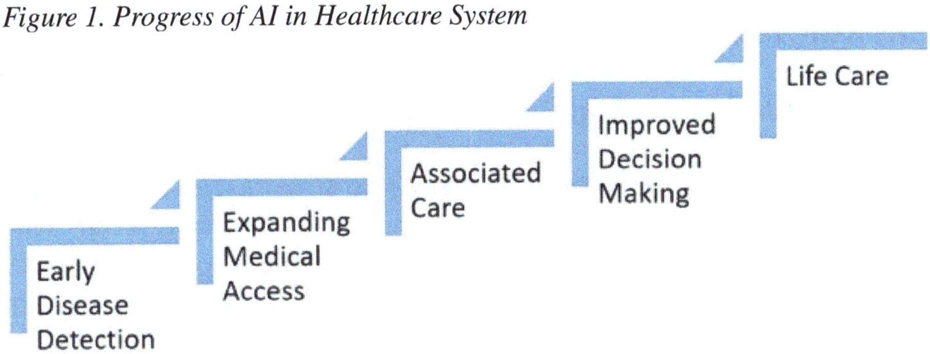

At the start of its development, AI systems relied on rule-based Clinical Decision Support Systems (CDSS) which followed pre-established clinical guidelines for making recommendations to healthcare professionals. The healthcare systems used by clinicians enable them to follow best practices by delivering medication error warnings and chronic condition management through alert tools and reminders. Predictive models have become standard practice in modern healthcare to forecast patient results and disease movement trajectories and identify admittance possibilities and create prevention-focused care approaches (Shan, & Li, 2024). Using AI technologies allows physicians to examine patient data along with laboratory results that identify individuals prone to developing sepsis, enabling medical staff to intervene early and save lives.

Modern healthcare systems have adopted generative AI technology that permits the generation of fresh content including synthetic medical pictures as well as clinical summaries and new drug compounds. Large language models in generative models help health practitioners develop medical reports as well as patient care guidelines and combine different sources of information to support clinical decisions (Ravichandran et al., 2024). Advanced healthcare systems move beyond support functions to enable healthcare professionals to work together with the platform for developing care delivery and research while engaging patients through unexplored means.

The primary objective of this chapter is to explore the evolving role of human-AI collaboration in healthcare and medicine, emphasizing the delicate balance between technological innovation and compassionate patient care. The chapter aims to provide a comprehensive understanding of how artificial intelligence can augment clinical decision-making, streamline administrative workflows, and enhance diagnostic accuracy while maintaining the human touch that is essential in patient-centered care. By the end of the chapter, readers should gain actionable insights into leveraging AI responsibly while preserving the compassionate essence of medical practice.

BACKGROUND

The Role of AI in Clinical Decision Making

Artificial Intelligence, through its transformative power, enhances clinical decision-making through accurate, expedited and standardized diagnosis and treatment determination processes. Doctors use established data insights to make better decisions, which involves both recognizing silent signs of disease and picking correct treatment solutions as well as forecasting possible medical complications. The artificial intelligence system functions as an intelligent tool that assists healthcare providers while avoiding the substitution of their professional medical decisions. The most extensive practical use of AI in clinical choice making occurs through medical imaging applications (Giordano et al., 2021). Deep learning systems achieve accurate disease diagnosis through their analysis of big datasets which contain X-ray and MRI and CT scan images to detect tumors, fractures and hemorrhages. The imaging systems provide additional human-like analysis capabilities for radiologists to help cut diagnostic errors while optimizing workflow management. Under emergency conditions, AI algorithms operate to determine patient emergency levels, helping accredited personnel perform triage and respond swiftly.

AI tools used in oncology react with molecular markers to find out which patients will benefit best from individual chemotherapy regimens or immunotherapies. Throughout healthcare facilities, AI delivers essential support through clinical decision systems that unite and supply appropriate guidelines along with drug-interaction reports with evidence-based recommendations during point-of-care interactions (Khalifa et al., 2024). The mission of AI implementation in healthcare should focus on supporting medical practitioners by revealing comprehensive information while eliminating ambiguity to generate and improve diagnosis quality and generate superior healthcare results for patients.

Diagnostic Support System

AI applications for diagnostic support through Diagnostic Support Systems (DSS) constitute the foundational technology for human-AI cooperation in healthcare. The diagnostic support systems help clinicians make their diagnostic assessments through patient data analysis including symptoms, along with lab results and imaging tests and medical records and generate possible diagnoses and suggested tests (Prathaban et al., 2024). Such capabilities substantially boost medical diagnosis reliability together with standardization performance for both rare and complex medical conditions. The diagnostic support systems of today operate with machine learning along with deep learning algorithms which use new data to gain knowledge and enhance their capabilities. The performance capabilities of AI models compare equally to expert radiologists when they evaluate lung nodules and fractures in addition to intracranial hemorrhages through radiological imaging. AI technology in dermatological practice helps medical staff perform diagnosis by categorizing skin lesions and identifying possible melanoma onset.

The Food and Drug Administration has approved AI technology for independent diagnosis of diabetic retinopathy using retinal imagery in ophthalmology practice (Bright et al., 2012). These diagnostic systems enable medical staff to detect diseases early while lowering diagnostic mistakes while providing automated assistance to handle lengthy tasks, which enhances their ability to deliver better patient care. To achieve effectiveness in clinical settings, diagnostic support systems should collaborate with human judgment instead of interfering with it. Healthcare professionals need systems with clear interfaces coupled with explanations and complete transparency in order to develop their trust. The clinical professional keeps the decision-making authority following AI recommendation outputs yet maintains their complete control over preserving human values and ethical care in every patient interaction. The use of diagnostic support systems demonstrates how artificial intelligence strengthens human medical practice instead of substituting human presence in healthcare, thus creating a system which combines technological assistance and compassionate care with clinical experience.

Prognostic Modeling and Risk Stratification

Modern healthcare requires accurate risk assessments from prognostic models, so AI tools continue to aid healthcare providers in improving diagnosis accuracy to support clinical practice. The goal of prognostic models involves forecasting disease progression through determinations of survival duration as well as recurrence prospects and complication susceptibility. Through risk stratification, medical staff group patients into categories according to their predicted vulnerability to enable specific treatment approaches and care order selection along with better resource management (Thurtle et al., 2019).

AI risk models in cardiology can determine heart failure and sudden cardiac arrest probabilities before events, thus enabling sooner treatment care and constant patient monitoring. Research models in oncology create survival prediction estimates together with therapy response forecasts from cancer characteristics as well as clinical patient information. Modern healthcare claims of AI use prognostic showing and risk stratification schemes to expect patient abilities while creating classes for patient assemblies based on forecast condition-development probabilities. Machine learning procedures analyze large EHRs together with genomic evidence and lifestyle drifts and imaging products to produce forecasts about disease development as well as action responses organized with probable health difficulties. Figure 2 shows the role and the steps involved in the progress of AI in clinical diagnosis.

Figure 2. Steps involved in the flow of the decision support system

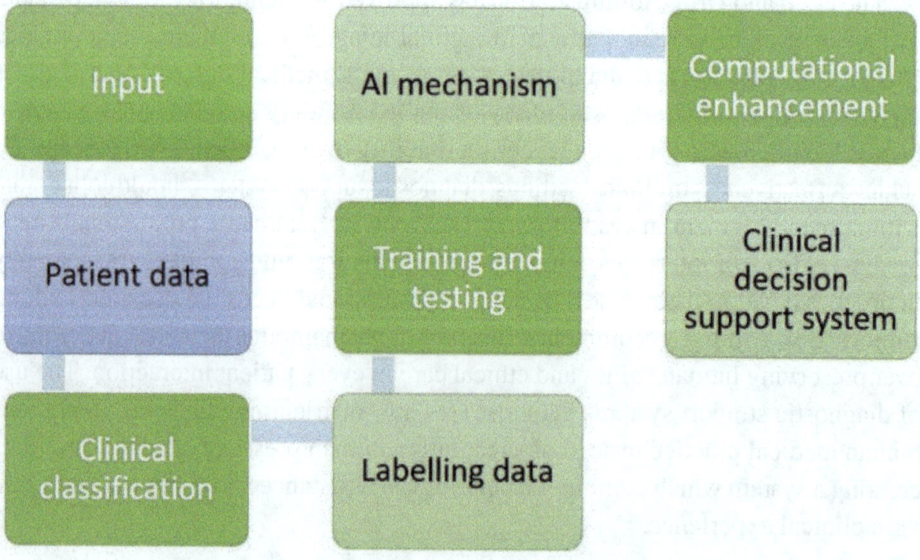

The early detection of patients who face increased danger of adverse events helps clinicians execute preemptive interventions to enhance treatment performance and achieve better results. AI predictive analysis provides exceptional value to medical management of continuing diseases such as diabetes, heart conditions and cancer. The integration of AI in oncological diagnostics uses previous patient data together with present diagnostic outcomes to forecast tumor recurrence as well as patient survival statistics. Cardiology services benefit from predictive models that analyze heart failure and stroke possibilities to identify risks which healthcare providers use for directing appropriate preventive care strategies. The obtained insights guide healthcare providers to make better treatment-related decisions regarding intensity levels as well as follow-up scheduling and resource distribution. The relationship between AI systems and healthcare providers in prognostic modeling enhances clinical judgment rather than substituting it.

AI tools help healthcare providers through evidence-based risk assessments that function as a secondary support mechanism to assist clinical practitioners in delivering targeted, timely and effective care. The implementation of AI into prognostic workflows establishes precise medicine and creates proactive healthcare systems which result in improved patient care alongside optimized healthcare resource management. Such patient information enables healthcare providers to build treatment strategies while supporting discussions concerning expected outcomes and family care objectives with patients. Stratification through AI technology serves as a common operational method for preventive medicine practice alongside population health management. Predictive analytics helps health systems detect high-risk patients facing diabetes or stroke as well as hospital readmission and thus enables specific preventive interventions and customized care plans (Rengaramanujam et al., 2026). These tools need to maintain a transparent system to allow clinicians a full understanding of risk prediction rationales.

AI in Drug Discovery and Personalized Treatment Planning

Through AI technologies, drug discovery processes now experience faster identification and development together with accelerated testing of new pharmaceutical compounds (Gauthaman, S. A. et al., 2026). Standard drug development recurs as a prolonged, high-cost procedure which demands years and multiple billions to create a single new medicine. Machine learning software analyzes simulated drug-biological interactions during development to detect detrimental effects which occur before marketing and creates new promising chemical drug structures (Muniasamy, A. et al., 2026). The utilization of AI in pharmaceutical discovery leads to shorter drug development periods and cuts down on expenses and risks during the drug discovery phase.

AI demonstrates its most significant value in drug utilization by finding new applications for approved medications. AI uses analysis of previous unrelated genetic-clinical data patterns to identify new therapeutic uses for approved drugs which proved critical in the COVID-19 pandemic. Programs of Artificial Intelligence programs work actively to enhance personalized therapy approaches which match well with precision medicine principles (Yogeshappa et al., 2024). AI tools combine multiple patient-related data groups such as genomic information, daily routines, existing health conditions, and treatment course history to deliver treatments that match effectiveness against tolerance. The implementation of AI in drug development and tailored medicine therapy enables medical staff to produce patient-tailored evidence-based care that provides maximum benefit to patients. Human-AI collaborative practices create the perfect framework for healthcare by strengthening medical professionals to make wise and understanding decisions through computational support that converts complex information into therapeutic medical actions.

Augmented Intelligence in Enhancement and Not Replacement

Human-AI collaboration in healthcare applications depends on augmented intelligence because artificial intelligence aims to improve medical expertise rather than assume clinical responsibilities. The approach known as augmented intelligence stands against automation employment narratives because it enables systems to act as supportive tools that boost the abilities of medical experts while enhancing both their professional expertise and operational efficiency as well as their decision-making capabilities (Naim, A., et al. (2026). AI tools within this approach support clinicians as co-pilots that present data insights while assisting with automated tasks and cutting clinician's mental workload.

AI systems operating in diagnostic imaging applications have the ability to highlight potential abnormalities in X-rays or MRIs, which directs radiologists toward essential study regions and prevents them from disregarding faint findings. Human experts maintain authority in final interpretations because they must combine clinical understanding of patients alongside their medical history and professional assessment of situations (Sadiku et al., 2021). Robotic systems with AI guidance lead to better control and precision in surgery even though skilled surgeons direct their operation. AI applications at healthcare organizations operate with human caregivers who maintain control of empathetic care decisions as well as ethical medical practice divisions.

Definition of Augmented Intelligence

The design philosophy of Augmented Intelligence combines human and machine interaction to enhance human intellectual capacities rather than attempting to take human roles. Augmented intelligence stands apart from regular AI since it employs artificial intelligence technologies to work as supporting systems which help human professionals make decisions and expand their cognitive powers and productivity levels. By uniting human capabilities with machine abilities, organizations achieve better results for both accuracy and human empathy while generating the most effective outcomes.

Healthcare applications of augmented intelligence combine AI technology with medical professionals to enhance clinical diagnosis along with treatment development and health services administration and patient service delivery (Zheng et al., 2017). Healthcare systems supply medical professionals with predictive analytics and useful suggestions in addition to practical insights which keep healthcare decisions as professional responsibilities. Through a collaborative process based on trust, technology becomes a tool that aids compassionate ethical patient-specific medical practices. In the healthcare evolution of tomorrow, augmented intelligence will extend human capabilities instead of substituting them to create superior clinical results for scientific and compassionate care.

Augmented intelligence functions to build a healthcare system that operates both efficiently and with higher degrees of humanism. When AI handles administrative work, it provides healthcare professionals with extra time to establish human connections with patients, thereby addressing their emotional and psychological requirements as well as developing therapeutic relationships. The inclusion of AI in decision support systems helps clinicians keep their medical knowledge up-to-date while providing them with better confidence in evidence-based practice. Augmented intelligence creates pathways for technological enhancement to support compassionate care in order to change healthcare into an intelligent system that meets the unique requirements of individual patients.

Co-Pilot Models in Diagnostics and Surgery

Co-pilot systems in healthcare diagnostics and surgery are transforming medical performance through AI system-MD collaborative approaches in the developing healthcare field. The designed systems serve medical personnel by boosting their capabilities instead of taking over their duties because they function as smart task-support tools to help with diagnosis processes and procedural work. Radiologists receive support from AI systems which detect abnormalities in medical images prior to human expert perception in radiological fields. The AI system's operational structure consists of detecting relevant regions alongside proposing potential diagnostic results, yet the radiologist utilizes these inputs to make a complete clinical assessment before reaching a final diagnosis. By integrating clinical strategies, medical practitioners can enhance disease detection and decrease professional exhaustion to maintain their ability to detect relevant medical signals.

AI systems enable surgical staff to access real-time data evaluation features for tissue analysis and blood flow examination and surgical field awareness during procedural tasks. During operative procedures, surgeons retain control by applying their clinical experience to patient needs and make final choices after AI offers supporting recommendations. Medical practitioners receiving assistance from co-pilot artificial intelligence systems gain two advantages from their data processing capabilities for both small and large information sets, so clinicians can focus on essential patient engagement and complex medical choices. Healthcare providers can improve patient care by partnering with AI technology while decreasing errors and preserving the use of compassionate care throughout the system instead of replacing one-on-one clinical care.

Empathy in AI-Driven Care

Artificial intelligence (AI) achieves considerable gains in healthcare which allows improved patient care over better diagnostics and modified treatment strategies. Medical professionals must consider essential questions about preserving empathy together with following ethical standards as AI emerges in healthcare delivery. The precise data-processing capabilities of AI systems do not encompass human capabilities for empathy and ethical judgment in healthcare, together with compassion for patients' care needs. Healthcare professionals must use AI tools to augment human qualities in care provision because this stance enables ethical and compassionate healthcare delivery.

The practice of healthcare empathy extends beyond familiarizing oneself with patient conditions to include detecting psychological and emotional and social requirements through compassionate treatment measures. The remarkable data processing capabilities of AI systems do not include genuine understanding of patient emotions and emotional support delivery capabilities. Regardless of its capabilities to identify diabetes risk through patient data, AI lacks essential human traits for consoling patients which healthcare providers provide through diagnosis communications (Rubin et al., 2024). Healthcare professionals need to remain present in medical interactions because AI systems cannot provide direct patient care even though they assist with diagnosis and administrative work.

The implementation of AI in healthcare creates substantial ethical problems pertaining to patient privacy protection alongside issues about patient independence, alongside issues involving fair medical treatment and provider responsibility. Data biases that remain unidentified and unaddressed enable AI to generate healthcare inequalities which specifically impact minority and underrepresented patient populations. The deployment of ethical AI health systems should establish transparent processes which provide patients and clinicians with visible explanations about decision methods and recommendation development. Patient consent and data security matters stand as essential matters during these situations. Every patient must get full information regarding data processing in addition to having inviolable privacy rights.

The implementation of empathy alongside ethical standards in health services requires partnership between healthcare professionals and AI technologies. The data-based solutions provided by AI to medical services need to orient their decision support toward comprehensive healthcare outcomes. The healthcare system relies on AI technology to identify medical threats while healthcare staff maintain complete responsibility to determine the patient's value system and lifestyle preferences when creating treatment protocols. Healthcare practitioners use technology as a tool to deliver customized care of superior ethical quality while showing empathy.

Ethical Considerations in Patient Care

The evolving medical environment necessitates healthcare ethics as an essential principle to protect patient care by letting artificial intelligence operate alongside compassion and fairness and respect (Muniasamy, A. eta l., 206; Rengaramanujam 2026). Standard ethical principles provide healthcare staff with guidance to make professional choices which protect their patients' welfare and identity and self-reliance and maintain trust and open understanding between providers and those they serve. Every medical aspect of AI decision-making, from diagnosis to treatment planning to care management, needs ethical consideration because it affects the core values of medical practice.

Autonomy and Informed Consent

The increasing healthcare decision-making role of AI systems necessitates proper accountability mechanisms to be established. The ethical standard of patient healthcare requires unambiguous responsibility for AI-assisted clinical decisions. The decision-making process must have clinicians standing at its center while AI serves to provide them with information as a supporting system rather than controlling healthcare decisions (Chervenak & McCullough, 2021). The need for transparency requires AI systems to provide clear explanations which allow healthcare professionals to understand the process of building their clinical decisions. Openness in AI technology systems creates mutual faith between patients along with medical professionals and the healthcare sector, which makes the technology serve as an assistance component rather than an autonomous decision machine.

Privacy and Confidentiality

The core ethical principle in healthcare focuses on patient-centered care and mandates treating patients with dignity because it requires respect and empathy. The power of artificial intelligence to advance healthcare must not lead to dismissing human aspects, which include emotional support, communication and compassion in medical care. AI systems must be ethically assessed by healthcare providers to preserve their patient trust-building capacity through establishing relationships with medical clients. Healthcare professionals must engage in significant patient-family dialogues alongside offering emotional support that exceeds AI system capabilities when AI systems affect major treatment decisions, including end-of-life choices and cancer interventions.

Bias and Fairness

Medical ethics protects patient decision-making power through patient autonomy as its core principle in preventing healthcare control losses. Medical practitioners must support their patients' treatment freedom by learning their beliefs together with their values and preferences. Patient autonomy remains crucial at this stage of artificial intelligence development since it enables healthcare recipients to preserve their freedom to choose medical options beyond AI-generated diagnostics and plans of care. Patient care experiences both quality and equity to a vast extent based on how bias and fairness are handled. Judgment and decision-making happen unintentionally, yet bias works as a predetermination or prejudice.

Various types of biases affect healthcare delivery, which include racial, gender-based, socioeconomic, age-related and bias through emerging technologies such as artificial intelligence. Healthcare disparities emerge because these biases result in mismatches between how medical professionals diagnose patients and what treatment options they receive and the methods they use for pain control and the health results patients obtain. The lack of proper pain medication delivery to Black patients remains a problem because medical professionals falsely believe there are biological differences between races. Medical professionals frequently overlook and diagnose incorrectly the symptoms that women present with disease manifestations, particularly in heart disease cases. Patients who belong to lower income groups are potentially at risk of insufficient healthcare treatment because of socioeconomic bias. Older adults together with disabled individuals, encounter discrimination while healthcare providers often grant some interventions to them at reduced priority levels.

Accountability and Transparency

Many healthcare choices between physicians and their patients are based on a shared decision-making process. The decision-making process should always include clinicians who will use AI tools to enhance their judgments instead of giving technology complete control. The shared decision-making model determines healthcare choices between physicians and their patients, but all decision-making activities must include clinicians who use AI tools to improve their judgments instead of giving technology control. The concept of fairness within patient care requires equal treatment and health services without discrimination based on social attributes. Fairness implementation demands recognition of biases across both personal and organizational systems. Healthcare professionals need individual training that enables them to detect and minimize implicit bias through cultural competence together with empathy skills.

Healthcare institutions need to develop inclusive policies alongside the implementation of diverse clinical trials programs that provide both resources and technologies to all patients equally. The integration of AI and machine learning tools in medical practice requires consistent evaluation because these systems need to avoid maintaining current biases. The process requires using diverse datasets and developing fairness testing and transparency methods for algorithms. A fair patient care approach produces better health results together with stronger relationships between patients and health providers, which strengthens a just and effective healthcare system. Modern medicine requires both moral and practical reasons to address bias.

Patient-Centered Care and Compassion

Healthcare delivery should prioritize patient-centered care because physicians must show both respect and dignity while demonstrating genuine empathy to their patients. As a tool to enhance medical services effectiveness, healthcare technology needs to maintain human emotional support as the most important and fundamental priority in patient care. Healthcare providers should maintain their key responsibility to build trusting patient relationships because ethical guidelines demand AI systems support human judgments rather than substitute physician interaction. When AI contributes to life-changing healthcare choices such as cancer therapies or end-of-life approaches, healthcare providers need to conduct personal discussions and offer aid which surpasses AI capabilities with patients and their families.

Patient Autonomy and shared Decision-making

The fundamental concept of medical ethics stresses the healthcare personal right to independently decide what medical choices they need. Healthcare providers must show respect for patients who want to decide their treatment options through decisions validated by their personal beliefs and values and individual preferences. The principle holds significant importance at present when healthcare professionals integrate AI systems and analytical data because it establishes patient control over care decisions regardless of AI recommendations. The healthcare decision-making process requires clinicians and patients to team up as they identify an appropriate medical course of action (Serrano et al., 2016). Medical professionals possess medication expertise, but patients maintain an exclusive understanding of personal life experiences and personal preferences and values. SDM establishes a system where healthcare providers assist patients in exploring their treatment options by clarifying the corresponding risks and advantages as well as the unknown elements while adapting solutions to their personal health needs.

Shared decision-making holds additional importance in AI-driven care because AI tools will produce data-based recommendations and prediction results yet remain incapable of grasping patient decision factors shaped by emotional and psychological aspects. The most statistically advantageous cancer treatment suggested by an AI algorithm clashes with a patient's individual choices, which include life quality and family commitments above numerical recommendations. The decoding of AI-generated information must be done by healthcare providers while keeping patient values as key factors in clinical choice processes.

Through shared decision-making models, patients who have multiple treatment choices alongside ambiguity about their treatments can keep control of their decision-making process. Medical systems utilize AI to produce clinical assessments which physicians use to direct healthcare choices, yet they must receive human-based recommendation delivery for cases with multiple treatment options. The review of drug options recommended by AI in chronic disease management requires clinical staff to include patients' perspectives on side effects and lifestyle limitations together with their emotional reactions to diagnoses.

Medical care providers must deliver simple explanations regarding AI-based support systems to patients to achieve successful patient autonomy integration alongside shared decision-making. AI-driven systems need to provide transparent explanations because both patients and clinicians should know how decisions are made along with what determining variables exist. The ethical application of artificial intelligence depends on patients being completely informed about data usage as well as AI's possible effects on their health treatment direction. Patient autonomy aligns perfectly with shared decision-making methods to preserve human care qualities while technology strengthens healthcare capabilities. The healthcare process allows patients both autonomy over decision-making and empowerment through complete system respect and active listening.

MAIN FOCUS OF THE CHAPTER

Human-AI Communication

The relationship between humans using artificial intelligence systems for assisting human decision-making constitutes Human-AI communication. Healthcare operations benefit from this communication when healthcare personnel join with AI technologies to improve both patient results and workplace productivity (Mou & Xu, 2017). Processing large data sets together with pattern analysis remains possible for AI systems. However, effective human-machine interaction ensures proper utilization of systems together with ethical operations and clear system visibility. Figure 3 shows the interaction between the human AI collaboration systems.

Figure 3. Human AI collaboration systems

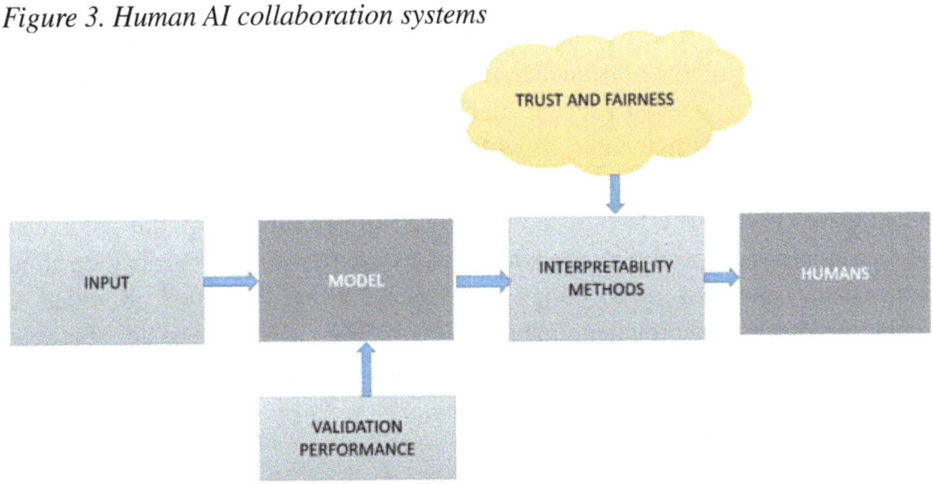

Clear and Transparent Communication

Human-AI communication encounters a principal obstacle because users need to understand and experience immediate clarity from the interaction. Medical AI systems, including diagnostic programs, provide complex decisions that require detailed explanation by healthcare staff along with treatment recommendation platform users to understand their reasoning processes effectively. True effectiveness in AI requires it to explain its logical steps, show how conclusions form as well as state prediction or recommendation confidence levels. AI's effectiveness depends on healthcare providers understanding how it generates its results, since clinicians must base their medical choices on them. An AI diagnostic tool examines radiological images to discover potential issues which could exist in the data. The AI platform requires delivering diagnostic findings to medical staff by presenting anomaly types together with its diagnostic reasoning alongside its evaluation accuracy. Healthcare professionals can access explanations from AI systems while asking needed questions, which enables them to use AI outputs as support mechanisms that reinforce their clinical competence instead of believing machine decisions.

Empathy and Contextual Awareness

Human interaction using empathy remains essential for healthcare AI functions when treating patients because it needs both analysis processing together with compassionate communication. Despite medical conversation facilitation capabilities, AI lacks full competence in both human clinician empathy and emotional intelligence. Clinicians delivering compassionate care can use AI frameworks for automated response recommendations as well as standardized compassionate information delivery together with patient concern analysis through data analysis. An AI-assisted chatbot system interacts with patients through an automatic service that delivers information about symptoms alongside therapeutic alternatives together with details about side effects. The patient support system through this automated service employs supportive dialog which guides users through their situation along with assurances about forthcoming medical procedures. The information that AI provides to healthcare providers enables them to achieve a suitable balance between delivering medical care alongside sensitive patient communication.

Real-time Collaboration

The operation of AI systems requires continuous connection with medical staff in the clinical domains to deliver speedy and precise healthcare decisions. The detector systems and adaptive recommendation features of AI tools give continuous feedback by allowing healthcare providers to modify patient data starting from vital signs to laboratory results. AI monitoring of critical care patients permits healthcare staff to detect early warnings that trigger efficient clinical intervention. The presentation of real-time information by AI systems must use display methods which help healthcare staff execute appropriate responses. AI systems should analyze alert importance then present critical information following actionable methods with treatment pathways for clinicians to use. This information delivery has become vital for human medical decisions in urgent situations demanding immediately effective responses to life and death.

Patient-Clinician-AI Interaction

The integration of AI systems into healthcare has created circumstances where patients receive AI-enabled services through both virtual assistants and telemedicine platforms and health monitoring devices during patient interactions. Both patients and users need to maintain easy access to AI system communications which always focuses on patient care needs. The system needs to present medical concepts using familiar vocabulary which enables the direction of healthcare actions together with the delivery of health-related information in a welcoming format.

AI-assisted healthcare delivery needs particular educational interventions to clarify medical system roles for patients and their effects on clinical decision-making processes. The operations of BI need transparency through a clear description of all healthcare provider-essential procedures and processes which include patient information investment steps. AI acts as an informational tool that extends human interaction between health practitioners and their patients through essential clinical information needed for confident medical decisions.

Addressing Ethical and Social Implications

Human-AI communication succeeds when healthcare providers work to fix the ethical problems which AI brings to medical systems in their interactions with patients. Healthcare providers need to explain their AI training methodologies to patients while ensuring equality in patient care without neglecting discrimination potential discrimination factors that arise from AI-generated suggestions. The ethical execution of AI technology must provide decision support that shows equality for every individual in society. Both healthcare providers and patients should obtain this guarantee.

Medical institutions need human-AI communication as a fundamental requirement to integrate AI systems effectively in their healthcare delivery model. The implementation of clear and empathetic AI interaction procedures enables healthcare providers to enhance patient outcomes through improved clinical effects while maintaining patient trust in AI-assisted medicine. Patient-focused medical care that promotes compassion benefits from artificial intelligence as a technological aid system when medical staff exchange information successfully with AI systems.

Designing Interpretable and Explainable AI Systems

The increasing use of artificial intelligence systems across multiple fields requires these systems to show their accuracy through explainable and interpretable mechanisms, particularly in critical domains such as healthcare. Such transparency is essential because medical staff, together with patients and regulatory bodies, require both faith and clarity in AI-based choices. The development of interpretable and explainable AI systems produces models which generate comprehensible insights that reveal decision processes, so users maintain transparent access to accountable processes. The highest risk context of healthcare demands essential systems' development because these systems help improve medical decision quality while sustaining ethical medical practices.

The design of interpretable AI systems requires builders to make models which display insight regarding their decision-making patterns, so humans can comprehend them. Decision trees and linear regression models maintain high interpretability because their design is basic, and their organizational processes remain easy to understand. Neural networks and deep learning algorithms reserve a "black box" function. Therefore, users lack perceptibility into the derivation method for precise results. Various methods have been created to show why complex models make decisions because of their unexplained reasoning process (Mohseni et al., 2021). Medical experts can explain individual predictions through tools like SHAP and LIME, which reveal what elements led to decision outcomes. These methods enable full clarity about decisive outcome factors when patients and medical staff use sophisticated AI systems.

The creation of explainable AI models demands that explanation outputs must be both relevant and understandable to users. Medical staff working with AI tools in healthcare need to fully comprehend the reasoning process which led to diagnostic results and treatment suggestions. Healthcare providers need user-friendly visualizations and clear, simple interfaces to understand information that underlies AI technology because they lack advanced technical knowledge in AI. Featured importance graphs together with saliency maps enable medical experts to better understand AI decision-making processes, which improve their evidence-based decision-making practices. The application of lay term explained concepts enables patients to better understand how AI contributes to their healthcare while promoting collaboration between providers and patients during decision-making sessions.

The development of explainable AI systems requires both ethical principles and their integration throughout the entire system design process. The systematic development requires AI models to demonstrate their clear explanations and maintain their integrity and openness and their capability to face questions of responsibility. The primary ethical problem lies in preventing AI from repeating discriminating patterns. AI systems developed using restricted information about specific population groups create results which create possible harm to these marginalized communities. AI system models with built-in bias-detection software and fairness algorithms developed by developers ensure equal treatment in choice execution processes. The ability to detect sources of incorrect or dangerous AI recommendations becomes possible through explainable systems which healthcare personnel can track for error identification. Ethical decision-making in AI-assisted healthcare depends on this system, which helps maintain accountability standards.

As a necessary step, AI technologies must become interpretable and explainable to achieve trustworthy and ethical healthcare use. The development of transparent, explainable and relevant models enables developers to heighten decision support and clinical quality outcomes while maintaining patient autonomy and providing fair healthcare services. AI's success in healthcare will rest on its ability to effectively explain its reasoning as technology assumes a more important position in healthcare delivery.

Communicating AI-Generated Recommendations to Patients

It is essential to deliver AI-recommended information to patients because this practice empowers both patients and providers to understand healthcare decisions while maintaining their role in care management. The recommendations provided by AI systems stem from complicated data evaluation processes that might make it challenging for patients to understand the reasoning behind decisions. The healthcare provider needs to convert the insights from AI algorithms into understandable language which patients can easily comprehend. Healthcare providers need to explain the AI-recommended diagnosis through the examination of patient medical records together with lifestyle information and test findings (Kreps, & Neuhauser, 2017). The simplification of AI recommendations produces an understanding for patients which enables them to trust their treatment options.

Natural communication between providers and patients demands both emotional support and deep emotional understanding. The combination of AI recommendations produces an overwhelming effect because patients face difficult medical conditions along with significant treatment choices. The healthcare provider must start these discussions by showing concern for patients' feelings while responding to their worries and providing assurance. Healthcare providers must recognize the importance of emotional aspects of patient decisions and clarify that AI provides assistance in ongoing collaborative decision-making in which medical professionals maintain their authority alongside patient beliefs. The involvement of patients through this process produces trust together with satisfied patients because they receive both support and hearing and active participation in decisions.

Healthcare patients need to understand that artificial intelligence serves as an aid in improving clinical decisions rather than functioning as a substitution for human medical expertise. The practitioners must show transparency about the AI system while revealing its operational processes, including used data and definable limitations within recommendations. The practice of correctly presenting AI systems leads patients to make better decisions about their healthcare despite potential worries regarding artificial intelligence. The presentation of AI as a dependable enhancement tool which supports healthcare relationships will help medical professionals gain acceptance and stronger partnership between patients and AI programs.

Trust-Building Between Patients, Clinicians and AI Tools

Trust formation between patients, clinicians and AI tools creates a necessary condition for AI system success in healthcare. Healthcare organizations must establish widespread acceptance of AI through trust between patients and clinicians because these systems perform diagnostic assessments and provide recommendations for treatments and monitor patients' conditions. Create trust by maintaining transparency along with precise communication and demonstrating reliable performance through demonstrated successful results of AI tools (Bergquist et al., 2024). Patients and healthcare personnel experience more trust in technology measurement when medical professionals provide detailed explanations about AI system decision processes and show how system recommendations comply with official medical benchmarks.

Empathy and collaboration play key roles in trust-building. Human expertise together with emotional intelligence should remain as essential elements since they cannot be substituted by AI data-driven insights. Some clinical staff should rely on AI technology solely for supportive functions without it becoming a replacement alternative in their delivery practices. Healthcare providers improve patient satisfaction by including patients in decision discussions featuring both AI recommendations and personal patient preferences. The joint work between clinicians and AI produces a model for responsibility sharing which leads to optimal patient outcomes. When clinicians utilize AI technology to extend their capabilities instead of handing over control to them, it leads to improved patient trust in healthcare AI.

An ethical standards framework enables trust development between three core groups which consist of patients and AI systems as well as clinicians. Healthcare workers need to take charge of personal data security concerns as well as discrimination issues while performing their responsibility to maintain data clarity. Healthcare providers should show patients the details of their data handling procedures to show their HIPAA compliance. The patient requires complete information surrounding the AI learning approaches to model training and dataset application alongside the bias elimination techniques. The combination of high-quality data and optimal

AI functionality protects the unbiased nature of recommendations for healthcare providers to establish trust in AI systems for responsible treatment management.

SOLUTIONS AND RECOMMENDATIONS

Human-Centered AI Design

Artificial Intelligence product design focused on human needs results in systems that assist the expectations and values but also life circumstances of everyone in healthcare. The goal in AI system development involves increasing human capability and delivering enhanced outcomes alongside vital human characteristics that underpin care delivery, like providing real care and fair medical treatment. Healthcare developers build AI system technologies through human-centered practices to enhance diagnostic choices between human operators and machines and therefore drive better patient outcomes.

During structure development phases, the process of planning AI requires user participation and response because of its importance for human-oriented approaches. The design process for AI healthcare tools requires involvement from both clinicians and patients in addition to other stakeholders from the start, according to Shneiderman et al. (2020). Software developers, able to analyze user needs and work routines, develop systems that present clear solutions which address original specifications. The workflow integration of clinical AI systems stands as the primary requirement for practitioners as patients seek AI tools to convey medical data through easily understandable actionable information. System design through standard user interaction methods leads to technical operational success with uniform user accessibility from the end-user perspective.

Healthcare AI applications require empathy and faith to be essential ingredients in human-oriented design procedures to stop emotional connections between healthcare providers and patients from diminishing. AI systems require methods of clear explanation to make it possible for medical staff to understand diagnostic suggestions and treatment proposals for presenting them to patients in a compassionate manner. Patients must actively take part in their care choices by themselves, since automated healthcare support should never eliminate human medical interaction. By placing a focus on human-centered AI, both human expert skills and technology will complement each other to create healthcare settings that best utilize their combined capabilities.

User Centric Design in Medical Tools

Medical tool development follows user-centric design principles because it directs development work toward comprehending healthcare worker needs and patient needs. The impact of medical tools on patient outcomes is what directs design solutions toward usability, accessibility first and then effectiveness in healthcare delivery. Through this approach, healthcare instruments integrate compatible advanced technologies that directly address user-base interaction requirements.

The approach of user-centric design prompts clinicians to create tools that suit their professional activities in medical workplaces. The delivery of straightforward operations and precise actionable results needs to be a standard requirement for all medical tools such as EHR systems and diagnostic devices and AI-assisted decision-making platforms. The interface system needs to use layouts that enhance mental processing through simplified procedures and decreased the need for user system travel. The diagnostic functionality powered by AI should display only essential information to healthcare staff during crucial decision points. The design process also requires medical staff participation to create tools which meet their practical requirements and support actual healthcare operations.

The approach of user-centric design for healthcare patients requires developers to create systems that increase patient autonomy during medical treatment. The design team works to create medical tools which display information through simple interfaces using non-specialized medical terminology. A mobile health application used by patients to track their chronic disease must offer instant feedback while reminding them about their medical data while presenting graphical representations of their health numbers for better care plan adherence (Arsand, & Demiris, 2008). Medical devices need ergonomic evaluation alongside easy usability, especially because senior citizens with disabilities sometimes encounter physical constraints. Trust-building needs medical organizations to start transparency while bringing customized supervision as fundamental basics for better patient interaction and service fulfillment.

A user-centric method builds patient trust in medical technology. Thus, patients follow their treatment plans better and achieve better health results. Modern medical tools that put users first enable healthcare providers to work more efficiently alongside better patient experiences, thus achieving greater patient care outcomes. Developers who focus on building medical tools through usability improvements and end-user accessibility and collaboration create resources which optimize performance standards and give patients and clinicians the power to make well-informed, confident healthcare decisions.

Accessibility and Usability for Both Clinicians and Patients

Healthcare medical tools along with technologies achieve success by offering easy accessibility to clinicians and patients. These two factors help to establish practical medical tools which reach their targets effectively while improving healthcare delivery as a whole. The quality of accessibility and usability creates major operational impacts on clinical workflows together with patient treatment decisions and delivery of healthcare services for clinical staff members. Patient factors which originate from accessibility and usability promote their health-related participation and better patient compliance with their treatment programs while producing superior health results.

In tool development for clinicians, designers concentrate on creating interfaces that offer smooth integration within their work space and maintain simplicity. The coverage consists of electronic health records systems as well as diagnostic tools and platforms powered by AI technology (Anderson et al., 2014). The tools used by clinicians for complex quick decisions need to be simple to use and require basic training because difficult interfaces diminish work efficiency. The design of user-friendly interfaces with low navigation complexity represents usability in interface creation. An effective AI diagnostic tool design must present vital information using unassuming displays that label essential data points in a straightforward and readable manner. The accessibility of tools refers to making these resources easily available through different clinical platforms to offer ready access for healthcare professionals. The integration of mobile devices and computers ensures doctors can obtain patient data and generate decisions both in stressful situations and when working with portable devices.

Users alongside healthcare patients require equally vital features of convenient access and usable interfaces which determine their ability to work with their healthcare plans and disease management strategies. Patients need to encounter digital health tools that function easily, and they must be able to understand clear instructions through visual aids which simplify complex medical information. A health app with effective design features should use tracking technology and present understandable feedback to users without medical training. Patients need accessible health tools which must be provided to everyone, including disabled users. Healthcare engineers create mobile devices alongside medical instruments with text size adjustability and screen reader access and verbal command capabilities to suit diverse patients experiencing physical restrictions and visual limitations. Accessibility for patients improves when tools operate on multiple operating systems and devices, especially when patients have restricted access to advanced technology.

The drive to make both medical personnel and patients comfortable with technology aims to establish a platform that will boost patient care quality while improving healthcare outcomes. Simple and adjustable medical implements calculated for healthcare providers bring better efficacy alongside low patient blocking levels and larger patient participation proportions. The integration of effective medical technology use by both clinical personnel and their patients leads to substantial enhancements in both patient health outcomes and health service operational efficiency.

FUTURE RESEARCH DIRECTIONS

Remote Monitoring and Virtual Health Assistants

Virtual health supporters organized with remote persistent observing tools create a healthcare innovation by permitting consistent fitness metric tracking and adapted non-clinic patient assistance. Remote monitoring allows patients to use wearable devices and sensors that measure their vital signs for health providers to monitor continuously. Through remote monitoring, healthcare professionals obtain the capability to both preventively handle chronic diseases and identify health problems before they become severe cases (Kalusivalingam et al., 2021)). Virtual health assistants fortified with AI skills aid patients through modified services, including real-time feedback maintenance, treatment alerts, symptom-tracking structures and health query answers. Remote tools connect patients with their care providers in new ways that boost practitioner-patient contact while patients follow care instruction more effectively, leading to lower requirements for repeated office visits, thus making medical services easily available to people with restricted mobility and those living in distant areas. The joint application of remote monitoring systems with virtual assistants enables ongoing care delivery which results in better health outcomes while helping bring about patient-centric healthcare practices.

AI-Assisted Surgeries With Real-Time Feedback

AI arrangements with machine learning abilities together with processer vision knowledge improve surgical accuracy over live monitoring during actions. Medical processes gain thorough operational feedback through schemes that analyze diagnostic sensor data and medicinal imaging as well as other analytical tools by running algorithms. AI expertise allows healthcare providers to classify essential organizations and show areas that need consideration while predicting possible surgical problems, thus boosting surgeons' capacity to make informed choices. Feedback mechanisms that operate in real time enhance diagnostic accuracy through decreased healthcare personnel errors when delivering specific interventions to anatomical structures (Trujillo et al., 2024). Through AI optimization, physicians can improve tool functionality and monitor process development while suggesting optimal surgical approaches which amalgamate to make superior outcomes and reduced recovery time and decreased medical liabilities. Surgeons can offer better and secure medical treatments that uphold precise accuracy due to AI incorporation in operating rooms.

AI Chatbots With Human Oversight

Healthcare organizations depend on AI chatbots supervised by humans to extend patient access to information and perform symptom assessment and provide healthcare assistance during all hours. Hospital supervise and organize chatbots using natural language treating composed with machine learning that grip routine queries and achieve healthcare calculations for patients and accomplish managerial tasks such as development appointments. Human intervention is mandatory to guarantee both safety and high-quality patient healthcare (Necz, 2024). When AI chatbots face complicated or sensitive healthcare situations, healthcare professionals need to step in to supervise the discussion and provide individualized treatment to patients. Specialists who use this mixture of AI-based schemes with their therapeutic knowledge attain enhanced patient interface while preserving quality care.

Integrating AI Literacy Healthcare Into Medical Education

A basic understanding of AI which must be taught within medical training programs helps future health practitioners to implement and manage AI technology systems when providing clinical care. AI systems continue to dominate medical diagnostics and treatment planning and patient management, so healthcare providers, along with medical students, need comprehensive knowledge about these technologies' operational principles and their ethical and practical and clinical consequences. The educational framework of AI should include basic AI concepts about machine learning together with natural language processing and data analytics, while demonstrating their practical applications in medical facilities. All training programs should teach the actual boundaries of AI technology while also instructing clinicians about human judgment situations (Jamal et al., 2023). Utilizing AI within medical education allows health professionals to develop improved comprehension of AI technology as well as champion its appropriate utilization, so this technology enhances patient results without sacrificing the human focus needed in healthcare delivery. The combined approach will teach upcoming medical professionals interdisciplinary abilities necessary for success in a technology-dominated healthcare system.

Data Privacy and Security Concerns

Healthcare's acceptance of AI and digital skills has made data privacy and security main problems that healthcare administrations must address. Because patient data represents sensitive information, the extensive quantities of personal health details within electronic health records (EHRs) together with wearables and artificial intelligence systems expose potential security breaches. Unauthorized access to patient data or data breaches or patient information misuse causes grave risks of identity theft alongside discrimination against patients and damages confidence in healthcare delivery systems. The fortification of patient privacy depends on AI implements following strict privacy rules such as U.S., HIPAA, and EU GDPR.

The effective operation of AI healthcare tools demands huge quantities of data, yet this process hampers patient ownership of healthcare data and their ability to provide consent and prevent personal information exposure. The medical camp must inform patients completely about their data usage in order to maintain transparency when AI drives medical research or clinical decisions. To guard sensitive well-being information from cyberattacks, AI schemes necessitate strong safety features, comprising encryption and multifactor verification (Jain et al., 2016). Unsecure AI systems create the possibility that attackers will discover their weak points, thus enabling them to breach patient privacy and cause service interruptions in medical facilities. The privacy and safety of patient data remain vulnerable when AI-driven tools are deployed, so healthcare organizations, together with technology developers, need to keep updating their security protocols.

Real Life Implementations Showing Human-AI Collaboration

Medical practices and patient care benefit from the current integration of human-AI collaboration in healthcare, which reveals the extensive medical potential when humans partner with AI systems. AI plays a major role in radiological diagnosis practices. AI algorithms designed for medical image analysis through image recognition programs help radiologists to accelerate their detection of medical abnormalities, including tumors and fractures and irregular patterns in X-rays and CT scans and MRIs. The AI technology functions alongside radiologists to mark specific regions which need closer investigation, although it does not perform tasks that only humans can handle. AI tools augment medical experts in their diagnostic activities, thus leading to swifter, accurate decisions that enhance both patient results and limit healthcare professionals' mistakes.

The da Vinci Surgical System represents an existing AI-assisted technology that gives surgeons live feedback while performing surgical operations. The arrangement improves surgical precision, permitting medical physicians to conduct negligibly invasive measures by improving their control and precision (Jiang et al., 2023). AI tools enable clinicians to obtain real-time analysis including vital signs checking and surgical movement optimization, thereby allowing surgeons to perform critical decisions under time constraints. Involving surgeon skill with AI data handling power indorses improved patient outcomes with diminutive recovery stages as it shows how social knowledge pools meritoriously with artificial intelligence abilities.

AI has recognized itself as an important element for modified medical care over genetic examination and lifestyle valuation and disease history investigation. AI analysis coupled with inherited testing data in microelectronic health records and additional datasets generates time-consuming complex personalized therapies which humans can successfully execute. The application of AI technologies allows oncologists to create specialized treatment plans that address distinct genetic abnormalities within individual patient tumors. The current scenarios serve medical staff as evidence that AI serves to assist clinical personnel instead of replacing them. Healthcare will be improved through the current combination of AI computational resources with human clinical expertise for delivering care virtually, so medical professionals can use advanced capabilities to create efficient healthcare systems.

CONCLUSION

Healthcare professionals participate in an industry revolution by implementing AI because it enables superior medical choices and persistent healthcare services along with specific treatment solutions. The great advantage of teamwork between humans and AI systems emerges from enabling medical staff to develop professionally by utilizing AI functions that aid them rather than doing their jobs themselves. The integration of AI tools in diagnosis alongside operations and modified medicine technology leads to better diagnostic outcomes and treatment results for real-world healthcare scenarios. This successful teamwork depends on total operational openness and protected patient information privacy and ethical standards while human decision-makers maintain their central position. AI develops into an advantageous healthcare resource through system development based on principles focused on human requirements for healthcare professionals and medical patients. Medical organizations need to offer accessible interfaces between AI tools and established operational systems to enable user access. The practice of dealing with and appropriately using AI technologies requires medical workers to acquire fundamental knowledge of Artificial Intelligence.

REFERENCES

Anderson, J. A., Godwin, K. M., Saleem, J. J., Russell, S., Robinson, J. J., & Kimmel, B. (2014). Accessibility, usability, and usefulness of a web-based clinical decision support tool to enhance provider–patient communication around self-management to prevent (STOP) stroke. *Health Informatics Journal*, *20*(4), 261–274. DOI: 10.1177/1460458213493195 PMID: 24352597

Arsand, E., & Demiris, G. (2008). User-centered methods for designing patient-centric self-help tools. *Informatics for Health & Social Care*, *33*(3), 158–169. DOI: 10.1080/17538150802457562 PMID: 18850399

Bergquist, M., Rolandsson, B., Gryska, E., Laesser, M., Hoefling, N., Heckemann, R., Schneiderman, J. F., & Björkman-Burtscher, I. M. (2024). Trust and stakeholder perspectives on the implementation of AI tools in clinical radiology. *European Radiology*, *34*(1), 338–347. DOI: 10.1007/s00330-023-09967-5 PMID: 37505245

Bright, T. J., Wong, A., Dhurjati, R., Bristow, E., Bastian, L., Coeytaux, R. R., Samsa, G., Hasselblad, V., Williams, J. W., Musty, M. D., Wing, L., Kendrick, A. S., Sanders, G. D., & Lobach, D. (2012). Effect of clinical decision-support systems: A systematic review. *Annals of Internal Medicine*, *157*(1), 29–43. DOI: 10.7326/0003-4819-157-1-201207030-00450 PMID: 22751758

Chervenak, F. A., & McCullough, L. B. (2021). Ethical considerations. In *Clinical Maternal-Fetal Medicine* (pp. 42–1). CRC Press. DOI: 10.1201/9781003222590-39

Diaz-Flores, E., Meyer, T., & Giorkallos, A. (2022). Evolution of artificial intelligence-powered technologies in biomedical research and healthcare. In *Smart Biolabs of the Future* (pp. 23–60). DOI: 10.1007/10_2021_189

Gauthaman, S. A. (2026). Introduction to machine learning and optimization in healthcare. In Muniasamy, A. (Ed.), *Integrative machine learning and optimization algorithms for disease prediction* (pp. 1–34). IGI Global. DOI: 10.4018/979-8-3373-1087-9.ch001

Gauthaman, S. A., Muniasamy, A., & Karunakaran, G. (2026). Current challenges in the pharmaceutical industry and AI's role in addressing them. In Muniasamy, A., & Karunakaran, G. (Eds.), *Applications of artificial intelligence in pharmaceuticals* (pp. 1–26). IGI Global. DOI: 10.4018/979-8-3373-2043-4.ch001

Giordano, C., Brennan, M., Mohamed, B., Rashidi, P., Modave, F., & Tighe, P. (2021). Accessing artificial intelligence for clinical decision-making. *Frontiers in Digital Health*, *3*, 645232. DOI: 10.3389/fdgth.2021.645232 PMID: 34713115

Jain, P., Gyanchandani, M., & Khare, N. (2016). Big data privacy: A technological perspective and review. *Journal of Big Data*, *3*(1), 1–25. DOI: 10.1186/s40537-016-0059-y

Jamal, A., Solaiman, M., Alhasan, K., Temsah, M. H., Sayed, G., & Soliman, M. (2023). Integrating ChatGPT in medical education: Adapting curricula to cultivate competent physicians for the AI era. *Cureus*, *15*(8). Advance online publication. DOI: 10.7759/cureus.43036 PMID: 37674966

Jiang, N., Liu, X., Liu, H., Lim, E. T. K., Tan, C. W., & Gu, J. (2023). Beyond AI-powered context-aware services: The role of human–AI collaboration. *Industrial Management & Data Systems*, *123*(11), 2771–2802. DOI: 10.1108/IMDS-03-2022-0152

Kalusivalingam, A. K., Sharma, A., Patel, N., & Singh, V. (2021). Enhancing patient care through IoT-enabled remote monitoring and AI-driven virtual health assistants: Implementing machine learning algorithms and natural language processing. *International Journal of Artificial Intelligence and Machine Learning*, *2*(3).

Khalifa, M., Albadawy, M., & Iqbal, U. (2024). Advancing clinical decision support: The role of artificial intelligence across six domains. *Computer Methods and Programs in Biomedicine Update*, *5*, 100142. DOI: 10.1016/j.cmpbup.2024.100142

Kreps, G. L., & Neuhauser, L. (2013). Artificial intelligence and immediacy: Designing health communication to personally engage consumers and providers. *Patient Education and Counseling*, *92*(2), 205–210. DOI: 10.1016/j.pec.2013.04.014 PMID: 23683341

Maadi, M., Akbarzadeh Khorshidi, H., & Aickelin, U. (2021). A review on human–AI interaction in machine learning and insights for medical applications. *International Journal of Environmental Research and Public Health*, *18*(4), 2121. DOI: 10.3390/ijerph18042121 PMID: 33671609

Mohseni, S., Zarei, N., & Ragan, E. D. (2021). A multidisciplinary survey and framework for design and evaluation of explainable AI systems. *ACM Transactions on Interactive Intelligent Systems*, *11*(3-4), 1–45. DOI: 10.1145/3387166

Mou, Y., & Xu, K. (2017). The media inequality: Comparing the initial human-human and human-AI social interactions. *Computers in Human Behavior*, *72*, 432–440. DOI: 10.1016/j.chb.2017.02.067

Muniasamy, A. (2026). Quantum computing in drug discovery: Revolutionizing pharmaceutical research. In Muniasamy, A., & Karunakaran, G. (Eds.), *Applications of artificial intelligence in pharmaceuticals* (pp. 59–96). IGI Global.

Muniasamy, A., & Karunakaran, G. (2026). Challenges and future directions: Emerging trends and limitations in ML and optimization for healthcare. In Muniasamy, A. (Ed.), *Integrative machine learning and optimization algorithms for disease prediction* (pp. 339–368). IGI Global.

Muniasamy, A., Tabassam, S., Hussain, M. A., Sultana, H., Muniasamy, V., & Bhatnagar, R. (2020). Deep learning for predictive analytics in healthcare. In Hassanien, A., Azar, A., Gaber, T., Bhatnagar, R., & Tolba, M. F. (Eds.), *The International Conference on Advanced Machine Learning Technologies and Applications (AMLTA2019)*. Springer. DOI: 10.1007/978-3-030-14118-9_4

Naim, A. (2026). AI-driven smart manufacturing and automation in pharmaceutical production. In Muniasamy, A., & Karunakaran, G. (Eds.), *Applications of artificial intelligence in pharmaceuticals* (pp. 157–194). IGI Global.

Necz, D. (2024). Rules over words: Regulation of chatbots in the legal market and ethical considerations. *Hungarian Journal of Legal Studies*, *64*(3), 472–485. DOI: 10.1556/2052.2023.00472

Prathaban, B. P., Subash, R., & Ashwini, A. (2024, October). AI based mental health assisted chatbot system. In *2024 International Conference on Power, Energy, Control and Transmission Systems (ICPECTS)* (pp. 1-6). IEEE. DOI: 10.1109/ICPECTS62210.2024.10780017

Ravichandran, P., Machireddy, J. R., & Rachakatla, S. K. (2024). Harnessing generative AI for automated data analytics in business intelligence and decision-making. *Hong Kong Journal of AI and Medicine*, *4*(1), 122–145.

Rengaramanujam, K., & Muniasamy, A. (2026). AI in hospital administration and formulary design: Optimizing resource allocation and patient flow. In Muniasamy, A., & Karunakaran, G. (Eds.), *Applications of Artificial Intelligence in Pharmaceuticals* (pp. 215–246). IGI Global.

Reverberi, C., Rigon, T., Solari, A., Hassan, C., Cherubini, P., & Cherubini, A. (2022). Experimental evidence of effective human–AI collaboration in medical decision-making. *Scientific Reports*, *12*(1), 14952. DOI: 10.1038/s41598-022-18751-2 PMID: 36056152

Rubin, M., Arnon, H., Huppert, J. D., & Perry, A. (2024). Considering the role of human empathy in AI-driven therapy. *JMIR Mental Health*, *11*(1), e56529. DOI: 10.2196/56529 PMID: 38861302

Sadiku, M. N., Musa, S. M., Sadiku, M. N., & Musa, S. M. (2021). Augmented intelligence. In *A primer on multiple intelligences* (pp. 191–199). DOI: 10.1007/978-3-030-77584-1_15

Serrano, N., Chang, M., Rogers, C. L., Orton, M., Mannino, R., Grob, M., & Moghanaki, D. (2016). Patient autonomy and shared decision-making in the management of urethral cancer. *Practical Radiation Oncology*, *6*(1), 66–70. DOI: 10.1016/j.prro.2015.09.002 PMID: 26577009

Shan, S., & Li, Y. (2024). Research on the application framework of generative AI in emergency response decision support systems for emergencies. *International Journal of Human-Computer Interaction*, 1–18.

Shneiderman, B. (2020). Human-centered artificial intelligence: Three fresh ideas. *AIS Transactions on Human-Computer Interaction*, *12*(3), 109–124. DOI: 10.17705/1thci.00131

Thurtle, D., Rossi, S. H., Berry, B., Pharoah, P., & Gnanapragasam, V. J. (2019). Models predicting survival to guide treatment decision-making in newly diagnosed primary non-metastatic prostate cancer: A systematic review. *BMJ Open*, *9*(6), e029149. DOI: 10.1136/bmjopen-2019-029149 PMID: 31230029

Trujillo, C. J., Ulloa, J. V., Vivas, G. E., Escobar, E. G., Gutiérrez, I. V., Tirado, P. A., & Cohen, J. V. (2024). Surgeons vs ChatGPT: Assessment and feedback performance based on real surgical scenarios. *Journal of Surgical Education*, *81*(7), 960–966. DOI: 10.1016/j.jsurg.2024.03.012 PMID: 38749814

Yogeshappa, V. G. (2024). AI-driven precision medicine: Revolutionizing personalized treatment plans. *International Journal of Computer Engineering and Technology*, *15*(5), 455–474.

Zheng, N. N., Liu, Z. Y., Ren, P. J., Ma, Y. Q., Chen, S. T., Yu, S. Y., & Wang, F. Y. (2017). Hybrid-augmented intelligence: Collaboration and cognition. *Frontiers of Information Technology & Electronic Engineering*, *18*(2), 153–179. DOI: 10.1631/FITEE.1700053

KEY TERMS AND DEFINITIONS

Chronic Healthcare Management: The ongoing monitoring, treatment, and coordination of care for patients with long-term health conditions, aiming to improve quality of life and reduce complications.

Digital Twin Technology: A virtual replica of a physical system or process that uses real-time data to simulate, predict, and optimize performance.

Disease Progression: The course and development of a disease over time, including changes in symptoms, severity, and impact on patient health.

IoT-Medical Tool: A medical device connected to the Internet of Things (IoT) that collects, transmits, and analyzes health data to support diagnosis, monitoring, and treatment.

Virtual Replica: A digital representation of a physical object, process, or system used for simulation, analysis, or predictive modeling.

Wearable Devices: Electronic devices worn on the body, such as smartwatches or biosensors, that monitor physiological parameters and provide health-related data.

Chapter 15
The Human Factor:
Evaluating the Impact of AI on Hospital Staff and Patient Care

P. Kirubanantham
https://orcid.org/0009-0005-6697-0178
SRM Institute of Science and Technology, Kattankulathur, India

Saranya A.
Amity University, Mumbai, India

M. Revathi
SRM Institute of Science and Technology, Kattankulathur, India

M. Sayeekumar
Jain University, India

Suresh Anand M.
https://orcid.org/0000-0002-1055-6083
SRM Institute of Science and Technology, Kattankulathur, India

ABSTRACT

This chapter examines how human factors shape the impact of artificial intelligence (AI) on hospital staff and patient healthcare outcomes. As AI technologies expand in healthcare, their influence on human interactions, workflows, and treatment results require thorough analysis. AI-driven clinical support systems, diagnostic tools, and patient interaction technologies enhance healthcare practitioners' competence but also raise concerns about trust, communication, and job satisfaction. AI simultaneously boosts clinical efficiency and reshapes how professionals engage with patients. Using real-world examples and research findings, this chapter explores AI's effects on hospital staff workloads, decision-making, and patient experiences.

DOI: 10.4018/979-8-3373-2787-7.ch015

It also addresses algorithmic bias and underscores the need for human-centered AI implementation. Regular evaluation systems are crucial for assessing AI's impact on staff and evolving technology. By fostering AI-professional collaboration, hospitals can improve patient outcomes and satisfaction.

INTRODUCTION

Artificial intelligence (AI) is reshaping healthcare in terms of providing better diagnostics, effectiveness of operations, and delivering care to patients (Sharma, B. K., 2025; Rengaramanujam et al., 2026).). Artificial Intelligence (AI): AI can be defined as a mimicry of human intelligence in machines that can think with capabilities of learning and decision-making. Human Factors Engineering (HFE): An interdisciplinary approach devoted to the effort to design a better relationship between humans and technology by looking at design efforts as applied to psychology, ergonomics, and engineering. Clinical Decision Support Systems (CDSS): The prospective brainchild of any AI, CDSS are systems that support clinicians in making informed clinical judgments by examining medical information and presenting recommendations. Whereas AI technology in the form of predictive analytics and administrative automation is reasonably transforming clinical processes, there is a dearth of research in the area of human-oriented outcomes. There is a fear of adapting to a changing workforce, loss of professional autonomy, and maintaining patient care. Medical workers should learn to combine their knowledge in dealing with AI technologies with efficient interpersonal communication. Even as there is much written about the technical aspects of AI, there is little that speaks to the implications of AI on provider roles, job satisfaction, skill development, and patient-provider relationships. This "gap" in the literature is what this chapter will seek to fill by discussing the impact that AI has on both hospital staff and patients, and why more morally and human-focused approaches to integration are necessary.

Most AI-related systems in the health industry favor the performance of machines at the expense of individuals, and thus, implementing them could be difficult. Resistance on the part of clinicians to bad interface design, lack of transparency, and/or insufficient training are among the key barriers. These issues are reflected in the failure of IBM Watson for Oncology, as its restricted diversity of training data and involvement of clinicians resulted in a decrease in trust (Shorrock, S., & Williams, C., 2016). Future AI systems will need to be more inclusive, transparent, and have an emotional aspect to caring to address ethical issues such as algorithmic bias, data privacy, and accountability.

This chapter contributes to other studies because it highlights the implications of the role of AI in personnel and relations between the hospitals and the patients, but not its technicalities. It looks into the way AI is changing the role, communications, and the quality of care, and seeks to support a human factors perspective that seeks to assure that technology does not act as a replacement for caring, patient-centered healthcare delivery.

BACKGROUND

Recent literature on Artificial Intelligence (AI) in healthcare is broad and explores the following areas in probing diagnostic imaging, predictive analytics, robotic surgery, and administrative efficiency. Research indicates that AI-based algorithms are frequently as precise as human specialists in identifying the presence of abnormalities in medical images, and in some cases, more accurate than humans in detecting some conditions, such as tumors, abnormalities of the neck, spinal cord, and conditions related to do with neurological diseases. Predictive analytics enables healthcare providers to actively deal with the high-risk patients and manage them to achieve positive results (Shneiderman, B., 2022). Administrative tasks such as appointment and billing, as well as EHR management, can also be handled with the help of AI, which can diminish the workloads that clinicians are exposed to and can also boost their service capacity. Many of the studies published, however, pay more attention to the technical performance of AI, as opposed to organizational, social, and ethical consequence considerations. There is a lack of research focusing on the impact of increasing AI on the role of healthcare workers, their trust in technology, or patient-provider communication. Besides, the issues associated with algorithmic bias, the lack of transparency, and ethical responsibility are understudied. This is the gap that shows the importance of conducting research focusing on human aspects to achieve AI integration in healthcare.

Understanding Human Factors in AI Implementation

AI in healthcare should be implemented effectively, and in order to do so, human factors must be well understood, as they dramatically improve human outcomes and performance rates (Holden et al., 2013). All of those things that are controversial in psychology, engineering, and design facilitate interactions between the medical personnel and systems. A lot of medical errors are based on system flaws and not people making decisions, which is why AI should be easy to use. In Figure 1, the user interface design can be a factor that causes major mistakes in critical moments. An approach based on human factors principles can help developers design AI tools that can simplify clinicians' work routines, improve situation awareness, and decrease the complexity of the work. Managing cognitive load is essential because stress and fatigue affect decision-making in a negative manner. Strategies that have been found to help combat burnout include those that simplify details and automate tasks (Mitchell, et al., 2014). Organizational training is necessary to provide the employees with the knowledge and skills in AI to achieve a harmonious combination of technology and human skills, contributing to safe and efficient care that is delivered with compassion.

Figure 1. Human Factors in AI Implementation

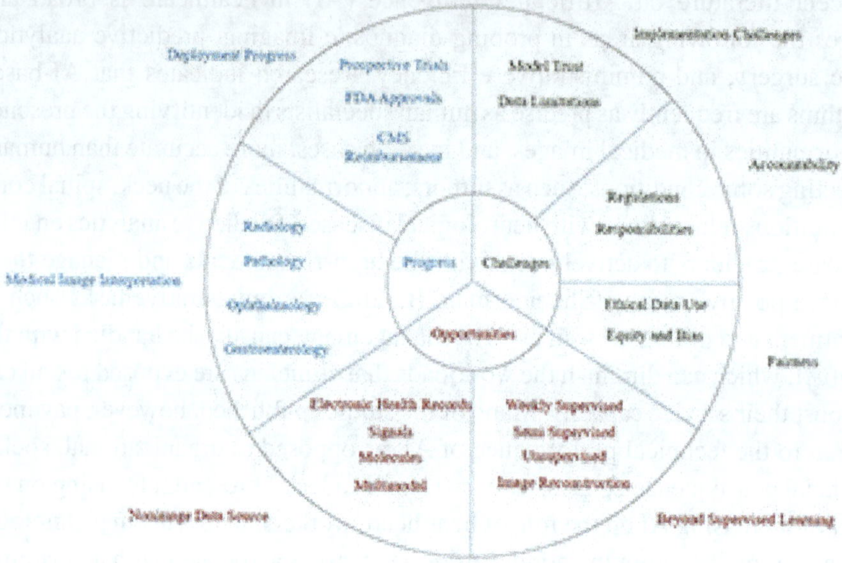

Definition and Scope

Appreciation of the human element in the implementation of AI healthcare supports a successful integration in that it enhances keeping the process safe and efficient (Cacciabue, & Vella, 2010). Being a multidisciplinary program, it deals with the interaction of systems in high-risk medical settings. In Figure 2, Inadequate AI design subjects people to an unmanageable cognitive load, which results in mistakes. By paying attention to human factors, it is easier to figure out workflow, communication, and interface problems and address them. The scope of human factors in AI implementation encompasses several key areas:

- **Usability**: High-pressure situations will be safer when AI systems maintain usability features that create intuitive operations for users.

- **Training**: The healthcare sector needs to train its professionals correctly to operate AI systems with proper knowledge about system constraints.
- **Workflow Integration**: Workflow Integration represents the process of designing AI tools to harmonize with existing clinical procedures so medical staff can achieve operational efficiency through maintaining current organizational procedures.
- **Patient Interaction**: Healthcare providers need to assess both the impact AI has on doctor-patient interactions and make sure technological advancements enhance human connection in medical practice.

Figure 2. Human Factor in Healthcare

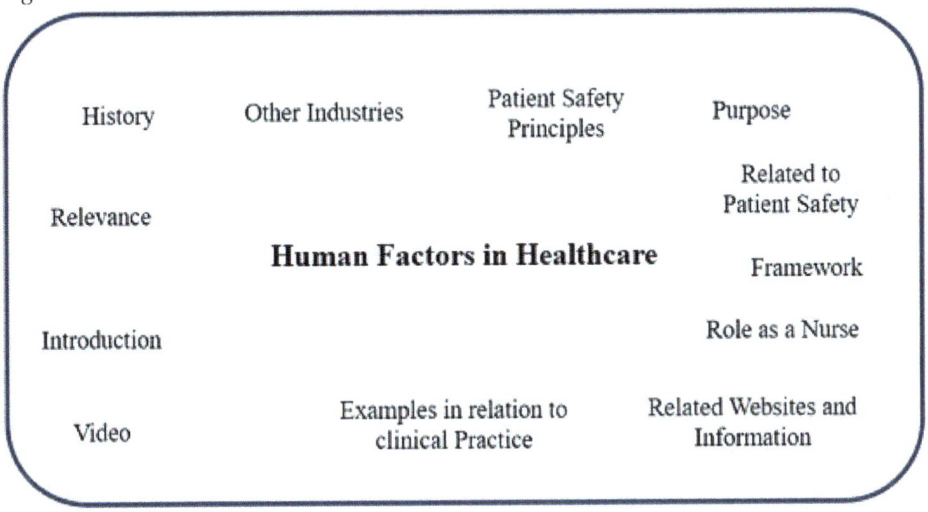

Key Principles of Human Factors Engineering

HFE has a crucial role in the optimization of the interaction of systems and people, especially in high-risk healthcare environments (Chignell, 2023). Its fundamental postulates include heightening safety, efficiency, and system performance through the drawing of tools that resonate with the capabilities and limitations, humans have in the workplace. HFE focuses on designing systems that will be convenient to use and will satisfy the needs and preferences of healthcare professionals to avoid making errors and facilitate the natural use of the system. Familiarity with human behavior forms a core issue as practitioners examine the interaction of the users to determine possible weaknesses of a particular system. The standardization increases reliability and decreases the requirement of training for the users and also has inbuilt feedback mechanisms such as visual or audible feedback, so that the user monitors the status of the system, validates what actions that he/she has taken, and detects errors (Nordlinger et al., 2020; Gauthaman, S. A., et al., 2026).

Impact of AI on Hospital Staff

Healthcare institutions are transforming work duties and organizational processes through Artificial Intelligence implementation, which produces both advantageous outcomes and implementation difficulties. Below are the key impacts:

Reduced Administrative Burden: More than two-thirds of repetitive activities, such as managing, scheduling, billing, and coding data, are simplified with the help of AI implementation (Praveen, & Kumar, 2024; Rengaramanujam, K., & Muniasamy, A.,2026). This saves clinicians and nurses from burnout, and they have time to concentrate on the patients. Better accuracy and efficiency in documentation lead to improved satisfaction among staff and help hospitals to cope with staff shortages by more efficient use of resources.

Enhanced Clinical Decision-Making: AI decision-making systems help the medical staff provide them with timely insights to identify a possible error or risk of making a wrong diagnosis. Improved diagnostics and predictive models help to detect disease earlier, so staff members need to be trained and provided with awareness about AI systems' functionality and weaknesses.

Workforce Adaptation and Skill Development: This would entail investing in the training of the workforce to acquire digital skills and create awareness of AI tools (Aminizadeh, 2024; Muniasamy, A., & Karunakaran, G., 2026). The continual education process helps employees understand the AI recommendations and improve the quality of care by utilizing best practices in the moment.

Addressing Workforce Shortages: AI saves time that could be utilized in menial duties; hence, employee retention. Such tools as the patient flow prediction, virtual assistants, and telemedicine enhance the distribution of resources, minimise delays, and alleviate the strains of healthcare workers in underserved regions.

Ethical and Operational Challenges: AI can increase the productivity of nurses by 30 to 50 percent, but issues such as algorithm bias and privacy problems still exist. You need to uphold empathy, and this demands ethical education as well as cultural adjustment and adjustment to technology, so as to maintain both in equal proportion, upholding the principle of care provided towards the patient.

Modeling the Impact of AI on Hospital Staff and Patient-Centered Outcomes

In this chapter, special attention is paid to the consideration of the humanistic aspects of the implementation of Artificial Intelligence (AI) in the hospital environment. Whereas technical and theoretical sections focused upon, here the main model of the research is introduced, and practical relevance thereof is addressed.

Proposed Schematic Model: Human-Centered AI Integration in Healthcare

In Figure 3, the model is composed of four interrelated parts that are all turned in the direction of Balanced AI Implementation, which will contribute to effectiveness without saying goodbye to compassion and trust in patient care.

a. AI-Driven Clinical Functions: The application of AI in clinical functions is an important part of modern medicine as it improves the accuracy of diagnosis and clinical choices. Technologies such as diagnostic imaging, clinical decision support systems (CDSS), and predictive analytics enable early data collection on diseases, individualized care planning, and the proactive management of patients, resulting in improved outcomes and increased efficiency in healthcare.

b. Operational Efficiency Tools: AI-based operational efficiency tools also automate administrative processes, including electronic health record (EHR) and scheduling, and billing. Such systems streamline operations within the hospital, decrease the number of working hours, and improve productivity. Ensuring that healthcare providers spend less time on routine processes also helps to ensure a higher quality of service delivery because providers have an increased amount of time dedicated to direct patient care.

c. Human Factor Considerations: Human factor considerations of the successful implementation of AI in healthcare (Bridger, et al., 2017). This would entail clinician trainings, AI literacy, an easy-to-grasp interface, and compatibility with clinical processes. Focusing on emotional intelligence and the cognitive burden of use guarantees the safety, user-friendliness of AI tools, and the facilitation of staff performance, instead of worsening clinical judgment and well-being.

d. Patient-Centered Impact: Patient-centered impact is based on the importance of strong doctor-patient communication, the development of trust, and transparency in the use of AI. It isn't a shallow, technology-first-only expense; emotional/empathetic care isn't sacrificed, and the priority is that technology enables rather than displaces human interaction. Preserving the relationality of healthcare, AI is able to increase the ethical standards and enrich the emotional connection between the patients and their healthcare providers.

Figure 3. Proposed Model for Human-Centered AI Integration in Healthcare

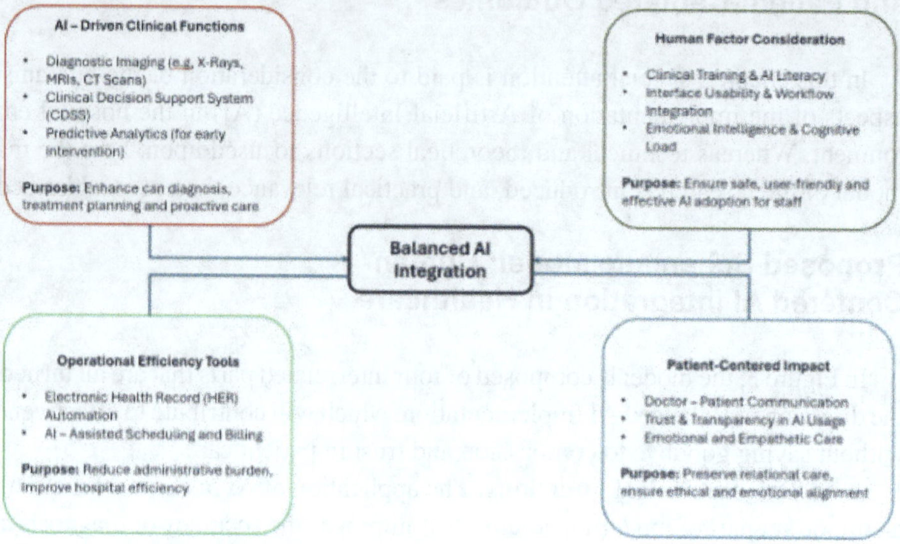

Practical Application of Findings

In a bid to effectively integrate AI in healthcare, hospitals are advised to focus on collaborative design by incorporating the end users, such as clinicians and administrators. Training should be given continually; ethical auditing and the feedback of patients are crucial to the achievement of transparency and accountability (Wiczorek, 2024). Automating is a tradeoff between maintenance and human interaction, whereby empathy and compassionate care are supported with responsible and humane adoption of AI.

Changes in Workload and Responsibilities

Hospital staff experiences major changes in their work responsibilities and workload due to the establishment of artificial intelligence systems in healthcare institutions. In Figure 4, the Healthcare professionals experience operational changes when artificial intelligence systems become increasingly common because these systems simplify healthcare operations.

Reduction of Administrative Tasks: AI has shown itself to be instrumental in decreasing the amount of administrative tasks hospital staff must handle. Healthcare practitioners dedicate about 70% of their daily work to documentation responsibilities, along with administrative duties at the expense of providing direct care to patients

(Rubeis, 2024). The automation of clinical workflow activities by AI improves operational efficiency since staff members dedicate their time to clinical services. AI-enabled digital medical workers process patient encounter documentation, which enables healthcare providers to provide better care directly to patients.

Shift in Clinical Responsibilities: The implementation of AI enables the automation of regular tasks, but it modifies medical staff duties to include different types of responsibilities. Healthcare providers now deal with more intricate cases beyond their standard duties because they must demonstrate critical thinking abilities and advanced problem-solving competencies. Staff who experience intellectual stimulation from this shift might also develop increased stress levels when they stay under constant high-pressure situations without sufficient less demanding activities.

Need for New Skill Sets: Healthcare professionals must learn new skill sets because the use of AI technology is emerging in health systems. Caring staff need complete training for using AI tools, along with training to understand and convert AI-generated information into decisions (Guastello, 2023). Staff members face extra work because they need continuous education about technology updates, as they work through these changes when performing their clinical responsibilities.

Potential for Burnout: The streamlining benefits AI offers healthcare institutions could lead to more extensive work stress among medical professionals who need to handle challenging cases that require ongoing system adjustments. Internal struggle to handle complex medical situations combined with insufficient assistance results in reduced job contentment which subsequently causes professional exhaustion.

Figure 4. Impacts of AI on Hospital Management Systems

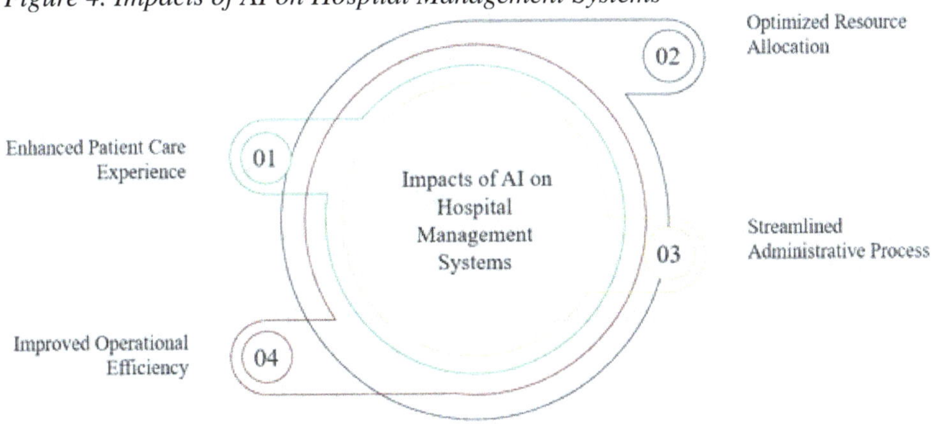

Training and Adaptation to AI Tools

The successful integration of artificial intelligence (AI) tools in healthcare settings hinges significantly on the training and adaptation of hospital staff. In Figure 5, Healthcare professionals need to learn essential skills for effective usage of AI tools in their work because AI technologies expand within healthcare systems.

Personalized Training Approaches: HCWs receive individualized educational programs through training systems enriched by AI technology at an increasing rate. The programs use machine learning algorithms to evaluate both personal learning characteristics along free and limited skills, which enables customized educational materials (Dewasiri et al., 2025; Naim, A., et al., 2026). Through AI-powered virtual reality (VR) simulations, healthcare staff can replicate real-life clinical experiences in which they can develop their procedural abilities and decision-making competencies through simulated controlled environments. The interactive training delivery method strengthens both nursing skills and the development of teamwork abilities, which nurses need to deliver quality patient care.

Curriculum Development: Educational institutions, together with healthcare facilities, must create extensive teaching programs that combine basic AI knowledge education for healthcare professionals. Healthcare workers need to learn about AI system abilities, together with principles of data protection and the prevention of bias in medical algorithms. All healthcare programs should teach the necessity of using AI-generated knowledge alongside medical professional experience to keep patient-directed care as the central focus of medical practices.

Ongoing Support and Resources: An organizational training approach must exist as a continuous learning cycle beyond single initial sessions. Healthcare workers need to participate in regular educational programs because the AI system technology changes quickly. Healthcare facilities should establish scheduled workshops together with periodic refresher courses that provide staff with internet-based resources to stay updated about modern AI applications in medical care (Kumar et al., 2024). Healthcare institutions that establish ongoing learning programs provide staff members the capability to adopt new tools effectively.

Collaboration with IT Experts: Healthcare providers need to work together with IT professionals to successfully adapt to AI tools in their practice. Participation of multidisciplinary teams throughout AI system development and implementation helps hospitals create technology that suits actual clinical workflows and addresses healthcare personnel's needs. By working together, healthcare institutions achieve better integration of AI technology along with increased clinical staff willingness to adopt these systems (Govindaraj et al., 2024; Muniasamy, 2025). The complete implementation of training with adaptation strategies remains vital for hospitals to achieve maximum AI tool benefits. Organizations that establish training to provide healthcare professionals with the required skills and knowledge produce healthcare environments that are at once efficient and effective, together with being compassionate.

Figure 5. AI used in Healthcare Applications

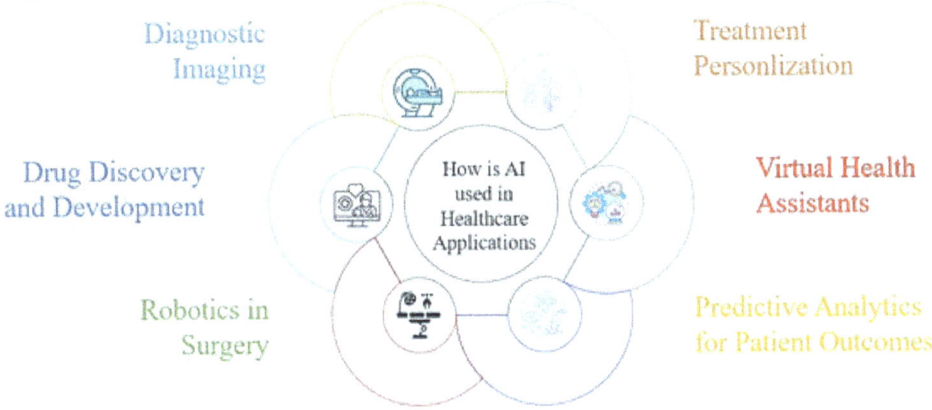

Trust and Acceptance Among Staff

The effective application of AI in hospitals requires trust and acceptance by the staff, which, in turn, affects their activity and the level of their reliance on AI tools.

Factors Influencing Trust: A more transparent approach towards the functioning of the systems used by artificial intelligence helps healthcare staff trust those systems more. The confidence grows due to a clear description and adherence to clinical judgment (Alowais et al., 2023; Gauthaman, S. A., et al., 2026). Knowledge gained by training and practicing handles and repeated learning lowers the fear and uncertainty, providing opportunities to become more comfortable with the successful adoption of AI tools into everyday healthcare routines and decision-making.

Impact on Professional Autonomy: Applying AI results in trust, which is influenced by how professional autonomy is affected. There might be fears of a provider losing clinical relevance, and therefore, it must be convincingly positioned as an aid with no threat of replacement, as this would go further in allaying the fears and provoke use.

Addressing Ethical Concerns: Confidence in AI is based on the need to solve ethical issues, such as privacy and algorithm bias. Since developing effective ethical frameworks, adequate communication, and decision-making with team members can help ensure staff acceptance, they are encouraged to trust AI as a useful resource in improving the quality of care.

AI's Role in Patient Care

In Figure 6, the introduction of AI has changed correct hospital patient care very fast, where advanced algorithms and data analysis enhance diagnostics, planned treatment, engagement with the patient, and product delivery of general health care.

Enhanced Diagnostics: AI is much more accurate in diagnostics, time-saving, and even faster in analyzing medical imaging than a human specialist (Shaheen et al., 2025; Gauthaman, S. A., et al., 2026). Its capacity to detect conditions with much time still left makes the early interventions possible, and clinicians appreciate that the AI can study large volumes of clinical data.

Remote Monitoring and Telemedicine: With the AI-powered remote health systems and telemedicine, and wearable devices, it will be possible to continuously monitor vital parameters and give early warnings, which will be used both to intervene in time and help decrease hospital visits, increase the convenience of patients, and deeper result in adherence to treatment plans.

AI-Powered Virtual Assistants: AI-enabled virtual health assistants provide round-the-clock services such as making inquiries about their conditions, scheduling appointments, and reminders of medication, boosting patient function, and increasing efficiency in linkages between patients and the healthcare specialists.

Operational Efficiency: AI can make hospitals more efficient by streamlining the process of scheduling, billing, and documentation, leaving the providers to concentrate on patient care (Youssef et al., 2025). It promotes individualized care and diagnostics, telecoaching, and making sure that technology is an accessory, not a substitute, in terms of the focus on the human element as the approach to the delivery of healthcare.

Figure 6. AI's Role in Healthcare

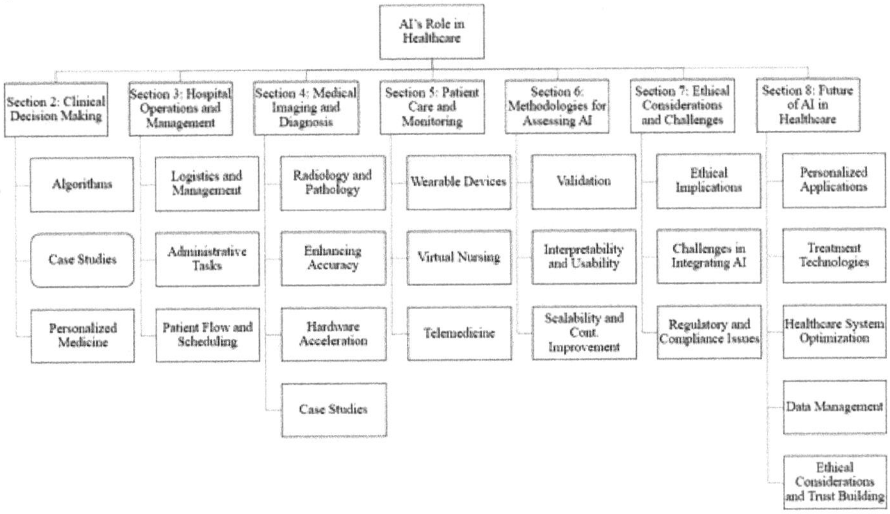

Enhancements in Patient Diagnostics and Treatment

AI is changing the face of healthcare by providing an added touch to precision in diagnosis and treatment, making patient care better and their stay at the hospital smoother with algorithms.

Enhanced Diagnostic Accuracy: The most profound use case of AI in healthcare is the improvement of diagnosis, particularly with regard to medical imaging (Zahlan, et al., 2023; Gauthaman, S. A., et al., 2026). AI is trained to be better at detecting such conditions as breast cancer and lung nodules than even specialists because it is trained not only on patterns but also on anomalies, and therefore can alert and diagnose much earlier when still in its early stages that the human eye would have failed to detect.

Speeding Up Diagnostic Processes: The area of application of AI in medicine is the diagnosis of certain issues, resulting in the improvement of accuracy and a faster evaluation of the process. Conventional diagnostics are long-term, so it takes time to treat the patient. AI-based analytics decrease the analysis time up to 70 percent, meaning there will be quicker diagnoses and, in turn, early interventions that can greatly increase patient survival rates.

Personalized Treatment Plans: AI is not limited to diagnostics; however, it is also used to develop individual treatment plans based on genomic data, history of illness, and lifestyle. In oncology, AI can personalize medication to the tumor characteristics, and this has been widely used in partnerships such as IBM Watson Health, providing better patient outcomes (Rani et al.,2025; Muniasamy, A. et al., 2020).

Predictive Analytics for Preventive Care: The AI predictive tools are employed by healthcare providers who diagnose risky patients prior to the onset of symptoms. AI helps to facilitate the prevention of diseases, eliminate readmissions, and enhance long-term results by analyzing large collections of data and existing health indicators of patients.

Addressing Health Disparities: Healthcare providers should take care of the issues of biases involved with AI algorithms to experience all the benefits it has in terms of diagnostics and treatment. Having a variety of training data ensures equal care. AI can increase accuracy, speed up processes, and make treatment more personal and predictive (Secinaro, et al., 2021; Gauthaman, S. A., et al., 2026). It will lead to a change towards patient-focused care when dealing with complicated medical conditions.

Patient Engagement through AI Tools

AI makes the patient more engaged, as it promotes communication, agency, and compliance with treatment and lifestyle management.

Improved Communication: Chatbots and virtual assistants can help patients at any time, remind them to take medicine, and support several interactions, adding to the engagement of patients, the level of care not achieved, and provider efficiency (Xu et al., 2023).

Personalized Patient Experience: Individualized patient engagement AI offers integrated healthcare messages and guidance that is specific to a person and their history, which improves compliance, the quality of care, and health outcomes through more precise communication and follow-ups.

Predictive Analytics for Proactive Care: Predictive analytics in AI recognizes health trends, predicts patient risks, can take early action, lessen hospitalization, and speed up supportive care, which makes patient outcomes and quality of life better and increases.

Efficiency and Cost-Effectiveness: Instead, AI can increase efficiency in costs and patient engagement processes by automatically receiving bookings and inquiries, thus liberating employee time, facilitating diagnosis early, and ensuring orderliness of treatment to enhance healthcare outcomes (Rasheed, et al., 2022).

Empowering Patients: The AIs grant patients' agency by providing them with the ability to receive individualized health data, enabling their understanding and control over care. A high level of engagement will result in better communication, better results, and facilitated custom and predictive care and healthcare progress across the systems.

Ethical Considerations in Patient Interactions

Healthcare organizations must proficiently handle ethical challenges stemming from AI patient interaction to sustain trustful and equitable human-centered medical care. Below are key considerations:

Patient Privacy and Data Security: Medical AI systems are dependent on large datasets, and depending on that, there must be a stringent protocol to protect the privacy of the patients in data collection, storage, and sharing (Dinesh, et al. 2025; Abdullah et al., 2025). The robust encryption, anonymization, and open management, per GDPR and HIPAA, are the touchstones of a trust between patients.

Informed Consent and Transparency: The patients have the right to know of the presence of AI in care delivery and have the right to refuse. Clear definitions of AI, functions, limitations, and risks are necessary to provide valid consent and correct treatment decisions.

Algorithmic Bias and Equity: This bias in training data creates a disparity among minority groups in the processes of diagnosis, treatment, and access to care. To solve this, there will be a need to use various datasets, conduct periodic audits, and incorporate a fairness-conscious approach to algorithms to adequately provide fair access to AI tools and their results for all patients.

Preserving Humanistic Care: Overuse of AI can make the treatment dehumanized since there is nothing AI can offer beyond human empathy (Crowther et al., 2025; Naim, A., et al., 2026).). The emotional restrictions of chatbots point to the necessity to combine them with human approval; artificial intelligence to improve costs, but not to lose the attitude of care and patience with patients in medical environments.

CASE STUDIES

Healthcare institutions use artificial intelligence deployment to show technology as the driving force, which advances clinical outcomes while also enhancing organizational performance. Proficient information technology research shows how artificial intelligence deployments shaped both medical staff operations and patient treatment quality in healthcare settings.

Enhanced Efficiency and Patient Outcomes: Boston Children's Hospital achieved workflow streamlining through the integration of virtual nursing assistants powered by AI, which enabled nurses to dedicate additional attention to patients and strengthen care delivery (Nordlinger et al., 2020; Gauthaman, S. A., et al., 2026). The improved patient satisfaction levels created fewer demands on nursing staff while simultaneously increasing their productivity. George Eliot Hospital employed AI technology to automate CT scan analysis, thus radiologists received both time-saving benefits alongside enhanced diagnostic precision through anomaly detection features that promoted patient safety throughout the process (Rani et al., 2025).

Predictive Analytics in Patient Management: Using Microsoft Azure AI healthcare software, Johns Hopkins Hospital developed predictive tools that assisted professionals in anticipating patient results while predicting readmission potential (Xu et al., 2023). The proactive care strategy allowed healthcare providers to build patient-specific interventions, leading to enhanced care quality and reduced complications during treatment. Chronic patients benefit from time-aware disease management systems that produce personalized therapeutic methods leading to improved health management outcomes.

Successful Implementations of AI in Hospitals

The successful use of artificial intelligence in healthcare shows how these systems can boost medical care standards and operational effectiveness and enable medical staff to flourish. The following section presents substantial case studies that demonstrate these implementation advantages.

A. University of Rochester Medical Center

The University of Rochester Medical Center (URMC) partnered with Butterfly Network to expand patient imaging capabilities through the Butterfly IQ probe technology deployment (Crowther et al., 2025). The portable ultrasound equipment with AI-based imaging features detects cholecystitis and bladder problems more rapidly and precisely. Since their implementation at URMC, ultrasound charge capture has grown by 116% while the number of scanning sessions has expanded by 74%. The achievement of this project demonstrates how AI technology enhances medical diagnosis quality and operational performance in healthcare establishments.

B. Valley Medical Center

The Dragonfly Utilize platform from Xsolis operated at Valley Medical Center by using AI to generate medical necessity scores that maximized patient observation rates (Rasheed et al., 2022). The medical team working under this system developed the ability to refer patients to physician advisory services during their first month at deployment, thus optimizing their case handling process. The reported data showed that the center achieved a 100% increase in their case reviews, and their observation rate for discharged patients improved to 13%. The healthcare profession gains AI-driven power from the technology that strengthens clinical decisions, together with better patient treatment results.

C. Healthfirst

Healthfirst encountered obstacles within their existing machine learning operations, so they chose to work with ClosedLoop for a solution that could scale. Due to their partnership with ClosedLoop, Healthfirst executed automation on data cleaning processes, including normalization and model training procedures, which reduced operational strain (Govindaraj et al., 2024; Muniasamy, 2025). The organization implemented 17 predictive models that analyze various outcomes and made many customized machine learning features. AI technology delivers operational enhancements that generate useful clinical findings to improve healthcare results.

D. Johns Hopkins Hospital

Through their alliance with Microsoft Azure AI, Johns Hopkins Hospital reached patient outcome forecasts by analyzing large-scale datasets from electronic health records together with genomic information. Healthcare providers now use this initiative to make knowledgeable decisions about disease development and treatment effects. The hospital uses history-based data patterns to enhance its preventive intervention capabilities, which streamlines treatment delivery to specific patient types.

E. University of Alabama at Birmingham Medicine

The Sickbay platform, created by Medical Informatics, allowed UAB Medicine to build a model that facilitated dynamic data collection and synchronization during heart surgeries. The system enables continuous patient monitoring through which anaesthesiology teams correlate patient information with their surgical treatment plans and administer medications (Dinesh et al., 2025). The performed implementation resulted in better patient information acquisition, together with extended operational visibility of patient health throughout surgical procedures.

LESSONS LEARNED FROM AI FAILURES

Healthcare systems fail to implement artificial intelligence technology successfully due to various critical challenges, which serve as essential learning material for future AI deployment in healthcare facilities. The identification of failed AI systems represents essential knowledge for medical facilities attempting to achieve AI potential while safeguarding against potential hazards. This document includes important knowledge derived from well-known AI implementation setbacks in healthcare systems.

A. IBM Watson for Oncology

Following much fanfare as a leading AI tool for cancer recommendations, IBM Watson for Oncology ended its operation due to critical setbacks. Recommendations provided by the system proved to be inconsistent with local clinical guidelines and real-world cases due to its dependence on restricted training data from Memorial Sloan Kettering Cancer Center's practices. Healthcare professionals expressed doubt after reports showed Watson making unsafe and improper medical suggestions. The failure demonstrates why AI systems require training data repositories diverse enough to handle different clinical situations and practice standards.

B. Google's Verily Health Sciences

The field trial at a facility in Thailand was developed by Google's Verily Health Sciences to utilize their AI system for diagnosing diabetic retinopathy. The system faced difficulties with subpar lighting conditions and unclear images, because of which technicians experienced a 21% rejection rate on their submissions. The AI system demonstrated much weaker results when tested in clinical situations as opposed to its lab-tested performance. The case demonstrates why strong tests across various clinical conditions remain essential for ensuring safe AI system implementation in medical operations.

C. Predictive Algorithms with Incomplete Data

A predictive algorithm produced dangerous results for a young man by showing healthy statistics from laboratory tests, prompting many to use incomplete data with caution. The algorithm did not incorporate patient family cardiac history, leading to a fatal cardiac arrest that occurred weeks afterward. This tragic event shows why AI models must integrate complete patient background information and why their algorithms should handle different risk variables.

D. Lack of User Engagement

AI systems frequently provide substandard performance because health practitioners failed to take part in the system development process. The interface of Watson received negative feedback because clinicians reported that it disrupted their workflow and was difficult to use. User engagement during the design process leads to tools that successfully meet user needs and integrate well with existing practice methods. The lesson demonstrates the necessity to include healthcare practitioners during both development and testing cycles of AI systems for obtaining satisfactory user outcomes.

E. Ethical and Accountability Issues

The failure of AI systems creates daunting ethical problems because responsibility remains difficult to determine. The responsibility for negative consequences from AI recommendations remains unclear, as developers, healthcare providers, and institutions might share responsibility for these situations. AI technology requires defined jurisdictions of responsibility to gain practitioner trust while also defining necessary actions to take when errors occur. AI deployment in healthcare requires essential lessons about comprehensive testing alongside ethical rules for AI system development, along with diverse data usage and medical staff involvement.

CHALLENGES AND BARRIERS TO EFFECTIVE INTEGRATION

Multiple obstacles and challenges concerning artificial intelligence deployment exist within hospital settings, which block its productive deployment. The identification of these barriers stands as vital for healthcare organizations that desire to use artificial intelligence technologies to enhance their patient services and operational excellence.

Broad Barriers to Implementation

A. Data Interoperability and Standardization

The main obstacle to AI implementation in healthcare systems stems from the need for compatible data. Patient medical records exist across different electronic health record (EHR) systems, which fail to follow uniform standards and protocols. The fragmented manner in which patient data exists makes data sharing plus integration unnecessarily hard for AI systems trying to access complete medical records. Different healthcare institutions employ various coding methods along with divergent medical terminology systems that cause problems when analyzing data due to inconsistent results. To overcome this challenge, healthcare systems need standardized data formatting features with interoperability frameworks like HL7 FHIR to establish simple system-to-system communication.

B. Resistance to Change

Healthcare organizations function under a traditional culture that prefers current operational practices instead of implementing new technological solutions. Medical organization staff, such as physicians and administrators, often create barriers when it comes to AI technology adoption because they resist its implementation. The practice of AI adoption faces resistance mainly from healthcare professionals who question the usefulness of AI technology, while doubting its ability to maintain both business operations and employment positions.

C. Lack of Technical Expertise

Organizations must develop specialized expertise and the ability to implement AI healthcare solutions effectively because most of them currently lack these competencies. Healthcare organizations encounter substantial challenges because they cannot find enough talent to develop, maintain, and implement AI systems. Top-class AI professionals are difficult for hospitals to acquire because they cannot fund adequate training measures for their existing workforce. Healthcare teams need essential expertise, so healthcare organizations must invest in educational and training measures.

D. Unclear Return on Investment (ROI)

Healthcare executives demonstrate instability regarding the profitability that AI technologies create. Healthcare executives show reluctance to fund AI developments because they have difficulty measuring the many benefits these technologies provide. It is essential to create defined metrics to assess AI application performance, which proves their value to stakeholders.

E. Integration with Existing Systems

The deployment of AI solutions requires full integration with existing HIS systems and EHRs to achieve desired results. The integration of modern healthcare solutions is prevented by technical limitations, which demand that hospital staff change their infrastructure, making it unacceptable for hospitals with limited adaptability. Present AI applications mostly function autonomously without the ability to connect smoothly with clinical workflow systems.

Resistance to Change Among Staff

The successful implementation of AI requires healthcare staff acceptance because they constitute a major barrier to integrating AI in hospitals. The success of innovation alongside patient care enhancement requires hospitals to understand resistance factors along implement suitable strategies.

A. Fear of Job Displacement

The main issue leading to resistance stems from healthcare professionals' concerns about job termination in their positions. Healthcare staff worry that AI systems will eliminate their positions, especially when used for diagnostic functions and administrative operations. Fearful attitudes create doubt regarding the advantages of AI technology thus establishing distrust between people. The challenges of fear need a solution through hospital leadership, who should clearly state that AI brings support for human experts. Organizations can decrease existing job concerns by showing how their AI tools function as decision-making support systems for clinicians.

B. Lack of Familiarity with Technology

Healthcare professionals resist AI technologies because they lack sufficient knowledge about them. The fast movement of healthcare technologies leaves numerous medical workers unsure about properly implementing these systems into their present operational routines. Organizations need to develop complete education about AI technology tools and clinical application knowledge for patient treatment to build confidence within their medical staff. Staff involvement in implementation reduces technology resistance because it builds their sense of ownership toward new systems.

C. Concerns About Workflow Disruption

Medical staff perceive artificial intelligence integration as likely to disrupt tested medical workflows, which produce operational problems and elevated workplace tension. New technology implementation easily leads workers to think that the solution adds more work instead of being beneficial. The planning phase of AI implementation should include staff involvement to help workers express concerns while designing workflows that can efficiently integrate AI functions. The team-based implementation delivers staff member validation, which leads to better staff adaptability.

D. Trust Issues with AI Systems

AI systems require maximum trust from users to succeed in adoption. The fear of inaccurate predictions combined with possible biases and accountability concerns prompts numerous healthcare staff to avoid algorithm usage. Professional medical personnel will not effectively employ AI technology when they do not have faith in its generated recommendations. Organizations should establish complete transparency regarding AI system development processes and implementation while showing their reliability through methodical tests and clinical research. The implementation of regular audits together with updates strengthens trust because it proves organizations' commitment to holding onto high-quality standards.

E. Change Management Strategies

Successful change management strategies stand in the way of employee acceptance when integrating artificial intelligence systems. Leaders need to present a transparent description of AI benefits focused on staff and patient welfare because this shows that advanced technology functions to improve care delivery rather than serving as a danger. Healthcare staff members should have designated open forums to voice their questions and concerns, which will build collaborative and trusting relationships. Healthcare staff need effective strategies to address change resistance because it determines AI integration success in hospitals.

Data Privacy and Security Concerns

The implementation of artificial intelligence systems in healthcare leads to major benefits, but simultaneously generates essential problems with protecting private medical data. Hospitals need to understand the challenges facing their patient data security because they depend on AI systems to handle patient information, which requires proper protection for delivering high-quality care.

A. Data Security Risks

Because AI systems analyze large collections of confidential patient data, they become powerful targets for cyber attackers. The comprehensive data present in Electronic Health Records (EHRs) includes full health records, together with patient identification data, along financial documentation. Attacks from cybercriminals occur when they discover weaknesses in either the AI algorithm programming or in the storage infrastructure running those algorithms, which results in compromised data security. To sustain the protection and fidelity of patient information, hospitals must put into practice sophisticated security protocols, which combine encryption methods alongside secure access protocols, along with scheduled audit systems.

B. Compliance with Regulations

The Health Insurance Portability and Accountability Act (HIPAA), together with the General Data Protection Regulation (GDPR), operate as strict confidentiality regulations that safeguard patient privacy for health organizations in both Europe and the United States. Healthcare entities must handle patient data properly, while patients need to approve its use under the regulations. The practice of non-compliance brings about severe consequences, while patients lose their trust in healthcare systems. The medical industry requires AI tools to respect all regulations since such compliance helps maintain healthcare standards that align with ethical and legal requirements.

C. Patient Consent and Transparency

Healthcare decisions made by AI systems will make the consent process for patients more complicated. The informed consent process for patients includes disclosure regarding the way their data will be utilized, together with information about diagnostic assessments and treatment suggestions driven by AI systems. Patients develop trust by understanding how AI supports their medical care, thus allowing them to have a comfortable relationship with the technology. The patient's trust in AI systems depends heavily on clear disclosure of their decision-making algorithms.

D. Minimizing Data Collection

AI systems need to operate using larger datasets, yet collecting large amounts of information creates heightened chances of vulnerability breaches during security incidents. Healthcare organizations should practice data minimization by gathering only those patient records needed to fulfill particular operational needs. The approach fulfills both risk reduction mandates and regulatory provisions that defend patient privacy.

E. Third-Party Vendor Risks

As various healthcare organizations acquire their Artificial Intelligence solutions from external vendors, these organizations become exposed to new security risks and vulnerabilities. For these vendors, healthcare organizations need to verify strict security standards and full compliance with relevant regulations. medical staff members need to have their data protection obligations specifically detailed in contractual agreements that also schedule regular security assessment activities.

F. Ethical Considerations

Healthcare AI deployments generate effects that exceed their technical aspects in their ethical dimension. The patient outcomes are at risk when AI systems utilize unrepresentative dataset training methods to develop algorithms that exhibit bias. Healthcare delivery maintains its equity by ensuring fairness is a basic requirement within AI applications. Hospitals need to prioritize data privacy and security measures when they implement AI systems to operate within their healthcare facilities.

Regulatory and Compliance Issues

Healthcare organizations need to solve several artificial intelligence (AI)-related regulatory and compliance problems which both protect patient safety while maintaining ethical standards. Medical organizations struggle to follow multiple regulations when they integrate AI systems into their clinical operations because AI technologies increasingly appear in healthcare workflows.

A. Evolving Regulatory Frameworks

Healthcare institutions currently operate without established guidelines that address AI usage specifically for healthcare purposes. The HIPAA in the United States, alongside the GDPR in Europe, present guidelines about data privacy and security, yet they do not resolve the particular difficulties created by AI technology implementation. The absence of appropriate regulations concerning AI needs new standards to emerge, which address the unique threats that AI creates, like biases in algorithms and unclear decision-making methods.

B. Compliance with Data Protection Regulations

The deployment of AI systems by healthcare organizations needs to follow strict data protection rules that apply to their operations. All organizations that handle HIPAA data need to establish strong security measures because patient information requires the highest level of protection against potential breaches. GDPR requires organizations to provide patients full data control through explicit consent procedures for every AI program that utilizes health-related sensitive information. Organizations that fail to meet these regulations risk steep financial consequences and affected patient relationships.

C. Accountability and Liability Issues

AI implementation creates challenging legal situations during errors, since the determination of accountability and responsibility becomes complex. It becomes hard to identify responsibility when an AI system provides incorrect advice that results in unfavorable treatment outcomes because developers and medical teams share accountability with health institutions. The essential responsibility of establishing clear accountability will give patients proper access to seek redress when AI-driven decisions result in harm.

D. Continuous Monitoring and Evaluation

The regulatory authorities now place rising importance on auditing and testing AI systems throughout their operational period. The evaluation of algorithms over time enables organizations to uncover biases or insufficient accuracy that emerge through data addition. Healthcare organizations require established systems to perform continuous monitoring of standards evolution because these systems ensure patient safety during compliance enforcement.

E. Engaging Stakeholders

Healthcare organizations need to effectively tackle regulatory challenges through stakeholder collaborations between regulatory bodies, along with compliance officers, clinicians, and patients during discussions on AI implementation procedures. The creation of guidelines through collaborative work enables organizations to manage the relationship between innovation and safety, together with ethical requirements.

SOLUTIONS AND RECOMMENDATIONS

To facilitate AI deployment in the hospital system, its functions should correspond to human-based care. The clinical and administrative workforce should be involved in the design or implementation process to gain efficacy and credibility. Lifelong learning is the need of the hour to make AI safe and deployable in real situations at the right time. There are key ethical issues that should be considered, including transparency, data privacy, and explainable. Utilization of the AI technologies should evolve through input and support; it does not replace the humane labor. The hope is that a balanced environment where AI increases the efficiency of hospitals without sacrificing the key aspects of empathy, safety, and human connection can be created.

Several essential best practices should guide the proper implementation of AI in healthcare practices:

- Start the integration by identifying particular problems that AI addresses, then create quantifiable targets for system deployment. When organizational needs become clear, it establishes a path that technology needs to follow.
- An organization must establish an approach to maintain both high-quality data standards and secure all information that enters AI platforms. Healthcare organizations should develop data cleaning and storage protocols alongside protocols to achieve HIPAA compliance for safeguarding patient privacy.
- Involving stakeholders alongside clinicians at the beginning of development allows for gathering opinions and resolving their issues. Staff insights help developers adjust AI solutions so they match the operational processes in healthcare effectively.
- The organization should evaluate multiple AI technologies through machine learning and natural language processing before selecting the ones that align with their business goals.
- Staff receive continuous support alongside training, which helps them embrace new AI tools through the development of an innovative work culture while minimizing their reluctance to change.

FUTURE RESEARCH DIRECTIONS

Artificial intelligence (AI) will completely transform healthcare operations by bringing together better patient healthcare solutions and improved operational productivity. The hospital landscape of AI is set to experience significant changes, which will become apparent during the year 2025.

BROAD PRACTICE TRANSFORMATIONS

A. Personalized Medicine

Advanced data analysis through artificial intelligence allows exact treatment regime creation by processing medical records together with genomic data and life habits of specific patients. Healthcare providers gain the ability to create personalized treatment plans because of this capability, thus delivering efficient therapeutics combined with reduced adverse effects. Researchers utilize AI to estimate treatment results for certain medications based on genetic characteristics that lead to enhanced therapeutic approaches.

B. Advanced Diagnostics

The discovery of medical conditions during early stages will undergo revolutionary change because of artificial intelligence diagnostics tools. New imaging enhancements enable faster, more precise image analysis of X-rays alongside MRIs and related medical images, which leads to a reduction in misdiagnosis occurrences. Hospitals can achieve workflow efficiency and speed up the test processing of critical tests through the implementation of predictive analytics in clinical settings.

C. Direct-to-Patient Models

Healthcare providers will transform their service delivery models through direct-to-patient (DTP) models that AI fuels. The improved model designs generate individualized assistance structures that enhance patient abilities to follow treatment instructions, therefore leading to improved clinical outcomes

D. Multimodal AI Solutions

AI systems will evolve into multi-source analytics that amalgamate medical pictures with EHRs along with genetic data to deliver extensive medical insights about patient well-being. A comprehensive approach under this system will enable medical practitioners to generate better decisions that lead to improved treatment designs.

E. Enhanced Workflow Efficiency

The automation capacity of AI technology will decrease healthcare practitioners' workload, thus enabling them to spend more time assisting patients. Healthcare operations will run more efficiently because of this administrative process improvement, which leads to higher staff satisfaction throughout facilities. The healthcare field of the future shows great promise to develop better patient care results alongside increased operational effectiveness.

Innovations on the Horizon

Artificial intelligence (AI) innovations currently under development will create major changes in healthcare service delivery and operational productivity. Doctors believe various essential developments will appear between 2025 and 2030.

A. Autonomous Patient Management

New agent AI systems will enable automatic chronic disease supervision and management tasks. Under such systems, computer systems will examine current patient information to modify treatment strategies while also prompting healthcare providers to intervene as needed, so constant medical attention remains available even in limited resource areas.

B. Integration of Generative AI

Generative AI stands as a central component for clinical documentation and supportive functions because it helps health professionals by completing administrative work so they can dedicate more time to patient care. Intelligent chatbots coupled with virtual assistants through this technology will help providers and patients improve their communication systems.

C. Enhanced Patient Engagement

Digital health innovations will give patients better management of their health through enhanced control over their healthcare processes. A combination of wearable technology with individualized software programs improves patient surveillance in real-time, thus boosting medical monitoring quality along with patient health outcomes. The benefits of artificial intelligence to redefine healthcare services into more effective patient-oriented care can be demonstrated through new product developments by 2025.

This chapter concludes on the significance of the consideration of human-related aspects in implementing AI in the context of hospitals, and formulates the research priorities that need to be elaborated in the future. There must be long-term research to measure the impact of AI in terms of the workload of clinicians, patient outcomes, and efficiency. Additional research must focus on the influence of cultural and organizational environments on AI adoption. The research should also be done on how empathy and emotional intelligence can be improved through AI in care delivery. To ensure sound merging of AI to healthcare practice, interdisciplinary collaboration and the development of standardized measures of usability, trust, and cognitive loads are necessary to provide coherent and coherent ethical, effective, and sustainable AI implementation.

CONCLUSION

This chapter discussed the disruptive importance of Artificial Intelligence (AI) in hospital settings, both in terms of the technology and the human-related issues that it poses. It has detailed the capability of AI in enhancing the diagnostic precision, predictive analysis, administrative effectiveness, and drug discovery rate, supporting the fact that it possesses the ability to increase the volume of the overall healthcare achievements. In addition to technical aspects, the chapter has highlighted that the need to examine human factors regarding clinical responsibilities, training requirements, emotional intelligence, and trust is a crucial element of the issue. The conceptual framework was introduced as a model for four major domains of AI assimilation: clinical functionality, operational efficiency, human considerations, and patient impact. In this light, the discussion has provided helpful guidelines on reasonable ways of implementing ethical AI, such as involving users, continuous education, and transparency of the systems. It suggested the areas of future research, too, the focus of which was to assess the long-term impact and to promote interdisciplinary design. In conclusion, the chapter remarks that sustainable integration of AI advisory needs the balanced treatment; the treatment that puts primary focus on human values, clinical practice augmentation, and empathy protection in patient care.

REFERENCES

Abdullah, R. M., Saad, L. A., Alasmari, Z. M., Ali, G. A., & Muniasamy, A. (2025). Human disease prediction mobile application using machine learning. In Alareeni, B., & Hamdan, A. (Eds.), *IoT and digital transformation: Innovating business models for the connected world (ICBT 2024). Lecture notes in networks and systems* (Vol. 1575). Springer. DOI: 10.1007/978-3-032-00450-5_19

Alowais, S. A., Alharbi, A. A., Alshammari, M. M., Alshammari, A. S., & Alenezi, M. N. (2023). Revolutionizing healthcare: The role of artificial intelligence in clinical practice. *BMC Medical Education*, *23*(1), 689. DOI: 10.1186/s12909-023-04698-z PMID: 37740191

Aminizadeh, S., Xu, H., Rani, M., & Bridger, R. (2024). Opportunities and challenges of artificial intelligence and distributed systems to improve the quality of healthcare service. *Artificial Intelligence in Medicine*, *149*, 102779. DOI: 10.1016/j.artmed.2024.102779 PMID: 38462281

Bridger, R. (2017). *Introduction to human factors and ergonomics*. CRC Press.

Cacciabue, P. C., & Vella, G. (2010). Human factors engineering in healthcare systems: The problem of human error and accident management. *International Journal of Medical Informatics*, *79*(4), e1–e17. DOI: 10.1016/j.ijmedinf.2008.10.005 PMID: 19101197

Chignell, M., Tong, T., Mizobuchi, S., Valdez, R. S., & Morita, P. (2023). The evolution of HCI and human factors: Integrating human and artificial intelligence. *ACM Transactions on Computer-Human Interaction*, *30*(2), 1–30. DOI: 10.1145/3557891

Crowther, D., Goh, K., Rauf, A., & Wang, Y. (2025). Assessing the impact of artificial intelligence on healthcare sector for enhancing sustainability. In *Transforming the healthcare sector through artificial intelligence and environmental sustainability* (pp. 3–21). Springer Nature Singapore. DOI: 10.1007/978-981-97-9555-0_1

Crowther, D., Goh, K., Rauf, A., & Wang, Y. (2025). *Transforming healthcare sector through AI*. Springer., DOI: 10.1007/978-981-97-9555-0

Dewasiri, N. J., Rathnasiri, M. S. H., & Karunarathna, K. S. S. N. (2025). Artificial intelligence-driven technologies for environmental sustainability in the healthcare industry. In *Transforming healthcare sector through artificial intelligence and environmental sustainability* (pp. 67–87). Springer Nature Singapore. DOI: 10.1007/978-981-97-9555-0

Dinesh, R. A., Shanmugam, J., & Biswas, K. (2025). AI for application solutions for healthcare services using AI detection and diagnosis of different diseases: A special emphasis on neuro-oncology. In *Radiomics and radiogenomics in neuro-oncology* (pp. 241–275). Academic Press. DOI: 10.1016/B978-0-443-18509-0.00009-8

Dinesh, R. A., Shanmugam, J., & Biswas, K. (2025). Radiogenomics in neuro-oncology. In *Radiomics and radiogenomics in neuro-oncology* (pp. 241–275). Academic Press. DOI: 10.1016/B978-0-443-18509-0.00009-8

Gauthaman, S. A. (2026). Introduction to machine learning and optimization in healthcare. In Muniasamy, A. (Ed.), *Integrative machine learning and optimization algorithms for disease prediction* (pp. 1–34). IGI Global. DOI: 10.4018/979-8-3373-1087-9.ch001

Govindaraj, M., Rajendran, R., Balasubramani, R., & Venkatraman, V. (2024). Revolutionizing healthcare: The transformative impact of artificial intelligence. In *Revolutionizing the healthcare sector with AI* (pp. 54–78). IGI Global Scientific Publishing. DOI: 10.4018/979-8-3693-3731-8.ch003

Guastello, S. J. (2023). *Human factors engineering and ergonomics: A systems approach*. CRC Press. DOI: 10.1201/9781003359128

Holden, R. J., Carayon, P., Gurses, A. P., Hoonakker, P., Hundt, A. S., Ozok, A. A., & Rivera-Rodriguez, A. J. (2013). SEIPS 2.0: A human factors framework for studying and improving the work of healthcare professionals and patients. *Ergonomics*, *56*(11), 1669–1686. DOI: 10.1080/00140139.2013.838643 PMID: 24088063

Kumar, R., Gupta, K., & Singh, R. (2024). Application of artificial intelligence in the healthcare sector: A critical analysis. In *Comparative law: Unraveling global legal systems* (pp. 387–412). Springer Nature Singapore. DOI: 10.1007/978-981-97-7815-7_23

Mitchell, R. J., Williamson, A. M., Molesworth, B., & Chung, A. Z. Q. (2014). A review of the use of human factors classification frameworks that identify causal factors for adverse events in the hospital setting. *Ergonomics*, *57*(10), 1443–1472. DOI: 10.1080/00140139.2014.933886 PMID: 24992815

Muniasamy, A. (2025). Revolutionizing health monitoring: Integrating transformer models with multi-head attention for precise human activity recognition using wearable devices. *Technology and Health Care*, *33*(1), 395–409. DOI: 10.3233/THC-241064 PMID: 39269866

Muniasamy, A., & Karunakaran, G. (2026). Challenges and future directions: Emerging trends and limitations in ML and optimization for healthcare. In Muniasamy, A. (Ed.), *Integrative machine learning and optimization algorithms for disease prediction* (pp. 339–368). IGI Global. DOI: 10.4018/979-8-3373-1087-9.ch012

Muniasamy, A., Tabassam, S., Hussain, M. A., Sultana, H., Muniasamy, V., & Bhatnagar, R. (2020). Deep learning for predictive analytics in healthcare. In Hassanien, A., Azar, A., Gaber, T., Bhatnagar, R., & Tolba, M. F. (Eds.), *The International Conference on Advanced Machine Learning Technologies and Applications (AMLTA2019)*. Springer. DOI: 10.1007/978-3-030-14118-9_4

Naim, A. (2026). AI-driven smart manufacturing and automation in pharmaceutical production. In Muniasamy, A., & Karunakaran, G. (Eds.), *Applications of artificial intelligence in pharmaceuticals* (pp. 157–194). IGI Global. DOI: 10.4018/979-8-3373-2043-4.ch006

Nordlinger, B., Villani, C., & Rus, D. (2020). *Healthcare and artificial intelligence*. Springer., DOI: 10.1007/978-3-030-32161-1

Praveen, R. V. S., & Kumar, M. L. (2024). *Artificial intelligence in healthcare: Revolutionizing clinical decision making and patient care*. Addition Publishing House. Retrieved from https://lnkd.in/g5mxjfsG

Rani, N., Kumar, A., & Bhardwaj, A. K. (2025). Machine and deep learning techniques for smart healthcare industry: Big picture and open research challenges. *Intelligent Biomedical Technologies and Applications for Healthcare*, *5*(0), 255–275. DOI: 10.1016/B978-0-443-22038-8.00017-9

Rani, N., Sharma, R., Gupta, P., & Kumar, M. (2025). Machine and deep learning in smart healthcare. *AIMS Public Health*. Advance online publication. DOI: 10.3934/publichealth.2024004

Rasheed, K., Qayyum, A., Ghalib, A., & Razzak, I. (2022). Explainable, trustworthy, and ethical machine learning for healthcare: A survey. *Computers in Biology and Medicine*, *149*, 106043. DOI: 10.1016/j.compbiomed.2022.106043 PMID: 36115302

Rengaramanujam, K., & Muniasamy, A. (2026). AI in hospital administration and formulary design: Optimizing resource allocation and patient flow. In Muniasamy, A., & Karunakaran, G. (Eds.), *Applications of artificial intelligence in pharmaceuticals* (pp. 215–246). IGI Global. DOI: 10.4018/979-8-3373-2043-4.ch008

Rubeis, G. (2024). *Ethics of medical AI*. Springer. DOI: 10.1007/978-3-031-55744-6

Secinaro, S., Calandra, D., Secinaro, A., Muthurangu, V., & Biancone, P. (2021). The role of artificial intelligence in healthcare: A structured literature review. *BMC Medical Informatics and Decision Making*, *21*(1), 1–23. DOI: 10.1186/s12911-021-01488-9 PMID: 33836752

Shaheen, R., & Salim, H. (2025). Role of artificial intelligence in healthcare. In *Intersection of human rights and AI in healthcare* (pp. 173–200). IGI Global Scientific Publishing. DOI: 10.4018/979-8-3693-7051-3.ch004

Sharma, B. K. (2025). AI managed hospital workforce. In *Role of artificial intelligence, telehealth, and telemedicine in medical virology* (pp. 221–251). Springer Nature Singapore. DOI: 10.1007/978-981-97-2938-8_11

Shneiderman, B. (2022). *Human-centered AI*. Oxford University Press. DOI: 10.1093/oso/9780192845290.001.0001

Shorrock, S., & Williams, C. (2016). *Human factors and ergonomics in practice: Improving system performance and human well-being in the real world*. CRC Press. DOI: 10.1201/9781315587332

Wiczorek, R. (2024). Human-centered design of AI in healthcare and the role of older patients. In *Advances in intelligent healthcare delivery and management: Research papers in honour of Professor Maria Virvou for invaluable contributions* (pp. 37–47). Springer Nature Switzerland. DOI: 10.1007/978-3-031-65430-5_2

Xu, Q., Li, Y., Chen, J., Zhang, L., & Wang, H. (2023). Interpretability of clinical decision support systems based on artificial intelligence from technological and medical perspective: A systematic review. *Journal of Healthcare Engineering*, *2023*(1), 9919269. DOI: 10.1155/2023/9919269 PMID: 36776958

Youssef, E.-R., Meriem, M., & Ait-Lemqeddem, H. (2025). ChatGPT and ethics in healthcare facilities: An overview and innovations in technical efficiency analysis. *AI and Ethics*, *5*(4), 1–18. DOI: 10.1007/s43681-025-00672-1

Zahlan, A., Ranjan, R. P., & Hayes, D. (2023). Artificial intelligence innovation in healthcare: Literature review, exploratory analysis, and future research. *Technology in Society*, *74*, 102321. DOI: 10.1016/j.techsoc.2023.102321

ADDITIONAL READING

Nordlinger, B., Villani, C., & Rus, D. (Eds.). (2020). *Healthcare and Artificial Intelligence*. Springer., DOI: 10.1007/978-3-030-32161-1

Shneiderman, B. (2020). Human-Centered Artificial Intelligence: Reliable, Safe & Trustworthy. *International Journal of Human-Computer Interaction*, *36*(6), 495–504. DOI: 10.1080/10447318.2020.1741118

Shneiderman, B. (2022). *Human-Centered AI*. Oxford University Press. DOI: 10.1093/oso/9780192845290.001.0001

KEY TERMS AND DEFINITIONS

Algorithmic Bias: Algorithmic bias is a systematic error in AI systems that results in unfair or inaccurate outcomes, often caused by non-representative, incomplete, or faulty training data.

Cognitive Load: Cognitive load represents the amount of mental effort required to process information; in healthcare, AI can help reduce unnecessary cognitive burden on clinicians, enabling them to focus on critical decision-making.

Electronic Health Records (EHRs): Electronic health records are digital versions of patients' medical charts that store information such as medical history, diagnoses, medications, treatment plans, immunization records, and test results.

Ethical AI: Ethical AI refers to the development and deployment of artificial intelligence systems in ways that respect fairness, transparency, accountability, privacy, and human rights within healthcare environments.

Generative AI: Generative AI comprises models capable of producing new content such as text, images, or clinical notes, which can assist in documentation, communication, and decision support in healthcare.

Healthcare Interoperability: Healthcare interoperability is the ability of different healthcare systems, software applications, and facilities to exchange, analyze, and use data securely and seamlessly across platforms.

Human Factors: Human factors is a multidisciplinary field that studies how people interact with systems, technologies, and environments, with the goal of maximizing performance, safety, and well-being in complex settings such as hospitals.

Human-Centered Design: Human-centered design is a development approach that places human needs, behaviors, and experiences at the core of designing healthcare technologies to ensure usability, acceptance, and effectiveness.

Predictive Analytics: Predictive analytics involves applying statistical techniques and artificial intelligence to historical and real-time healthcare data to forecast patient outcomes, disease risks, and hospital process efficiency.

Telemedicine: Telemedicine is the delivery of healthcare services such as diagnosis and treatment through telecommunications technology, which can be enhanced by AI-driven monitoring and communication tools to support remote patient care.

Virtual Assistants: Virtual assistants are AI-powered conversational interfaces that support healthcare providers and patients by assisting with tasks such as appointment scheduling, reminders, medication management, and information retrieval.

Workflow Optimization: Workflow optimization refers to improving the efficiency and effectiveness of healthcare processes, often through AI-enabled automation, to reduce administrative burdens and support more effective patient care.

Chapter 16
Ethical and Regulatory Evaluation of Autonomous AI Systems in Surgical Practices

S. Ida Evangeline
https://orcid.org/0000-0003-2997-7897
Government College of Engineering, Tirunelveli, India

ABSTRACT

Autonomous artificial intelligence (AI) systems are transforming surgical practice, enabling enhanced precision, efficiency, and personalization. Yet, their integration introduces critical ethical and regulatory challenges. This chapter explores current applications of AI in surgical settings—preoperative planning, intraoperative decision-making, and postoperative monitoring—highlighting clinical benefits alongside risks such as algorithmic bias and lack of explainability. Key ethical issues are examined, including informed consent, moral responsibility, and data privacy. The chapter also evaluates global regulatory responses, such as the FDA's Total Product Lifecycle model and the EU's Artificial Intelligence Act. Case studies, including the da Vinci Surgical System and the Smart Tissue Autonomous Robot, illustrate real-world implications. The chapter concludes with forward-looking recommendations emphasizing adaptive regulation, interdisciplinary collaboration, and human-centered design to responsibly guide AI's role in surgical care.

DOI: 10.4018/979-8-3373-2787-7.ch016

INTRODUCTION

The rapid advancement of artificial intelligence technologies is revolutionizing the landscape of modern medicine, particularly in surgical practices. Autonomous AI systems are increasingly being integrated into the surgical workflow—augmenting human decision-making, enhancing precision, and enabling minimally invasive procedures that were once considered unattainable. Robotic assisted operations, AI enabled diagnostic imaging and intraoperative guidance are among the technologies that hold the promise of a paradigm change in the way surgical care is rendered offering a potential to improve patient outcome, decrease the surgical errors, and increase the efficiency of the healthcare systems (Guni et al., 2024).

However, the integration of autonomous AI into surgical environments does not come without profound ethical and regulatory challenges. Surgical decision-making is a high-stakes endeavor, often involving life-or-death consequences, where the application of AI must be approached with extreme caution. There are urgent ethical questions around patient safety, liability attribution, informed consent, algorithmic bias, and transparency (Muniasamy et al. 2026; Gauthaman, S. A., et al. 2026; Gauthaman et al., 2026). In the case where AI systems make mistakes in their decisions who is at fault? When patients cannot understand non-human agents' decision processes, can they really consent to procedures guided by such agents? What safeguards are needed in order for these technologies to not perpetuate or worsen already existing disparities, or introduce new risks? (Morris et al. 2024)

Moreover, the regulatory ecosystem has struggled to keep pace with the accelerating development of surgical AI technologies. Traditional frameworks for medical device approval and oversight are often ill-suited to address the adaptive and opaque nature of machine learning algorithms (Muniasamy et al. 2026; Gauthaman, S. A., et al. 2026; Gauthaman et al., 2026). However, with continuous learning after deployment, the need for dynamic and proactive regulatory mechanisms increases. While a patchwork of guidelines—regulatory approach by the U.S. Food and Drug Administration (FDA) to the European Union's (EU) Artificial Intelligence Act—is emerging, there is no cohesive and globally harmonized framework (Iftikhar et al. 2024).

This chapter provides a structured and critical examination of the ethical and regulatory dimensions associated with the deployment of autonomous AI systems in surgical settings. The discussion will begin by mapping the current capabilities and applications of AI in surgical practice, followed by an exploration of the core ethical dilemmas that arise from its use. Then, it will discuss explainability and why interpretable AI models are needed in clinical settings. We will present a detailed analysis of the global regulatory landscape, including policy gaps, liability concerns, and emerging legal precedents. We will then discuss the promise and peril of autonomous surgical AI using case studies. Finally, the chapter will suggest the ways of responsible innovation in the future and such innovations should be conducted with the coordination among developers, clinicians, ethicists and policymakers.

The chapter attempts to unpack these complex issues and thus provide a useful perspective to the ongoing research on responsible AI deployment in hospitals. In the transition from innovation to implementation of surgical AI, ethical integrity and regulatory foresight must be pillars of the future it builds for technology that does not merely supplement patient care, but instead compliments it.

BACKGROUND

AI in Surgical Practice: Landscape and Applications

The integration of artificial intelligence into surgical practice marks a transformative moment in the evolution of modern medicine, as shown in Figure 1. It is increasingly evident that AI technologies including machine learning algorithms, deep learning networks, and computer vision systems are being integrated into the surgical workflow, from preoperative diagnostics and intraoperative guidance to postoperative monitoring. These systems are becoming decision making agents that can augment, and in some cases even replace, parts of human clinical judgment.

Figure 1. AI-Integrated Surgical Workflow

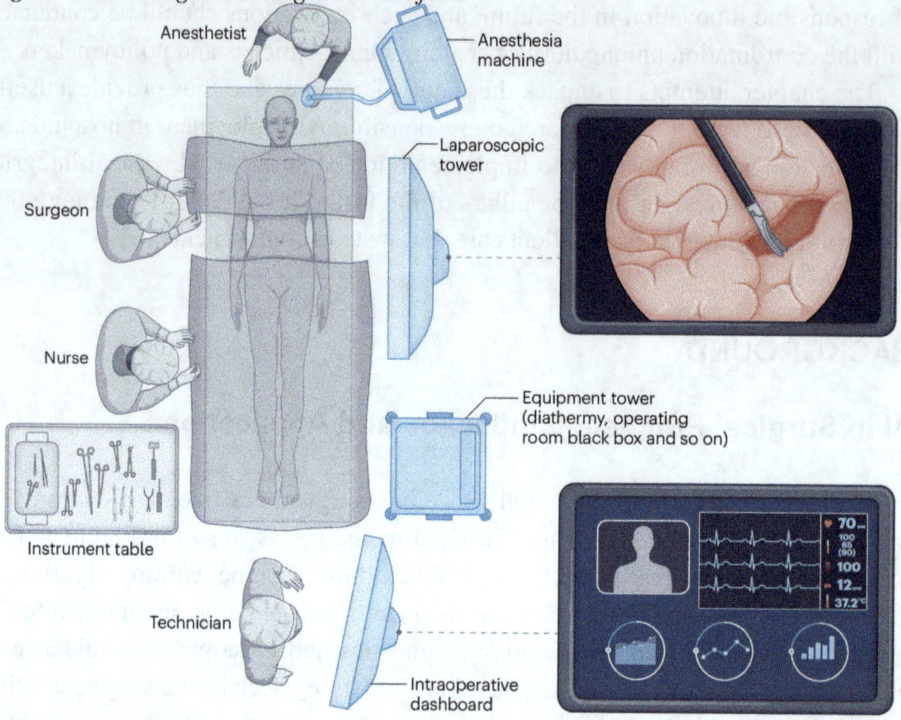

(Varghese et al. 2024)

In the preoperative phase, AI has demonstrated significant value in enhancing surgical planning. Predictive models trained on large volumes of patient data can evaluate individual surgical risks, recommend personalized procedural strategies, and anticipate potential complications. Convolutional neural networks in image-based AI can then interpret complex diagnostic scans, such as CT and MRI, and generate detailed three-dimensional reconstructions of anatomical structures. These reconstructions allow the surgeon to identify critical regions, improve their navigation, and select the best incision points. This preparatory phase is also supported by natural language processing tools which synthesize unstructured clinical notes, patient histories and comorbidity data to provide a more complete preoperative assessment (Arjmandnia & Alimohammadi, 2024).

During surgery, the role of AI extends into the operating theatre itself. Robotic-assisted surgical systems such as the da Vinci platform have become standard in many high-volume surgical centers, facilitating precise, minimally invasive procedures. Although such systems are currently semi-autonomous and heavily reliant on human control, AI modules embedded within them are being trained to perform specific surgical tasks with increasing levels of independence. Instrument tracking and tissue recognition are performed with real time computer vision and decision support algorithms monitor procedural progress and provide intraoperative alerts when deviations from standard surgical protocols are detected. Specifically, systems like the Smart Tissue Autonomous Robot have shown that supervised autonomous performance of certain surgical tasks, like soft tissue suturing, is possible in a manner that matches or surpasses the performance of human surgeons. This transition to AI as a surgical actor in its own right will be gradual (Tsai et al. 2024).

Postoperative care is also being reshaped by AI. Predictive analytics systems are now used to monitor patient recovery trajectories, detect early signs of complications, and anticipate readmission risks. Such systems integrate data from electronic health records, wearable sensors, and real time vital monitoring to alert clinicians to deviations from expected recovery patterns before clinical symptoms become apparent. Additionally, AI driven risk stratification models are being used to inform individualized postoperative care plans and long term prognostic assessments i.e. predicting tumor recurrence or functional recovery after orthopedic surgeries (Hashimoto et al. 2024).

While the integration of AI into surgical environments presents substantial opportunities for improving patient outcomes, enhancing procedural precision, and increasing healthcare efficiency, it also introduces significant challenges. One of the most pressing concerns is the issue of algorithmic bias. Datasets not representative of diverse patient populations can lead to skewed predictions and outcomes of AI systems that harm marginalized groups. In addition, technical failures, faulty sensor input, and use of opaque 'black box' models increase risk of unintended harm. In scenarios in which an AI system has a determinative role in surgical decision making, especially in the case of a negative outcome, the question of accountability is a pressing one (Lee et al. 2024).

With each advancement of AI technologies in surgery, the boundary between assistive tools and autonomous agents is becoming more and more indistinct. This evolving role necessitates a deeper examination of ethical boundaries, the distribution of responsibility, and the frameworks for clinical validation and oversight. The following sections examine these critical dimensions, first through an ethical analysis of the ramifications of using AI in high stakes surgical contexts, and then through a discussion of the potential to automate the surgical task in certain situations.

Ethical Considerations in Autonomous Surgical AI

The integration of autonomous AI systems into surgical practice raises a spectrum of ethical challenges that go beyond technical performance and clinical outcomes. These systems are able to influence or execute decisions that could drastically affect people's lives and they challenge basic principles of medical ethics, such as autonomy, beneficence, non-maleficence, and justice. As critical decisions are delegated to non human agents in high stakes environments such as the operating theatre, the ethical scrutiny of this delegation must be rigorous so as not to compromise the core values of medical practice in the name of technological efficiency, as shown in 2 (Power, 2024).

Figure 2. Ethical Dilemmas in Autonomous Surgical AI

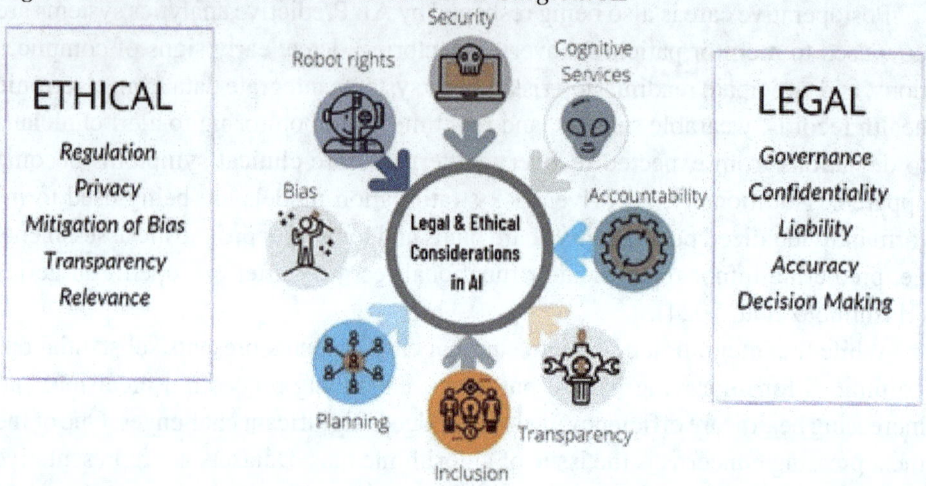

(Naik et al. 2022)

One of the primary ethical concerns is informed consent. Traditionally, patients provide consent for procedures based on their understanding of risks, benefits, and the nature of the intervention, all communicated by a human physician. This process is complicated by the involvement of AI, especially when their decision making mechanisms are opaque or even clinicians cannot fully explain. Can a patient be said to have truly given informed consent if they don't know how the system functions or the nature of its recommendations, if an AI system recommends or executes part of a surgical procedure? The implications of this are profound in terms of transparency and explainability in clinical AI systems, and whether existing consent practices are sufficient in an environment of algorithmically guided care (Rivero-Moreno et al. 2024).

Closely linked to the issue of consent is the question of responsibility. In conventional surgical practice, liability for clinical decisions lies with the operating surgeon. Yet, when AI systems take an increasingly active role—choosing procedural pathways, adjusting surgical parameters or even autonomous tasks—the moral and legal responsibility for the actions of the system is questioned. We do not know who is accountable in the case of an adverse outcome or a surgical error, the clinician, the institution, the AI system developer, or some combination thereof. The diffusion of responsibility undermines existing legal frameworks and moral reasoning about agency, particularly in probabilistic models rather than deterministic logic (Pressman et al. 2024).

Another critical ethical dilemma concerns algorithmic bias. AI models are trained on datasets that often reflect existing disparities in healthcare delivery. These biases can then be embedded into AI systems such that patients of different races, gender, socioeconomic status, or other demographic variables receive differential treatment outcomes. In a surgical setting, biased algorithms can lead to the prioritizing of patients for procedures, suggest different approaches based on demographic trends, or make less accurate predictions for underrepresented groups. Such perpetuation of inequities in AI systems goes against the ethical commitment to justice and equity in healthcare, and thus algorithms should undergo bias audits, have diverse datasets, and equitable model development (Snyder et al. 2024).

Another issue is data privacy. The effective functioning of AI systems is dependent on vast amounts of patient data. This data is often highly sensitive biometric and behavioral information, and ethical concerns relate to consent, confidentiality and data ownership in the collection, storage and processing of it. In addition, real time monitoring and continuous data feeds for postoperative care could blur the line between clinical necessity and invasive surveillance (Vakili Ojarood, Mohebbi, & Akbari, 2024).

Philosophical debate also exists on the moral agency of AI systems themselves. Unlike AI, which lacks consciousness or intentionality, the fact that it can influence outcomes in complex environments means that we need to revisit our ethical frameworks. Other scholars have suggested defining AI as "moral instruments" rather than moral agents, such that the ethical assessment depends on the design, deployment, and use of the system, rather than on the system's internal states. This viewpoint supports the ethical responsibility of designers, regulators, and clinicians to guarantee that AI frameworks mirror and reinforce human values instead of working in unmapped moral area (Kothinti, 2024).

Last, the ethical challenge is oversight of dynamic, evolving AI. While traditional surgical tools are static after approval, the AI systems may continue to learn and adapt in real time, leading to changes which were not part of the original validation process (Muniasamy et al. 2026; Gauthaman, S. A., et al. 2026; Gauthaman et al., 2026). Such a continuous evolution calls for new ethical oversight models that do not hinge on a single point of approval, but rather include constant monitoring, real world performance evaluation and ethical review in the course of the operational life of the system (Fangerau, 2024).

As AI systems become increasingly capable of assuming more and more responsibilities in the surgical context, the ethical discourse must develop in tandem. Not only is this a regulatory challenge, but it is a profound moral imperative to ensure that these technologies serve patients in the best possible ways, preserve human dignity, and uphold professional integrity. The second section will extend these concerns to the technical and ethical import of explainability in clinical AI within the context of high stakes surgical care.

Explainability and Transparency in AI Systems

As artificial intelligence systems increasingly influence decisions in surgical practice, the demand for transparency and explainability becomes both a technical necessity and an ethical imperative. The degree of explainability, or the level to which the internal mechanics of an AI system can be interpreted and understood by humans, is key not only to clinical accountability, but also to the adherence of providers to AI systems. The ability to comprehend and dissect the rationale behind the AI generated recommendation or actions is critical in surgical environments where the outcomes may be irreversible and life altering, not only for informed clinical decision making, but also in order to garner trust from patients and practitioners (Patidar et al. 2024).

Modern AI, particularly models based on deep learning architectures, often operate as "black boxes." These systems process massive datasets through layers of abstraction, making it difficult to trace the logic that underpins a specific prediction or surgical recommendation. Although such models can achieve high accuracy in, for instance, detecting anomalies on imaging scans or choosing incision paths, they lack interpretability, which is a severe limitation in clinical settings. Unlike data scientists, surgeons must justify their decisions in real time and to multiple stakeholders (patients, colleagues, legal authorities, and regulatory bodies). If the rationale behind a decision cannot be articulated, the legitimacy of the decision, as well as the AI system that made it, is questionable (Muthusubramanian et al. 2024).

The ethical implications of opacity in surgical AI are substantial. If a system misclassifies an anatomical structure or recommends an unsafe procedural step without an interpretable rationale, clinicians may find it difficult to override the system's output or explain their course of action. It can erode clinical autonomy, undermine professional judgment and introduce ambiguity in cases of surgical complications or litigation. In such scenarios, informed consent becomes more problematic as patients may be unwilling to entrust their care to systems whose operations are not only opaque to outsiders but also even to the surgical team using them (Olateju et al. 2024).

Explainability is also critical in the context of algorithmic auditing and continuous learning. Many AI systems deployed in healthcare are adaptive, meaning they evolve based on new data collected during their use. Healthcare institutions may not be aware of shifts in performance or emerging patterns of error without clear documentation of how changes in the system's behavior occur over time. On the other hand, transparent AI systems allow traceability, i.e., each decision can be traced back to the identifiable inputs which can be rigorously analyzed post hoc and subjected to meaningful quality assurance (Sasikala & Sachan, 2024).

In recent years, technical efforts have been made to increase the interpretability of AI systems in healthcare. To make deep learning models more understandable, techniques like attention mapping, saliency visualization and feature attribution models like SHAP (Shapley Additive Explanations) and LIME (Local Interpretable Model-Agnostic Explanations) are being employed. As given in Table 1, these tools can be used in surgical applications to highlight which anatomical features led to a certain classification, or which sensor inputs were most important for a robotic decision. These approaches provide some transparency, but they are not without limitations, such as oversimplifying the underlying complexity or providing shallow clarity without deep interpretive insight (Goktas, 2024).

Table 1. Comparison of explainability techniques in surgical AI

Method	Description	Strengths	Limitations	Example Application
SHAP	Shapley Additive Explanations quantify each feature's contribution to a prediction.	Theoretically grounded, consistent explanations.	Computationally intensive; assumes model additivity.	Identifying key risk factors in postop complications
LIME	Local Interpretable Model-Agnostic Explanations approximate a model locally with simpler models.	Model-agnostic, intuitive explanations.	Instability; explanations may vary with sampling.	Interpreting incision suggestions from black-box models
Attention Maps	Highlight input regions that the model focuses on during decision-making.	Native to deep models, aligns with human intuition.	May not always correlate with causal importance.	Visualizing focus areas in surgical image segmentation
Saliency Maps	Show which parts of input data most influence model output gradients.	Fast to compute, good for initial diagnostics.	Sensitive to input noise; lacks consistency across samples.	Detecting anomalies in intraoperative imaging

Furthermore, the demand for explainability must be balanced with the practical constraints of surgical environments. Overly complex explanations can actually get in the way of clinical decision making in high pressure situations. This means that explainable AI systems must be designed to be relevant, concise, and appropriate to context. Instead of striving for full transparency of all system operations, transparency should be focused on providing actionable, comprehensible and clinically meaningful insights (Marey et al. 2024).

There is also a cultural dimension to the pursuit of transparency in AI. Trust in medical technology is not built solely on performance metrics, but also on the perceived integrity, fairness, and accountability of the system. This trust is fostered by explainability, which aligns AI behavior with human ethical expectations, reinforces the clinician as a responsible agent, and protects patient autonomy. In such a sense, transparency is not just a technical feature, but a necessary condition for ethical AI design and deployment (Barnes & Hutson, 2024).

With AI systems becoming more deeply embedded in surgical practice, a functional standard of explainability will be central to the ethical acceptance and regulatory approval of such systems. The following section will explore how these concerns are being addressed by different jurisdictions and regulatory bodies, and how legal frameworks are adapting to ensure that transparency, accountability, and safety remain fundamental principles in surgical AI adoption.

MAIN FOCUS OF THE CHAPTER

Global Regulatory Frameworks for AI in Surgery

As autonomous AI systems become increasingly prevalent in surgical practice, the development of robust regulatory frameworks has emerged as a central concern for ensuring their safe, effective, and ethically aligned deployment. AI systems, and particularly those that are based on machine learning, are by nature complex, adaptable, and opaque in a way that traditional medical devices are not. These attributes are at odds with the existing ways of regulating tools that learn, evolve, and dynamically interact with clinical environments. Currently, regulatory bodies around the world are faced with the task of evaluating and authorizing AI surgical systems, including those that demonstrate some degree of autonomy (Maher & Chang, 2024).

In the United States, the FDA has taken significant steps toward formalizing a regulatory pathway for AI and machine learning-enabled software as a medical device. Because these systems can change over time, the FDA proposed a Total Product Lifecycle approach. The regulatory oversight envisioned by this model does not end with the one time approval, but rather extends through premarket review, real world performance monitoring and post market modifications. The FDA's Predetermined Change Control Plan proposal would allow AI developers to define beforehand the changes their system could undergo, so the agency could approve future algorithmic updates without having to resubmit again and again. This approach recognizes that AI is adaptive, but it also requires greater transparency and documentation from developers to determine how updates will be validated and monitored (Smith et al. 2022).

In Europe, the regulatory landscape is evolving under the European Union Artificial Intelligence Act (AIA), which adopts a risk-based classification system for AI systems. Surgical AI, given its high-stakes implications for health and safety, is typically categorized as "high-risk," subjecting it to stringent compliance requirements. They also include requirements for robustness, transparency, human oversight, data quality, and post market monitoring. The AIA stresses the human in the loop oversight principle, that is, if a decision is critical, such as in patient care, it must remain under meaningful human control. Moreover, the Act requires high risk AI systems to be assessed for conformity, and registered in a public EU database, which increases traceability and accountability (Meszaros et al. 2022).

The United Kingdom, after its departure from the EU, is developing its own AI governance strategy through the Medicines and Healthcare products Regulatory Agency (MHRA). The UK's vision for regulation is adaptive with a sandbox environment for developers to trial AI systems without full approval under regulatory guidance. The goal of this approach is to achieve a tradeoff between safety and flexibility, especially in rapidly changing domains such as surgical robotics and AI guided interventions (Rana et al. 2025).

Other jurisdictions are similarly active. Japan's Pharmaceuticals and Medical Devices Agency has a collaborative model for assessing AI-enabled surgical tools, in which academic institutions are often included in the review. Both Canada and Australia have updated their medical device regulations to include AI software, with post market surveillance requirements particular to systems with learning components (Joshi et al. 2024).

Across these frameworks, several common themes emerge. First, there is a universal recognition of the need for continuous oversight rather than static approval. Second, transparency is not only in how decisions are made by AI systems but also in how they are communicated to regulators and clinical users when changes are made to the systems. Third, there is a growing recognition by all major jurisdictions that interdisciplinary collaboration is necessary in the design and review of AI systems, including ethicists, clinicians, engineers, and legal experts. Lastly, there is increasing interest in developing international standards for clinical AI (e.g. from the International Medical Device Regulators Forum and the International Organization for Standardization (ISO)) to harmonise evaluation criteria across borders (O'Sullivan et al. 2019).

Yet, despite these promising developments, significant gaps remain. Most regulatory frameworks are still better suited for rule-based or static AI systems than for fully autonomous and adaptive surgical agents. There is no uniform validation metric, the risk classification is uneven, and there are inconsistent enforcement mechanisms across jurisdictions, which results in fragmented regulatory environment. Additionally, the legal provisions that are currently in force do not take into account the subtleties of liability and professional responsibility in the situations where human surgeons and autonomous systems make decisions together (Wah, 2025).

In the absence of a globally unified framework, hospitals and health systems deploying surgical AI must navigate a complex patchwork of regulatory obligations and ethical expectations. As a result, some institutions have created in house governance protocols, such as AI ethics boards and oversight committees, to assess the technical validity and ethical consequences of applying AI to surgery. In that sense, these local initiatives can be viewed as precursors of more comprehensive and harmonized models of AI regulation in the future (Kovacs et al. 2025).

With the advancement of AI, especially towards greater autonomy in a surgical setting, regulatory frameworks will need to keep pace. We must simultaneously pursue safety, accountability, and innovation, and we must do so dynamically, allowing for the speed and complexity of AI in healthcare.

Legal and Policy Challenges

The growing integration of autonomous AI systems in surgical environments presents complex legal and policy challenges that strain the boundaries of existing medical jurisprudence. These systems will move from passive decision support tools to active participants in clinical procedures, and the frameworks that have guided liability, professional responsibility, and insurance coverage in the healthcare setting will need to be rethought. The resolution of these challenges is not theoretical but foundational to the operationalization of AI in high risk medical settings and necessary to sustain public trust, institutional accountability, and ethical coherence of surgical practice (Wang & Ma, 2025).

Foremost among the legal concerns is the issue of liability. Surgical practice has long been governed by well-established principles of medical malpractice, wherein a human clinician is held responsible for errors or negligence that result in patient harm. The model described above becomes problematic, however, with the introduction of AI, especially autonomous systems that make or implement critical intraoperative decisions. However, if an AI system misidentifies an anatomical structure, suggests an incorrect incision path, or performs a surgical maneuver that results in adverse outcomes, the question of assigning fault is difficult. Was this error an algorithm bug? A failure in system integration by the hospital? A lack of oversight by the surgeon? Or something more systemic, related to regulatory approval? (Ferreres, 2025)

This diffusion of agency across multiple stakeholders introduces the notion of shared liability, wherein responsibility is distributed among the AI developers, clinical users, device manufacturers, and the institutions deploying the technology. However, as of now, this model is underdeveloped in legal practice. There are no established clear standards of causation and fault by courts or regulatory bodies to evaluate the role of an AI driven decision in surgical harm. Without precedent, litigation in this space can be inconsistent and various jurisdictions may interpret negligence and accountability according to differing interpretations (Naili et al. 2025).

Closely linked to liability is the question of informed consent, which in the age of AI demands redefinition. Traditional informed consent assumes that clinicians understand the intervention well enough to explain its nature, benefits, risks, and alternatives to the patient. In cases of complex AI systems that are informed by machine learning, clinicians themselves may not have a full understanding of how specific recommendations or decisions are generated. This opacity poses the question of how informed consent can be, if it is built upon the outputs of systems whose internal workings are even hidden from expert users. AI-specific consent protocols have been argued for by ethical and legal scholars to be incorporated in which patients are expressly informed about the nature and boundaries of the technologies used in their care (Corfmat et al 2025).

Another emerging concern is regulatory lag, whereby existing legal frameworks fail to keep pace with technological advancement. The current medical device laws were created for static instruments, not for systems that update themselves based on new data. Therefore, a significant portion of AI tools exists in a grey zone where its post deployment evolution is not fully captured by regulatory oversight. Such regulation creates potential liability for system failures as well as for the regulatory bodies that approved their use without clear mechanisms for ongoing evaluation. Dynamic licensing and adaptive compliance regimes are being explored by policymakers as new legislative models, but these are nascent and lacking in harmonization across the globe (ElHassan & Arabi, 2025).

The implications of these challenges extend to the insurance industry, which must adapt to a landscape where surgical errors may stem from algorithmic decision-making rather than clinician negligence. Such incidents may not be covered by traditional malpractice insurance designed for human professional actions. The discussions surrounding AI specific insurance models have been prompted, where liability premiums are based on algorithmic risk profiles, training data integrity and system transparency. AI systems may also have to provide more detailed logs and audit trails to insurers to assist risk assessment retrospectively and assigning fault in the case of litigation. Nevertheless, the actuarial science supporting such insurance models is underdeveloped and healthcare institutions are not equipped to deal with the legal murkiness that AI caused errors could bring (Yin, 2025).

To address these gaps, a number of hospitals and healthcare systems are starting to put in place internal policy frameworks to manage legal exposure and provide ethical oversight ((Rengaramanujam et al., 2026; Muniasamy et al. 2026; Gauthaman, S. A., et al. 2026; Gauthaman et al., 2026). AI risk assessment protocols, data governance boards, interdisciplinary ethics committees, etc., all of which are deployed to assess if new AI technologies are ready and safe. Though these measures show institutional initiative, they also highlight the necessity for more defined national and international policies with the ability to provide standardized legal protections, ethical guidelines, and operational safeguards (Xue & Weng, 2025).

Finally, the legal and policy environment in which autonomous surgical AI will be developed is still largely in flux. As these technologies develop and become further embedded within surgical workflows, the law must adapt to new forms of harm, new liability models, and prevent innovation from outrunning accountability. For the future to be one of AI-driven surgery that is not only technologically effective, but also legally and ethically sound, we will need to develop clear legal definitions, codify duties of care, and facilitate multi stakeholder dialogue.

Case Studies in Autonomous Surgical AI Deployment

To understand the real-world implications of ethical, regulatory, and legal challenges discussed in prior sections, it is essential to examine actual deployments of autonomous and semi-autonomous AI systems in surgical practice. These case studies give insight into the transformative potential as well as the complex risks of AI in the operating theatre. Empirical examples make it clear that the incorporation of AI into surgery is not a smooth process which is uniform but is characterized by institutional variation, evolving technological capability and varying approaches to governance and clinical validation (Khanna et al 2025).

One of the most widely recognized platforms in the field of surgical robotics is the da Vinci Surgical System, developed by Intuitive Surgical. While not fully autonomous, da Vinci represents a foundational example of how AI-driven robotics have reshaped minimally invasive surgery. Robotic arms, magnified 3D visualization and tremor filtration enhance the surgeon's dexterity and precision. The platform contains embedded AI components that help with optimal instrument positioning and movement prediction. Da Vinci has been used in over 10 million procedures over the years in urological, gynecological and cardiac surgeries. While its success has helped robotic surgery gain broader institutional acceptance, the fact that it still relies on human control shows that the industry is still wary of full autonomy. However, da Vinci systems have been adopted widely, despite mechanical failures and surgical complications, which have resulted in investigations into regulatory lapses and questions about human and machine accountability (Liu et al. 2025).

In contrast to da Vinci's surgeon-controlled model, the Smart Tissue Autonomous Robot (STAR) project has pushed the boundaries of autonomy in surgical

AI. STAR was developed by researchers at Johns Hopkins University, and was able to autonomously perform soft tissue suturing with an accuracy comparable to that of experienced human surgeons. In 2022, in a landmark study, STAR performed laparoscopic intestinal anastomosis on pigs with minimal human interaction using computer vision, force feedback and AI based path planning. This was one of the first times a robot acted autonomously completing a complex surgical task. Implications of this performance of STAR are broad: it confirms the feasibility of autonomous execution of surgery, but at the same time raises fundamental ethical and regulatory issues related to oversight, fail safe mechanisms, and surgeon involvement in autonomous workflows. Although STAR is still in experimental phases, it represents the technological horizon of autonomous AI in operative settings (Panesar et al. 2019).

A different model of AI integration is found in systems designed for AI-assisted surgical planning and triage. One such example is the use of AI by the Mayo Clinic, where machine learning models are applied to imaging and patient data to recommend surgical interventions or non-invasive alternatives. They help predict postoperative outcomes and identify patients with high risk for complications. While these tools do not directly intervene during surgery, they have a strong impact on surgical decision making and demonstrate the range of AI involvement from preoperative analytics to intraoperative execution. Strong interdisciplinary governance structures, such as AI ethics boards and algorithm performance review, have been key to successful deployment at the Mayo Clinic, as these innovations are brought in line with patient centered care principles (Caine et al. 2022).

Karolinska University Hospital in Sweden has tried out AI systems that monitor intraoperative metrics and predict deviations to expected surgical paths internationally. Although still being evaluated, these systems are intended as safety layers, alerting surgical teams to subtle signs of complications before they become apparent. To incorporate AI ethics into clinical practice, the hospital has been progressive, and any AI system deployed must undergo a thorough ethical review involving patient representatives, ethicists, and medical professionals (Elemento et al. 2021).

The FDA's approval of AI-based imaging and diagnostic tools like the Viz.ai platform for stroke detection has also given momentum to AI adoption in the surgical specialties indirectly. Although these systems do not perform surgery per se, they show how AI's predictive power is trusted in time sensitive, high risk medical scenarios. However, the successful approval and adoption of such systems demonstrate the possibility of extending AI into operative contexts, as long as there are solid evidence and validation protocols (Milam & Koo, 2023).

Conversely, there have been cautionary cases where insufficient validation led to suboptimal outcomes. In 2019, the UK's National Health Service (NHS) paused the deployment of an AI-powered diagnostic support system after findings that the tool underperformed on minority populations and presented uncalibrated recommendations during surgical planning. In this case, the need for representativeness in training datasets, the dangers of algorithmic bias, and the perils of launching systems without appropriate ethical or regulatory oversight were on display. Together, these case studies demonstrate the breadth of the surgical AI ecosystem, from how it is developed, to how it is validated, and how it is deployed. It shows the different levels of autonomy, the significance of contextual governance, and the practical difficulties to guarantee the ethical integrity and patient safety in intricate clinical settings. These examples illustrate important lessons about what constitutes responsible and accountable implementation in the field (and where caution is still advised) while the field is still evolving (Goktas & Grzybowski, 2025).

Ethical AI Governance

As autonomous AI systems continue to evolve and integrate more deeply into surgical environments, the future of their development and deployment will be shaped not only by technological progress, but by the frameworks of ethical governance and interdisciplinary collaboration that emerge alongside them. The increasing realization that the long term success and societal acceptance of AI in surgery will rely on our ability to innovate in ways that are safe, equitable, accountably, and human centered. Finally, the ethical and regulatory questions that have arisen in recent years are not temporary obstacles but permanent challenges that will determine what role AI will play in modern surgical practice and whether that role will be legitimate and sustainable (Dasgupta & Raison, 2025).

One of the most significant future directions is the move toward adaptive and anticipatory regulation. Static approval models, once sufficient for traditional medical devices, are poorly suited to AI systems that evolve over time through machine learning((Muniasamy et al. 2026; Gauthaman, S. A., et al. 2026; Gauthaman et al., 2026). Regulators have started to realize that there is a need for dynamic oversight structures that permit continuous post market evaluation, algorithmic transparency, and ability to revoke or revise approvals based on real world performance data. Automated reporting systems, real time validation protocols, and robust auditing mechanisms to identify drift in system behavior or emergent risks in different clinical contexts will likely be part of future regulatory frameworks. As AI systems adapt, these mechanisms must track technical performance but also that the AI systems continue to operate within ethical boundaries (Ahern, 2025).

In parallel with regulatory innovation, the role of interdisciplinary collaboration is poised to become a central pillar of ethical AI governance. Surgical AI systems sit at the intersection of medicine, engineering, ethics, and law((Muniasamy et al. 2026; Gauthaman, S. A., et al. 2026; Gauthaman et al., 2026). The responsible development of AI for healthcare requires close cooperation with AI developers, clinicians, biomedical engineers, healthcare administrators, legal experts and patient advocates. Leading institutions should standardize the practice of multidisciplinary ethics committees, which are already emerging, to evaluate AI tools before clinical deployment. These committees can then assess technical validity, as well as broader ethical implications, such as patient autonomy, fairness and broader societal impact. In particular, patient voices will be included in these evaluations, as patients are often excluded from decision making processes that will impact them the most (Li et al. 2025).

Another important trajectory is the design and implementation of ethical AI frameworks tailored to healthcare. Existing models of ethical AI—while valuable—are often too abstract or generalized to capture the high-stakes, context-specific nature of surgical practice. Future frameworks must acknowledge the complexity of surgical decision making, the particular vulnerabilities of patients under anesthesia, and the relational dynamics of clinicians and AI systems. These frameworks should delineate clear boundaries of permissible degrees of autonomy, norms of informed consent for AI driven procedures and requirements for safeguarding human agency within the surgical workflow. In the case of AI, ethical principles must be operationalized by technical design: interpretability, accountability, and fail-safe mechanisms should be built into the very architecture of the AI systems (Jha et al. 2025).

Central to future governance models is a shift in perspective—one that reframes AI not as a replacement for clinicians but as a collaborative partner. "AI as a collaborator" is a concept that encourages a hybrid decision-making model where AI complements human cognition and makes precision possible without replacing clinical judgment." This model assumes that human oversight is not a formality, but an active and informed interaction with AI outputs. To enable this paradigm, surgeons need to be educated and trained in the use of AI. In the future, clinicians will not only need to know how to operate AI tools, but also how to read, critique, and intervene in their outputs. Therefore, ethical governance needs to be extended to professional development and institutional culture (Wah, 2025).

Equity and access is a further consideration for future directions. The development and deployment of advanced surgical AI systems in high income healthcare systems is a concern because it may exacerbate global health disparities. Access to AI technologies must be equitable and the infrastructural capacity to validate, deploy, and maintain them must become a central concern of international governance. Creating open source AI tools, promoting transparency in training datasets, and building local capacity in under resourced settings will be essential to spread the benefits of AI widely rather than having them concentrated among the few (Hemmatyar et al. 2025).

Finally, the future of AI in surgery will depend on the development of international norms and collaborative policy-making. Regional regulatory bodies are moving forward, but the transnational nature of AI development and data flows requires a global approach. It is necessary for international bodies like the World Health Organization (WHO), the International Medical Device Regulators Forum, and ISO to harmonize the standards of safety, efficacy and ethical compliance. By coordinating this, regulatory fragmentation will be reduced, cross border approval processes will be streamlined and a shared commitment to responsible innovation (Parveen et al. 2025) will be encouraged.

In sum, the ethical and regulatory future of autonomous surgical AI lies in building governance ecosystems that are flexible, inclusive, and forward-looking. The advancement of technology must be matched by the readiness of institutions and ethical resolve. If we embed these values into the systems we create and the structures that oversee them, then the next generation of surgical innovation will be smarter, safer, fairer, and fundamentally human centered.

SOLUTIONS AND RECOMMENDATIONS

The responsible integration of autonomous AI systems in surgical practice requires coordinated action across ethical design, regulatory innovation, legal reform, and institutional governance. Drawing on the analysis presented in previous sections, this chapter offers the following actionable recommendations:

1. **Adopt Adaptive Regulatory Frameworks**

Regulators should transition from static, one-time approval models to dynamic, lifecycle-based oversight. Mechanisms such as real-time monitoring, continuous learning validation, and pre-approved change control plans (as piloted by the FDA) should be institutionalized for AI-enabled surgical systems.

2. **Mandate Contextual Explainability Standards**

AI systems used in surgery must meet domain-specific interpretability criteria. Developers should employ explainability techniques—such as SHAP, LIME, and attention maps—while ensuring outputs are meaningful and actionable for clinicians in high-stakes environments.

3. **Institutionalize AI Ethics Committees**

Hospitals and healthcare systems should establish multidisciplinary ethics boards to evaluate AI tools prior to deployment (Rengaramanujam et al., 2026). These committees should include surgeons, engineers, ethicists, patient advocates, and legal experts to ensure broad and accountable oversight.

4. **Develop Clear Liability and Insurance Models**

Legal systems must redefine responsibility in the era of autonomous surgical AI. Shared liability frameworks involving developers, clinicians, and healthcare institutions should be piloted, and insurance systems adapted to reflect algorithmic risk profiles and system-level accountability.

5. **Embed Equity and Bias Auditing in AI Design**

To prevent algorithmic harm, developers must use diverse, representative datasets and conduct systematic bias assessments. International funding and collaboration should support AI adaptation for under-resourced healthcare settings, preventing global disparities in surgical AI access.

6. **Integrate AI Literacy into Surgical Training**

Medical education must evolve to prepare surgeons for collaborative decision-making with AI systems. Training should include not only operational proficiency but also ethical awareness, interpretability critique, and system limitations.

7. **Promote International Harmonization**

Global agencies such as the WHO, ISO, and the International Medical Device Regulators Forum (IMDRF) should collaborate to establish cross-border standards for surgical AI. A harmonized framework would accelerate safe innovation and streamline global approvals.

FUTURE RESEARCH DIRECTIONS

As autonomous AI systems continue to evolve within surgical practice, several critical research gaps remain. Advancing the field requires interdisciplinary inquiry that not only deepens technological capabilities but also anticipates societal, ethical, and legal impacts. This section outlines key areas where future research is urgently needed:

1. **Dynamic Validation Models for Continuous Learning Systems**

Most AI regulatory frameworks remain predicated on static models. Future research must explore dynamic validation protocols capable of assessing AI systems that adapt post-deployment—especially in high-stakes surgical contexts.

2. **Causal Explainability in Complex Surgical Environments**

Current explainability tools provide correlational insights. There is a pressing need for research into causal models that explain *why* an AI system recommends a surgical action, not just *how* it arrived there, to better support clinical accountability.

3. **Context-Aware Ethical Algorithms**

Investigations into ethics-aware design are still nascent. Future work should develop models that can recognize and respond to context-specific ethical boundaries, such as those involving vulnerable patient populations, emergency scenarios, or cross-cultural sensitivities.

4. **Shared Agency and Decision-Making Frameworks**

New conceptual frameworks are needed to define and operationalize "shared decision-making" between humans and AI in surgery. This includes empirical studies on how clinicians interact with AI systems under pressure, and how responsibility is negotiated in real time.

5. **AI Performance in Underrepresented Populations and Global South Settings**

Research must examine how surgical AI performs across different demographic groups, healthcare infrastructures, and cultural contexts. This includes data equity studies, field deployments in low-resource environments, and frameworks for context-specific adaptation.

6. **Legal Precedents and Policy Prototypes**

Legal scholars and ethicists should collaborate on generating model legislation and liability test cases to guide courts and regulators. Empirical studies of AI litigation, insurance design, and professional accountability in surgical harm cases are critical.

7. **Societal Perception and Trust-Building Mechanisms**

Longitudinal research on public perception, patient trust, and clinician acceptance of surgical AI is needed. This includes psychological, sociological, and media studies to inform design choices and governance strategies that foster legitimacy and public engagement.

CONCLUSION

The emergence of autonomous AI systems in surgical practice represents one of the most profound transformations in the history of modern medicine. These technologies promise to revolutionize surgical care through enhanced precision, consistency, and adaptability, yet they also pose significant ethical, legal, and regulatory challenges. This chapter has demonstrated that the integration of AI in the surgical domain is not only about technical advance, but also a paradigm change that calls for a complete reevaluation of responsibility, accountability, and human agency in the clinical setting.

Beginning with an exploration of AI's expanding role in preoperative planning, intraoperative guidance, and postoperative monitoring, we established that the scope of surgical AI is both wide-reaching and rapidly evolving. This evolution brings with it new ethical dilemmas, including those surrounding informed consent and moral accountability, algorithmic bias, data privacy, and the risk of eroding patient autonomy. Many AI systems, especially deep learning based, are highly complex and opaque, which is a major concern for explainability, with ramifications for both clinical decision making and public trust.

In regulatory terms, the chapter has demonstrated that while national and regional bodies such as the FDA, the European Union, and the UK's MHRA are beginning to construct frameworks for AI oversight, these efforts remain fragmented and incomplete. Most current approaches fail to account for the adaptive and autonomous nature of modern AI systems. Additionally, the global regulatory ecosystem is inconsistent, which leads to a lack of uniformity in safety and ethical compliance standards across jurisdictions. The legal uncertainties around liability and professional responsibility make the adoption of surgical AI all the more complicated, particularly when human and machine share—or, rather, blur—the decision making.

Through real-world case studies such as the da Vinci Surgical System and the STAR robot, we observed both the promise and the perils of AI deployment in operative settings. The examples highlighted the need for rigorous validation, continuous oversight and institutional readiness. The paper also calls attention to the increasing need for systems thinking in governance, in which ethical reflection, legal clarity, and technical excellence are not isolated efforts, but parts of a whole governance strategy.

Looking ahead, the future of ethical and regulatory evaluation in autonomous surgical AI hinges on several critical imperatives. They include the institution of adaptive, lifecycle oriented regulatory models, the institutionalization of interdisciplinary ethics oversight, and the development of international standards that will both encourage innovation and equity. All of these are centered on the understanding that AI should not be thought of as a substitute for human clinicians, but instead as a partner that must be designed, governed, and evaluated with the full complexity of human centered care in mind.

This chapter has aimed to provide not only an overview of current ethical and regulatory challenges, but also a framework for thinking about how surgical AI can be responsibly integrated into hospital systems worldwide. The way forward for researchers, healthcare professionals, policymakers and developers is to build intelligent, adaptive systems of governance that are as smart as the technologies they aim to control.

REFERENCES

Ahern, D. (2025). The new anticipatory governance culture for innovation: Regulatory foresight, regulatory experimentation and regulatory learning. *arXiv preprint arXiv:2501.05921.*

Arjmandnia, F., & Alimohammadi, E. (2024). The value of machine learning technology and artificial intelligence to enhance patient safety in spine surgery: A review. *Patient Safety in Surgery*, *18*(1), 11. DOI: 10.1186/s13037-024-00393-0 PMID: 38528562

Barnes, E., & Hutson, J. (2024). Navigating the complexities of AI: The critical role of interpretability and explainability in ensuring transparency and trust. *International Journal of Multidisciplinary and Current Educational Research*, *6*(3).

Caine, N. A., Ebbert, J. O., Raffals, L. E., Philpot, L. M., Sundsted, K. K., Mikhail, A. E., & Shah, V. H. (2022, July). A 2030 vision for the Mayo Clinic Department of Medicine. [Elsevier.]. *Mayo Clinic Proceedings*, *97*(7), 1232–1236.

Corfmat, M., Martineau, J. T., & Régis, C. (2025). High-reward, high-risk technologies? An ethical and legal account of AI development in healthcare. *BMC Medical Ethics*, *26*(1), 4.

Dasgupta, P., & Raison, N. (2025). AI in surgery. In *Artificial Intelligence in Urology* (pp. 237–248). Academic Press.

Elemento, O., Leslie, C., Lundin, J., & Tourassi, G. (2021). Artificial intelligence in cancer research, diagnosis, and therapy. *Nature Reviews. Cancer*, *21*(12), 747–752.

ElHassan, B. T., & Arabi, A. A. (2025). Ethical forethoughts on the use of artificial intelligence in medicine. *International Journal of Ethics and Systems*, *41*(1), 35–44.

Fangerau, H. (2024). Artificial intelligence in surgery: Ethical considerations in the light of social trends in the perception of health and medicine. *EFORT Open Reviews*, *9*(5), 323–328.

Ferreres, A. R. (2025). Ethical and legal issues regarding artificial intelligence (AI) and management of surgical data. *European Journal of Surgical Oncology*, *51*(1), 108279.

Gauthaman, S. A. (2026). Introduction to machine learning and optimization in healthcare. In Muniasamy, A. (Ed.), *Integrative Machine Learning and Optimization Algorithms for Disease Prediction* (pp. 1–34). IGI Global.

Gauthaman, S. A., Muniasamy, A., & Karunakaran, G. (2026). Current challenges in the pharmaceutical industry and AI's role in addressing them. In Muniasamy, A., & Karunakaran, G. (Eds.), *Applications of Artificial Intelligence in Pharmaceuticals* (pp. 1–26). IGI Global.

Goktas, P. (2024). Ethics, transparency, and explainability in generative AI decision-making systems: A comprehensive bibliometric study. *Journal of Decision Systems*, 1–29.

Goktas, P., & Grzybowski, A. (2025). Shaping the future of healthcare: Ethical clinical challenges and pathways to trustworthy AI. *Journal of Clinical Medicine*, *14*(5), 1605.

Guni, A., Varma, P., Zhang, J., Fehervari, M., & Ashrafian, H. (2024). Artificial intelligence in surgery: The future is now. *European Surgical Research*, *65*(1), 22–39.

Hashimoto, D. A., Varas, J., & Schwartz, T. A. (2024). Practical guide to machine learning and artificial intelligence in surgical education research. *JAMA Surgery*, *159*(4), 455–456.

Hemmatyar, A., Soleymani, S., Khosravi-Mashizi, M., Saberi, A., Shirinzadeh-Dastgiri, A., Naseri, A., & Neamatzadeh, H. (2025). Ethical considerations in the use of the da Vinci Surgical System in modern surgery. *Indian Journal of Surgical Oncology*, 1–20.

Iftikhar, M., Saqib, M., Zareen, M., & Mumtaz, H. (2024). Artificial intelligence: Revolutionizing robotic surgery. *Annals of Medicine and Surgery (London)*, *86*(9), 5401–5409.

Jha, D., Durak, G., Sharma, V., Keles, E., Cicek, V., Zhang, Z., & Bagci, U. (2025). A conceptual framework for applying ethical principles of AI to medical practice. *Bioengineering (Basel, Switzerland)*, *12*(2), 180.

Joshi, G., Jain, A., Araveeti, S. R., Adhikari, S., Garg, H., & Bhandari, M. (2024). FDA-approved artificial intelligence and machine learning (AI/ML)-enabled medical devices: An updated landscape. *Electronics (Basel)*, *13*(3), 498.

Khanna, R., Raison, N., Martinez, A. G., Ourselin, S., Montorsi, F., Briganti, A., & Dasgupta, P. (2025). At the cutting edge: The potential of autonomous surgery and challenges faced. *BMJ Surgery, Interventions, & Health Technologies*, *7*(1), e000338.

Kothinti, R. R. (2024). Artificial intelligence in healthcare: Revolutionizing precision medicine, predictive analytics, and ethical considerations in autonomous diagnostics. *World Journal of Advanced Research and Reviews*, *19*(3), 3395–3406.

Kovacs, D. G., Ladefoged, C. N., Rosenkjær, J. B., Mawassi, F., Hingelberg, L. A., Laursen, A. O. A., Fischer, B. M., & Andersen, F. L. (2025). Is the clinical implementation of in-house artificial intelligence–developed algorithms happening? *Journal of Nuclear Medicine*, *66*(2), 183–185. DOI: 10.2967/jnumed.124.268156 PMID: 39667815

Lee, Y., Shin, T., Tessier, L., Javidan, A., Jung, J., Hong, D., & Force, D. S. T. (2024). Harnessing artificial intelligence in bariatric surgery: Comparative analysis of ChatGPT-4, Bing, and Bard in generating clinician-level bariatric surgery recommendations. *Surgery for Obesity and Related Diseases*, *20*(7), 603–608. DOI: 10.1016/j.soard.2024.03.011 PMID: 38644078

Li, H., Han, Z., Wu, H., Musaev, E. R., Lin, Y., Li, S., Makatsariya, A. D., Chekhonin, V. P., Ma, W., & Zhang, C. (2025). Artificial intelligence in surgery: Evolution, trends, and future directions. *International Journal of Surgery*, *111*(2), 2101–2111. DOI: 10.1097/JS9.0000000000002159 PMID: 39693484

Liu, Y., Ku, Y. C., Zhang, J., Ding, H., Kazanzides, P., & Armand, M. (2025). dARt Vinci: Egocentric data collection for surgical robot learning at scale. *arXiv preprint arXiv:2503.05646*.

Maher, K., & Chang, A. C. (2024). Regulatory frameworks for artificial intelligence in cardiovascular medicine and surgery. In *Intelligence-Based Cardiology and Cardiac Surgery* (pp. 421–426). Academic Press. DOI: 10.1016/B978-0-323-90534-3.00026-3

Marey, A., Arjmand, P., Alerab, A. D. S., Eslami, M. J., Saad, A. M., Sanchez, N., & Umair, M. (2024). Explainability, transparency and black box challenges of AI in radiology: Impact on patient care in cardiovascular radiology. *The Egyptian Journal of Radiology and Nuclear Medicine*, *55*(1), 183. DOI: 10.1186/s43055-024-01356-2

Meszaros, J., Minari, J., & Huys, I. (2022). The future regulation of artificial intelligence systems in healthcare services and medical research in the European Union. *Frontiers in Genetics*, *13*, 927721. DOI: 10.3389/fgene.2022.927721 PMID: 36267404

Milam, M. E., & Koo, C. W. (2023). The current status and future of FDA-approved artificial intelligence tools in chest radiology in the United States. *Clinical Radiology*, *78*(2), 115–122. DOI: 10.1016/j.crad.2022.08.135 PMID: 36180271

Morris, M. X., Fiocco, D., Caneva, T., Yiapanis, P., & Orgill, D. P. (2024). Current and future applications of artificial intelligence in surgery: Implications for clinical practice and research. *Frontiers in Surgery*, *11*, 1393898. DOI: 10.3389/fsurg.2024.1393898 PMID: 38783862

Muniasamy, A., & Karunakaran, G. (2026). Challenges and future directions: Emerging trends and limitations in ML and optimization for healthcare. In Muniasamy, A. (Ed.), *Integrative Machine Learning and Optimization Algorithms for Disease Prediction* (pp. 339–368). IGI Global.

Muthusubramanian, M., Jangoan, S., Sharma, K., & Krishnamoorthy, G. (2024). Demystifying explainable AI: Understanding, transparency and trust. *International Journal for Multidisciplinary Research*, *6*(2), 1–13.

Naik, N., Hameed, B. M., Shetty, D. K., Swain, D., Shah, M., Paul, R., Aggarwal, K., Ibrahim, S., Patil, V., Smriti, K., Shetty, S., Rai, B. P., Chlosta, P., & Somani, B. K. (2022). Legal and ethical consideration in artificial intelligence in healthcare: Who takes responsibility? *Frontiers in Surgery*, *9*, 862322. DOI: 10.3389/fsurg.2022.862322 PMID: 35360424

Naili, Y. T., Mangkunegara, I. S., Purwono, P., & Baballe, M. A. (2025). Regulatory challenges in AI-based diagnostics: Legal implications of AI use in medical diagnostics. In *BIO Web of Conferences, 152*, 01034. EDP Sciences.

O'Sullivan, S., Nevejans, N., Allen, C., Blyth, A., Leonard, S., Pagallo, U., Holzinger, K., Holzinger, A., Sajid, M. I., & Ashrafian, H. (2019). Legal, regulatory, and ethical frameworks for development of standards in artificial intelligence (AI) and autonomous robotic surgery. *International Journal of Medical Robotics and Computer Assisted Surgery*, *15*(1), e1968. DOI: 10.1002/rcs.1968 PMID: 30397993

Olateju, O., Okon, S. U., Olaniyi, O. O., Samuel-Okon, A. D., & Asonze, C. U. (2024). Exploring the concept of explainable AI and developing information governance standards for enhancing trust and transparency in handling customer data. Available at *SSRN*. DOI: 10.2139/ssrn.4879025

Panesar, S., Cagle, Y., Chander, D., Morey, J., Fernandez-Miranda, J., & Kliot, M. (2019). Artificial intelligence and the future of surgical robotics. *Annals of Surgery*, *270*(2), 223–226. DOI: 10.1097/SLA.0000000000003262 PMID: 30907754

Parveen, S., Amjad, M., Rauf, S. A., Arbab, S., Jamalvi, S. A., Saleem, S. E. U. R., & Haque, M. A. (2025). Surgical decision-making in the digital age: The role of telemedicine–a narrative review. *Annals of Medicine and Surgery (London)*, *87*(1), 242–249.

Patidar, N., Mishra, S., Jain, R., Prajapati, D., Solanki, A., Suthar, R., & Patel, H. (2024). Transparency in AI decision making: A survey of explainable AI methods and applications. *Advances of Robotic Technology*, *2*(1), xx–xx.

Power, D. (2024). Ethical considerations in the era of AI, automation, and surgical robots: There are plenty of lessons from the past. *Discover Artificial Intelligence*, *4*(1), 65.

Pressman, S. M., Borna, S., Gomez-Cabello, C. A., Haider, S. A., Haider, C., & Forte, A. J. (2024, April). AI and ethics: A systematic review of the ethical considerations of large language model use in surgery research. [MDPI.]. *Health Care*, *12*(8), 825.

Rana, S. S. S., Ghahremani, J. S., & Navarro, R. A. (2025). The future of Food and Drug Administration regulation on artificial intelligence–enabled medical devices: An orthopedic surgeon's guide. *Journal of Shoulder and Elbow Surgery*, *34*(1), 260–264.

Rengaramanujam, K., & Muniasamy, A. (2026). AI in hospital administration and formulary design: Optimizing resource allocation and patient flow. In Muniasamy, A., & Karunakaran, G. (Eds.), *Applications of Artificial Intelligence in Pharmaceuticals* (pp. 215–246). IGI Global.

Rivero-Moreno, Y., Rodriguez, M., Losada-Muñoz, P., Redden, S., Lopez-Lezama, S., Vidal-Gallardo, A., & Teran, S. M. (2024). Autonomous robotic surgery: Has the future arrived? *Cureus*, *16*(1), xx–xx.

Sasikala, B., & Sachan, S. (2024). Decoding decision-making: Embracing explainable AI for trust and transparency. *Exploring the Frontiers of Artificial Intelligence and Machine Learning Technologies*, *42*, xx–xx.

Smith, T. G., Norasi, H., Herbst, K. M., Kendrick, M. L., Curry, T. B., Grantcharov, T. P., & Cleary, S. P. (2022). Creating a practical transformational change management model for novel artificial intelligence–enabled technology implementation in the operating room. *Mayo Clinic Proceedings. Innovations, Quality & Outcomes*, *6*(6), 584–596.

Snyder, K. B., Stewart, R. A., & Hunter, C. J. (2024). Ethical considerations for the application of artificial intelligence in pediatric surgery. *AI and Ethics*, 1–8.

Tsai, A. Y., Carter, S. R., & Greene, A. C. (2024, February). Artificial intelligence in pediatric surgery. [WB Saunders.]. *Seminars in Pediatric Surgery*, *33*(1), 151390.

Vakili-Ojarood, M., Naseri, A., Shirinzadeh-Dastgiri, A., & Saberi, A., HaghighiKian, S. M., Rahmani, A., … Neamatzadeh, H. (2024). Ethical considerations and equipoise in cancer surgery. *Indian Journal of Surgical Oncology*, *15*(Suppl 3), 363–373.

Varghese, C., Harrison, E. M., O'Grady, G., & Topol, E. J. (2024). Artificial intelligence in surgery. *Nature Medicine*, *30*(5), 1257–1268.

Wah, J. N. K. (2025). Revolutionizing surgery: AI and robotics for precision, risk reduction, and innovation. *Journal of Robotic Surgery*, *19*(1), 1–15.

Wang, Y., & Ma, Z. (2025). Ethical and legal challenges of medical AI on informed consent: China as an example. *Developing World Bioethics*, *25*(1), 46–54.

Xue, J., & Weng, S. (2025). Navigating the legal complexities of telesurgery in China: An assessment of tort liability and the path forward. *Medicine, Science, and the Law*, *65*(1), 15–22.

Yin, E. T. (2025). Regulation and ethical issues of artificial intelligence in Ghana: Towards a harmonious AI law. In *Exploring AI Implications on Law, Governance, and Industry* (pp. 119–156). IGI Global Scientific Publishing.

KEY TERMS AND DEFINITIONS

AI Ethics Committee: A multidisciplinary institutional body composed of clinicians, ethicists, engineers, and patient representatives that evaluates AI systems for ethical, clinical, and societal impact prior to deployment in healthcare settings.

Algorithmic Bias: Describes systemic and unfair outcomes produced by AI systems due to biased data, model architecture, or development practices. In surgery, such bias can manifest as unequal treatment efficacy across demographic groups.

Autonomous Surgical AI: Refers to artificial intelligence systems that can independently perform surgical tasks with minimal or no human intervention. These systems typically utilize real-time data, machine learning, and robotic integration to make intraoperative decisions.

Black Box Model: An AI system whose internal workings are not transparent or interpretable, making it difficult to understand how decisions are made. Such models are problematic in surgical contexts where accountability and rationale are essential.

Ethical Oversight: The structured process of assessing whether an AI system aligns with ethical principles such as beneficence, non-maleficence, justice, and respect for patient autonomy. It is often conducted by interdisciplinary review boards.

Explainability: The degree to which the internal decision-making processes of an AI system can be understood and interpreted by human users. High explainability is essential in clinical settings to support trust, accountability, and informed decision-making.

Informed Consent: A foundational principle in medical ethics and law, referring to the process by which a patient voluntarily agrees to a procedure after receiving sufficient information about its risks, benefits, and alternatives. The introduction of AI complicates this process when decision mechanisms are not transparent.

Lifecycle Regulation: A regulatory philosophy that emphasizes ongoing evaluation and monitoring of AI systems beyond initial approval. It accounts for the adaptive and evolving nature of machine learning in clinical environments.

Shared Liability: A legal concept wherein responsibility for an adverse event or error is distributed across multiple stakeholders, including clinicians, AI developers, manufacturers, and healthcare institutions. This approach is becoming increasingly relevant in AI-assisted surgical care.

Total Product Lifecycle (TPLC): A regulatory approach used by the U.S. Food and Drug Administration to monitor AI-enabled medical devices throughout their development, deployment, and post-market updates. It emphasizes continuous oversight and accountability.

Compilation of References

Abdullah, R. M., Saad, L. A., Alasmari, Z. M., Ali, G. A., & Muniasamy, A. (2025). Human disease prediction mobile application using machine learning. In Alareeni, B., & Hamdan, A. (Eds.), *IoT and digital transformation: Innovating business models for the connected world (ICBT 2024). Lecture notes in networks and systems* (Vol. 1575). Springer., DOI: 10.1007/978-3-032-00450-5_19

Abraham, S. (2024). Challenges in the implementation of technology in effective hospital management system: A quantitative study. *Journal of Informatics Education and Research.*

Abràmoff, M. D., Tarver, M. E., Loyo-Berrios, N., Trujillo, S., Char, D., Obermeyer, Z., Eydelman, M. B., & Maisel, W. H. (2023). Considerations for addressing bias in artificial intelligence for health equity. *NPJ Digital Medicine*, *6*(1), 170. DOI: 10.1038/s41746-023-00913-9 PMID: 37700029

Ahern, D. (2025). The new anticipatory governance culture for innovation: Regulatory foresight, regulatory experimentation and regulatory learning. *arXiv preprint arXiv:2501.05921.*

Ahmad, K., Khan, K., & Al-Fuqaha, A. (2020). Intelligent fusion of deep features for improved waste classification. *IEEE Access : Practical Innovations, Open Solutions*, *8*, 1–12. DOI: 10.1109/ACCESS.2020.2995681

Al Kuwaiti, A., Nazer, K., Al-Reedy, A., Al-Shehri, S., Al-Muhanna, A., Subbarayalu, A. V., Al Muhanna, D., & Al-Muhanna, F. A. (2023). A review of the role of artificial intelligence in healthcare. *Journal of Personalized Medicine*, *13*(6), 951. DOI: 10.3390/jpm13060951 PMID: 37373940

Ala, A., & Chen, F. (2022). Appointment scheduling problem in complexity systems of the healthcare services: A comprehensive review. *Journal of Healthcare Engineering*, *2022*(1), 5819813. DOI: 10.1155/2022/5819813 PMID: 35281532

Alahmed, Y., Abadla, R., & Ansari, M. J. (2024). Enhancing safety in autonomous vehicles through advanced AI-driven perception and decision-making systems. In *2024 Fifth International Conference on Intelligent Data Science Technologies and Applications (IDSTA)* (pp. 208–217). DOI: 10.1109/IDSTA62194.2024.10746990

Alasmari, A., & Muniasamy, A. (2025). Integrating Bayesian and convolution neural network for uncertainty estimation of cataract from fundus images. *Computer Modeling in Engineering & Sciences, 143*(1), 569–592. DOI: 10.32604/cmes.2025.060484

Albahri, A. S., Duhaim, A. M., Fadhel, M. A., Alnoor, A., Baqer, N. S., Alzubaidi, L., Albahri, O. S., Alamoodi, A. H., Bai, J., Salhi, A., Santamaría, J., Ouyang, C., Gupta, A., Gu, Y., & Deveci, M. (2023). A systematic review of trustworthy and explainable artificial intelligence in healthcare: Assessment of quality, bias risk, and data fusion. *Information Fusion, 96*, 156–191. DOI: 10.1016/j.inffus.2023.03.008

Ali, F., El-Sappagh, S., Islam, S. R., Kwak, D., Ali, A., Imran, M., & Kwak, K.-S. (2020). A smart healthcare monitoring system for heart disease prediction based on ensemble deep learning and feature fusion. *Information Fusion, 63*, 208–222. DOI: 10.1016/j.inffus.2020.06.008

Almalawi, A., Khan, A. I., Alsolami, F., Abushark, Y. B., & Alfakeeh, A. S. (2023). Managing security of healthcare data for a modern healthcare system. *Sensors (Basel), 23*(7), 3612. DOI: 10.3390/s23073612 PMID: 37050672

Alowais, S. A., Alghamdi, S. S., Alsuhebany, N., Alqahtani, T., Alshaya, A. I., Almohareb, S. N., Aldairem, A., Alrashed, M., Bin Saleh, K., Badreldin, H. A., Al Yami, M. S., Al Harbi, S., & Albekairy, A. M. (2023). Revolutionizing healthcare: The role of artificial intelligence in clinical practice. *BMC Medical Education, 23*(1), 689. DOI: 10.1186/s12909-023-04698-z PMID: 37740191

Alpaydin, E. (2020). *Introduction to machine learning*. MIT Press.

Alves, M., Seringa, J., Silvestre, T., & Magalhães, T. (2024). Use of artificial intelligence tools in supporting decision-making in hospital management. *BMC Health Services Research, 24*(1), 24. DOI: 10.1186/s12913-024-11602-y PMID: 39456040

Amann, J., Blasimme, A., Vayena, E., Frey, D., & Madai, V. I. (2020). Explainability for artificial intelligence in healthcare: A multidisciplinary perspective. *BMC Medical Informatics and Decision Making, 20*(1), 1–9. DOI: 10.1186/s12911-020-01332-6

Amershi, S., Begel, A., Bird, C., DeLine, R., Gall, H., Kamar, E., & Zimmermann, T. (2019). Software engineering for machine learning: A case study. *Proceedings of the 41st International Conference on Software Engineering: Software Engineering in Practice*, 291–300. DOI: 10.1109/ICSE-SEIP.2019.00042

Aminizadeh, S., Xu, H., Rani, M., & Bridger, R. (2024). Opportunities and challenges of artificial intelligence and distributed systems to improve the quality of healthcare service. *Artificial Intelligence in Medicine*, *149*, 102779. DOI: 10.1016/j.artmed.2024.102779 PMID: 38462281

Amisha, , Malik, P., Pathania, M., & Rathaur, V. K. (2019). Overview of artificial intelligence in medicine. *Journal of Family Medicine and Primary Care*, *8*(7), 2328–2331. DOI: 10.4103/jfmpc.jfmpc_440_19 PMID: 31463251

Anderson, J. A., Godwin, K. M., Saleem, J. J., Russell, S., Robinson, J. J., & Kimmel, B. (2014). Accessibility, usability, and usefulness of a web-based clinical decision support tool to enhance provider–patient communication around self-management to prevent (STOP) stroke. *Health Informatics Journal*, *20*(4), 261–274. DOI: 10.1177/1460458213493195 PMID: 24352597

An, Y., Zhang, H., Sheng, Y., Wang, J., & Chen, X. (2021). MAIN: Multimodal attention-based fusion networks for diagnosis prediction. In *2021 IEEE International Conference on Bioinformatics and Biomedicine (BIBM)* (pp. 809–816). IEEE. https://doi.org/DOI: 10.1109/BIBM52615.2021.9669634

Ardila, D., Kiraly, A. P., Bharadwaj, S., Choi, B., Reicher, J. J., Peng, L., Tse, D., Etemadi, M., Ye, W., Corrado, G., Naidich, D. P., & Shetty, S. (2019). End-to-end lung cancer screening with three-dimensional deep learning on low-dose chest computed tomography. *Nature Medicine*, *25*(6), 954–961. DOI: 10.1038/s41591-019-0447-x

Arigbabu, A. T., Olaniyi, O. O., Adigwe, C. S., Adebiyi, O. O., & Ajayi, S. A. (2024). Data governance in AI-enabled healthcare systems: A case of the Project Nightingale. *Asian Journal of Research in Computer Science*, *17*(5), 85–107. DOI: 10.9734/ajrcos/2024/v17i5441

Arjmandnia, F., & Alimohammadi, E. (2024). The value of machine learning technology and artificial intelligence to enhance patient safety in spine surgery: A review. *Patient Safety in Surgery*, *18*(1), 11. DOI: 10.1186/s13037-024-00393-0 PMID: 38528562

Arsand, E., & Demiris, G. (2008). User-centered methods for designing patient-centric self-help tools. *Informatics for Health & Social Care*, *33*(3), 158–169. DOI: 10.1080/17538150802457562 PMID: 18850399

Athish, V. P., SS, S. N., & Rajeswari, D. (2023). Cirrhosis prediction in chronic liver disease patients using machine learning techniques.In Proceedings of the 3rd International Conference on Pervasive Computing and Social Networking (ICPCSN) (pp. 437–441). IEEE.

Ayemowa, M. O., Ibrahim, R., & Khan, M. M. (2024). Analysis of recommender system using generative artificial intelligence: A systematic literature review. SSRN *Electronic Journal,* 1–20. DOI: 10.2139/ssrn.4922584

Bahrami, M., & Forouzanfar, M. (2022). Sleep apnea detection from single-lead ECG: A comprehensive analysis of machine learning and deep learning algorithms. *IEEE Transactions on Instrumentation and Measurement*, *71*, 4003011. DOI: 10.1109/TIM.2022.3151947

Bajwa, J., Munir, U., Nori, A., & Williams, B. (2021). Artificial intelligence in healthcare: Transforming the practice of medicine. *Future Healthcare Journal*, *8*(2), e188–e194. DOI: 10.7861/fhj.2021-0095 PMID: 34286183

Baltazar, L. R., Manzanillo, M. G., Gaudillo, J., Viray, E. D., Domingo, M., Tiangco, B., & Albia, J. (2021). Artificial intelligence on COVID-19 pneumonia detection using chest X-ray images. *PLoS One*, *16*(10), e0257884. DOI: 10.1371/journal.pone.0257884 PMID: 34648509

Bandla, M. S., Liju, A. M., Luharia, A., & Mishra, G. V. (2023). Artificial intelligence in healthcare with special consideration in radio imaging. In *2023 1st DMIHER International Conference on Artificial Intelligence in Education and Industry 4.0 (IDICAIEI)* (Vol. 1, pp. 1–5). DOI: 10.1109/IDICAIEI58380.2023.10406913

Bardhan, I., Chen, H., & Karahanna, E. (2020). Connecting systems, data, and people: A multidisciplinary research roadmap for chronic disease management. *Management Information Systems Quarterly*, *44*(1), 185–200. DOI: 10.25300/MISQ/2020/14644

Barnes, E., & Hutson, J. (2024). Navigating the complexities of AI: The critical role of interpretability and explainability in ensuring transparency and trust. *International Journal of Multidisciplinary and Current Educational Research*, *6*(3).

Barocas, S., Hardt, M., & Narayanan, A. (2019). Fairness and machine learning. fairmlbook.org.

Bartsch, G.Jr, Mitra, A. P., Mitra, S. A., Almal, A. A., Steven, K. E., Skinner, D. G., Fry, D. W., Lenehan, P. F., Worzel, W. P., & Cote, R. J. (2016). Use of artificial intelligence and machine learning algorithms with gene expression profiling to predict recurrent nonmuscle invasive urothelial carcinoma of the bladder. *The Journal of Urology*, *195*(2), 493–498. DOI: 10.1016/j.juro.2015.09.090 PMID: 26459038

Beam, A. L., & Kohane, I. S. (2018). Big data and machine learning in health care. *Journal of the American Medical Association*, *319*(13), 1317–1318. DOI: 10.1001/jama.2017.18391 PMID: 29532063

Begum, A., Muniasamy, A., Sabahath, A., Yaqub, H., & Karunakaran, G. (2024). Coronary heart disease classification using deep learning approach with feature selection for improved accuracy. *Technology and Health Care*, *32*(3), 1991–2007. DOI: 10.3233/THC-231807 PMID: 38339946

Bekbolatova, M., Mayer, J., Ong, C., & Toma, M. (2024). Transformative potential of AI in healthcare: Definitions, applications, and navigating the ethical landscape and public perspectives. *Health Care*, •••, 12. PMID: 38255014

Benneh Mensah, G., & Dutta, P. K. (2024). Evaluating if Ghana's Health Institutions and Facilities Act 2011 (Act 829) sufficiently addresses medical negligence risks from integration of artificial intelligence systems. *Mesopotamian Journal of Artificial Intelligence in Healthcare*, 35–41.

Bergquist, M., Rolandsson, B., Gryska, E., Laesser, M., Hoefling, N., Heckemann, R., Schneiderman, J. F., & Björkman-Burtscher, I. M. (2024). Trust and stakeholder perspectives on the implementation of AI tools in clinical radiology. *European Radiology*, *34*(1), 338–347. DOI: 10.1007/s00330-023-09967-5 PMID: 37505245

Bhatnagar, R., Muniasamy, A., & Muniasamy, V. (2021). Predictive analytics for cardiovascular disease diagnosis using machine learning techniques. In Hassanien, A., Bhatnagar, R., & Darwish, A. (Eds.), *Advanced machine learning technologies and applications (AMLTA 2020). Advances in intelligent systems and computing* (Vol. 1141). Springer., DOI: 10.1007/978-981-15-3383-9_45

Bica, I., Alaa, A. M., Lambert, C., & Van Der Schaar, M. (2021). From real-world patient data to individualized treatment effects using machine learning: Current and future methods to address underlying challenges. *Clinical Pharmacology and Therapeutics*, *109*(1), 87–100. DOI: 10.1002/cpt.1907 PMID: 32449163

Blease, C., Bernstein, M. H., Gaab, J., Kaptchuk, T. J., & Locher, C. (2019). Computerization and the future of primary care: A survey of general practitioners in the UK. *BMJ Open*, *9*(11), e031160. DOI: 10.1136/bmjopen-2019-031160

Blease, C., Kharko, A., Bernstein, M. H., Gaab, J., Kaptchuk, T. J., & DesRoches, C. M. (2019). Artificial intelligence and the future of primary care: Exploratory qualitative study of UK general practitioners' views. *Journal of Medical Internet Research*, *21*(3), e12802. DOI: 10.2196/12802

Bleher, H., & Braun, M. (2022). Diffused responsibility: Attributions of responsibility in the use of AI-driven clinical decision support systems. *AI and Ethics*, *2*(4), 747–761. DOI: 10.1007/s43681-022-00135-x PMID: 35098247

Bohr, A., & Memarzadeh, K. (2020). *Artificial Intelligence in Healthcare*. Academic Press., DOI: 10.1016/C2018-0-04097-9

Boonstra, A., & Laven, M. (2022). Influence of artificial intelligence on the work design of emergency department clinicians: A systematic literature review. *BMC Health Services Research*, *22*(1), 669. DOI: 10.1186/s12913-022-08070-7 PMID: 35585603

Bouguettaya, A., Team, V., Stuart, E. M., & Aboujaoude, E. (2025). AI-driven report-generation tools in mental healthcare: A review of commercial tools. *General Hospital Psychiatry*, *94*, 150–158. DOI: 10.1016/j.genhosppsych.2025.02.018 PMID: 40088857

Bressman, E., Long, J. A., Honig, K., Zee, J., McGlaughlin, N., Jointer, C., Asch, D. A., Burke, R. E., & Morgan, A. U. (2022). Evaluation of an automated text message–based program to reduce use of acute health care resources after hospital discharge. *JAMA Network Open*, *5*(10), e2238293. DOI: 10.1001/jamanetworkopen.2022.38293 PMID: 36287564

Bridger, R. (2017). *Introduction to human factors and ergonomics*. CRC Press.

Bright, T. J., Wong, A., Dhurjati, R., Bristow, E., Bastian, L., Coeytaux, R. R., Samsa, G., Hasselblad, V., Williams, J. W., Musty, M. D., Wing, L., Kendrick, A. S., Sanders, G. D., & Lobach, D. (2012). Effect of clinical decision-support systems: A systematic review. *Annals of Internal Medicine*, *157*(1), 29–43. DOI: 10.7326/0003-4819-157-1-201207030-00450 PMID: 22751758

Brynjolfsson, E., & McAfee, A. (2014). *The second machine age: Work, progress, and prosperity in a time of brilliant technologies*. WW Norton & Company.

Buess, L., Keicher, M., Navab, N., Maier, A., & Arasteh, S. T. (2025). From large language models to multimodal AI: A scoping review on the potential of generative AI in medicine. *arXiv preprint* arXiv:2502.09242. https://doi.org//arXiv.2502.09242DOI: 10.48550

Business Insider. (2025). *Check out the exclusive 11-slide pitch deck startup Doctronic used to raise $5 million for its AI agents to replace 'Dr. Google*. Author.

Bzdok, D., & Meyer-Lindenberg, A. (2018). Machine learning for precision psychiatry: Opportunities and challenges. *Biological Psychiatry: Cognitive Neuroscience and Neuroimaging*, *3*(3), 223–230. DOI: 10.1016/j.bpsc.2017.11.007 PMID: 29486863

Cabitza, F., Rasoini, R., & Gensini, G. F. (2017). Unintended consequences of machine learning in medicine. *Journal of the American Medical Association*, *318*(6), 517–518. DOI: 10.1001/jama.2017.7797 PMID: 28727867

Cacciabue, P. C., & Vella, G. (2010). Human factors engineering in healthcare systems: The problem of human error and accident management. *International Journal of Medical Informatics*, *79*(4), e1–e17. DOI: 10.1016/j.ijmedinf.2008.10.005 PMID: 19101197

Caine, N. A., Ebbert, J. O., Raffals, L. E., Philpot, L. M., Sundsted, K. K., Mikhail, A. E., & Shah, V. H. (2022, July). A 2030 vision for the Mayo Clinic Department of Medicine. [Elsevier.]. *Mayo Clinic Proceedings*, *97*(7), 1232–1236.

Callahan, T. J., Kahn, M. G., Barnard, J., Bauck, A. E., Brown, J., Davidson, B. N., ... & Meeker, D. (2016). A harmonized data quality assessment terminology and framework for the secondary use of electronic health record data. eGEMs (Generating Evidence & Methods to improve patient outcomes), 4(1), 18. DOI: 10.13063/2327-9214.1244

Carvalho, D. V., Pereira, E. M., & Cardoso, J. S. (2019). Machine learning interpretability: A survey on methods and metrics. *Electronics (Basel)*, *8*(8), 832. DOI: 10.3390/electronics8080832

Challen, R., Denny, J., Pitt, M., Gompels, L., Edwards, T., & Tsaneva-Atanasova, K. (2019). Artificial intelligence, bias and clinical safety. *BMJ Quality & Safety*, *28*(3), 231–237. DOI: 10.1136/bmjqs-2018-008370 PMID: 30636200

Char, D. S., Shah, N. H., & Magnus, D. (2018). Implementing machine learning in health care—Addressing ethical challenges. *The New England Journal of Medicine*, *378*(11), 981–983. DOI: 10.1056/NEJMp1714229 PMID: 29539284

Chatterjee, A., Pahari, N., & Prinz, A. (2022). HL7 FHIR with SNOMED-CT to achieve semantic and structural interoperability in personal health data: A proof-of-concept study. *Sensors (Basel)*, *22*(10), 3756. DOI: 10.3390/s22103756 PMID: 35632165

Chen, J., Liu, X., Li, L., Yu, P. S., & Gao, Y. (2020). Data drift detection via model uncertainty. *Proceedings of the AAAI Conference on Artificial Intelligence*, *34*(04), 6992–6999.

Chervenak, F. A., & McCullough, L. B. (2021). Ethical considerations. In *Clinical Maternal-Fetal Medicine* (pp. 42–1). CRC Press. DOI: 10.1201/9781003222590-39

Chignell, M., Tong, T., Mizobuchi, S., Valdez, R. S., & Morita, P. (2023). The evolution of HCI and human factors: Integrating human and artificial intelligence. *ACM Transactions on Computer-Human Interaction*, *30*(2), 1–30. DOI: 10.1145/3557891

Choudhry, M. D., Sundarrajan, M., & Sundaram, K. (2024). Bias and fairness in generative AI. In *Generative AI and LLMs: Natural language processing and generative adversarial networks* (p. 177). DOI: 10.1515/9783111425078-009

Clifton, D. A. (2016). *Machine Learning for Healthcare Technologies*. IET., DOI: 10.1049/PBHE002E

Cohen, I. G., & Mello, M. M. (2018). HIPAA and protecting health information in the 21st century. *Journal of the American Medical Association*, *320*(3), 231–232. DOI: 10.1001/jama.2018.5630 PMID: 29800120

Corfmat, M., Martineau, J. T., & Régis, C. (2025). High-reward, high-risk technologies? An ethical and legal account of AI development in healthcare. *BMC Medical Ethics*, *26*(1), 4.

Coronato, A., Naeem, M., De Pietro, G., & Paragliola, G. (2020). Reinforcement learning for intelligent healthcare applications: A survey. *Artificial Intelligence in Medicine*, *109*, 101964. DOI: 10.1016/j.artmed.2020.101964 PMID: 34756216

Cortez, N. (2018). Digital health: Scaling healthcare to the world. In *Springer* (pp. 249–269). Springer.

Crowther, D., Goh, K., Rauf, A., & Wang, Y. (2025). Assessing the impact of artificial intelligence on healthcare sector for enhancing sustainability. In *Transforming the healthcare sector through artificial intelligence and environmental sustainability* (pp. 3–21). Springer Nature Singapore. DOI: 10.1007/978-981-97-9555-0_1

Crowther, D., Goh, K., Rauf, A., & Wang, Y. (2025). *Transforming healthcare sector through AI*. Springer., DOI: 10.1007/978-981-97-9555-0

D'Agostino, M., & Vázquez, M. (2021). Adversarial robustness of deep neural networks: A survey. *Information Fusion*, *70*, 106–123.

Dasgupta, P., & Raison, N. (2025). AI in surgery. In *Artificial Intelligence in Urology* (pp. 237–248). Academic Press.

Davenport, T. H. (2018). *The AI advantage: How to put the artificial intelligence revolution to work*. MIT Press. DOI: 10.7551/mitpress/11781.001.0001

Davenport, T., & Kalakota, R. (2019). The potential for artificial intelligence in healthcare. *Future Healthcare Journal*, *6*(2), 94–98. DOI: 10.7861/futurehosp.6-2-94 PMID: 31363513

Delahanty, R. J., Alvarez, J., Flynn, L. M., Sherwin, R. L., & Jones, S. S. (2019). Development and evaluation of a machine learning model for the early identification of sepsis in pediatric patients. *JAMA Network Open*, *2*(10), e1914377. DOI: 10.1001/jamanetworkopen.2019.14377

Denecke, K., May, R., & Rivera-Romero, O. (2024). Transformer models in healthcare: A survey and thematic analysis of potentials, shortcomings and risks. *Journal of Medical Systems*, *48*(1), 23. DOI: 10.1007/s10916-024-02043-5 PMID: 38367119

Dhade, P., & Shirke, P. (2024). Federated learning for healthcare: A comprehensive review. *Engineering Proceedings*, *59*(1), 230.

Diaz-Flores, E., Meyer, T., & Giorkallos, A. (2022). Evolution of artificial intelligence-powered technologies in biomedical research and healthcare. In *Smart Biolabs of the Future* (pp. 23–60). DOI: 10.1007/10_2021_189

Dilsizian, S. E., & Siegel, E. L. (2014). Artificial intelligence in medicine and cardiac imaging: Harnessing big data and advanced computing to provide personalized medical diagnosis and treatment. *Current Cardiology Reports*, *16*(1), 441. DOI: 10.1007/s11886-013-0441-8 PMID: 24338557

Dinesh, R. A., Shanmugam, J., & Biswas, K. (2025). AI for application solutions for healthcare services using AI detection and diagnosis of different diseases: A special emphasis on neuro-oncology. In *Radiomics and radiogenomics in neuro-oncology* (pp. 241–275). Academic Press. DOI: 10.1016/B978-0-443-18509-0.00009-8

Domingues, C., Jarak, I., Veiga, F., Dourado, M., & Figueiras, A. (2023, October 6). Pediatric Drug Development: Reviewing Challenges and Opportunities by Tracking Innovative Therapies. *Pharmaceutics*, *15*(10), 2431. DOI: 10.3390/pharmaceutics15102431 PMID: 37896191

Doshi-Velez, F., & Kim, B. (2017). Towards a rigorous science of interpretable machine learning. arXiv preprint arXiv:1702.08608.

DuBois, K. N. (2019). Deep medicine: How artificial intelligence can make healthcare human again. *Perspectives on Science and Christian Faith*, *71*, 199–201.

Elemento, O., Leslie, C., Lundin, J., & Tourassi, G. (2021). Artificial intelligence in cancer research, diagnosis, and therapy. *Nature Reviews. Cancer*, *21*(12), 747–752.

Elgin, C. Y., & Elgin, C. (2024). Ethical implications of AI-driven clinical decision support systems on healthcare resource allocation: A qualitative study of healthcare professionals' perspectives. *BMC Medical Ethics*, *25*(1), 148. DOI: 10.1186/s12910-024-01151-8 PMID: 39707327

Elhaddad, M., & Hamam, S. (2024). AI-driven clinical decision support systems: An ongoing pursuit of potential. *Cureus*, 16. DOI: 10.7759/cureus.57728 PMID: 38711724

ElHassan, B. T., & Arabi, A. A. (2025). Ethical forethoughts on the use of artificial intelligence in medicine. *International Journal of Ethics and Systems*, *41*(1), 35–44.

Eloranta, S., & Boman, M. (2022). Predictive models for clinical decision making: Deep dives in practical machine learning. *Journal of Internal Medicine*, *292*(2), 278–295. DOI: 10.1111/joim.13483 PMID: 35426190

Eslamitabar, S., Lame, E., Rouzbahani, A., & Roozbahani, Z. (2024). *Legal and ethical challenges of artificial intelligence applications in healthcare*. Health Technology Assessment in Action. DOI: 10.18502/htaa.v7i4.14653

Esteva, A., Kuprel, B., Novoa, R. A., Ko, J., Swetter, S. M., Blau, H. M., & Thrun, S. (2017). Dermatologist-level classification of skin cancer with deep neural networks. *Nature*, *542*(7639), 115–118. DOI: 10.1038/nature21056 PMID: 28117445

Esteva, A., Robicquet, A., Ramsundar, B., Kuleshov, V., DePristo, M., Chou, K., Cui, C., Corrado, G., Thrun, S., & Dean, J. (2019). A guide to deep learning in healthcare. *Nature Medicine*, *25*(1), 24–29. DOI: 10.1038/s41591-018-0316-z PMID: 30617335

European Commission. (2020). White Paper on Artificial Intelligence: A European approach to excellence and trust. https://ec.europa.eu/info/publications/white-paper-artificial-intelligence-european-approach-excellence-and-trust_en

Evidence.care(n.d).About the top health care analytics tools Retrieved June 6, 2020 https://evidence.care/top-healthcare-analytics-tools

Eyers, T., & Krastev, Y. (2020). Ethics in surgical innovations from the patient perspective. *Yearbook of Medical Informatics*, *29*(01), 169–175. DOI: 10.1055/s-0040-1701994 PMID: 32823312

Familoni, B. T. (2024). Ethical frameworks for AI in healthcare entrepreneurship: A theoretical examination of challenges and approaches. *International Journal of Frontiers in Biology and Pharmaceutical Research*, *5*(1), 57–65.

Fangerau, H. (2024). Artificial intelligence in surgery: Ethical considerations in the light of social trends in the perception of health and medicine. *EFORT Open Reviews*, *9*(5), 323–328.

Fan, Y., Long, E., Cai, L., Cao, Q., Wu, X., & Tong, R. (2021). Machine learning approaches to predict risks of diabetic complications and poor glycemic control in nonadherent type 2 diabetes. *Frontiers in Pharmacology*, *12*, 665951. DOI: 10.3389/fphar.2021.665951 PMID: 34239440

Feldman, M., Friedler, S. A., Moeller, J., Scheidegger, C., & Venkatasubramanian, S. (2015). Certifying and removing disparate impact. *Proceedings of the 21st ACM SIGKDD International Conference on Knowledge Discovery and Data Mining*, 259–268.

Feng, Y., Ting, J. S. Z., Xu, X., Bee, C. K., En, O. T., Hendra, T. W. J. I., Ting, Y., Lei, X., Chen, W.-X., Wang, Y., Li, S., Cui, Y., Wang, Z., Zhen, L., Liu, Y., Goh, R. S. M., & Tan, C. H. (2023). Deep neural network augments performance of junior residents in diagnosing COVID-19 pneumonia on chest radiographs. *Diagnostics (Basel)*, *13*(8), 1433. DOI: 10.3390/diagnostics13081397 PMID: 37189498

Ferreres, A. R. (2025). Ethical and legal issues regarding artificial intelligence (AI) and management of surgical data. *European Journal of Surgical Oncology*, *51*(1), 108279.

Finlayson, S. G., Subbaswamy, A., Singh, K., Bowers, J., Kupke, A., Zittrain, J., Kohane, I. S., & Saria, S. (2021). The clinician and dataset shift in artificial intelligence. *The New England Journal of Medicine*, *385*(3), 283–286. DOI: 10.1056/NEJMc2104626 PMID: 34260843

Fjeld, J., Achten, N., Hilligoss, H., Nagy, A. C., & Srikumar, M. (2020). Principled Artificial Intelligence: Mapping consensus in ethical and rights-based approaches to principles for AI. Berkman Klein Center for Internet & Society.

Friedman, A. B., Delgado, M. K., & Weissman, G. E. (2024). Artificial intelligence for emergency care triage—Much promise, but still much to learn. *JAMA Network Open*, *7*(5), e248857. DOI: 10.1001/jamanetworkopen.2024.8857 PMID: 38713470

Gama, J., Žliobaitė, I., Bifet, A., Pechenizkiy, M., & Bouchachia, A. (2014). A survey on concept drift adaptation. *ACM Computing Surveys*, *46*(4), 44. DOI: 10.1145/2523813

GarillColes et al. (2010). Three kinds of proactive risk analyses for health care. The Joint Commission Journal on Quality and Patient Safety, 36(8), 365–375, AP1–AP3.

Gautam, R., & Sharma, M. (2020). Prevalence and diagnosis of neurological disorders using different deep learning techniques: A meta-analysis. *Journal of Medical Systems*, *44*(2), 49. DOI: 10.1007/s10916-019-1519-7 PMID: 31902041

Gauthaman, S. A. (2026). Introduction to machine learning and optimization in healthcare. In Muniasamy, A. (Ed.), *Integrative Machine Learning and Optimization Algorithms for Disease Prediction* (pp. 1–34). IGI Global.

Gauthaman, S. A., (2026). Introduction to machine learning and optimization in healthcare. In Muniasamy, A. (Ed.), *Integrative machine learning and optimization algorithms for disease prediction* (pp. 1–34). IGI Global., DOI: 10.4018/979-8-3373-1087-9.ch001

Gauthaman, S. A., Muniasamy, A., & Karunakaran, G. (2026). Current challenges in the pharmaceutical industry and AI's role in addressing them. In Muniasamy, A., & Karunakaran, G. (Eds.), *Applications of Artificial Intelligence in Pharmaceuticals* (pp. 1–26). IGI Global., DOI: 10.4018/979-8-3373-2043-4.ch001

Gerke, S., Minssen, T., & Cohen, G. (2020). Ethical and legal challenges of artificial intelligence-driven healthcare. *Cambridge Quarterly of Healthcare Ethics*, *29*(1), 67–82.

Gerke, S., Minssen, T., & Cohen, I. G. (2020). Ethical and legal challenges of artificial intelligence-driven healthcare. In *Artificial intelligence in healthcare* (pp. 295–336). Academic Press., DOI: 10.1016/B978-0-12-818438-7.00012-5

Ghassemi, M., Oakden-Rayner, L., & Beam, A. L. (2021). The false hope of current approaches to explainable artificial intelligence in health care. *The Lancet. Digital Health*, *3*(11), e745–e750. DOI: 10.1016/S2589-7500(21)00208-9

Giordano, C., Brennan, M., Mohamed, B., Rashidi, P., Modave, F., & Tighe, P. (2021). Accessing artificial intelligence for clinical decision-making. *Frontiers in Digital Health*, *3*, 645232. DOI: 10.3389/fdgth.2021.645232 PMID: 34713115

Goktas, P. (2024). Ethics, transparency, and explainability in generative AI decision-making systems: A comprehensive bibliometric study. *Journal of Decision Systems*, 1–29.

Goktas, P., & Grzybowski, A. (2025). Shaping the future of healthcare: Ethical clinical challenges and pathways to trustworthy AI. *Journal of Clinical Medicine*, *14*(5), 1443. DOI: 10.3390/jcm14051605 PMID: 40095575

Google, A. I. (2021). Model Cards for Model Reporting. https://modelcards.withgoogle.com/

Gorrepati, L. (2024). Integrating AI with electronic health records (EHRs) to enhance patient care. *International Journal of Health Sciences*, *7*(8), 38–50. DOI: 10.47941/ijhs.2368

Govindaraj, M., Rajendran, R., Balasubramani, R., & Venkatraman, V. (2024). Revolutionizing healthcare: The transformative impact of artificial intelligence. In *Revolutionizing the healthcare sector with AI* (pp. 54–78). IGI Global Scientific Publishing. DOI: 10.4018/979-8-3693-3731-8.ch003

Graham, S., Depp, C., Lee, E. E., Nebeker, C., Tu, X., Kim, H.-C., & Jeste, D. V. (2019). Artificial intelligence for mental health and mental illnesses: An overview. *Current Psychiatry Reports*, *21*(11), 116. DOI: 10.1007/s11920-019-1094-0 PMID: 31701320

Graziani, M., Dutkiewicz, L., Calvaresi, D., Amorim, J. P., Yordanova, K., Mor, V., Nair, R., Abreu, P. H., Blanke, T., Pulignano, V., Prior, J. O., Lauwaert, L., Reijers, W., Depeursinge, A., Andrearczyk, V., & Müller, H. (2023). A global taxonomy of interpretable AI: Unifying the terminology for the technical and social sciences. *Artificial Intelligence Review*, *56*(4), 3473–3504. DOI: 10.1007/s10462-022-10256-8 PMID: 36092822

Greenhalgh, T., Wherton, J., Papoutsi, C., Lynch, J., Hughes, G., A'Court, C., Hinder, S., Fahy, N., Procter, R., & Shaw, S. (2017). Beyond adoption: A new framework for theorizing and evaluating nonadoption, abandonment, and challenges to the scale-up, spread, and sustainability of health and care technologies. *Journal of Medical Internet Research*, *19*(11), e367. DOI: 10.2196/jmir.8775

Guastello, S. J. (2023). *Human factors engineering and ergonomics: A systems approach*. CRC Press. DOI: 10.1201/9781003359128

Guni, A., Varma, P., Zhang, J., Fehervari, M., & Ashrafian, H. (2024). Artificial intelligence in surgery: The future is now. *European Surgical Research*, *65*(1), 22–39.

Gunning, D., & Aha, D. (2019). DARPA's Explainable Artificial Intelligence (XAI) Program. *AI Magazine*, *40*(2), 44–58. DOI: 10.1609/aimag.v40i2.2850

Guo, H., Wu, Y., Zhao, R., Yang, X., Peyrodie, L., Nianga, J., & Wang, Z. (2024). Leveraging AI for strategic management in healthcare: Enhancing operational and financial performance. *Journal of Intelligence and Knowledge Engineering*.

Gupta, A., Gupta, A., Soanki, S., & Kishore, J. (2025). AI and medical imaging: The next era of radiology and pathology detection. In *2025 First International Conference on Advances in Computer Science, Electrical, Electronics, and Communication Technologies (CE2CT)* (pp. 103–108). DOI: 10.1109/CE2CT64011.2025.10939755

Gupta, R., Srivastava, D., Sahu, M., Tiwari, S., Ambasta, R. K., & Kumar, P. (2021). Artificial intelligence to deep learning: Machine intelligence approach for drug discovery. *Molecular Diversity*, *25*(3), 1315–1360. DOI: 10.1007/s11030-021-10217-3 PMID: 33844136

Gurovich, Y., Hanani, Y., Bar, O., Nadav, G., Fleischer, N., Gelbman, D., & Kamphausen, S. B. (2019). Identifying facial phenotypes of genetic disorders using deep learning. *Nature Medicine*, *25*(1), 60–64. DOI: 10.1038/s41591-018-0279-0 PMID: 30617323

Hanguang, X., Feizhong, Z., Xingyue, L., Tianqi, L., Zhipeng, L., Xin, L., & Xiaoxuan, H. (2025). A comprehensive survey of large language models and multimodal large language models in medicine. *Information Fusion*, *117*, 102888. DOI: 10.1016/j.inffus.2024.102888

Hantel, A., Walsh, T. P., Marron, J. M., Kehl, K. L., Sharp, R., Van Allen, E., & Abel, G. A. (2024). Perspectives of oncologists on the ethical implications of using artificial intelligence for cancer care. *JAMA Network Open*, *7*(3), e244077. DOI: 10.1001/jamanetworkopen.2024.4077 PMID: 38546644

Harris, J. E. (2022). COVID-19 Incidence and hospitalization during the delta surge were inversely related to vaccination coverage among the most populous US Counties. *Health Policy and Technology*, *11*(2), 100583. DOI: 10.1016/j.hlpt.2021.100583 PMID: 34868833

Hartsock, I., & Rasool, G. (2024). Vision-language models for medical report generation and visual question answering: A review. *Frontiers in Artificial Intelligence*, *7*, 1430984. DOI: 10.3389/frai.2024.1430984 PMID: 39628839

Hashimoto, D. A., Rosman, G., Rus, D., & Meireles, O. R. (2018). Artificial intelligence in surgery: Promises and perils. *Annals of Surgery*, *268*(1), 70–76. DOI: 10.1097/SLA.0000000000002693 PMID: 29389679

Hashimoto, D. A., Varas, J., & Schwartz, T. A. (2024). Practical guide to machine learning and artificial intelligence in surgical education research. *JAMA Surgery*, *159*(4), 455–456.

Hassan, E. A., & El-Ashry, A. M. (2024). Leading with AI in critical care nursing: Challenges, opportunities, and the human factor. *BMC Nursing*, *23*(1), 752. DOI: 10.1186/s12912-024-02363-4 PMID: 39402609

Hasselgren, C., & Oprea, T. I. (2024). Artificial intelligence for drug discovery: Are we there yet? *Annual Review of Pharmacology and Toxicology*, *64*(1), 527–550. DOI: 10.1146/annurev-pharmtox-040323-040828 PMID: 37738505

He, J., Baxter, S. L., Xu, J., Xu, J., Zhou, X., & Zhang, K. (2019). The practical implementation of artificial intelligence technologies in medicine. *Nature Medicine*, *25*(1), 30–36. DOI: 10.1038/s41591-018-0307-0 PMID: 30617336

Hemmatyar, A., Soleymani, S., Khosravi-Mashizi, M., Saberi, A., Shirinzadeh-Dastgiri, A., Naseri, A., & Neamatzadeh, H. (2025). Ethical considerations in the use of the da Vinci Surgical System in modern surgery. *Indian Journal of Surgical Oncology*, 1–20.

Hendrycks, D., & Gimpel, K. (2017). A baseline for detecting misclassified and out-of-distribution examples in neural networks. *International Conference on Learning Representations (ICLR).*

Hezam, I. M., Ali, A. M., Alshamrani, A. M., Gao, X., & Abdel-Basset, M. (2024). Artificial intelligence's impact on drug delivery in healthcare supply chain management: Data, techniques, analysis, and managerial implications. *Journal of Big Data*, *11*(1), 177. DOI: 10.1186/s40537-024-01049-7

Higgins, D., & Madai, V. I. (2020). From bit to bedside: A practical framework for artificial intelligence product development in healthcare. *Advanced Intelligent Systems*, *2*(10), 2000052. DOI: 10.1002/aisy.202000052

Hinton, G. (2018). Deep learning—A technology with the potential to transform health care. *Journal of the American Medical Association*, *320*(11), 1101–1102. DOI: 10.1001/jama.2018.11100 PMID: 30178065

Holden, R. J., Carayon, P., Gurses, A. P., Hoonakker, P., Hundt, A. S., Ozok, A. A., & Rivera-Rodriguez, A. J. (2013). SEIPS 2.0: A human factors framework for studying and improving the work of healthcare professionals and patients. *Ergonomics*, *56*(11), 1669–1686. DOI: 10.1080/00140139.2013.838643 PMID: 24088063

Holstein, K., Wortman Vaughan, J., Daumé, H.III, Dudik, M., & Wallach, H. (2019). Improving fairness in machine learning systems: What do industry practitioners need? *Proceedings of the 2019 CHI Conference on Human Factors in Computing Systems*, 1–16. DOI: 10.1145/3290605.3300830

Hosny, A., Parmar, C., Quackenbush, J., Schwartz, L. H., & Aerts, H. J. (2018). Artificial intelligence in radiology. *Nature Reviews. Cancer*, *18*(8), 500–510. DOI: 10.1038/s41568-018-0016-5 PMID: 29777175

Hossen, M., Majid, E., Kashem, S. B. A., Khandakar, A., Nashbat, M., Ashraf, A., Hasan-Zia, M., Kunju, A. K. A., Kabir, S., & Chowdhury, M. E. H. (2024). A reliable and robust deep learning model for effective recyclable waste classification. *IEEE Access : Practical Innovations, Open Solutions*, *12*, 1–15. DOI: 10.1109/ACCESS.2024.3354774

Howard, F. M., Gao, C. A., & Sankey, C. (2020). Implementation of an automated scheduling tool improves schedule quality and resident satisfaction. *PLoS One*, *15*(8), e0236952. DOI: 10.1371/journal.pone.0236952 PMID: 32780751

Hu, Y., Kothapalli, S. V., Gan, W., Sukstanskii, A. L., Wu, G. F., Goyal, M., Yablonskiy, D. A., & Kamilov, U. S. (2023). DiffGEPCI: 3D MRI synthesis from mGRE signals using 2.5D diffusion model. *arXiv*, arXiv:2311.18073.

Huang, S., Yang, J., Fong, S., & Zhao, Q. (2020). Artificial intelligence in cancer diagnosis and prognosis: Opportunities and challenges. *Cancer Letters*, *471*, 61–71. DOI: 10.1016/j.canlet.2019.12.007 PMID: 31830558

IBM. (2023). AI in Healthcare: Transforming Patient Care. https://www.ibm.com/watson-health

Ibrahim, A. M., Abdel-Aziz, H. R., Mohamed, H. A. H., Zaghamir, D. E. F., Wahba, N. M. I., Hassan, G. A., Shaban, M., EL-Nablaway, M., Aldughmi, O. N., & Aboelola, T. H. (2024). Balancing confidentiality and care coordination: Challenges in patient privacy. *BMC Nursing*, *23*(1), 564. DOI: 10.1186/s12912-024-02231-1 PMID: 39148055

Iftikhar, M., Saqib, M., Zareen, M., & Mumtaz, H. (2024). Artificial intelligence: Revolutionizing robotic surgery. *Annals of Medicine and Surgery (London)*, *86*(9), 5401–5409. DOI: 10.1097/MS9.0000000000002426 PMID: 39238994

In, E., Geçkil, A. A., Kavuran, G., Şahin, M., Berber, N. K., & Kuluöztürk, M. (2022). Using artificial intelligence to improve the diagnostic efficiency of pulmonologists in differentiating COVID-19 pneumonia from community-acquired pneumonia. *Journal of Medical Virology*, *94*(8), 3698–3705. DOI: 10.1002/jmv.27777 PMID: 35419818

Ippolito, D., Maino, C., Gandola, D., Franco, P. N., Miron, R., Barbu, V., Bologna, M., Corso, R., & Breaban, M. E. (2023). Artificial intelligence applied to chest X-ray: A reliable tool to assess the differential diagnosis of lung pneumonia in the emergency department. *Diseases (Basel, Switzerland)*, *11*(4), 171. DOI: 10.3390/diseases11040171 PMID: 37987282

Jain, P., Gyanchandani, M., & Khare, N. (2016). Big data privacy: A technological perspective and review. *Journal of Big Data*, *3*(1), 1–25. DOI: 10.1186/s40537-016-0059-y

Jamal, A., Solaiman, M., Alhasan, K., Temsah, M. H., Sayed, G., & Soliman, M. (2023). Integrating ChatGPT in medical education: Adapting curricula to cultivate competent physicians for the AI era. *Cureus*, *15*(8). Advance online publication. DOI: 10.7759/cureus.43036 PMID: 37674966

Jandoubi, B., & Akhloufi, M. A. (2025). Multimodal artificial intelligence in medical diagnostics. *Information (Basel)*, *16*(7), 591. DOI: 10.3390/info16070591

Jeyaraman, M., Balaji, S., Jeyaraman, N., & Yadav, S. (2023). Unraveling the ethical enigma: Artificial intelligence in healthcare. *Cureus*, *15*(8), e43262. DOI: 10.7759/cureus.43262 PMID: 37692617

Jha, D., Durak, G., Sharma, V., Keles, E., Cicek, V., Zhang, Z., Srivastava, A., Rauniyar, A., Hagos, D. H., Tomar, N. K., Miller, F. H., Topcu, A., Yazidi, A., Håkegård, J. E., & Bagci, U. (2025). A conceptual framework for applying ethical principles of AI to medical practice. *Bioengineering (Basel, Switzerland)*, *12*(2), 152. DOI: 10.3390/bioengineering12020180 PMID: 40001699

Jha, S., Menzies, T., & Chen, T. Y. (2020). Fairness in machine learning: A survey. *ACM Computing Surveys*, *53*(6), 1–40.

Jha, S., Topol, E. J., & Adashi, E. Y. (2020). Disruptive innovation and the future of healthcare workforce. *Journal of the American Medical Association*, *323*(21), 2117–2118. DOI: 10.1001/jama.2020.6509

Jia, L.-L., Zhao, J.-X., Pan, N.-N., Liu-Yan, S., Zhao, L.-P., Tian, J.-H., & Huang, G. (2022). Artificial intelligence model on chest imaging to diagnose COVID-19 and other pneumonias: A systematic review and meta-analysis. *European Journal of Radiology Open*, *9*, 100438. DOI: 10.1016/j.ejro.2022.100438 PMID: 35996746

Jiang, F., Jiang, Y., Zhi, H., Dong, Y., Li, H., Ma, S., Wang, Y., Dong, Q., Shen, H., & Wang, Y. (2017). Artificial intelligence in healthcare: Past, present and future. *Stroke and Vascular Neurology*, *2*(4), 230–243. DOI: 10.1136/svn-2017-000101 PMID: 29507784

Jiang, N., Liu, X., Liu, H., Lim, E. T. K., Tan, C. W., & Gu, J. (2023). Beyond AI-powered context-aware services: The role of human–AI collaboration. *Industrial Management & Data Systems*, *123*(11), 2771–2802. DOI: 10.1108/IMDS-03-2022-0152

Jian, Y., Pasquier, M., Sagahyroon, A., & Aloul, F. (2021). A machine learning approach to predicting diabetes complications. *Health Care*, *9*, 1712. PMID: 34946438

Johnson, A. E. W., Pollard, T. J., Shen, L., Lehman, L. H., Feng, M., Ghassemi, M., Moody, B., Szolovits, P., Anthony Celi, L., & Mark, R. G. (2016). MIMIC-III, a freely accessible critical care database. *Scientific Data*, *3*(1), 160035. DOI: 10.1038/sdata.2016.35 PMID: 27219127

Johnson, K. B., Wei, W. Q., Weeraratne, D., Frisse, M. E., Misulis, K., Rhee, K., & Denny, J. C. (2018). Precision medicine, AI, and the future of personalized health care. *Clinical Pharmacology and Therapeutics*, *103*(3), 362–364. DOI: 10.1002/cpt.1015

Joshi, G., Jain, A., Araveeti, S. R., Adhikari, S., Garg, H., & Bhandari, M. (2024). FDA-approved artificial intelligence and machine learning (AI/ML)-enabled medical devices: An updated landscape. *Electronics (Basel)*, *13*(3), 498.

Kagiyama, N., Shrestha, S., Farjo, P. D., & Sengupta, P. P. (2019). Artificial intelligence: Practical primer for clinical research in cardiovascular disease. *Journal of the American Heart Association*, *8*(17), e012788. DOI: 10.1161/JAHA.119.012788 PMID: 31450991

Kairouz, P., McMahan, H. B., Avent, B., Bellet, A., Bennis, M., Bhagoji, A. N., ... & Zhao, S. (2021). Advances and open problems in federated learning. Foundations and Trends® in Machine Learning, 14(1–2), 1–210.

Kairouz, P., McMahan, H. B., Avent, B., et al. (2021). Advances and open problems in federated learning. *Foundations and Trends® in Machine Learning, 14*(1–2), 1–210. https://doi.org/DOI: 10.1561/2200000083

Kaissis, G. A., Makowski, M. R., Rückert, D., & Braren, R. F. (2020). Secure, privacy-preserving and federated machine learning in medical imaging. *Nature Machine Intelligence*, *2*(6), 305–311. DOI: 10.1038/s42256-020-0186-1

Kalusivalingam, A. K., Sharma, A., Patel, N., & Singh, V. (2021). Enhancing patient care through IoT-enabled remote monitoring and AI-driven virtual health assistants: Implementing machine learning algorithms and natural language processing. *International Journal of Artificial Intelligence and Machine Learning*, *2*(3).

Karargyris, A., Umeton, R., Sheller, M. J., Aristizabal, A., George, J., Wuest, A., Pati, S., Kassem, H., Zenk, M., Baid, U., Narayana Moorthy, P., Chowdhury, A., Guo, J., Nalawade, S., Rosenthal, J., Kanter, D., Xenochristou, M., Beutel, D. J., Chung, V., & Mattson, P. (2023). Federated benchmarking of medical artificial intelligence with MedPerf. *Nature Machine Intelligence*, *5*(7), 799–810. DOI: 10.1038/s42256-023-00652-2 PMID: 38706981

Karri, H. K., Begum, A., & George, L. (2024). Optimizing Healthcare Efficiency: The Role of Artificial Intelligence in Medical Records Management. *International Journal of Engineering and Management Research*, *14*(6), 55–67. DOI: 10.31033/ijemr.14.6.55-67

Kaur, S., Singla, J., Nkenyereye, L., Jha, S., Prashar, D., Joshi, G. P., El-Sappagh, S., Islam, M. S., & Islam, S. R. (2020). Medical diagnostic systems using artificial intelligence (AI) algorithms: Principles and perspectives. *IEEE Access : Practical Innovations, Open Solutions*, *8*, 228049–228069. DOI: 10.1109/ACCESS.2020.3042273

Kawazoe, Y., Shibata, D., Shinohara, E., Aramaki, E., & Ohe, K. (2021). A clinical specific BERT developed using a huge Japanese clinical text corpus. *PLoS One*, *16*(11), e0259763. DOI: 10.1371/journal.pone.0259763 PMID: 34752490

Kelly, C. J., Karthikesalingam, A., Suleyman, M., Corrado, G., & King, D. (2019). Key challenges for delivering clinical impact with artificial intelligence. *BMC Medicine*, *17*(1), 195. DOI: 10.1186/s12916-019-1426-2 PMID: 31665002

Keshta, I. (2022). AI-driven IoT for smart health care: Security and privacy issues. *Informatics in Medicine Unlocked*, *30*, 100903. DOI: 10.1016/j.imu.2022.100903

Keshta, I., & Odeh, A. (2021). Security and privacy of electronic health records: Concerns and challenges. *Egyptian Informatics Journal*, *22*(2), 177–183. DOI: 10.1016/j.eij.2020.07.003

Khalifa, M., Albadawy, M., & Iqbal, U. (2024). Advancing clinical decision support: The role of artificial intelligence across six domains. *Computer Methods and Programs in Biomedicine Update*, *5*, 100142. DOI: 10.1016/j.cmpbup.2024.100142

Khamaj, A. (2025). AI-enhanced chatbot for improving healthcare usability and accessibility for older adults. *Alexandria Engineering Journal*, *116*, 202–213. DOI: 10.1016/j.aej.2024.12.090

Khanna, R., Raison, N., Martinez, A. G., Ourselin, S., Montorsi, F., Briganti, A., & Dasgupta, P. (2025). At the cutting edge: The potential of autonomous surgery and challenges faced. *BMJ Surgery, Interventions, & Health Technologies*, *7*(1), e000338.

Khouibiri, N., Farhaoui, Y., & Allaoui, A. (2023). Design and analysis of a recommendation system based on collaborative filtering techniques for big data. *Intelligent and Converged Networks*, *4*(4), 296–304. DOI: 10.23919/ICN.2023.0024

Kim, M., Sohn, H., Choi, S., & Kim, S. (2023). Requirements for trustworthy artificial intelligence and its application in healthcare. *Healthcare Informatics Research*, *29*(4), 315–322. DOI: 10.4258/hir.2023.29.4.315 PMID: 37964453

Kothinti, R. R. (2024). Artificial intelligence in healthcare: Revolutionizing precision medicine, predictive analytics, and ethical considerations in autonomous diagnostics. *World Journal of Advanced Research and Reviews*, *19*(3), 3395–3406.

Kotter, E., & Ranschaert, E. (2021). Challenges and solutions for introducing artificial intelligence (AI) in daily clinical workflow. *European Radiology*, *31*(1), 5–7. DOI: 10.1007/s00330-020-07148-2 PMID: 32797308

Kovacs, D. G., Ladefoged, C. N., Rosenkjær, J. B., Mawassi, F., Hingelberg, L. A., Laursen, A. O. A., Fischer, B. M., & Andersen, F. L. (2025). Is the clinical implementation of in-house artificial intelligence–developed algorithms happening? *Journal of Nuclear Medicine*, *66*(2), 183–185. DOI: 10.2967/jnumed.124.268156 PMID: 39667815

Kreps, G. L., & Neuhauser, L. (2013). Artificial intelligence and immediacy: Designing health communication to personally engage consumers and providers. *Patient Education and Counseling*, *92*(2), 205–210. DOI: 10.1016/j.pec.2013.04.014 PMID: 23683341

Krittanawong, C., (2021). Artificial Intelligence in Precision Cardiovascular Medicine. *Journal of the American College of Cardiology*, *77*(23), 2921–2930. DOI: 10.1234/placeholder07 PMID: 28545640

Kruse, C. S., Frederick, B., Jacobson, T., & Monticone, D. K. (2017). Cybersecurity in healthcare: A systematic review of modern threats and trends. *Technology and Health Care*, *25*(1), 1–10. DOI: 10.3233/THC-161263 PMID: 27689562

Kumar, R., Gupta, K., & Singh, R. (2024). Application of artificial intelligence in the healthcare sector: A critical analysis. In *Comparative law: Unraveling global legal systems* (pp. 387–412). Springer Nature Singapore. DOI: 10.1007/978-981-97-7815-7_23

Kwon, J. M., Kim, K. H., Jeon, K. H., & Lee, S. Y. (2020). A machine learning algorithm to predict hypokalemia in patients using routine blood tests and ECGs. *Journal of Electrocardiology*, *59*, 95–100. DOI: 10.1016/j.jelectrocard.2020.01.002

Kwon, J., & Johnson, M. E. (2014). Proactive Versus Reactive Security Investments in the Healthcare Sector. *Management Information Systems Quarterly*, *38*(2), 451–472. DOI: 10.25300/MISQ/2014/38.2.06

Lawry, T. (2020). *AI in Health: A Leader's Guide to Winning in the New Age of Intelligent Health Systems*. CRC Press., DOI: 10.4324/9780429321214

LeCun, Y., Bengio, Y., & Hinton, G. (2015). Deep learning. *Nature*, *521*(7553), 436–444. DOI: 10.1038/nature14539 PMID: 26017442

Lee, Y., Shin, T., Tessier, L., Javidan, A., Jung, J., Hong, D., & Force, D. S. T. (2024). Harnessing artificial intelligence in bariatric surgery: Comparative analysis of ChatGPT-4, Bing, and Bard in generating clinician-level bariatric surgery recommendations. *Surgery for Obesity and Related Diseases*, *20*(7), 603–608. DOI: 10.1016/j.soard.2024.03.011 PMID: 38644078

Letourneau-Guillon, L., Camirand, D., Guilbert, F., & Forghani, R. (2020). Artificial intelligence applications for workflow, process optimization and predictive analytics. *Neuroimaging Clinics of North America*, *30*(4), e1–e15. DOI: 10.1016/j.nic.2020.08.008 PMID: 33039002

Li, H., Han, Z., Wu, H., Musaev, E. R., Lin, Y., Li, S., Makatsariya, A. D., Chekhonin, V. P., Ma, W., & Zhang, C. (2025). Artificial intelligence in surgery: Evolution, trends, and future directions. *International Journal of Surgery*, *111*(2), 2101–2111. DOI: 10.1097/JS9.0000000000002159 PMID: 39693484

Lin, X., Quan, Z., Wang, Z.-J., Ma, T., & Zeng, X. (2020). KGNN: Knowledge graph neural network for drug-drug interaction prediction. In *IJCAI* (pp. 2739–2745). IJCAI. DOI: 10.24963/ijcai.2020/380

Liu, Y., Ku, Y. C., Zhang, J., Ding, H., Kazanzides, P., & Armand, M. (2025). dARt Vinci: Egocentric data collection for surgical robot learning at scale. *arXiv preprint arXiv:2503.05646*.

Liu, X., Rivera, S. C., & Faes, L. (2019). Reporting guidelines for clinical trial reports for interventions involving artificial intelligence: The CONSORT-AI extension. *Nature Medicine*, *26*(9), 1364–1374. DOI: 10.1038/s41591-020-1034-x PMID: 32908283

Liu, Y., Cao, X., Chen, T., Jiang, Y., You, J., Wu, M., Wang, X., Feng, M., Jin, Y., & Chen, J. (2025). From screens to scenes: A survey of embodied AI in healthcare. *Information Fusion*, *119*, 103033. DOI: 10.1016/j.inffus.2025.103033

London, A. J. (2019). Artificial Intelligence and Black-Box Medical Decisions: Accuracy versus Explainability. *The Hastings Center Report*, *49*(1), 15–21. DOI: 10.1002/hast.973 PMID: 30790315

Low, D. M., Bentley, K. H., & Ghosh, S. S. (2020). Automated assessment of psychiatric disorders using speech: A systematic review. *Laryngoscope Investigative Otolaryngology*, *5*(1), 96–116. DOI: 10.1002/lio2.354 PMID: 32128436

Maadi, M., Akbarzadeh Khorshidi, H., & Aickelin, U. (2021). A review on human–AI interaction in machine learning and insights for medical applications. *International Journal of Environmental Research and Public Health*, *18*(4), 2121. DOI: 10.3390/ijerph18042121 PMID: 33671609

Maddox, T. M., Rumsfeld, J. S., & Payne, P. R. (2019). Questions for artificial intelligence in health care. *Journal of the American Medical Association*, *321*(1), 31–32. DOI: 10.1001/jama.2018.18932

Maher, K., & Chang, A. C. (2024). Regulatory frameworks for artificial intelligence in cardiovascular medicine and surgery. In *Intelligence-Based Cardiology and Cardiac Surgery* (pp. 421–426). Academic Press. DOI: 10.1016/B978-0-323-90534-3.00026-3

Maleki Varnosfaderani, S., & Forouzanfar, M. (2024). The role of AI in hospitals and clinics: Transforming healthcare in the 21st century. *Bioengineering (Basel, Switzerland)*, *11*(4), 337. DOI: 10.3390/bioengineering11040337 PMID: 38671759

Mandl, K. D., (2020). The Evolution of the Learning Health System. *Health Affairs*, *39*(7), 1171–1177. DOI: 10.1377/hlthaff.2020.00818

Marey, A., Arjmand, P., Alerab, A. D. S., Eslami, M. J., Saad, A. M., Sanchez, N., & Umair, M. (2024). Explainability, transparency and black box challenges of AI in radiology: Impact on patient care in cardiovascular radiology. *The Egyptian Journal of Radiology and Nuclear Medicine*, *55*(1), 183. DOI: 10.1186/s43055-024-01356-2

Mariscal-Harana, J., et al. (2022). An AI tool for automated analysis of large-scale unstructured clinical cine CMR databases.

Markus, A. F., Kors, J. A., & Rijnbeek, P. R. (2021). The role of explainability in creating trustworthy artificial intelligence for health care: A comprehensive survey of the terminology, design choices, and evaluation strategies. *Journal of Biomedical Informatics*, *113*, 103655. DOI: 10.1016/j.jbi.2020.103655 PMID: 33309898

Marsha, R., (2021). Proactive Measures to Mitigate Cyber Security Challenges in IoT based Smart Healthcare Networks. 2021 IEEE International IOT, *Electronics and Mechatronics Conference (IEMTRONICS)*. https://doi.org/DOI: 10.1109/IEMTRONICS52119.2021

Masters, K. (2019). Artificial intelligence in medical education. *Medical Teacher, 41*(9), 976–980. DOI: 10.1080/0142159X.2019.1595557

Matheny, M. E., (2019). Artificial Intelligence in Health Care: Applications and Challenges. *Journal of the American College of Radiology, 16*(9), 1318–1326. DOI: 10.1234/placeholder05

McCorduck, P., & Cfe, C. (2004). *Machines who think: A personal inquiry into the history and prospects of artificial intelligence.* CRC Press. DOI: 10.1201/9780429258985

McKinney, S. M., Sieniek, M., Godbole, V., Godwin, J., Antropova, N., Ashrafian, H., Back, T., Chesus, M., Corrado, G. S., Darzi, A., Etemadi, M., Garcia-Vicente, F., Gilbert, F. J., Halling-Brown, M., Hassabis, D., Jansen, S., Karthikesalingam, A., Kelly, C. J., King, D., & Shetty, S. (2020). International evaluation of an AI system for breast cancer screening. *Nature, 577*(7788), 89–94. DOI: 10.1038/s41586-019-1799-6 PMID: 31894144

Mehta, N., Pandit, A., & Shukla, S. (2019). Transforming healthcare with big data analytics and artificial intelligence: A systematic mapping study. *Journal of Biomedical Informatics, 100*, 103311. DOI: 10.1016/j.jbi.2019.103311 PMID: 31629922

Meskó, B., Hetényi, G., & Győrffy, Z. (2018). Will artificial intelligence solve the human resource crisis in healthcare? *BMC Health Services Research, 18*(1), 545. DOI: 10.1186/s12913-018-3359-4 PMID: 30001717

Meszaros, J., Minari, J., & Huys, I. (2022). The future regulation of artificial intelligence systems in healthcare services and medical research in the European Union. *Frontiers in Genetics, 13*, 927721. DOI: 10.3389/fgene.2022.927721 PMID: 36267404

Michelmore, R., & Hoi, S. C. H. (2020). Real-time drift detection for data streams. *IEEE Transactions on Neural Networks and Learning Systems, 31*(8), 2809–2822.

Microsoft Responsible, A. I. (2023). Responsible AI principles and practices. https://www.microsoft.com/en-us/ai/responsible-ai

Milam, M. E., & Koo, C. W. (2023). The current status and future of FDA-approved artificial intelligence tools in chest radiology in the United States. *Clinical Radiology, 78*(2), 115–122. DOI: 10.1016/j.crad.2022.08.135 PMID: 36180271

Mitchell, M., Wu, S., Zaldivar, A., Barnes, P., Vasserman, L., Hutchinson, B., & Gebru, T. (2019). Model cards for model reporting. *Proceedings of the Conference on Fairness, Accountability, and Transparency*, 220–229. DOI: 10.1145/3287560.3287596

Mitchell, R. J., Williamson, A. M., Molesworth, B., & Chung, A. Z. Q. (2014). A review of the use of human factors classification frameworks that identify causal factors for adverse events in the hospital setting. *Ergonomics*, *57*(10), 1443–1472. DOI: 10.1080/00140139.2014.933886 PMID: 24992815

Mittelstadt, B. D., Allo, P., Taddeo, M., Wachter, S., & Floridi, L. (2016). The ethics of algorithms: Mapping the debate. *Big Data & Society*, *3*(2), 2053951716679679. DOI: 10.1177/2053951716679679

Moghadasi, N., Valdez, R. S., Piran, M., Moghaddasi, N., Linkov, I., Polmateer, T. L., Loose, D. C., & Lambert, J. H. (2024). Risk analysis of artificial intelligence in medicine with a multilayer concept of system order. *Systems*, *12*(2), 47. DOI: 10.3390/systems12020047

Mohsen, F., Ali, H., El Hajj, N., & Shah, Z. (2022). Artificial intelligence-based methods for fusion of electronic health records and imaging data. *Scientific Reports*, *12*(1), 17981. DOI: 10.1038/s41598-022-22514-4 PMID: 36289266

Mohseni, S., Zarei, N., & Ragan, E. D. (2021). A multidisciplinary survey and framework for design and evaluation of explainable AI systems. *ACM Transactions on Interactive Intelligent Systems*, *11*(3-4), 1–45. DOI: 10.1145/3387166

Moradveisi, B., Muwakkit, S., Zamani, F., Ghaderi, E., Mohammadi, E., & Zgheib, N. K. (2019, August 27). *ITPA, TPMT*, and *NUDT15* Genetic Polymorphisms Predict 6-Mercaptopurine Toxicity in Middle Eastern Children With Acute Lymphoblastic Leukemia. *Frontiers in Pharmacology*, *10*, 916. DOI: 10.3389/fphar.2019.00916 PMID: 31507415

Moreno-Sánchez, P. A. (2023). Data-driven early diagnosis of chronic kidney disease: Development and evaluation of an explainable AI model. *IEEE Access : Practical Innovations, Open Solutions*, *11*, 38359–38369. DOI: 10.1109/ACCESS.2023.3264270

Morley, J., Floridi, L., Kinsey, L., & Elhalal, A. (2020). From what to how: An initial review of publicly available AI ethics tools, methods and research to translate principles into practices. *Science and Engineering Ethics*, *26*(4), 2141–2168. DOI: 10.1007/s11948-019-00165-5 PMID: 31828533

Morley, J., Machado, C. C. V., Burr, C., Cowls, J., Joshi, I., Taddeo, M., & Floridi, L. (2020). The ethics of AI in health care: A mapping review. *Social Science & Medicine*, *260*, 113172. DOI: 10.1016/j.socscimed.2020.113172 PMID: 32702587

Morris, M. X., Fiocco, D., Caneva, T., Yiapanis, P., & Orgill, D. P. (2024). Current and future applications of artificial intelligence in surgery: Implications for clinical practice and research. *Frontiers in Surgery*, *11*, 1393898. DOI: 10.3389/fsurg.2024.1393898 PMID: 38783862

Mou, Y., & Xu, K. (2017). The media inequality: Comparing the initial human-human and human-AI social interactions. *Computers in Human Behavior*, *72*, 432–440. DOI: 10.1016/j.chb.2017.02.067

Munavalli, J. R., Boersma, H. J., Rao, S. V., & Van Merode, G. G. (2020). Real-time capacity management and patient flow optimization in hospitals using AI methods. In *Artificial intelligence and data mining in healthcare* (pp. 55–69). Springer.

Muniasamy, A. Muniasamy, Sabahath A., Begum, A., Yaqub, H., & Karunakaran, G. (2023). Lung cancer histopathology image classification using transfer learning with convolution neural network model. *Technology and Health Care,*33, 1–12. https://content.iospress.com/articles/technology-and-health-care/thc231029

Muniasamy, A. (2025). Revolutionizing health monitoring: Integrating transformer models with multi-head attention for precise human activity recognition using wearable devices. *Technology and Health Care*, *33*(1), 395–409. https://content.iospress.com/articles/technology-and-health-care/thc241064. DOI: 10.3233/THC-241064 PMID: 39269866

Muniasamy, A. (2026). Quantum computing in drug discovery: Revolutionizing pharmaceutical research. In Muniasamy, A., & Karunakaran, G. (Eds.), *Applications of artificial intelligence in pharmaceuticals* (pp. 59–96). IGI Global., DOI: 10.4018/979-8-3373-2043-4.ch003

Muniasamy, A., & Asiri, F. (2025). Advanced human activity recognition on wearables with multi-scale sparse attention. *Multimedia Tools and Applications*, *84*(30), 36623–36652. Advance online publication. DOI: 10.1007/s11042-024-20475-6

Muniasamy, A., Bhatnagar, R., & Karunakaran, G. (2021). Predicting COVID-19 spread in Saudi Arabia using artificial intelligence techniques—Proposing a shift towards a sustainable healthcare approach. In Hassanien, A., Bhatnagar, R., & Darwish, A. (Eds.), *Artificial intelligence for sustainable development: Theory, practice and future applications. Studies in computational intelligence* (Vol. 912). Springer., DOI: 10.1007/978-3-030-51920-9_6

Muniasamy, A., Tabassam, S., Hussain, M. A., Sultana, H., Muniasamy, V., & Bhatnagar, R. (2020). Deep learning for predictive analytics in healthcare. In Hassanien, A., Azar, A., Gaber, T., Bhatnagar, R., & Tolba, M. F. (Eds.), *The International Conference on Advanced Machine Learning Technologies and Applications (AMLTA2019)* (pp. xx-xx). Springer. https://doi.org/DOI: 10.1007/978-3-030-14118-9_4

Murdoch, B. (2021). Privacy and artificial intelligence: Challenges for protecting health information in a new era. *BMC Medical Ethics*, *22*(1), 122. DOI: 10.1186/s12910-021-00687-3 PMID: 34525993

Murdoch, W. J., Singh, C., Kumbier, K., Abbasi-Asl, R., & Yu, B. (2019). Definitions, methods, and applications in interpretable machine learning. *Proceedings of the National Academy of Sciences of the United States of America*, *116*(44), 22071–22080. DOI: 10.1073/pnas.1900654116

Murphy, K., Di Ruggiero, E., Upshur, R., Willison, D. J., Malhotra, N., Cai, J. C., Lui, V., & Gibson, J. (2021). Artificial intelligence for good health: A scoping review of the ethics literature. *BMC Medical Ethics*, *22*(1), 14. DOI: 10.1186/s12910-021-00577-8 PMID: 33588803

Murugan, S., Venkatesan, C., Sumithra, M., Gao, X.-Z., Elakkiya, B., Akila, M., & Manoharan, S. (2021). DEMNET: A deep learning model for early diagnosis of Alzheimer diseases and dementia from MR images. *IEEE Access : Practical Innovations, Open Solutions*, *9*, 90319–90329. DOI: 10.1109/ACCESS.2021.3090474

Muthusubramanian, M., Jangoan, S., Sharma, K., & Krishnamoorthy, G. (2024). Demystifying explainable AI: Understanding, transparency and trust. *International Journal for Multidisciplinary Research*, *6*(2), 1–13.

Nagabushanam, P., Thomas George, S., & Radha, S. (2020). EEG signal classification using LSTM and improved neural network algorithms. *Soft Computing*, *24*(13), 9981–10003. DOI: 10.1007/s00500-019-04515-0

Naik, N., Hameed, B. M., Shetty, D. K., Swain, D., Shah, M., Paul, R., Aggarwal, K., Ibrahim, S., Patil, V., Smriti, K., Shetty, S., Rai, B. P., Chlosta, P., & Somani, B. K. (2022). Legal and ethical consideration in artificial intelligence in healthcare: Who takes responsibility? *Frontiers in Surgery*, *9*, 862322. DOI: 10.3389/fsurg.2022.862322 PMID: 35360424

Naili, Y. T., Mangkunegara, I. S., Purwono, P., & Baballe, M. A. (2025). Regulatory challenges in AI-based diagnostics: Legal implications of AI use in medical diagnostics. In *BIO Web of Conferences, 152*, 01034. EDP Sciences.

Nair, M., Svedberg, P., Larsson, I., & Nygren, J. M. (2024). A comprehensive overview of barriers and strategies for AI implementation in healthcare: Mixed-method design. *PLoS One*, *19*(8), e0305949. DOI: 10.1371/journal.pone.0305949 PMID: 39121051

Nasarian, E., Alizadehsani, R., Acharya, U. R., & Tsui, K.-L. (2024). Designing interpretable ML system to enhance trust in healthcare: A systematic review to proposed responsible clinician-AI-collaboration framework. *Information Fusion*, *108*, 102412. DOI: 10.1016/j.inffus.2024.102412

Nasrullah, S., & Jalali, A. (2022). Detection of types of mental illness through the social network using ensembled deep learning model. *Computational Intelligence and Neuroscience*, *2022*, 9404242. DOI: 10.1155/2022/9404242 PMID: 35378814

Navath, S. (2023). Transforming healthcare: The impact and future of artificial intelligence in healthcare. *Journal of Artificial Intelligence and Machine Learning*, *1*(1), 16–21. DOI: 10.55124/jaim.v1i1.234

Necz, D. (2024). Rules over words: Regulation of chatbots in the legal market and ethical considerations. *Hungarian Journal of Legal Studies*, *64*(3), 472–485. DOI: 10.1556/2052.2023.00472

Nemati, S., Holder, A., Razmi, F., Stanley, M. D., Clifford, G. D., & Buchman, T. G. (2018). An interpretable machine learning model for accurate prediction of sepsis in the ICU. *Critical Care Medicine*, *46*(4), 547–553. DOI: 10.1097/CCM.0000000000002936

Nezamabadi, K., Sardaripour, N., Haghi, B., & Forouzanfar, M. (2022). Unsupervised ECG analysis: A review. *IEEE Reviews in Biomedical Engineering*, *16*, 208–224. DOI: 10.1109/RBME.2022.3154893 PMID: 35226604

Nguyen, D. C., Pham, Q. V., Pathirana, P. N., Ding, M., Seneviratne, A., Lin, Z., Dobre, O., & Hwang, W. J. (2022). Federated learning for smart healthcare: A survey. *ACM Computing Surveys*, *55*(3), 1–37. DOI: 10.1145/3501296

NHS England. (2023). Artificial Intelligence: How AI is transforming the NHS. https://www.england.nhs.uk/aifuture/

Nordlinger, B., Villani, C., & Rus, D. (2020). *Healthcare and artificial intelligence*. Springer., DOI: 10.1007/978-3-030-32161-1

Novillo-Ortiz, D., Marin, H. D. F., & Saigí-Rubió, F. (2018). The role of digital health in supporting the achievement of the Sustainable Development Goals (SDGs). *International Journal of Medical Informatics*, *114*, 106–107. DOI: 10.1016/j.ijmedinf.2018.03.011 PMID: 29602629

O'Sullivan, S., Nevejans, N., Allen, C., Blyth, A., Leonard, S., Pagallo, U., Holzinger, K., Holzinger, A., Sajid, M. I., & Ashrafian, H. (2019). Legal, regulatory, and ethical frameworks for development of standards in artificial intelligence (AI) and autonomous robotic surgery. *International Journal of Medical Robotics and Computer Assisted Surgery, 15*(1), e1968. DOI: 10.1002/rcs.1968 PMID: 30397993

Obermeyer, Z., & Emanuel, E. J. (2016). Predicting the Future — Big Data, Machine Learning, and Clinical Medicine. *The New England Journal of Medicine, 375*(13), 1216–1219. DOI: 10.1056/NEJMp1606181 PMID: 27682033

Odofin, O. T., Abayomi, A. A., Uzoka, A. C., Adekunle, B. I., Agboola, O. A., & Owoade, S. (2023). AI-based automation framework for laboratory diagnostics in hospital information management systems. *International Journal of Management and Organizational Research.*

Okada, Y., Ning, Y., & Ong, M. E. H. (2023). Explainable artificial intelligence in emergency medicine: An overview. *Clinical and Experimental Emergency Medicine, 10*(4), 354–362. DOI: 10.15441/ceem.23.145 PMID: 38012816

Olateju, O., Okon, S. U., Olaniyi, O. O., Samuel-Okon, A. D., & Asonze, C. U. (2024). Exploring the concept of explainable AI and developing information governance standards for enhancing trust and transparency in handling customer data. Available at *SSRN*. DOI: 10.2139/ssrn.4879025

Olawade, D. B., David-Olawade, A. C., Wada, O. Z., Asaolu, A. J., Adereni, T., & Ling, J. (2024). Artificial intelligence in healthcare delivery: Prospects and pitfalls. *Journal of Medicine, Surgery, and Public Health, 3*, 100108. DOI: 10.1016/j.glmedi.2024.100108

Ouanes, K., & Farhah, N. (2024). Effectiveness of artificial intelligence (AI) in clinical decision support systems and care delivery. *Journal of Medical Systems, 48*(1), 74. DOI: 10.1007/s10916-024-02098-4 PMID: 39133332

Pandey, S., Chouhan, V., Verma, D., Rajrah, S., Alenezi, F., Saini, R., & Santosh, K. C. (2022). Do-it-yourself recommender system: Reusing and recycling with blockchain and deep learning. *IEEE Access : Practical Innovations, Open Solutions, 10*, 1–12. DOI: 10.1109/ACCESS.2022.3199661

Panesar, S., Cagle, Y., Chander, D., Morey, J., Fernandez-Miranda, J., & Kliot, M. (2019). Artificial intelligence and the future of surgical robotics. *Annals of Surgery, 270*(2), 223–226. DOI: 10.1097/SLA.0000000000003262 PMID: 30907754

Parkar, T. V., & Kamath, K. S. (2025). Next-gen healthcare: AI and IoT innovations and future trends in healthcare. In *Intelligent Systems and IoT Applications in Clinical Health* (pp. 219–242). IGI Global.

Parveen, S., Amjad, M., Rauf, S. A., Arbab, S., Jamalvi, S. A., Saleem, S. E. U. R., & Haque, M. A. (2025). Surgical decision-making in the digital age: The role of telemedicine–a narrative review. *Annals of Medicine and Surgery (London)*, *87*(1), 242–249.

Parvin, N., Joo, S. W., Jung, J. H., & Mandal, T. K. (2025). Multimodal AI in biomedicine: Pioneering the future of biomaterials, diagnostics, and personalized healthcare. *Nanomaterials (Basel, Switzerland)*, *15*(12), 895. DOI: 10.3390/nano15120895 PMID: 40559258

Patel, S., & Pandey, M. (2024). Skin cancer classification using CNN and transfer learning (TL). In *Proceedings of the 2024 International Conference on Inventive Computation Technologies (ICICT)*. IEEE. DOI: 10.1109/ICICT60155.2024.10544854

Patel, V. L., (2009). Translational cognition for decision support in biomedical and health care domains. *Journal of Biomedical Informatics*, *42*(2), 288–301. DOI: 10.1016/j.jbi.2008.08.004

Patidar, N., Mishra, S., Jain, R., Prajapati, D., Solanki, A., Suthar, R., & Patel, H. (2024). Transparency in AI decision making: A survey of explainable AI methods and applications. *Advances of Robotic Technology*, *2*(1), xx–xx.

Paul, D., Sanap, G., Shenoy, S., Kalyane, D., Kalia, K., & Tekade, R. K. (2021). Artificial intelligence in drug discovery and development. *Drug Discovery Today*, *26*(1), 80–93. DOI: 10.1016/j.drudis.2020.10.010 PMID: 33099022

Pepic, I., Feldt, R., Ljungström, L., Torkar, R., Dalevi, D., Maurin Söderholm, H., Andersson, L.-M., Axelson-Fisk, M., Bohm, K., Sjöqvist, B. A., & Candefjord, S. (2021). Early detection of sepsis using artificial intelligence: A scoping review protocol. *Systematic Reviews*, *10*(1), 28. DOI: 10.1186/s13643-020-01561-w PMID: 33453724

Pham, T. (2025). Ethical and legal considerations in healthcare AI: Innovation and policy for safe and fair use. *Royal Society Open Science*, *12*(5), 241873. DOI: 10.1098/rsos.241873 PMID: 40370601

Pierre, K., Haneberg, A. G., Kwak, S., Peters, K. R., Hochhegger, B., Sananmuang, T., . . . Forghani, R. (2023, April). Applications of artificial intelligence in the radiology roundtrip: process streamlining, workflow optimization, and beyond. In *Seminars in Roentgenology* (Vol. 58, No. 2, pp. 158-169). WB Saunders. DOI: DOI: 10.1053/j.ro.2023.02.003

Pinsky, M. R., Bedoya, A., Bihorac, A., Celi, L., Churpek, M., Economou-Zavlanos, N. J., Elbers, P., Saria, S., Liu, V., Lyons, P. G., Shickel, B., Toral, P., Tscholl, D., & Clermont, G. (2024). Use of artificial intelligence in critical care: Opportunities and obstacles. *Critical Care*, *28*(1), 113. DOI: 10.1186/s13054-024-04860-z PMID: 38589940

Poplin, R., Chang, P. C., Alexander, D., Schwartz, S., Colthurst, T., Ku, A., Newburger, D., Dijamco, J., Nguyen, N., Afshar, P. T., Gross, S. S., Dorfman, L., McLean, C. Y., & DePristo, M. A. (2018). A universal SNP and small-indel variant caller using deep neural networks. *Nature Biotechnology*, *36*(10), 983–987. DOI: 10.1038/nbt.4235 PMID: 30247488

Porto, B. M. (2024). Improving triage performance in emergency departments using machine learning and natural language processing: A systematic review. *BMC Emergency Medicine*, *24*(1), 219. DOI: 10.1186/s12873-024-01135-2 PMID: 39558255

Power, D. (2024). Ethical considerations in the era of AI, automation, and surgical robots: There are plenty of lessons from the past. *Discover Artificial Intelligence*, *4*(1), 65.

Powers, B., Obermeyer, Z., Vogeli, C., & Mullainathan, S. (2019). Dissecting racial bias in an algorithm used to manage the health of populations. *Science*, *366*(6464), 447–453. DOI: 10.1126/science.aax2342 PMID: 31649194

Prabhune, A. G., Priya, P. S. K., Chandra, R., Thakur, A., Srihari, V. R., & Bhat, S. S. (2025). A web-based platform for optimizing healthcare resource allocation and workload management using agile methodology and WISN theory. *BMC Health Services Research*, *25*(1), 400. DOI: 10.1186/s12913-025-12473-7 PMID: 40102889

Prathaban, B. P., Subash, R., & Ashwini, A. (2024, October). AI based mental health assisted chatbot system. In *2024 International Conference on Power, Energy, Control and Transmission Systems (ICPECTS)* (pp. 1-6). IEEE. DOI: 10.1109/ICPECTS62210.2024.10780017

Praveen, R. V. S., & Kumar, M. L. (2024). *Artificial intelligence in healthcare: Revolutionizing clinical decision making and patient care*. Addition Publishing House. Retrieved from https://lnkd.in/g5mxjfsG

Pressman, S. M., Borna, S., Gomez-Cabello, C. A., Haider, S. A., Haider, C., & Forte, A. J. (2024, April). AI and ethics: A systematic review of the ethical considerations of large language model use in surgery research. [MDPI.]. *Health Care*, *12*(8), 825.

PubMed. (2023). Enhancing human-AI collaboration: The case of colonoscopy. *PubMed ID: 37940501*.

Pugazhendi, D., (2020). Remote health monitoring using IoT and cloud integration. Journal of Computer Networks and Communications. *Article ID, 923817*. Advance online publication. DOI: 10.1234/placeholder06

Quan, M. K., Nguyen, D. C., Nguyen, V.-D., Wijayasundara, M., Setunge, S., & Pathirana, P. N. (2024). Toward privacy-preserving waste classification in the Internet of Things. *IEEE Internet of Things Journal*, *11*(14), 24814–24825. DOI: 10.1109/JIOT.2024.3386727

Raghupathi, W., & Raghupathi, V. (2014). Big data analytics in healthcare: Promise and potential. *Health Information Science and Systems*, *2*(1), 3. DOI: 10.1186/2047-2501-2-3 PMID: 25825667

Rahman, A., Debnath, T., Kundu, D., Khan, M. S., Aishi, A. A., Sazzad, S., Sayduzzaman, M., & Band, S. S. (2024). Machine learning and deep learning-based approach in smart healthcare: Recent advances, applications, challenges and opportunities. *AIMS Public Health*, *11*(1), 58–109. DOI: 10.3934/publichealth.2024004 PMID: 38617415

Rajeswari, D. (2023). Application of Bayes rule for precise analysis of class-imbalanced stroke data. In *Proceedings of the 2023 International Conference on Innovative Computing, Intelligent Communication and Smart Electrical Systems (ICSES)*. IEEE.

Rajkomar, A., Dean, J., & Kohane, I. (2019). Machine learning in medicine. *The New England Journal of Medicine*, *380*(14), 1347–1358. DOI: 10.1056/NEJMra1814259 PMID: 30943338

Rajkomar, A., Hardt, M., Howell, M. D., Corrado, G., & Chin, M. H. (2018). Ensuring fairness in machine learning to advance health equity. *Annals of Internal Medicine*, *169*(12), 866–872. DOI: 10.7326/M18-1990 PMID: 30508424

Rajpurkar, P., Chen, E., Banerjee, O., & Topol, E. J. (2022). AI in health and medicine. *Nature Medicine*, *28*(1), 31–38. DOI: 10.1038/s41591-021-01614-0

Rajpurkar, P., Irvin, J., Ball, R. L., Zhu, K., Yang, B., Mehta, H., & Ng, A. Y. (2018). Deep learning for chest radiograph diagnosis: A retrospective comparison of the CheXNeXt algorithm to practicing radiologists. *PLoS Medicine*, *15*(11), e1002686. DOI: 10.1371/journal.pmed.1002686

Ramezani, M., Takian, A., Bakhtiari, A., Rabiee, H. R., Fazaeli, A. A., & Sazgarnejad, S. (2023). The application of artificial intelligence in health financing: A scoping review. *Cost Effectiveness and Resource Allocation : C/E*, *21*(1), 83. DOI: 10.1186/s12962-023-00492-2 PMID: 37932778

Rana, S. S. S., Ghahremani, J. S., & Navarro, R. A. (2025). The future of Food and Drug Administration regulation on artificial intelligence–enabled medical devices: An orthopedic surgeon's guide. *Journal of Shoulder and Elbow Surgery*, *34*(1), 260–264.

Rani, N., Kumar, A., & Bhardwaj, A. K. (2025). Machine and deep learning techniques for smart healthcare industry: Big picture and open research challenges. *Intelligent Biomedical Technologies and Applications for Healthcare*, *5*(0), 255–275. DOI: 10.1016/B978-0-443-22038-8.00017-9

Rasheed, K., Qayyum, A., Ghalib, A., & Razzak, I. (2022). Explainable, trustworthy, and ethical machine learning for healthcare: A survey. *Computers in Biology and Medicine*, *149*, 106043. DOI: 10.1016/j.compbiomed.2022.106043 PMID: 36115302

Rathore, F. A., & Rathore, M. A. (2023). The emerging role of artificial intelligence in healthcare. *JPMA. The Journal of the Pakistan Medical Association*, *73*(7), 1368–1369. DOI: 10.47391/JPMA.23-48 PMID: 37469045

Ravichandran, P., Machireddy, J. R., & Rachakatla, S. K. (2024). Harnessing generative AI for automated data analytics in business intelligence and decision-making. *Hong Kong Journal of AI and Medicine*, *4*(1), 122–145.

Razzak, M. I., Imran, M., & Xu, G. (2019). Big data analytics for preventive medicine. *Neural Computing & Applications*, *32*(9), 4417–4451. DOI: 10.1007/s00521-019-04095-y

Reddy, S.. (2020). Artificial intelligence in health care: Anticipating challenges to ethics, privacy, and bias. *Journal of the Royal Society of Medicine*, *113*(1), 20–22. DOI: 10.1177/0141076819898555

Reddy, S., Fox, J., & Purohit, M. P. (2019). Artificial intelligence-enabled healthcare delivery. *Journal of the Royal Society of Medicine*, *112*(1), 22–28. DOI: 10.1177/0141076818815510 PMID: 30507284

Research, I. B. M. (2020). AI Fairness 360: An extensible toolkit for detecting, understanding, and mitigating unwanted algorithmic bias. arXiv preprint arXiv:1810.01943.

Reverberi, C., Rigon, T., Solari, A., Hassan, C., Cherubini, P., & Cherubini, A. (2022). Experimental evidence of effective human–AI collaboration in medical decision-making. *Scientific Reports, 12*(1), 14952. DOI: 10.1038/s41598-022-18751-2 PMID: 36056152

Ribeiro, M. T., Singh, S., & Guestrin, C. (2016). "Why should I trust you?": Explaining the predictions of any classifier. Proceedings of the 22nd ACM SIGKDD International Conference on Knowledge Discovery and Data Mining, 1135–1144.

Rim, B., Sung, N.-J., Min, S., & Hong, M. (2020). Deep learning in physiological signal data: A survey. *Sensors (Basel), 20*(4), 969. DOI: 10.3390/s20040969 PMID: 32054042

Rivero-Moreno, Y., Rodriguez, M., Losada-Muñoz, P., Redden, S., Lopez-Lezama, S., Vidal-Gallardo, A., & Teran, S. M. (2024). Autonomous robotic surgery: Has the future arrived? *Cureus, 16*(1), xx–xx.

Rubeis, G. (2024). *Ethics of medical AI*. Springer. DOI: 10.1007/978-3-031-55744-6

Rubin, M., Arnon, H., Huppert, J. D., & Perry, A. (2024). Considering the role of human empathy in AI-driven therapy. *JMIR Mental Health, 11*(1), e56529. DOI: 10.2196/56529 PMID: 38861302

Rudin, C. (2019). Stop explaining black box models for high stakes decisions and use interpretable models instead. *Nature Machine Intelligence, 1*(5), 206–215. DOI: 10.1038/s42256-019-0048-x PMID: 35603010

Russell, R. G., Lovett Novak, L., Patel, M., Garvey, K. V., Craig, K. J. T., Jackson, G. P., Moore, D., & Miller, B. M. (2023). Competencies for the use of artificial intelligence-based tools by health care professionals. *Academic Medicine, 98*(3), 348–356. DOI: 10.1097/ACM.0000000000004963 PMID: 36731054

Russell, S. J., & Norvig, P. (2010). *Artificial intelligence: A modern approach*. Pearson.

Sabahath, A., Muniasamy, A., Begum, A., Yaqub, H., & Karunakaran, G. (2023). Lung cancer histopathology image classification using transfer learning with convolution neural network model. *Technology and Health Care, 33*, 1–12. https://content.iospress.com/articles/technology-and-health-care/thc231029

Sadiku, M. N., Musa, S. M., Sadiku, M. N., & Musa, S. M. (2021). Augmented intelligence. In *A primer on multiple intelligences* (pp. 191–199). DOI: 10.1007/978-3-030-77584-1_15

Sadybekov, A. V., & Katritch, V. (2023). Computational approaches streamlining drug discovery. *Nature*, *616*(7958), 673–685. DOI: 10.1038/s41586-023-05905-z PMID: 37100941

Saria, S., Butte, A., & Sheikh, A. (2021). Better medicine through machine learning: What's real, and what's artificial? *PLoS Medicine*, *18*(3), e1002721.

Sarvamangala, D., & Kulkarni, R. V. (2022). Convolutional neural networks in medical image understanding: A survey. *Evolutionary Intelligence*, *15*(1), 1–22. DOI: 10.1007/s12065-020-00540-3 PMID: 33425040

Sasikala, B., & Sachan, S. (2024). Decoding decision-making: Embracing explainable AI for trust and transparency. *Exploring the Frontiers of Artificial Intelligence and Machine Learning Technologies*, *42*, xx–xx.

Schuitmaker, L., Drogt, J., Benders, M., & Jongsma, K. (2025). Physicians' required competencies in AI-assisted clinical settings: A systematic review. *British Medical Bulletin*, *153*(1), 36–53. DOI: 10.1093/bmb/ldae025 PMID: 39821209

Sculley, D., Holt, G., Golovin, D., Davydov, E., Phillips, T., Ebner, D., & Dennison, D. (2015). Hidden technical debt in machine learning systems. *Advances in Neural Information Processing Systems*, *28*, 2503–2511.

Secinaro, S., Calandra, D., Secinaro, A., Muthurangu, V., & Biancone, P. (2021). The role of artificial intelligence in healthcare: A structured literature review. *BMC Medical Informatics and Decision Making*, *21*(1), 125. DOI: 10.1186/s12911-021-01488-9 PMID: 33836752

Sendak, M. P., D'Arcy, J., & Kashyap, S.. (2020). A path for translation of machine learning products into healthcare delivery. *NPJ Digital Medicine*, *3*, 90. DOI: 10.1038/s41746-020-00307-0

Sengupta, D. (2023). Artificial intelligence in diagnostic dermatology: Challenges and the way forward. *Indian Dermatology Online Journal*, *14*(6), 782–787. DOI: 10.4103/idoj.idoj_462_23 PMID: 38099026

Senior, A. W., Evans, R., Jumper, J., Kirkpatrick, J., Sifre, L., Green, T., Qin, C., Žídek, A., Nelson, A. W., Bridgland, A., Penedones, H., Petersen, S., Simonyan, K., Crossan, S., Kohli, P., Jones, D. T., Silver, D., Kavukcuoglu, K., & Hassabis, D. (2020). Improved protein structure prediction using potentials from deep learning. *Nature*, *577*(7792), 706–710. DOI: 10.1038/s41586-019-1923-7 PMID: 31942072

Serrano, N., Chang, M., Rogers, C. L., Orton, M., Mannino, R., Grob, M., & Moghanaki, D. (2016). Patient autonomy and shared decision-making in the management of urethral cancer. *Practical Radiation Oncology*, *6*(1), 66–70. DOI: 10.1016/j.prro.2015.09.002 PMID: 26577009

Shaheen, R., & Salim, H. (2025). Role of artificial intelligence in healthcare. In *Intersection of human rights and AI in healthcare* (pp. 173–200). IGI Global Scientific Publishing. DOI: 10.4018/979-8-3693-7051-3.ch004

Shan, S., & Li, Y. (2024). Research on the application framework of generative AI in emergency response decision support systems for emergencies. *International Journal of Human-Computer Interaction*, 1–18.

Sharma, B. K. (2025). AI managed hospital workforce. In *Role of artificial intelligence, telehealth, and telemedicine in medical virology* (pp. 221–251). Springer Nature Singapore. DOI: 10.1007/978-981-97-2938-8_11

Sheng, T. J., Islam, M. S., Misran, N., Baharuddin, M. H., Arshad, H., Islam, M. R., Rmili, H., & Islam, M. T. (2020). An Internet of Things-based smart waste management system using LoRa and TensorFlow deep learning model. *IEEE Access : Practical Innovations, Open Solutions*, *8*, 1–12. DOI: 10.1109/ACCESS.2020.3016255

Shickel, B., Tighe, P. J., Bihorac, A., & Rashidi, P. (2018). Deep EHR: A survey of recent advances in deep learning techniques for electronic health record (EHR) analysis. *IEEE Journal of Biomedical and Health Informatics*, *22*(5), 1589–1604. DOI: 10.1109/JBHI.2017.2767063

Shneiderman, B. (2020). Human-centered artificial intelligence: Three fresh ideas. *AIS Transactions on Human-Computer Interaction*, *12*(3), 109–124. DOI: 10.17705/1thci.00131

Shneiderman, B. (2022). *Human-centered AI*. Oxford University Press. DOI: 10.1093/oso/9780192845290.001.0001

Shorrock, S., & Williams, C. (2016). *Human factors and ergonomics in practice: Improving system performance and human well-being in the real world*. CRC Press. DOI: 10.1201/9781315587332

Shortliffe, E. H., & Sepúlveda, M. J. (2018). Clinical Decision Support in the Era of Artificial Intelligence. *Journal of the American Medical Association*, *320*(21), 2199–2200. DOI: 10.1001/jama.2018.17163 PMID: 30398550

Simon, B. D., Ozyoruk, K. B., Gelikman, D. G., Harmon, S. A., & Türkbey, B. (2025). The future of multimodal artificial intelligence models for integrating imaging and clinical metadata: A narrative review. *Diagnostic and Interventional Radiology (Ankara, Turkey)*, *31*(4), 303–312. DOI: 10.4274/dir.2024.242631 PMID: 39354728

Smith, T. G., Norasi, H., Herbst, K. M., Kendrick, M. L., Curry, T. B., Grantcharov, T. P., & Cleary, S. P. (2022). Creating a practical transformational change management model for novel artificial intelligence–enabled technology implementation in the operating room. *Mayo Clinic Proceedings. Innovations, Quality & Outcomes*, *6*(6), 584–596.

Snyder, K. B., Stewart, R. A., & Hunter, C. J. (2024). Ethical considerations for the application of artificial intelligence in pediatric surgery. *AI and Ethics*, 1–8.

Soenksen, L. R., Ma, Y., Zeng, C., Boussioux, L., Villalobos Carballo, K., Na, L., Wiberg, H. M., Li, M. L., Fuentes, I., & Bertsimas, D. (2022). Integrated multimodal artificial intelligence framework for healthcare applications. *NPJ Digital Medicine*, *5*(1), 149. DOI: 10.1038/s41746-022-00689-4 PMID: 36127417

Soltan, A. A., Kouchaki, S., Zhu, T., Kiyasseh, D., Taylor, T., Hussain, Z. B., Peto, T., Brent, A. J., Eyre, D. W., & Clifton, D. (2020). Artificial intelligence driven assessment of routinely collected healthcare data is an effective screening test for COVID-19 in patients presenting to hospital. *medRxiv*. https://doi.org/DOI: 10.1101/2020.07.07.20148361

Sosunova, I., & Porras, J. (2022). IoT-enabled smart waste management systems for smart cities: A systematic review. *IEEE Access : Practical Innovations, Open Solutions*, *10*, 73326–73363. DOI: 10.1109/ACCESS.2022.3188308

Strubell, E., Ganesh, A., & McCallum, A. (2019). Energy and policy considerations for deep learning in NLP. *Proceedings of the 57th Annual Meeting of the Association for Computational Linguistics*, 3645-3650. DOI: 10.18653/v1/P19-1355

Suresh, H., & Guttag, J. V. (2021). A framework for understanding unintended consequences of machine learning. *Communications of the ACM*, *64*(10), 66–75.

Suryawanshi, V., Kanyal, D., Sabale, S. R., & Bhoyar, V. (2024). *The role of AI in enhancing hospital operational efficiency and patient care*. Multidisciplinary Reviews. DOI: 10.31893/multirev.2025153

Tahernejad, A., Sahebi, A., Abadi, A. S. S., & Safari, M. (2024). Application of artificial intelligence in triage in emergencies and disasters: A systematic review. *BMC Public Health*, *24*(1), 3203. DOI: 10.1186/s12889-024-20447-3 PMID: 39558305

Thurtle, D., Rossi, S. H., Berry, B., Pharoah, P., & Gnanapragasam, V. J. (2019). Models predicting survival to guide treatment decision-making in newly diagnosed primary non-metastatic prostate cancer: A systematic review. *BMJ Open*, *9*(6), e029149. DOI: 10.1136/bmjopen-2019-029149 PMID: 31230029

Tonekaboni, S., Joshi, S., McCradden, M. D., & Goldenberg, A. (2019). What clinicians want: Contextualizing explainable machine learning for clinical end use. *Proceedings of the Machine Learning Research, 106*, 359–380. https://proceedings.mlr.press/v106/tonekaboni19a.html

Topol, E. (2019). *Deep medicine: how artificial intelligence can make healthcare human again*. Hachette UK. https://dl.acm.org/doi/10.5555/3350442

Topol, E. (2019). *Deep medicine: How artificial intelligence can make healthcare human again*. Basic Books.

Topol, E. (2019). *Deep Medicine: How Artificial Intelligence Can Make Healthcare Human Again*. Basic Books., DOI: 10.1234/placeholder03

Topol, E. J. (2019). High-performance medicine: The convergence of human and artificial intelligence. *Nature Medicine*, *25*(1), 44–56. DOI: 10.1038/s41591-018-0300-7 PMID: 30617339

Torfi, A., Fox, E. A., & Reddy, C. K. (2022). Differentially private synthetic medical data generation using convolutional GANs. *Information Sciences*, *586*, 485–500. DOI: 10.1016/j.ins.2021.12.018

Trebble, T. M., Hansi, N., Hydes, T., Smith, M. A., & Baker, M. (2010). Process mapping the patient journey: An introduction. *BMJ (Clinical Research Ed.)*, *341*(aug13 1), c4078. Advance online publication. DOI: 10.1136/bmj.c4078 PMID: 20709715

Trujillo, C. J., Ulloa, J. V., Vivas, G. E., Escobar, E. G., Gutiérrez, I. V., Tirado, P. A., & Cohen, J. V. (2024). Surgeons vs ChatGPT: Assessment and feedback performance based on real surgical scenarios. *Journal of Surgical Education*, *81*(7), 960–966. DOI: 10.1016/j.jsurg.2024.03.012 PMID: 38749814

Tsai, A. Y., Carter, S. R., & Greene, A. C. (2024, February). Artificial intelligence in pediatric surgery. [WB Saunders.]. *Seminars in Pediatric Surgery*, *33*(1), 151390.

Tsopra, R., Fernandez, X., Luchinat, C., Alberghina, L., Lehrach, H., Vanoni, M., Dreher, F., Sezerman, O. U., Cuggia, M., de Tayrac, M., Miklasevics, E., Itu, L. M., Geanta, M., Ogilvie, L., Godey, F., Boldisor, C. N., Campillo-Gimenez, B., Cioroboiu, C., Ciusdel, C. F., & Burgun, A. (2021). A framework for validating AI in precision medicine: Considerations from the European ITFoC consortium. *BMC Medical Informatics and Decision Making*, *21*(1), 274. DOI: 10.1186/s12911-021-01634-3 PMID: 34600518

Vakili-Ojarood, M., Naseri, A., Shirinzadeh-Dastgiri, A., & Saberi, A., HaghighiKian, S. M., Rahmani, A., … Neamatzadeh, H. (2024). Ethical considerations and equipoise in cancer surgery. *Indian Journal of Surgical Oncology*, *15*(Suppl 3), 363–373.

Van den Berg, M. P., Mulder, B. A., Klaassen, S. H., Maass, A. H., van Veldhuisen, D. J., van der Meer, P., Nienhuis, H. L. A., Hazenberg, B. P. C., & Rienstra, M. (2019). Heart failure with preserved ejection fraction, atrial fibrillation, and the role of senile amyloidosis. *European Heart Journal*, *40*(16), 1287–1293. DOI: 10.1093/eurheartj/ehz057 PMID: 30753432

Van Driest SL, McGregor TL. Pharmacogenetics in clinical pediatrics: challenges and strategies. Per Med. 2013 Sep;10(7):. .DOI: 10.2217/pme.13.70

van Wynsberghe, A. (2021). Sustainable AI: AI for sustainability and the sustainability of AI. *AI and Ethics*, *1*(3), 213–218. DOI: 10.1007/s43681-021-00043-6

Varghese, C., Harrison, E. M., O'Grady, G., & Topol, E. J. (2024). Artificial intelligence in surgery. *Nature Medicine*, *30*(5), 1257–1268.

Varshney, K. R. (2016). Engineering safety in machine learning. *Proceedings of the 2016 IEEE International Conference on Data Science and Advanced Analytics (DSAA)*, 615–622.

Vaswani, A., Shazeer, N., Parmar, N., Uszkoreit, J., Jones, L., Gomez, A. N., & Polosukhin, I. (2017). Attention is all you need. *Advances in Neural Information Processing Systems*, *30*. Advance online publication. DOI: 10.48550/arXiv.1706.03762

Veernapu, K. (2022). Artificial intelligence in processing medical insurance claims: Generating claim denial letters with deep learning and natural language processing algorithms. *International Journal of Multidisciplinary Research and Growth Evaluation*.

Verghese, A., Shah, N. H., & Harrington, R. A. (2018). What this computer needs is a physician: Humanism and artificial intelligence. *Journal of the American Medical Association*, *319*(1), 19–20. DOI: 10.1001/jama.2017.19198 PMID: 29261830

Vettoretti, M., Cappon, G., Facchinetti, A., & Sparacino, G. (2020). Advanced diabetes management using artificial intelligence and continuous glucose monitoring sensors. *Sensors (Basel), 20*(14), 3870. DOI: 10.3390/s20143870 PMID: 32664432

Vieira, S., Pinaya, W. H., & Mechelli, A. (2017). Using deep learning to investigate the neuroimaging correlates of psychiatric and neurological disorders: Methods and applications. *Neuroscience and Biobehavioral Reviews, 74*, 58–75. DOI: 10.1016/j.neubiorev.2017.01.002 PMID: 28087243

VV. Nagendra Kumar, and D. Rajeswari. "Analyzing Prognosis Methods Using Machine Learning Algorithms for Detecting Copd." *2022 International Conference on Applied Artificial Intelligence and Computing (ICAAIC)*. IEEE, 2022.

Wah, J. N. K. (2025). Revolutionizing surgery: AI and robotics for precision, risk reduction, and innovation. *Journal of Robotic Surgery, 19*(1), 1–15.

Wang, F., & Preininger, A. (2019). AI in health: State of the art, challenges, and future directions. *Yearbook of Medical Informatics, 28*(1), 16–26. DOI: 10.1055/s-0039-1677908 PMID: 31419814

Wang, J., & Liu, X. (2021). Medical image recognition and segmentation of pathological slices of gastric cancer based on Deeplab v3+ neural network. *Computer Methods and Programs in Biomedicine, 207*, 106210. DOI: 10.1016/j.cmpb.2021.106210 PMID: 34130088

Wang, Y., & Ma, Z. (2025). Ethical and legal challenges of medical AI on informed consent: China as an example. *Developing World Bioethics, 25*(1), 46–54.

Waring, J., Lindvall, C., & Umeton, R. (2020). Automated machine learning: Review of the state-of-the-art and opportunities for healthcare. *Artificial Intelligence in Medicine, 104*, 101822. DOI: 10.1016/j.artmed.2020.101822 PMID: 32499001

Weng, C., & Weiskopf, N. G. (2013). Methods and dimensions of electronic health record data quality assessment: Enabling reuse for clinical research. *Journal of the American Medical Informatics Association : JAMIA, 20*(1), 144–151. DOI: 10.1136/amiajnl-2011-000681 PMID: 22733976

WHO. (2021). Ethics and governance of artificial intelligence for health: WHO guidance. World Health Organization. https://www.who.int/publications/i/item/9789240029200

Wiczorek, R. (2024). Human-centered design of AI in healthcare and the role of older patients. In *Advances in intelligent healthcare delivery and management: Research papers in honour of Professor Maria Virvou for invaluable contributions* (pp. 37–47). Springer Nature Switzerland. DOI: 10.1007/978-3-031-65430-5_2

Wiens, J., Saria, S., Sendak, M., Ghassemi, M., Liu, V. X., Doshi-Velez, F., Jung, K., Heller, K., Kale, D., Saeed, M., Ossorio, P. N., Thadaney-Israni, S., & Goldenberg, A. (2019). Do no harm: A roadmap for responsible machine learning for health care. *Nature Medicine*, *25*(9), 1337–1340. DOI: 10.1038/s41591-019-0548-6 PMID: 31427808

Wilkinson, M. D., Dumontier, M., Aalbersberg, I. J., Appleton, G., Axton, M., Baak, A., Blomberg, N., Boiten, J.-W., da Silva Santos, L. B., Bourne, P. E., Bouwman, J., Brookes, A. J., Clark, T., Crosas, M., Dillo, I., Dumon, O., Edmunds, S., Evelo, C. T., Finkers, R., & Mons, B. (2016). The FAIR guiding principles for scientific data management and stewardship. *Scientific Data*, *3*(1), 160018. DOI: 10.1038/sdata.2016.18 PMID: 26978244

Williamson, S. M., & Prybutok, V. (2024). Balancing privacy and progress: A review of privacy challenges, systemic oversight, and patient perceptions in AI-driven healthcare. *Applied Sciences (Basel, Switzerland)*, *14*(2), 675. DOI: 10.3390/app14020675

Wong, A., (2018). Development and validation of a machine learning model to predict mortality risk in older adults using routine primary care data. *Age and Ageing*, *47*(2), 166–172. DOI: 10.1093/ageing/afx166 PMID: 28927235

World Health Organization (WHO). (2021). *Ethics and governance of artificial intelligence for health: WHO guidance*. https://www.who.int/publications/i/item/9789240029200

Wu, H., Lu, X., & Wang, H. (2023). The application of artificial intelligence in health care resource allocation before and during the COVID-19 pandemic: Scoping review. *JMIR AI*, *2*, e38397. DOI: 10.2196/38397

Wynants, L., Van Calster, B., Bonten, M. M., Collins, G. S., Debray, T. P., De Vos, M., & Damen, J. A. (2020). Prediction models for diagnosis and prognosis of COVID-19 infection: Systematic review and critical appraisal. *BMJ (Clinical Research Ed.)*, *369*, m1328. DOI: 10.1136/bmj.m1328

Xue, J., & Weng, S. (2025). Navigating the legal complexities of telesurgery in China: An assessment of tort liability and the path forward. *Medicine, Science, and the Law*, *65*(1), 15–22.

Xu, Q., Li, Y., Chen, J., Zhang, L., & Wang, H. (2023). Interpretability of clinical decision support systems based on artificial intelligence from technological and medical perspective: A systematic review. *Journal of Healthcare Engineering*, *2023*(1), 9919269. DOI: 10.1155/2023/9919269 PMID: 36776958

Xu, X., Li, J., Zhu, Z., Zhao, L., Wang, H., Song, C., & Pei, Y. (2024). A comprehensive review on synergy of multi-modal data and AI technologies in medical diagnosis. *Bioengineering (Basel, Switzerland), 11*(3), 219. DOI: 10.3390/bioengineering11030219 PMID: 38534493

Yadav, G. S., & Longhurst, C. A. (2025). Will AI make the electronic health record more efficient for clinicians? *NEJM AI, 2*(3). Advance online publication. DOI: 10.1056/AIe2500020

Yang, Y., Zhang, L., Du, M., Bo, J., Liu, H., Ren, L., Li, X., & Deen, M. J. (2021). A comparative analysis of eleven neural networks architectures for small datasets of lung images of COVID-19 patients toward improved clinical decisions. *Computers in Biology and Medicine, 139*, 104887. DOI: 10.1016/j.compbiomed.2021.104887 PMID: 34688974

Ye, J., Woods, D., Jordan, N., & Starren, J. (2024). The role of artificial intelligence for the application of integrating electronic health records and patient-generated data in clinical decision support. *AMIA Joint Summits on Translational Science Proceedings AMIA Summit on Translational Science, 2024*, 459–467. PMID: 38827061

Yeung, K., Howes, A., & Pogrebna, G. (2020). AI governance by human rights-centric design. *Nature Machine Intelligence, 2*(1), 1–3.

Yin, E. T. (2025). Regulation and ethical issues of artificial intelligence in Ghana: Towards a harmonious AI law. In *Exploring AI Implications on Law, Governance, and Industry* (pp. 119–156). IGI Global Scientific Publishing.

Yi, X., Walia, E., & Babyn, P. (2019). Generative adversarial network in medical imaging: A review. *Medical Image Analysis, 58*, 101552. DOI: 10.1016/j.media.2019.101552 PMID: 31521965

Yogeshappa, V. G. (2024). AI-driven precision medicine: Revolutionizing personalized treatment plans. *International Journal of Computer Engineering and Technology, 15*(5), 455–474.

Yoon, J. H., Pinsky, M. R., & Clermont, G. (2022). Artificial intelligence in critical care medicine. *Critical Care, 26*(1), 75. DOI: 10.1186/s13054-022-03915-3 PMID: 35337366

Youssef, E.-R., Meriem, M., & Ait-Lemqeddem, H. (2025). ChatGPT and ethics in healthcare facilities: An overview and innovations in technical efficiency analysis. *AI and Ethics, 5*(4), 1–18. DOI: 10.1007/s43681-025-00672-1

Yuan, X., Chen, J., Zhang, K., Wu, Y., & Yang, T. (2021). A stable AI-based binary and multiple class heart disease prediction model for IoMT. *IEEE Transactions on Industrial Informatics*, *18*(3), 2032–2040. DOI: 10.1109/TII.2021.3098306

Yu, K.-H., Beam, A. L., & Kohane, I. S. (2018). Artificial intelligence in healthcare. *Nature Biomedical Engineering*, *2*(10), 719–731. DOI: 10.1038/s41551-018-0305-z PMID: 31015651

Zahlan, A., Ranjan, R. P., & Hayes, D. (2023). Artificial intelligence innovation in healthcare: Literature review, exploratory analysis, and future research. *Technology in Society*, *74*, 102321. DOI: 10.1016/j.techsoc.2023.102321

Zaretsky, J., Kim, J. M., Baskharoun, S., Zhao, Y., Austrian, J., Aphinyanaphongs, Y., Gupta, R., Blecker, S. B., & Feldman, J. (2024). Generative artificial intelligence to transform inpatient discharge summaries to patient-friendly language and format. *JAMA Network Open*, *7*(3), e240357. DOI: 10.1001/jamanetworkopen.2024.0357 PMID: 38466307

Zayas-Cabán, T., Okubo, T. H., & Posnack, S. (2023). Priorities to accelerate workflow automation in health care. *Journal of the American Medical Informatics Association : JAMIA*, *30*(1), 195–201. DOI: 10.1093/jamia/ocac197 PMID: 36259967

Zhang, S., Yu, J., & Xu, X. (2023). Rethinking Human-AI Collaboration in Complex Medical Decision Making: A Case Study in Sepsis Diagnosis. *arXiv preprint arXiv:2309.12368.*

Zheng, N. N., Liu, Z. Y., Ren, P. J., Ma, Y. Q., Chen, S. T., Yu, S. Y., & Wang, F. Y. (2017). Hybrid-augmented intelligence: Collaboration and cognition. *Frontiers of Information Technology & Electronic Engineering*, *18*(2), 153–179. DOI: 10.1631/FITEE.1700053

Zhou, B., Yang, G., Shi, Z., & Ma, S. (2022). Natural language processing for smart healthcare. *IEEE Reviews in Biomedical Engineering*, *17*, 4–18. DOI: 10.1109/RBME.2022.3210270 PMID: 36170385

About the Contributors

Anandhavalli Muniasamy is an Associate Professor in the Department of Computer Science at King Khalid University, Saudi Arabia. She earned her Ph.D. in Computer Science and Engineering from Sikkim Manipal University, India. Her research expertise spans data mining, data analytics, artificial intelligence (AI), soft computing, and data science, with a strong focus on machine learning and deep learning for advanced data analysis. She has authored over 35 research papers and book chapters in reputed international journals. She has actively participated in more than 30 national and international conferences, contributing through presentations and edited book publications. She has led multiple research projects as Principal Investigator and Co-Principal Investigator, including a funded project supported by the All India Council for Technical Education (AICTE). Beyond research, she serves as a long-time manuscript reviewer for top-tier journals and a Ph.D. thesis examiner for several universities. She is frequently invited to deliver guest lectures and contributes as an editorial board member for reputed journals and conferences. She is a member of professional bodies including the International Association of Engineers (IAENG), the Computer Society of India (CSI), and the International Association of Computer Science and Information Technology (IACSIT). Her current research is centered on using AI technologies—particularly machine learning and deep learning—to address complex challenges in medical data analysis, aiming to deliver impactful, innovative solutions.

A. Prabhu Chakkaravarthy was born on 18th February 1985 in Tamilnadu, India. He received his Ph.D. in Computer Science and Engineering from Sathyabama Institute of Science and Technology, Chennai, India. He is graduated from Anna University, Chennai in 2007 with the Bachelor of Technology degree in Computer Science and Engineering. He received the Master of Technology degree in Computer Science and Engineering from Sathyabama University, Chennai in 2012 with Distinction. He is currently working as an Assistant Professor in Networking and Communications, SRM Institute of Science and Technology, Kattankulathur, Chennai, India. He is currently pursuing a postdoctoral fellowship at the National Kaohsiung University of Science and Technology, which is located in Kaohsiung, Taiwan. He has published more than 70 research papers in national, international conferences, journals including 8 in Science Citation Indexed journals. He has published 10 patents, 2 patents granted. His research interests include IOT, Artificial Intelligence, Deep Learning, Data Science, Signal Processing and Image Processing.

Dhanalakshmi J. was born on th September 1992 in Tamilnadu, India. She received the B.E. degree in Computer Science and Engineering and M.E. degree in Computer Science and Engineering from Anna University, Tamil Nadu, India. She was ranked 31st at Anna University for her Masters degree in Computer Science and Engineering. She was a software developer at Fermtronics Technology Solutions until 2018. She completed her Ph.D. degree at the School of Computer Science and Engineering in B.S. Abdur Rahman Crescent Institute of Science and Technology, located in Chennai, India. She is currently pursuing a postdoctoral fellowship at the National Kaohsiung University of Science and Technology, which is located in Kaohsiung, Taiwan. She is currently working as an Assistant Professor in Data Science and Business Systems, SRM Institute of Science and Technology, Kattankulathur, Chennai, India. She published more than 10 research papers in International, National Journals including Conferences and Book Chapter in SCI and Scopus Indexed. Her research interests include Energy Analytics, Artificial Intelligence, Deep Learning, Data Science, Internet of Things (IOT) and Machine Learning.

* * *

Ashwini A. received her Bachelor degree in Electronics and Communication Engineering and Master degree in Communication and Networking from Ponjesly College of Engineering, Nagercoil under Anna University, Chennai. She received her PhD degree in Anna University Chennai, India. She has published many papers in journal and participated in many International Conferences. Her research interests include Medical Image Processing, Nanotechnology, Image Segmentation, Cloud computing, Internet of Things. Email: a.aswiniur@gmail.com

Bindhu A. is an Assistant Professor of Computer Science with over 10 years of experience, passionate about research in science and technology. She is currently affiliated with Infant Jesus College of Arts and Science for Women in Kanniyakumari, where she has been an Assistant Professor and Head since 2019. She earned her Ph.D. in 2024 from Manonmaniam Sundaranar University

Tirunelveli, an M.Phil. in 2008 from Alagappa University, and an MCA in 1999 from Manonmaniam Sundaranar University. She is a prolific researcher, having published papers in Scopus journals. She has also authored a book titled "Cloud Computing". Her expertise lies in Image Processing, Machine Learning and Artificial Intelligence. She is a reviewer for prestigious journals like IEEE Access, Systems and Soft Computing and Computers in Biology and Medicine. Her patent, "IoT based Automatic detection and prevention of all types of leaf disease and other environmental factors using AI camera, WSN and Machine learning algorithms", was published on December 2022.

Mahadevan A. is working as an Assistant Professor in the Department of Electronics and Communication Engineering at Sri Venkateswara College of Engineering, has about 15 years of teaching experience. He received his B.E degree in Electronics and Communication Engineering from Madras Institute of Technology, Anna University and M.E. degree in Communication Systems from Adhiyamaan College of Engineering, Anna University. He has published around 3 research articles in various national and international journals. He authored for the book tilted "Mechatronics and IoT" for the benefit of UG students. His area of research includes Analog circuit design, Sensors, Digital Communication, Microwave Engineering, RF Design, IoT Applications, etc.

Devi Arumugam currently serves as an Associate Professor in the Department of ECE at IFET College of Engineering, Villupuram. She completed her PhD at Anna University, Chennai. ME in the stream of Embedded System Technologies and BE in the stream of Electronics and Communication Engineering. She is a senior member of IEEE and a permanent member of ISTE. She has supervised numerous projects and served as a resource person for project expos. Her research interests include machine learning, deep learning, and embedded systems. She has been recognized with prestigious awards, including the Best Project Award from IEEE and IETE. Her research contributions have been published in over 25 reputable journals and books.

Anorgul I. Ashirova is an Associate Professor working at the Department of General Professional Sciences, Mamun University, Khiva, Uzbekistan.

Zamira Atamuratova is working at the Department of Pedagogy and Psychology, Urgench State University, Urgench, Uzbekistan.

Rajeswari D. is currently working as a Professor in the Department of Data Science and Business Systems, School of Computing, College of Engineering and Technology, SRM Institute of Science and Technology, Kattankulathur, India. Received Ph.D. degree in 2017 from College of Engineering, Guindy, Anna

University under the guidance of Dr.V. Jawahar Senthilkumar, Professor, College of Engineering, Guindy, Anna University. Completed M.Tech., Information Technology in 2010 from PSG College of Technology, Coimbatore, Anna University. Received GATE stipend from 2008 to 2010 for completing M.Tech. Completed B.Tech., Information Technology in 2008 from Annai Mathammal Sheela Engineering College, Anna University. Received International Travel Support (ITS) from SERB to attend 2023 POMS Annual Conference from 21 May to 25 May in USA.

Shruthi Anadhavalli Gathaman is a final year MBBS student at Mahsa University, with a keen interest in integrating artificial intelligence into the medical field. She has contributed to significant research papers, including "Enhancing Medical Sector Efficiency: A Comprehensive Case Study Based on Data Visualization Tools for Business Applications" (DOI: 10.4018/979-8-3693-6537-3.ch011) and "Enhancing Business Applications in ENT Diseases Management Through Data Visualization" (DOI: 10.4018/979-8-3693-6537-3.ch010). Shruthi aims to leverage innovative technologies to improve healthcare delivery and patient outcomes.

Pawan Kumar Goel is an accomplished academician and researcher with 19.5 years of experience, is an Associate Professor at Raj Kumar Goel Institute of Technology, Ghaziabad. He holds a Ph.D. in Computer Science Engineering and is UGC NET qualified. His expertise spans various domains, including wireless sensor networks, cloud computing, and artificial intelligence. Dr. Goel has published extensively in prestigious journals and conferences, with notable papers on topics such as cybersecurity, IoT, and machine learning. He is an active member of numerous professional bodies, including the IEEE, Computer Society of India and the International Association of Engineers. Recognized for his contributions, he has received several awards and certificates of appreciation. Dr. Goel is dedicated to fostering industry-academia collaborations and has organized numerous workshops and seminars. He is also involved in various training programs, MOOCs, and NPTEL certifications, contributing significantly to the advancement of education and research in his field.

Mehrigul Hayitova is working in the Department of Medicine at Termez University of Economics and Service, Termez, Uzbekistan.

S. Ida Evangeline is presently working as an Assistant Professor in the Department of Electrical and Electronics Engineering at the Government College of Engineering, Tirunelveli, Tamilnadu, India. She obtained her Bachelor's in Electrical and Electronics Engineering from Manonmaniam Sundaranar University in 2003, and Master's in Power Systems Engineering from Anna University, Chennai,

Tamilnadu, India in 2005. She completed her PhD degree in 2023 at Anna University, Chennai, Tamilnadu, India. She has published six research papers in international journals. Her current research interests include optimal power flow, renewable energy, soft computing, machine learning, and deep learning.

Khusan Jurayev is Associate Professor and Head of the Department of Finance and Tourism atTermez University of Economics and Service, Uzbekistan.

Amala K. J. received the B.Tech. degree in Computer Science and Engineering from Cochin University of Science and Technology and the M.E. degree in Computer Science from Noorul Islam Centre for Higher Education. She is currently pursuing the Ph.D. degree in Computer Science and Engineering with the Data Science and Business Systems at SRM Institute of Science and Technology, Tamil Nadu, India. She has qualified for the University Grants Commission (UGC) National Eligibility Test (NET) and has over 12 years of teaching experience in undergraduate and postgraduate computer science education. Her research interests include Learning to Rank, Machine Learning and Artificial Intelligence. Her current research focuses on integrating contextual and positional biases into attention-based two-tower models for click prediction and modeling dynamic user behaviors using Bayesian nonparametric approaches.

Mohammed Wajid Khan completed his Ph.D. in 2023, with research contributions spanning artificial intelligence and its applications. He has published six papers in peer-reviewed journals and presented three papers at national and international conferences. His academic work reflects a strong commitment to advancing knowledge in emerging technologies and their real-world impact.

S.Kaja Mohideen received his Bachelor of Engineering Degree in Electronics and Communication Engineering from Thiagarajar College of Engineering, Madurai, in the year 1988. He did his Masters in M.E. Applied Electronics from Coimbatore Institute of Technology, Coimbatore, in the year 1991. He received his Ph.D Degree from Anna University, Chennai in 2008 for his research in the field of VLSI Design. He has got more than Thirty Years of Teaching Experience and currently is the Senior Professor, ECE Department & Controller of Examinations in B.S. Abdur Rahman Crescent Institute of Science & Technology, Chennai. His area of interest includes VLSI Design, Microcontroller based system design, IOT, Antenna Design, Image Processing. He is having 35 publications in International journals and more than 20 publications in National/ International conferences to his credit. He has produced 9 Doctorates and currently supervising 4 Research scholars.

Umamaheswari P. holds a B.E. in Information Technology from Periyar Maniammai College of Engineering and Technology (2003), an M.B.A. from Alagappa University, Karaikudi, Tamil Nadu (2006), and an M.Tech in Computer Science from SASTRA Deemed University, Thanjavur, Tamil Nadu (2011). She earned her Ph.D. in Computer Science and Engineering from SASTRA Deemed University. With two decades of experience, she has taught both undergraduate and postgraduate courses in Computer Science. She is currently an Assistant Professor in the Department of Computer Science and Engineering at SRC Campus, SASTRA University, Kumbakonam. Her research interests focus on Data Mining, Machine Learning, and Deep Learning. She has published numerous research papers in international conferences, SCI-indexed journals, Scopus, and book chapters.

Banu Priya Prathaban was born on 3rd February 1991 in Tamilnadu, India. She received her Ph.D. in Electronics and Communication Engineering from SRM Institute of Science and Technology, Chennai, India. She is graduated from Anna University, Chennai in 2012 with the Bachelor of Technology degree in Electronics and Communication Engineering. She received the Master of Technology degree in Embedded Systems Technologies from Anna University, Chennai in 2014 with gold medal. She is currently working as an Assistant Professor in Networking and Communications, SRM Institute of Science and Technology, Kattankulathur, Chennai, India. She has published more than 70 research papers in national, international conferences, journals including 8 in Science Citation Indexed journals with 103 citations. Her research interests include Embedded Systems, IoT, Artificial Intelligence, Deep Learning, Data Science, Signal Processing and Image Processing.

Ravikumar R. N. is an experienced academician with over 12+ years of teaching and research expertise across institutions in India, the UAE, and the Maldives. He currently serves as an Assistant Professor at Marwadi University, Rajkot, specializing in Machine Learning, Recommender Systems, and AI-driven applications in healthcare and security. He holds a Ph.D. in Machine Learning and Recommender Systems from Amity University, Jaipur, a Master of Engineering in CSE from VMRF University, Salem, and a Bachelor of Engineering in CSE from Anna University. He also has a MiniMBA from the Swiss eLearning Institute. Dr. Ravikumar has authored more than 8+ multiple SCIE/Scopus-indexed journal articles, 25+ IEEE/Springer conference papers, and co-authored a book on Artificial Intelligence. He has also published 9 patents and contributed 10+ book chapters in emerging domains such as Federated Learning, Blockchain, and Digital Twins for IGI Global, Wiley and Springer publisher. He actively mentors students through initiatives like the Research Activities Club (RAC) and Student Research Internship Training (SRIT), promoting innovation and research culture.

Arunkumar Ramamoorthy is working as Lecturer in Digital Forensics and Cyber Security at the University of South Wales, Treforest, United Kingdom. He completed his Doctorate in Computer Science and Engineering at Anna University, Chennai, where he also earned his M.Tech in Information Technology. His B.Eng in Computer Science and Engineering was awarded by Karunya University, Coimbatore, India. With 15 years of academic experience. He has contributed over 20 research articles in fields such as Information Security, Digital Forensics, Mobile Application Security, Artificial Intelligence, Deep Learning, and Network Security. He holds two Indian patents in neural networks and machine learning and one Australian patent in Cyber Security. Furthermore, he has published 2 book chapters, and a active reviewer for various International Journals like Springer, Elsevier, Taylor & Francis. He is a member of the Computer Society of India (CSI) and the Indian Society of Technical Education (ISTE).

Aarthi S. is a dedicated Assistant Professor in Computer Science with over six years of teaching experience. She is currently pursuing her Ph.D. at Marwadi University, Gujarat, and holds an M.Phil. and MCA from Bharathiar University, Tamil Nadu. Throughout her academic career, Aarthi has specialized in programming languages such as C++, Java, and C, and contributed to research in recommender systems and AI-related data privacy. She has published journal articles, contributed to book chapters, and actively participated in technical workshops. Known for her student mentorship and engagement in academic events, Aarthi remains committed to fostering innovation and excellence in computer science education.

Vinu S. is working as Assistant Professor in SRM Institute of Science and Technology, Kattankulathur, Chennai. He has completed his doctoral degree in Anna University. His areas of research includes Artificial Intelligence, Deep Learning and AR/VR.

Karthic Sundaram is working as Assistant Professor in SRM Institute of Science and Technology, Kattankulathur, Chennai. He has completed his doctoral degree in Anna University. His areas of research includes Artificial Intelligence, Deep Learning and Network Security.

Latha Tamilselvan received her B.E. in Electronics & Communication Engineering from Bharathidasan University in 1990, M.E. in Communication Systems from National Institute of Technology, Trichy in 1995 and Ph.D in Computer Science & Engineering (Protocols for Routing Security in Mobile Ad hoc Networks) from Anna University, Chennai in 2008. She has a teaching experience of more than 25 years. She is the Director, MIS in B.S. Abdur Rahman Crescent Institute of Science and Technology. She is also an academic council member, doctoral committee member and staff selection committee member at various other universities. She is a recognized supervisor for guiding Ph.D Scholars in the school of Computer Information and Mathematical Sciences at B.S. Abdur Rahman Crescent Institute of Science and Technology and she guided 8 scholars & is currently guiding 2 research scholars. Her area of research includes Mobile ad hoc networks, Network Security, Cloud Computing. She reviewed the book "Computer Networks" and "Computer and Telecommunication Networks" for McGraw-Hill Pub. She is a reviewer for the reputed journals. She has published around 50 Research papers, in international journals, International Conferences and National conferences. Her Papers have over 1100+ citations so far.

Athish Venkatachalam is a Graduate Student at Clemson University, pursuing a Master of Science in Computer Science. He completed his Bachelor of Technology in Computer Science and Business Systems at SRM Institute of Science and Technology (SRMIST), where he held leadership positions as Chairperson of SRM IET on Campus and Convener of the Technical Team at the Directorate of Student Affairs. Athish is recognized for his expertise in Cloud Computing, Distributed Computing, and DevOps, and earned accolades in various hackathons, including being a finalist in the All-India Level Smart India Hackathon 2022. At Clemson, Athish serves as a Graduate Research Assistant at the Human-AI Empowerment Lab, where he is dedicated to exploring AI for Social Good. In addition to his research work, Athish is the President of the Clemson Graduate Student Government, having previously served as the Director of Clemson Graduate Travel Grants. In this capacity, he plays an essential role in advocating for and supporting the graduate student community. Athish was also honored with the Best Outgoing Student award in 2023 by SRMIST for his exceptional academic achievements, leadership, and contributions to the university.

Syed Khaja Ahmedudin Zakir received Masters and Bachelor degree in Electronics & Communication Engineering in 2013 and 1999 respectively from Jawaharlal Nehru Technological University, Hyderabad, Telangana - India. Currently he is working as Lecturer in Electrical Engineering department, College of Engineering and Technology, University of Technology and Applied Sciences-Ibra. He has over 23 years of combined experience in Teaching (Graduate & Diploma Level) and IT industry. Skills in Embedded C, Application programming and MATLAB. He had published 13 papers in various conferences and journals. His area of interest includes IoT, Embedded Systems and the Communication Domain.

Index

A

B

C

N

O

P

R

S

V

W

www.ingramcontent.com/pod-product-compliance
Lightning Source LLC
LaVergne TN
LVHW061530290926
849162LV00004B/739